Herbal Medicine and Aging: Potential of Natural Treatment for Age-Related Diseases

Herbal Medicine and Aging: Potential of Natural Treatment for Age-Related Diseases

Editor: Evelyn Sharp

AMERICAN
MEDICAL PUBLISHERS
www.americanmedicalpublishers.com

AMERICAN
MEDICAL PUBLISHERS
www.americanmedicalpublishers.com

Cataloging-in-Publication Data

Herbal medicine and aging : potential of natural treatment for age-related diseases / edited by Evelyn Sharp.
p. cm.
Includes bibliographical references and index.
ISBN 978-1-63927-862-6
1. Older people--Diseases--Alternative treatment. 2. Geriatrics--Alternative treatment.
3. Herbs--Therapeutic use. 4. Older people--Diseases--Rehabilitation. 5. Aging. I. Sharp, Evelyn.
RC953.8.A48 H47 2023
615.547--dc23

American Medical Publishers,
41 Flatbush Avenue,
1st Floor, New York,
NY 11217, USA

ISBN 978-1-63927-862-6 (Hardback)

Contents

Preface IX

Chapter 1 **Improvement in Frailty in a Patient with Severe Chronic Obstructive Pulmonary Disease After Ninjin'yoeito Therapy** 1
Hirai Kuniaki, Tanaka Akihiko, Homma Tetsuya, Mikuni Hatsuko, Kawahara Tomoko, Ohta Shin, Kusumoto Sojiro, Yamamoto Mayumi, Yamaguchi Fumihiro, Suzuki Shintaro, Ohnishi Tsukasa and Sagara Hironori

Chapter 2 **Multifunctional Actions of Ninjin'yoeito, a Japanese Kampo Medicine: Accumulated Scientific Evidence Based on Experiments with Cells and Animal Models, and Clinical Studies** 5
Kanako Miyano, Miki Nonaka, Miaki Uzu, Kaori Ohshima and Yasuhito Uezono

Chapter 3 **Combined Use of Ninjin'yoeito Improves Subjective Fatigue Caused by Lenalidomide in Patients with Multiple Myeloma: A Retrospective Study** 12
Tomoki Ito, Akiko Konishi, Yukie Tsubokura, Yoshiko Azuma, Masaaki Hotta, Hideaki Yoshimura, Takahisa Nakanishi, Shinya Fujita, Aya Nakaya, Atsushi Satake, Kazuyoshi Ishii and Shosaku Nomura

Chapter 4 **Mesenchymal Stem Cell Therapy for Aging Frailty** 16
Ivonne Hernandez Schulman, Wayne Balkan and Joshua M. Hare

Chapter 5 **A Clinical Study of Ninjin'yoeito with Regard to Frailty** 26
Naoya Sakisaka, Kazuo Mitani, Sadahiro Sempuku, Tamaki Imai, Yoshinori Takemoto, Hiroaki Shimomura and Takahisa Ushiroyama

Chapter 6 **Kampo Medicines for Frailty in Locomotor Disease** 31
Hajime Nakae, Yuko Hiroshima and Miwa Hebiguchi

Chapter 7 **Frailty and *Caenorhabditis elegans* as a Benchtop Animal Model for Screening Drugs Including Natural Herbs** 36
Katsuyoshi Matsunami

Chapter 8 **Clinical Practice Guidelines and Evidence for the Efficacy of Traditional Japanese Herbal Medicine (Kampo) in Treating Geriatric Patients** 42
Shin Takayama, Ryutaro Arita, Akiko Kikuchi, Minoru Ohsawa, Soichiro Kaneko and Tadashi Ishii

Chapter 9 **Semen Cassiae Extract Improves Glucose Metabolism by Promoting GlUT4 Translocation in the Skeletal Muscle of Diabetic Rats** 53
Meiling Zhang, Xin Li, Hangfei Liang, Huqiang Cai, Xueling Hu, Yu Bian, Lei Dong, Lili Ding, Libo Wang, Bo Yu, Yan Zhang and Yao Zhang

Chapter 10 **The Modulatory Properties of Li-Ru-Kang Treatment on Hyperplasia of Mammary Glands Using an Integrated Approach**.....64
Shizhang Wei, Liqi Qian, Ming Niu, Honghong Liu, Yuxue Yang, Yingying Wang, Lu Zhang, Xuelin Zhou, Haotian Li, Ruilin Wang, Kun Li and Yanling Zhao

Chapter 11 **Antibacterial Activity and Mechanism of Action of Aspidinol Against Multi-Drug-Resistant Methicillin-Resistant *Staphylococcus aureus***.....74
Xin Hua, Qin Yang, Wanjiang Zhang, Zhimin Dong, Shenye Yu, Stefan Schwarz and Siguo Liu

Chapter 12 **Sirt1 Activation by Post-ischemic Treatment with Lumbrokinase Protects Against Myocardial Ischemia-Reperfusion Injury**.....86
Yi-Hsin Wang, Shun-An Li, Chao-Hsin Huang, Hsing-Hui Su, Yi- Hung Chen, Jinghua T. Chang and Shiang-Suo Huang

Chapter 13 **Aqueous Extract of Black Maca Prevents Metabolism Disorder via Regulating the Glycolysis/Gluconeogenesis-TCA Cycle and PPARα Signaling Activation in Golden Hamsters Fed a High-Fat, High-Fructose Diet**.....100
Wenting Wan, Hongxiang Li, Jiamei Xiang, Fan Yi, Lijia Xu, Baoping Jiang and Peigen Xiao

Chapter 14 **Mechanisms of Triptolide- Induced Hepatotoxicity and Protective Effect of Combined Use of Isoliquiritigenin: Possible Roles of Nrf2 and Hepatic Transporters**.....114
Zhenyan Hou, Lei Chen, Pingfei Fang, Hualin Cai, Huaibo Tang, Yongbo Peng, Yang Deng, Lingjuan Cao, Huande Li, Bikui Zhang and Miao Yan

Chapter 15 **Phospholipase Cγ2 Signaling Cascade Contribute to the Antiplatelet Effect of Notoginsenoside Fc**.....129
Yingqiu Liu, Tianyi Liu, Kevin Ding, Zengyuan Liu, Yuanyuan Li, Taotao He, Weimin Zhang, Yunpeng Fan, Wuren Ma, Li Cui and Xiaoping Song

Chapter 16 **Ninjin'yoeito Improves Behavioral Abnormalities and Hippocampal Neurogenesis in the Corticosterone Model of Depression**.....140
Kenta Murata, Nina Fujita, Ryuji Takahashi and Akio Inui

Chapter 17 **Protective Effects of Total Glycoside from *Rehmannia glutinosa* Leaves on Diabetic Nephropathy Rats via Regulating the Metabolic Profiling and Modulating the TGF-β1 and Wnt/β-Catenin Signaling Pathway**.....151
Xinxin Dai, Shulan Su, Hongdie Cai, Dandan Wei, Hui Yan, Tianyao Zheng, Zhenhua Zhu, Er-xin Shang, Sheng Guo, Dawei Qian and Jin-ao Duan

Chapter 18 **Tricaproin Isolated from *Simarouba glauca* Inhibits the Growth of Human Colorectal Carcinoma Cell Lines by Targeting Class-1 Histone Deacetylases**.....166
Asha Jose, Motamari V. N. L. Chaitanya, Elango Kannan and Subba Rao V. Madhunapantula

Chapter 19 **Inhibition of Akt/mTOR/p70S6K Signaling Activity with Huangkui Capsule Alleviates the Early Glomerular Pathological Changes in Diabetic Nephropathy**.....182
Wei Wu, Wei Hu, Wen-Bei Han, Ying-Lu Liu, Yue Tu, Hai-Ming Yang, Qi-Jun Fang, Mo-Yi Zhou, Zi-Yue Wan, Ren-Mao Tang, Hai-Tao Tang and Yi-Gang Wan

Chapter 20 **Identification of Steroidogenic Components Derived from *Gardenia jasminoides* Ellis Potentially Useful for Treating Postmenopausal Syndrome**......199
Xueyu Wang, Guo-Cai Wang, Jianhui Rong, Shi Wei Wang, Tzi Bun Ng, Yan Bo Zhang, Kai Fai Lee, Lin Zheng, Hei-Kiu Wong, Ken Kin Lam Yung and Stephen Cho Wing Sze

Chapter 21 **Anti-hyperplasia Effects of Total Saponins from Phytolaccae Radix in Rats with Mammary Gland Hyperplasia via Inhibition of Proliferation and Induction of Apoptosis**......218
Xiaoliang Li, Zhibin Wang, Yu Wang, Yanan Zhang, Xia Lei, Ping Xin, Xin Fu, Ning Gao, Yanping Sun, Yanhong Wang, Bingyou Yang, Qiuhong Wang and Haixue Kuang

Permissions

List of Contributors

Index

Preface

Herbal medicine refers to the practice of using plants to treat diseases and improve overall health and wellness. These medicines are available in the form of powders, tablets, extracts, capsules, teas, and dried or fresh plants. It also uses bee and fungal products, as well as shells, minerals and animal parts. There are several herbs that are frequently utilized in herbal medicine such as garlic, Echinacea, ginseng, dong quai, ginger, Hypericum perforatum, etc. Herbal medicine is considered to have various medicinal herbs that have anti-aging properties. The extracts of the basil plant and Momordica charantia can slow down the ageing process, as well as treat age-related diseases. Furthermore, extracts of Salvia miltiorrhiza, Curcumin longa and naringin found in grapes and citrus fruits hold significant potential in initiating differentiation capability and cumulative proliferation of stem cells. This book explores all the important aspects of herbal medicine and aging in the modern day. It provides significant information to help develop a good understanding of the potential of natural treatment for age-related diseases. The extensive content of this book provides the readers with a thorough understanding of the subject.

Significant researches are present in this book. Intensive efforts have been employed by authors to make this book an outstanding discourse. This book contains the enlightening chapters which have been written on the basis of significant researches done by the experts.

Finally, I would also like to thank all the members involved in this book for being a team and meeting all the deadlines for the submission of their respective works. I would also like to thank my friends and family for being supportive in my efforts.

Editor

1

Improvement in Frailty in a Patient with Severe Chronic Obstructive Pulmonary Disease After Ninjin'yoeito Therapy

Hirai Kuniaki, Tanaka Akihiko, Homma Tetsuya, Mikuni Hatsuko, Kawahara Tomoko, Ohta Shin, Kusumoto Sojiro, Yamamoto Mayumi, Yamaguchi Fumihiro, Suzuki Shintaro, Ohnishi Tsukasa and Sagara Hironori*

Division of Allergology and Respiratory Medicine, Department of Internal Medicine, Showa University School of Medicine, Tokyo, Japan

***Correspondence:**
Hirai Kuniaki
medi123@infoseek.jp

Frailty is a poor prognostic factor in patients with chronic obstructive pulmonary disease (COPD). Although various studies have assessed the effects of conventional treatment with bronchodilators, nutritional support, and pulmonary rehabilitation for frailty in patients with COPD, none have addressed the effects of traditional Japanese medicine (Kampo medicine). Herein, we report the successful management of frailty using Ninjin'yoeito therapy in a 76-year-old patient with COPD. Despite being prescribed multiple bronchodilators, nutritional supplement therapy, patient education, and pulmonary rehabilitation, the patient exhibited unintentional weight loss, low energy, and low physical activity. Ninjin'yoeito was prescribed and these subjective symptoms began to improve 1 month after treatment initiation. In 6 months, the patient reported no frailty, had increased muscle mass, and had achieved an almost normal healthy state. Ninjin'yoeito has been associated with both physical effects, such as improvement in overall physical strength and appetite, and reduction in fatigue, and psychological effects, such as greater motivation and reduction of depression and anxiety symptoms. Physicians have usually treated COPD primarily with organ-specific treatments, such as bronchodilators; however, addressing both the physiological and psychological vulnerability has been difficult. This case report illustrates the potential usefulness of Ninjin'yoeito treatment for frailty in patients with COPD.

Keywords: frailty, chronic obstructive pulmonary disease, Ninjin'yoeito therapy, Kampo medicine, anorexia

BACKGROUND

Frailty is defined as a non-specific state of physiological decline in advanced old age, characterized by vulnerability to adverse health issues, and it is a concept that has attracted the physicians' attention in patients with COPD. Many patients with COPD encounter frailty (1), and as frailty is expected to be reversible, particularly if addressed at an early stage, it is possible that the patients experience symptomatic improvement after appropriate interventions for correctable or removable factors (2). Various therapeutic methods, such as smoking cessation, pharmacologic therapy using bronchodilators, long term oxygen therapy, and pulmonary rehabilitation, showed efficacy in subsets of COPD comorbid patients (3). However, there are many patients with severe COPD who do not show improvement in frailty despite applying adequate treating strategies.

Traditional Japanese medicine (Kampo medicine) is known to be effective for several respiratory diseases (4–6), but to the best of our knowledge, only few studies have examined the effects of traditional Japanese medicine on frailty in patients with COPD. Ninjin'yoeito is a traditional Japanese medicine derived from 12 crude drugs, i.e., rehmannia root, Japanese angelica root, atractylodes rhizome, *Poria sclerotium*, ginseng, cinnamon bark, polygala root, peony root, citrus unshiu peel, astragalus root, glycyrrhiza, and schisandra fruit. Ninjin'yoeito prescription was approved by the Japanese Ministry of Health, and as it is used to treat fatigue, anorexia, night sweats, and anemia, we hypothesized that it may be beneficial for frailty. Herein, we have described a unique case of a patient who showed no improvement in frailty after conventional treatment but recuperated after Ninjin'yoeito administration.

CASE REPORT

A 76-year-old man with severe chronic obstructive pulmonary disease (COPD) presented with a feeling of fatigue, weight loss, and reduced physical activities. He was diagnosed with COPD at the age of 69 years and had retired from work the following year. His smoking history included 40 cigarettes per day between the age of 14 and 69 years; his airflow limitation was classified as severe by the Global initiative for Chronic Obstructive Lung Disease; and a chest computed tomography (CT) scan showed severe emphysema. He had started long-term oxygen therapy at the age of 72 years and is currently inhaling 3 L/min of oxygen. Medical and family histories were otherwise unremarkable. Cardiac ultrasound excluded comorbid congestive heart failure or pulmonary hypertension, and CT pulmonary arteriography also excluded chronic pulmonary thromboembolism. As the patient had a history of acute exacerbations of COPD more than twice a year with extreme respiratory symptoms, he was prescribed a combination of inhaled long-acting antimuscarinic antagonist, long-acting beta2-agonist, corticosteroid, and oral carbocysteine, ambroxol, and theophylline. He reported symptoms of dyspnea on exertion, depression and anxiety, and a decrease in physical activity. He also experienced anorexia with a weight loss of more than 5 kg in a year, and no other possible causes of weight loss, such as tuberculosis and malignant tumor, were observed. Therefore, in addition to respiratory pharmacotherapy, we prescribed an antianxiety drug and provided nutritional supplement therapy, patient education, and pulmonary rehabilitation. However, the patient's mental and physical symptoms did not improve after 4 months. Furthermore, he exhibited deterioration in activities of daily living as well as physical and mental weakness; hospital visits were difficult and therefore, he considered home care. Persistent weight loss, poor endurance and energy, and low physical activity levels led to the diagnosis of physical frailty according to Fried's criteria (7). This vulnerability was supported by assessments using the Kihon Checklist (KCL) (8), the COPD Assessment Test (CAT) (9), and the Hospital Anxiety and Depression Scale (HADS) (10), all of which revealed high scores indicating inferior status. The KCL is a tool designed by a study group from the Japanese Ministry of Health, Labor and Welfare and comprises 25 items divided into seven categories: physical strength, nutritional status, oral function, socialization, memory, mood, and lifestyle. The KCL scores range from 0 (no frailty) to 25 (severe frailty); a previous study classified the patients' frailty status as non-frail (0–3), prefrail (4–7), and frail (8–25) (11). The CAT is a reliable tool that comprises eight items that assess the various COPD symptoms and is widely used in clinical practice. The CAT scores range from 0 to 40, with a score of 0 indicating no impairment. The HADS is also widely used to measure the level of anxiety and depression and comprises 14 items: 7 associated with anxiety (HADS-A) and 7 associated with depression (HADS-D). The HADS-A and HADS-D scores ranged from 0 to 21, and are in the range 8–10 for doubtful cases and ≥11 for definite cases. For the present case, we continued the pharmacological treatment, nutritional supplement therapy, patient education, and pulmonary rehabilitation and included 2.5 g of Ninjin'yoeito to be taken 3 times a day before meals.

After administration of Ninjin'yoeito, physical examination and blood tests such as electrolytes, liver function tests, and renal function test were performed to evaluate the side effects of Ninjin'yoeito administration. However, no side effects were detected. A significant improvement in symptoms, including increased appetite and alleviation of mood disorders and weight loss, was observed 1 month after initiating Ninjin'yoeito administration. Body weight and muscle mass continued to increase, and after 6 months of Ninjin'yoeito administration, the body weight increased by 8 kg compared with that prior to Ninjin'yoeito administration. Body composition assessed using bioelectrical impedance (InBody 720; Biospace, Tokyo, Japan) showed increasing muscle mass and no change in the body fat percentage (**Figure 1**). The patient's KCL, CAT, and HADS scores increased over time (**Figure 2**), and his status improved from frailty to non-frailty. Written informed consent was obtained from the participant for the publication of this case report.

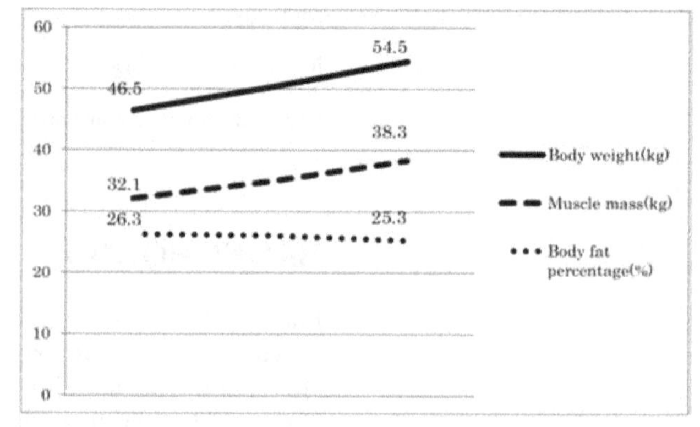

FIGURE 1 | Body composition changes during Ninjin'yoeito therapy. Body composition was assessed at the indicated time points using bioelectrical impedance. Ninjin'yoeito administration increased the body weight and muscle mass without affecting body fat percentage.

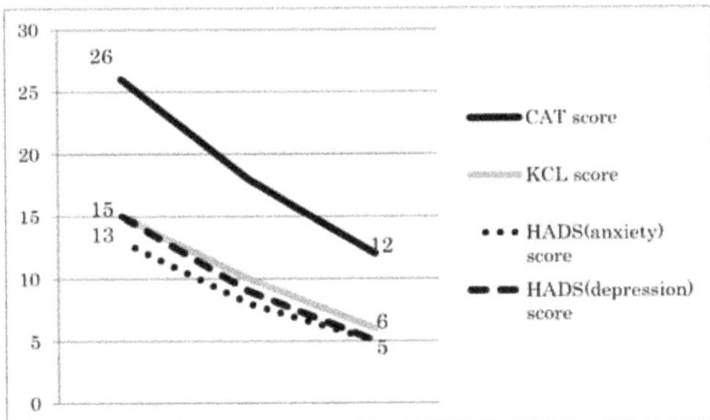

FIGURE 2 | Changes in important factors of frailty and COPD during Ninjin'yoeito therapy. Ninjin'yoeito administration improved the patient's KCL, CAT, and HADS scores. The KCL comprises 25 items divided into seven categories: physical strength, nutritional status, oral function, socialization, memory, mood, and lifestyle. The CAT comprises 8 items that assess the various COPD symptoms. The HADS is used to measure the level of anxiety and depression and comprises 14 items.

DISCUSSION

This case report revealed two major findings. First, in patients who do not recover with conventional management of COPD, Ninjin'yoeito can improve their physical status from frailty to non-frailty. Second, Ninjin'yoeito can improve psychological frailty.

Ninjin'yoeito can improve physical frailty. The patient was categorized as having physical frailty because he fulfilled three of Fried's criteria, i.e., weight loss, feeling of fatigue, and decreased physical activity. All the three symptoms improved, and he could be categorized as non-frail at 6 months after initiating Ninjin'yoeito administration. COPD has a high morbidity and mortality rate, and various prognostic factors are being considered for COPD. Importantly, each item of Fried's criteria on the frailty tool has been shown to be a risk factor for COPD (12–14). Various factors, such as systemic inflammation, hypoxemia, increased respiratory effort, and hormonal abnormality, have been reported to result in appetite reduction and weight loss in patients with COPD (15). Although several intervention studies on weight loss have been reported (16–18), weight loss still remains refractory in some patients. In recent years, pulmonary rehabilitation has been demonstrated to improve frailty in patients with COPD; however, pulmonary rehabilitation in patients with severe frailty is more difficult to complete (19), and treatment strategies in frail patients with COPD who do not respond to conventional treatment are not clear. Our case report suggests that Ninjin'yoeito is a promising drug for frailty in patients with COPD who cannot complete pulmonary rehabilitation.

Ninjin'yoeito can improve the psychological frailty. Treatment of anxiety and depression in patients with COPD is particularly important, because it has been reported that the risk of ineffectiveness of conventional therapies increases if patients with COPD have psychological comorbidities (20, 21). The beneficial effects of Ninjin'yoeito were mirrored by favorable changes in the patient's KCL score, CAT score reflecting quality of life, and HADS score reflecting anxiety and depression. In support of our findings, previous studies have reported that Ninjin'yoeito can improve the mental status in patients with Alzheimer's disease (22).

Increase in physical activities has been shown to be an important factor in patients with COPD (14), and a reduction in both physical capacity (23) and mental health contributes to the decline in physical activity (21). We propose that the Ninjin'yoeito was effective in this case because it has multiple effects that address both physiological and psychological issues. Ninjin'yoeito is composed of 12 crude drugs each of which has its own unique effect(s). For example, ginseng and schisandra fruit have an anti-fatigue effect (24); ginseng and citrus unshiu peel have an anti-anorectic effect; and ginseng and atractylodes rhizome possess antidepressant and anti-aging effects. Thus, Ninjin'yoeito can be expected to improve the physical activity levels in patients with COPD because it positively affects both the physical and psychological symptoms. Additionally, the pulmonary pharmacological approach addresses only the organ-specific concerns rather than the comprehensive status of the patient, e.g., bronchodilators are prescribed to increase the airflow in patients with COPD. Recently, the concept of frailty, which comprehensively evaluates the state of a patient, is gaining attention. Furthermore, frailty is a particularly important risk factor in COPD, and there are no specific or effective management strategies. Thus, herein, it is important to note that while Ninjin'yoeito did not improve the respiratory function, it was effective in alleviating depression and anxiety symptoms and improving the appetite and physical activity levels, thereby acting as a "remedy for frailty."

CONCLUDING REMARKS

This case report provides important preliminary evidence that Ninjin'yoeito therapy can improve frailty in patients with COPD. To the best of our knowledge, this is the first report of its kind. Future clinical studies are required to evaluate the effects of Ninjin'yoeito therapy on frailty in patients with COPD.

AUTHOR CONTRIBUTIONS

HK, TA, OS, OT, and SH designed this study. HK, HT, YF, and KS performed clinical, functional, and laboratory assessments. SS, YM, MH, KT, and SH were involved in revising the manuscript. HK and TA wrote the manuscript. All authors significantly contributed to the data interpretation and manuscript preparation.

ACKNOWLEDGMENTS

The authors are grateful to Yoshito Miyata and Megumi Jinno for their assistance in the interpretation of the results and critical review of the manuscript.

REFERENCES

Park SK, Richardson CR, Holleman RG, Larson JL. Frailty in people with COPD, using the National Health and Nutrition Evaluation Survey dataset (2003-2006). *Heart Lung* (2013) 423:163–70. doi: 10.1016/j.hrtlng.2012.07.004

Clegg A, Young J, Iliffe S, Rikkert MO, Rockwood K. Frailty in elderly people. *Lancet* (2013) 381:752–62. doi: 10.1016/S0140-6736(12)62167-9

Global Strategy for the Diagnosis. *Management and Prevention of COPD, Global Initiative for Chronic Obstructive Lung Disease (GOLD)* (2018). Available online at: http://goldcopd.org

Mukaida K, Hattori N, Kondo K, Morita N, Murakami I, Haruta Y, et al. A pilot study of the multiherb Kampo medicine bakumondoto for cough in patients with chronic obstructive pulmonary disease. *Phytomedicine* (2011)18:625–9. doi: 10.1016/j.phymed.2010.11.006

Urata Y, Yoshida S, Irie Y, Tanigawa T, Amayasu H, Nakabayashi M. Treatment of asthma patients with herbal medicine TJ-96: a randomized controlled trial. *Respir Med.* (2002) 96:469–74. doi: 10.1053/rmed.2002.1307

Tatsumi K, Shinozuka N, Nakayama K, Sekiya N, Kuriyama T, Fukuchi Y. Hochuekkito improves systemic inflammation and nutritional status in elderly patients with chronic obstructive pulmonary disease. *J Am Geriatr Soc.* (2009) 57:169–70. doi: 10.1111/j.1532-5415.2009.02034.x

Fried LP, Tangen CM, Walston J, Newman AB, Hirsch C, Gottdiener J. Frailty in older adults: evidence for a phenotype. *J Gerontol A Biol Sci Med Sci.* (2001) 56:M146–56. doi: 10.1093/gerona/56.3.M146

Sewo Sampaio PY, Sampaio RA, Yamada M, Arai H. Systematic review of the Kihon Checklist: Is it a reliable assessment of frailty? *Geriatr Gerontol Int.* (2016) 16:893–902. doi: 10.1111/ggi.12833

Jones PW, Harding G, Berry P, Wiklund I, Chen WH, Leidy NK. Development and first validation of the COPD Assessment Test. *Eur Respir J.* (2009) 34:648–54. doi: 10.1183/09031936.00102509

Zigmond AS, Snaith RP. The hospital anxiety and depression scale. *Acta Psychiatr Scand.* (1983) 67:361–70. doi: 10.1111/j.1600-0447.1983.tb09716.x

Satake S, Senda K, Hong YJ, Miura H, Endo H, Sakurai T, et al. Validity of the Kihon Checklist for assessing frailty status. *Geriatr Gerontol Int.* (2016) 16:709–15. doi: 10.1111/ggi.12543

Celli BR, Cote CG, Marin JM, Casanova C, Montes de Oca M, Mendez RA, et al. The body-mass index, airflow obstruction, dyspnea, and exercise capacity index in chronic obstructive pulmonary disease. *N Engl J Med.* (2004) 350:1005–12. doi: 10.1056/NEJMoa021322

Kovarik M, Joskova V, Patkova A, Koblizek V, Zadak Z, Hronek M. Hand grip endurance test relates to clinical state and prognosis in COPD patients better than 6-minute walk test distance. *Int J Chron Obstruct Pulmon Dis.* (2017) 12:3429–35. doi: 10.2147/COPD.S144566

Waschki B, Kirsten A, Holz O, Müller KC, Meyer T, Watz H, et al. Physical activity is the strongest predictor of all-cause mortality in patients with COPD: a prospective cohort study. *Chest* (2011) 140:331–42. doi: 10.1378/chest.10-2521

Raguso CA, Luthy C. Nutritional status in chronic obstructive pulmonary disease: role of hypoxia. *Nutrition* (2011) 27:138–43. doi: 10.1016/j.nut.2010.07.009

Yamaguchi Y, Hibi S, Ishii M, Hanaoka Y, Kage H, Yamamoto H, et al. Pulmonary features associated with being underweight in older men. *J Am Geriatr Soc.* (2011) 59:1558–60. doi: 10.1111/j.1532-5415.2011.03536.x

Collins PF, Elia M, Stratton RJ. Nutritional support and functional capacity in chronic obstructive pulmonary disease: a systematic review and meta-analysis. *Respirology* (2013) 18:616–29. doi: 10.1111/resp.12070

Ferreira IM, Brooks D, White J, Goldstein R. Nutritional supplementation for stable chronic obstructive pulmonary disease. *Cochrane Database Syst Rev.* (2012) 12:CD000998. doi: 10.1002/14651858.CD000998.pub3

Maddocks M, Kon SS, Canavan JL, Jones SE, Nolan CM, Labey A, et al. Physical frailty and pulmonary rehabilitation in COPD: a prospective cohort study. *Thorax* (2016) 71:988–95. doi: 10.1136/thoraxjnl-2016-208460

Wilson I. Depression in the patient with COPD. *Int J Chron Obstruct Pulmon Dis.* (2006) 1:61–4. doi: 10.2147/copd.2006.1.1.61

Maurer J, Rebbapragada V, Borson S, Goldstein R, Kunik ME, Yohannes AM, et al. Anxiety and depression in COPD: current understanding, unanswered questions, and research needs. *Chest* (2008) 134:43S–56S. doi: 10.1378/chest.08-0342

Kudoh C, Arita R, Honda M, Kishi T, Komatsu Y, Asou H, et al. Effect of ninjin'yoeito, a Kampo (traditional Japanese) medicine, on cognitive impairment and depression in patients with Alzheimer's disease: 2 years of observation. *Psychogeriatrics* (2016) 16:85–92. doi: 10.1111/psyg.12125

Belza B, Steele BG, Hunziker J, Lakshminaryan S, Holt L, Buchner DM. Correlates of physical activity in chronic obstructive pulmonary disease. *Nurs Res.* (2001) 50:195–202. doi: 10.1097/00006199-200107000-00003

Kim YJ, Yoo SR, Chae CK, Jung UJ, Choi MS. Omija fruit extract improves endurance and energy metabolism by upregulating PGC-1α expression in the skeletal muscle of exercised rats. *J Med Food* (2014) 17:28–35. doi: 10.1089/jmf.2013.3071

2

Multifunctional Actions of Ninjin'yoeito, a Japanese Kampo Medicine: Accumulated Scientific Evidence Based on Experiments with Cells and Animal Models, and Clinical Studies

*Kanako Miyano[1], Miki Nonaka[1], Miaki Uzu[1], Kaori Ohshima[1,2] and Yasuhito Uezono[1,3,4,5]**

[1] Division of Cancer Pathophysiology, National Cancer Center Research Institute, Tokyo, Japan, [2] Faculty of Pharmaceutical Sciences, Tokyo University of Science, Chiba, Japan, [3] Division of Supportive Care Research, Exploratory Oncology Research and Clinical Trial Center, National Cancer Center, Tokyo, Japan, [4] Innovation Center for Supportive, Palliative and Psychosocial Care, National Cancer Center Hospital, Tokyo, Japan, [5] Department of Comprehensive Oncology, Nagasaki University Graduate School of Biomedical Sciences, Nagasaki, Japan

***Correspondence:**
Yasuhito Uezono
yuezono@ncc.go.jp

Herbal medicines are currently employed for the treatment of several types of diseases, and also employed for the improvement of Quality of Life (QOL) of patients over the world, in particular, in Asian countries. In Japan, a Japanese herbal medicine namely kampo medicine has been prescribed for the improvement of QOL of patients. Ninjinyoeito (NYT), composed of 12 herbal plants, is one of kampo medicines and used for helping recovery of diseases and improving several symptoms that suffer patients such as anemia, anorexia and fatigue. Recent scientific research approaches to kampo medicines with cells and animal models enable to prove that NYT has multiple functions for improvement of symptoms. Also, clinical studies using NYT support such actions to be widely used for the improvement of symptoms that reduce the QOL of patients.

Keywords: herbal ingredient, kampo medicine, Ninjinyoeito, mixed ingredients, scientific evidence

INTRODUCTION

Ninjinyoeito (NYT) is a Japanese herbal medicine prescribed and clinically admired in Japan. NYT has multi-functional beneficial activities so that it is used for improvement of recovery from diseases or some symptoms (1–7). Further, NYT has been reported to have antiviral action on hepatitis C virus (HCV), antioxidant and immuno modulatory effects (8, 9). NYT is composed of 12 crude ingredients, including Rehmannia root, Japanese angelica root, Atractylodes rhizome, Poria sclerotium, Ginseng, Cinnamon bark, Polygala root, Peony root, Citrus unshiu peel, Astragalus root, Glycyrrhiza, and Schisandra fruit.

Recent scientific approaches to analyze the mechanism of action of kampo medicine including NYT enable to understand how kampo medicines act on patients and their functional sites of action (10–12). Further, understanding of the mechanism of action for each herbal ingredient composed of NYT help the mechanism of action of NYT. In this review, we introduce multifunctional actions of NYT by showing accumulated scientific evidence based on experiments with cells and animal models and also clinical studies using NYT.

ACTIONS OF NYT FOR THE IMPROVEMENT OF DISEASES OR SYMPTOMS

Because of multi components of NYT, NYT has a variety of sites of action so that it is widely used for improvement of several types of symptoms, as follows.

Contribution of NYT to Improve Neurodisorder

NYT has been postulated to contribute of improvement of symptoms of Alzheimer's disease patients (13). In an experiment with rat embryo astrocytes, Yabe reported that NYT and its constituent onjisaponins contained in the roots of polygala tenuifolia significantly elicited nerve growth factor (NGF) secretion, a neurotrophic peptide (14). NGF is well known to be associated with the development and maintenance of cholinergic neurons in basal forebrain (15).

Sato demonstrated that the γ chain of immunoglobulin Fc receptor (FcRγ) and Fyn protein tyrosine kinase (Fyn) signaling cascade is critically involved in cuprizone-induced demyelination without any lymphocytic response with a model for certain human demyelinationing disorders (4). They showed in the model that NYT administration recovered the demyelination in cuprizone-treated mice, and also showed the site of action of NYT is the FcRγ Fyn-Rho (Rac2)—p38 mitogen-activated protein kinase phosphorylated myelin basic protein signaling, which is working in the myelination process (4).

With olfactory bulb lesions injured by Zinc sulfate perfusion, Song investigated the effects of NYT on brain monoamine and NGF (16). They showed the reductions of dopamine and its metabolites, 5-HT and its metabolite in olfactory bulb, hippocampus and substantia nigra in the model, and NYT inhibited the reduction. As a result, NYT consequently recovered the learning and memory lowered by Zinc sulfate perfusion (16).

Myelopoiesis and Erythropoiesis

Hematopoiesis is the process whereby functional, mature hematopoietic cells (red blood cells (RBCs), leukocytes, and platelets) are generated from hematopoietic stem cells in bone marrow (BM). Erythropoiesis, one aspect of hematopoiesis in which erythroid progenitors, such as burst forming unit-erythroid (BFU-B) and colony forming unit-erythroid (CFU-E) cells, is initially generated and then gives rise to erythroblasts, reticulocytes, and finally RBCs, which contain hemoglobin functioning in oxygen transport (17, 18). Failure of erythropoiesis results in a shortage of or damage to RBCs and underlies anemia. NYT has been reported to overcome anemia resulting from anticancer therapies in humans (1). In mice treated with an anticancer drug 5-fluorouracil (5-FU) and received anemia due to 5-FU, oral administration of NYT protected against hematotoxicity and induced immature erythroid progenitor cells. Also, oral administration of NYT improved 5-FU-induced anemic conditions, determined by measurement of reticulocyte and RBC numbers, hemoglobin and hematocrit levels in peripheral blood, and increases in BFU-E and CFU-E in BM in mice (3).

Modulation of Immunoresponses

Takaku reported that NYT enhanced synergistically the antitumor vaccine effects induced by $CD8^+$ T cells. They demonstrated that NYT is a useful adjuvant herbal medicine for cancer immunotherapy (6).

Multiple myeloma (MM) is an incurable malignancy of plasma cells and includes the involvement of chemokines, cytokines and growth factors secreted from MM (19). For these patients over 65 years, Melphalan-prednisone (MP) therapy has been employed (5). In this study, MP treatment lowered the concentrations of several cytokines such as RANTES, sE-selectin, but not Ang-2 and VEGF. When treated together with NYT, it enhanced MP-associated reduction and also reduced Ang-2 and VEGF. During this combination therapy, immunoglobulin concentrations were significantly improved and improved general fatigue of patients, suggesting beneficial immunotherapeutic effects of NYT on MM patients (5).

Neuropathic Pain

NYT has been reported to have anticytotoxic activities. In neuron-like pheochromocytoma PC12 cells, an antitumor drug oxaliplatin induced neurodegeneration. With this model, NYT was found to prevent the neurodegenerative effects by oxaliplatin (20). Further, in mice model, the same authors reported that NYT and its gradient ginseng, in particular, ginsenoside Rg_3, suppressed oxaliplatin-induced neurite damage and neuropathic pain (7).

Scavenging Action of NYT on Several Types of Free Radicals

NYT has been reported to have scavenging activity of several types of radicals including 1,1-diphenyl-2-picrylhydrazyl (DPPH) radicals in *in vitro* system as well as ascorbic acid and α-tocopherol (8). They proposed that examination of radical scavenging ability of kampo medicines is a better method for evaluating the efficacy of kampo medicines (8). Actually, Hange-shasinto, a kampo medicine that is widely prescribed for therapeutic use of oral stomatitis, has been reported to have radical scavenging effects in six out of seven herbal ingredients consisting of Hange-shasinto (21).

Frailty in Locomotor Disease

Frailty is a syndrome that includes broad problems of senility and consists of three domains: physical, psychological, and social. Kampo medicines are used for intervention in cases of hypofunction in a mental or physical state (22). For frailty, NYT is useful in patients with symptoms of coldness or cutaneous dryness. NYT demonstrates hematopoietic activity and is effective for osteoporosis management (22). Also, NYT was effective for anorexia of aging in Alzheimer's disease (23).

ACCUMULATED EVIDENCE OF THE EFFECTS OF EACH HERBAL PLANTS CONSISTING OF NYT

Here we show the effects of each herbal ingredient that consist of NYT, as follows (**Table 1**).

Rehmannia Root

Rehmannia root has been reported to have antiosteoporotic and neuroprotective effects (25, 26). Catalpol, the main component in Rehmannia root, inhibited ischemia-induced promyelinating oligodendrocyte damage by the regulation of intracellular homeostasis through Na^+/Ca^+ exchanger 3 activity (27). Also, catalpol reduced insulin resistance caused by high-fat diet and inflammation of adipose tissues by the inhibition of the c-Jun N-terminal kinase and nuclear factor-κ B-induced signaling (24). Catalpol is presented as a potential therapeutic for neurodegenerative diseases (25).

Japanese Angelica Root

Japanese angelica root contains many of bioactive components. One of main components is ligustilide (30). Ligustilide has antiinflammatory and antinociceptive effects (28, 29). Qian reported that ligustilide ameliorated pain caused by inflammation and inhibited TLR4 upregulation in spinal astrocytes induced by injection of complete Freund's adjuvant (30).

Atractylodes Rhizome

For atractylenolide I (ATR) in Atractylodes rhizome, a pilot randomized study ($n = 11$) of ATR on cachexia patients with

TABLE 1 | Physiological functions of basic components from each ingredients in NYT.

	Herbal ingredients	Formula in NYT	Basic components	Physiological functions	References
1	Rehmannia Root	4.0 g	catalpol	• Antiosteoporotic • Antineurodegenerative • Regulation of Na^+/Ca^{2+} exchanger 3	(24–27)
2	Japanese Angelica Root	4.0 g	ligustilide	• Antiinflammatory	(28–30)
3	Atractylodes Rhizome	4.0 g	atractylenolides	• Improve symptom of cancer patients	(31)
4	Poria Sclerotium	4.0 g	pachymic acid	• Antitumor • Inhibition of enzymes from acyl ghrelin (active) to des-acyl ghrelin (inactive)	(32–37)
5	Ginseng	3.0 g	ginsenoside	• Antitumor • Antiinflammatory • Antioxidative	(7, 38–41)
6	Cinnamon Bark	2.5 g	cinnamaldehyde	• Antiinflammatory • Antioxidative • Antitumor • Neuroprotective	(42–46)
7	Polygala Root	2.0 g	tenuigenin	• Neuroprotective • Antiinflammatory	(47–49)
8	Peony Root	2.0 g	paeoniflorin	• Pain relief • Ca^{2+} channel inhibition	(50–52)
9	Citrus Unshiu Peel	2.0 g	hesperidine, hesperetin	• Neuroprotective • Antioxidant • Antiinflammatory	(53–56)
10	Astragalus Root	1.5 g	astragaloside, isoastragaloside	• Elevation of adiponectin production • Antitumor	(57–60)
11	Glycyrrhiza	1.0 g	glycyrrhizin, glycycoumarin	• Antiinflammatory • Antioxidative • Neuroparotective • Keep ghrelin levels as pachimic acid	(32, 61, 62)
12	Schisandra Fruit	1.0 g	schizandrin	• Antiinflammatory • Enhancement of skeletal muscle endurance	(63–65)

gastric cancer showed ATR was significantly more effective than fish-oil-enriched nutritional supplementation in improving appetite and Karnofski performance status, suggesting ATR might be beneficial in alleviating cachexic symptoms in gastric cancer patients (31).

Poria Sclerotium

Poria sclerotium has a long history as a herbal medicine and a wild spectrum of pharmacological activities such as antitumor, antioxidant, antiinflammatory effects (33). Pachymic acid, one of the main components of Poria sclerotium, has been reported to have antitumor effects to several types of tumor cells (34–37). On the other hand, Rikkunshito, a kampo medicine prescribed for gastrointestinal disorders, enhances orexigenic ghrelin-mediated signaling (10, 12). Acyl ghrelin is the active hormone and it degrades inactive form of des-acyl ghrelin by ghrelin deacylating enzymes (32). Pachymic acid in Poria sclerotium as well as glycycoumarin in Glycyrrhiza and 10-gingerol in Ginger inhibited this enzyme activity and kept circulating acyl ghrelin levels, thus maintaining the effect of ghrelin (32). NYT contains both Poria sclerotium and Glycyrrhiza, suggesting these two ingredients may involve the ghrelin-mediated signaling in NYT (12).

Ginseng

Ginseng has a wide range of pharmacological activities including antitumor, antiinflammatory, antioxidative and inhibition of cardiovascular diseases (40, 41). Further, the extract of Ginseng (Rg_3) showed a protective effect against neurite damage induced by oxaliplatin (7). Ginseng extracts partially relieved oxaliplatin-induced neuropathic pain (7). In the effect to central neurons system, many of studies suggest ginseng causes improvement in memory and learning in the aged or damaged brain in rats (38). Also, ginsenoside-Rg_2 from Panax ginseng protected memory impairment through antiapoptosis with a rat model having vascular dementia (39).

Cinnamon Bark

Cinnamon bark is widely used in food and traditional herbal medicine including NYT. Cinnamon has been reported to elicit diverse biological functions such as antiinflammatory (42) antioxidant (43), antimicrobial (43), and antitumor activity (44). A recent report showed that cinnamaldehyde has potent neuroprotective effects against oxidative stress and apoptosis induced by glutamate with rat pheochromocytoma PC12 cell as a neuron model (45). As for antioxidative effect of cinnamon bark, Sedighi recently reported that the extract of cinnamon bark with ethanol could protect the heart injured by ischemia–reperfusion probably because of its antioxidant properties (46).

Polygala Root

Tenuigenin in Polygala root has been reported to have neuroprotective effects. For example, it promoted hippocampal neural stem cell proliferation and differentiation (48) and it also has protective effects in cultured hippocampal neurons (47). Furthermore, tenuigenin has antiinflammatory effects and it inhibited lipopolysaccharide-induced inflammatory responses in microglia via activating the Nuclear factor E2-related factor 2-mediated heme oxygenase 1 signaling pathway (49).

Peony Root

Products from Peony root have been used for pain relief (52) and antispasmodic (51). Paeoniflorin, a glycoside isolated from Peony root, is reported to inhibit L-type Ca^{2+} currents in neuroblastoma NG108-15 cells (50). These effects may partially explain paeoniflorin or Peony root to cause neuronal or neuroendocrine inhibitory effects as well as pain relief (50).

Citrus Unshiu Peel

A flavonoid hesperetin in Citrus unshiu peel is reported to have a variety of biological activities, including anticancer, antiviral, antioxidant, neuroprotective and antiinflammatory properties (55). For example, hesperidin ameliorates cognitive dysfunction, oxidative stress and apoptosis against aluminum chloride induced rat model of Alzheimer's disease (56). Administration of citrus unshiu peel is reported to reverse age-induced demyelination (54). Also, restoration of FcRγ/Fyn signaling activated by citrus unshiu peel repaired central nervous system demyelination (53).

Astragalus Root

Main components in Astragalus root are astragaloside and isoastragaloside. Xu reported that astragaloside and isoastragaloside in Astragalus root by screening of 50 medical herbs elevated circulating adiponectin levels by enhancing adiponectin production in mouse adipocytes (60), a well-known hormone to reduce risk of obesity, cardiovascular, and diabetic pathophysiology (57, 58). Also, Astragalus extract was reported to inhibit destruction of gastric cancer cells to methothelial cells by antiapoptosis, suggesting that Astragalus root can be used an adjuvant chemotherapeutic agent in gastric cancer therapy (59).

Glycyrrhiza

Glycyrrhiza extracts such as glycyrrhizin has been reported to have a variety of biological activities such as antiinflammation, anticancer, antioxidative, antiviral, antimicrobial effects as well as neuroprotective and immunomodulatory effects (61, 62). Also, as mentioned in the above section of Poria sclerotium, glycycoumarin in Glycyrrhiza inhibited circulating deacylating enzymes to consequently enhance the ghrelin-mediated signaling (32).

Schisandra Fruit

Schisandra fruit has many of bioactive activities. Kim reported that its extracts improved endurance and energy metabolism by upregulation of proliferator-activated receptor γ coactivator-1α (PGC-1α) in the skeletal muscle of exercised rats (64). Moon reported schizandrin, a main component of Schisandra fruit had antiinflammatory effects and it could be useful for the inflammatory and atopic diseases (63). Further, schizandrin B, an extract from Schisandra fruit ameliorated the lipopolysaccharide-induced depressive-like behaviors by attenuation of inflammation in the hypothalamic paraventricular nucleus and central nucleus of the amygdala in mice (65).

CLINICAL STUDIES USING NYT

Although not so many, clinical studies regarding the effects of NYT on healthy human or patients have been conducted. Clinical reports showed that BT-11, the extract of dried roots of Polygala that is ingredient of NYT, had memory-enhancing effects in a randomized, placebo-controlled and double-blind study of BT-11 in healthy adults (66). The extract is also reported to have enhancing effects in cognition in elderly humans in a randomized, placebo-controlled and double-blind study (67).

In clinical study with Alzheimer's patients (23 patients) over 2-year period, two groups between donepezil (11 patients) and donepezil with NYT (12 patients) treatment were compared and assessed. Tests performed included Mini-Mental State Examination and the Alzheimer's Disease Assessment Scale-cognitive component-Japanese version for cognitive function (13). Further, the Neuropsychiatric Inventory was used to evaluate the patients' mood status at baseline and every 6 months for 2 years (13). Authors demonstrated that A 2-year follow-up of patients receiving donepezil with NYT treatment showed an improved cognitive outcome and alleviation of Alzheimer's disease-related depression, judged from several tests mentioned (13). Further, an open-label pilot study with frail Alzheimer's disease patients showed that NYT could be a new-type dementia therapeutic agent with low risk of adverse effects, which improves anorexia, apathy, and cognitive dysfunction (23).

Nowadays, complementary and alternative medicine such as traditional Chinese medicines and Japanese kampo medicines is frequently used together with western medicines for treatment of diseases including chronic kidney diseases (68). In an open-label clinical study, Hsiao reported that NYT could decrease chronic inflammation and increase QOL in 59 (27 NYT and 32 control) patients treated with hemodialysis due to chronic kidney diseases (68). In addition, a randomized controlled trial with NYT was conducted in patients receiving ribavirin, which shows a strong antiviral effect on hepatitis C. Ribavirin is known to cause serve anemia and this is the major problem. In the study, NYT was shown to ameliorate the anemia induced by ribavirin in patients with hepatitis C (1). Also, combination of a clinical study with hepatitis C patients and *in vitro* studies have shown that NYT and some of its ingredients were effective in the treatment of chronic hepatitis C (69). With regard to hepatocellular carcinoma, one study in cancer patients having advanced hepatocellular carcinoma, together with experimental study with a rat hepatocellular carcinoma model revealed that NYT could enable continuous administration of the anticancer drug sorafenib due to suppression of failure of liver functions and reduction of platelets (70). Lastly, a clinical I/II open-label study with NYT showed that NYT was safe and useful for improvement of fatigue in nonanemic cancer survivors (71).

CONCLUSION

Since NYT is consist of 12 herbal ingredients and each ingredient has potent improving activities of a variety of symptoms in patients with significant biological activities, the beneficial effect of NYT could be promising. Accordingly, not a few of clinical studies with NYT are now ongoing. In the near future we will recognize and understand the beneficial effects of NYT to patients suffering from many of unpleasant symptoms, owing to the progression of evidence-based scientific researches with NYT.

AUTHOR CONTRIBUTIONS

In this review, KM and YU mainly wrote and summarized the data of NYT. MN, MU and KO contributed to summarize the effects of each ingredient composed of NYT. As a results, all authors have made a substantial, direct and intellectual contribution to the work.

FUNDING

This work was supported by research grants from AMED under Grant Number 17lk0310037h0001, from Kracie Pharma, Ltd. and from Advanced Brain Research International, Inc.

REFERENCES

Motoo Y, Mouri H, Ohtsubo K, Yamaguchi Y, Watanabe H, Sawabu N. Herbal medicine Ninjinyoeito ameliorates ribavirin-induced anemia in chronic hepatitis C: a randomized controlled trial. *World J Gastroenterol.* (2005) 11:4013–7. doi: 10.3748/wjg.v11.i26.4013

Tanaka K, Sawamura S. Therapeutic effect of a traditional Chinese medicine, ren-shen-yang-rong-tang (Japanese name: Ninjin'yoeito) on nitric oxide-mediated lung injury in a mouse infected with murine cytomegalovirus. *Int Immunopharmacol.* (2000) 6:678–85. doi: 10.1016/j.intimp.2005. 10.011

Takano F, Ohta Y, Tanaka T, Sasaki K, Kobayashi K, Takahashi T, et al. Oral administration of Ren-Shen-Yang-Rong-Tang 'Ninjin'yoeito' protects against hematotoxicity and induces immature erythroid progenitor cells in 5- fluorouracil-induced anemia. *Evid Based Complement Alternat Med.* (2009) 6:247–56. doi: 10.1093/ecam/nem080

Sato N, Seiwa, C, Komatsu, Y, Kawakita, T, Asou H, Yasukawa A. A Kampo medicine Ninjin-Youei-To promotes recovery from demyelination by FcRγ/Fyn signaling. *J Traditional Veterinary Med.* (2008) 16:3–12.

Nomura S, Ishii K, Fujita Y, Azuma Y, Hotta M, Yoshimura Y, et al. Immunotherapeutic effects of Ninjin-youei-to on patients with multiple myeloma. *Curr Trends Immunol.* (2014) 15:19–27.

Takaku S, Shimizu M, Takahashi H. Japanese Kampo medicine ninjin'yoeito synergistically enhances tumor vaccine effects mediated by CD8+ T cells. *Oncol Lett.* (2017) 13:3471–8. doi: 10.3892/ol.2017.5937

Suzuki T, Yamamoto A, Ohsawa M, Motoo Y, Mizukami H, Makino T. Effect of ninjin'yoeito and ginseng extracts on oxaliplatin-induced neuropathies in mice. *J Nat Med.* (2017) 71:757–64. doi: 10.1007/s11418-017-1113-6

Egashira T, Takayama F, Komatsu Y. Changes of materials that scavenge 1,1-diphenyl-2-picrylhydrazyl radicals in plasma by per-oral administration of Kampo medicine, Ninjin-yoei-to in rats. *J Pharm Pharmacol.* (2003) 55:367–71. doi: 10.1211/002235702711

Nakada T, Watanabe K, Jin GB, Triizuk K, Hanawa T. Effect of ninjin-youei-to on Th1/Th2 type cytokine production in different mouse strains. *Am J Chin Med.* (2002) 30:215–23. doi: 10.1142/S0192415X0200034X

Fujitsuka N, Asakawa A, Uezono Y, Minami K, Yamaguchi T, Niijima A, et al. Potentiation of ghrelin signaling attenuates cancer anorexia-cachexia and prolongs survival. *Transl Psychiatry.* (2011) 1:e23. doi: 10.1038/tp.2011.25

Fujitsuka N, Asakawa A, Morinaga A, Amitani MS, Amitani H, Katsuura G, et al.

Increased ghrelin signaling prolongs survival in mouse models of human aging through activation of sirtuin1. *Mol Psychiatry.* (2016) 21:1613–23. doi: 10.1038/mp.2015.220

Uezono Y, Miyano K, Sudo Y, Suzuki M, Shiraishi S, Terawaki K. A review of traditional Japanese medicines and their potential mechanism of action. *Curr Pharm Des.* (2012) 18:4839–53. doi: 10.2174/138161212803216924

Kudoh C, Arita R, Honda M, Kishi T, Komatsu Y, Asou H, et al. Effect of ninjin'yoeito, a Kampo (traditional Japanese) medicine, on cognitive impairment and depression in patients with Alzheimer's disease: 2 years of observation. *Psychogeriatrics* (2016) 16:85–92. doi: 10.1111/psyg.12125

Yabe T, Tuchida H, Kiyohara H, Takeda T, Yamada H. Induction of NGF synthesis in astrocytes by onjisaponins of Polygala tenuifolia, constituents of kampo (Japanese herbal) medicine, Ninjin-yoei-to. *Phytomedicine* (2003) 10:106–14. doi: 10.1078/094471103321659799

Thoenen H. The changing scene of neurotrophic factors. *Trends Neurosci.* (1991) 14:165–70.

Song Q-H, Torizuka K, Iijima K, Watanabe K, Cyong J-C. Effects of Ninjin- yoei-to (Rensheng-Yangrong-Tang), a Kampo medicine, on brain monoamine and nerve growth factor contents in mice with olfactory bulb lesions. *J Traditional Med.* (2001) 18:64–70.

McGrath K, Palis J. Ontogeny of erythropoiesis in the mammalian embryo. *Curr Top Dev Biol.* (2008) 82:1–22. doi: 10.1016/S0070-2153(07)00001-4

Inoue T, Kulkeaw K, Muennu K, Tanaka Y, Nakanishi Y, Sugiyama D. Herbal drug ninjin'yoeito accelerates myelopoiesis but not erythropoiesis in vitro. *Genes Cells.* (2014) 19:432–40. doi: 10.1111/gtc.12143

Kyle RA, Therneau TM, Rajkumar SV, Offord JR, Larson DR, Plevak MF, et al. A long-term study of prognosis in monoclonal gammopathy of undetermined significance. *N Engl J Med.* (2002) 346:564–9. doi: 10.1056/NEJMoa01133202

Suzuki T, Yamamoto A, Ohsawa M, Motoo Y, Mizukami H, Makino T. Ninjin'yoeito and ginseng extract prevent oxaliplatin-induced neurodegeneration in PC12 cells. *J Nat Med.* (2015) 69:531–7. doi: 10.1007/s11418-015-0921-9

Matsumoto C, Sekine-Suzuki E, Nyui M, Ueno M, Nakanishi I, Omiya Y, et al. Analysis of the antioxidative function of the radioprotective Japanese traditional (Kampo) medicine, hangeshashinto, in an aqueous phase. *J Radiat Res.* (2015) 56:669–77. doi: 10.1093/jrr/rrv023

Nakae H, Hiroshima Y, Hebiguchi M. Kampo medicines for frailty in locomotor disease. *Front Nutr.* (2018) 5:31. doi: 10.3389/fnut.2018.00031

Ohsawa M, Tanaka Y, Ehara Y, Makita S, Onaka KA (2017). Possibility of simultaneous treatment with the multicomponent drug, Ninjin'yoeito, for anorexia, apathy, and cognitive dysfunction in frail Alzheimer's disease patients: an open-label pilot study. *J Alzheimer Dis Rep.* 1:229–235. doi: 10.3233/ADR-170026

Zhou J, Xu G, Ma S, Li F, Yuan M, Xu H, et al. Catalpol ameliorates high-fat diet-induced insulin resistance and adipose tissue inflammation by suppressing the JNK and NF-kB pathways. *Biochem Biophys Res Commun.* (2015) 467:853–8. doi: 10.1016/j.bbrc.2015.10.054

Jiang B, Shen RF, Bi J, Tian XS, Hinchliffe T, Xia Y. Catalpol: a following complete Freund's adjuvant peripheral injection. *Cell Mol Neurobiol.* (2016) 36:143–9. doi: 10.1007/s10571-015-0228-0

Liu C, Ma R, Wang L, Zhu R, Liu H, Guo Y, et al. Rehmanniae radix in osteoporosis: a review of traditional chinese medicinal uses, phytochemistry, pharmacokinetics and pharmacology. *J Ethnopharmacol.* (2017) 198:351–62. doi: 10.1016/j.jep.2017.01.021

Cai Q, Ma T, Tian Y, Li C, Li H. Catalpol inhibits ischemia-induced premyelinating oligodendrocyte damage through regulation of intercellular calcium homeostasis via Na+/Ca2+ exchanger 3. Int J Mol Sci. (2018) 19:E1925. doi: 10.3390/ijms19071925

Du J, Yu Y, Ke Y, Wang C, Zhu L, Qian ZM. Ligustilide attenuates pain behavior induced by acetic acid or formalin. *J Ethnopharmacol.* (2007) 112:211–4. doi: 10.1016/j.jep.2007.02.007

Liu Y, Jia Z, Dong L, Wang, R, Qiu G. A randomized pilot study of atractylenolide I on gastric cancer cachexia patients. *Evid Based Complement Alternat Med.* (2008) 5:337–44. doi: 10.1093/ecam/nem031

Sadakane C, Muto S, Nakagawa K, Ohnishi S, Saegusa Y, Nahata M, et al. 10-Gingerol, a component of rikkunshito, improves cisplatin-induced anorexia by inhibiting acylated ghrelin degradation. *Biochem Biophys Res Commun.* (2011) 412:506–11. doi: 10.1016/j.bbrc.2011.08.002

Wang YZ, Zhang J, Zhao YL, Li T, Shen T, Li JQ, et al. Mycology, cultivation, traditional uses, phytochemistry and pharmacology of *Wolfiporia cocos* (Schwein.) Ryvarden et Gilb.: a review. *J Ethnopharmacol.* (2013) 147:265–76. doi: 10.1016/j.jep.2013.03.027

Gao AH, Zhang L, Chen X, Chen Y, Xu ZZ, Liu YN, et al. Inhibition of ovarian cancer proliferation and invasion by pachymic acid. *Int J Clin Exp Pathol.* (2015) 8:2235–41.

Chen Y, Lian P, Liu Y, Xu K. Pachymic acid inhibits tumorigenesis in gallbladder carcinoma cells. *Int J Clin Exp Med.* (2015) 8:17781–8.

Wen H, Wu Z, Hu H, Wu Y, Yang G, Lu J, et al. The anti- tumor effect of pachymic acid on osteosarcoma cells by inducing PTEN and Caspase 3/7-dependent apoptosis. *J Nat Med.* (2018) 72:57–63. doi: 10.1007/s11418-017-1117-2

Sun KX, Xia HW. Pachymic acid inhibits growth and induces cell cycle arrest and apoptosis in gastric cancer SGC-7901 cells. *Oncol Lett.* (2018) 16:2517–24. doi: 10.3892/ol.2018.8899

Zhong Y-M, Nishijo H, Uwano T, Tamura R, Kawanishi K, Ono T, et al. Red ginseng ameliorated place navigation deficits in young rats with hippocampal lesions and aged rats. *Physiol Behav.* (2000) 69:511–25. doi: 10.1016/S0031-9384(00)00206-7

Zhang G, Liu A, Zhou Y, San X, Jin T, Jin Y. Panax ginseng ginsenoside-Rg2 protects memory impairment via anti-apoptosis in a rat model with vascular dementia. *J Ethnopharmacol.* (2008) 115:441–8. doi: 10.1016/j.jep.2007.10.026

Zheng M, Xin Y, Li Y, Xu F, Xi X, Guo H, et al. Ginsenosides: A potential neuroprotective agent. *Biomed Res Int.* (2018) 2018:8174345. doi: 10.1155/2018/8174345

Kim JH. Pharmacological and medical applications of Panax ginseng and ginsenosides: a review for use in cardiovascular diseases. *J Ginseng Res.* (2018) 42:264–9. doi: 10.1016/j.jgr.2017.10.004

Lee SH, Lee SY, Son DJ, Lee H, Yoo HS, Song S, et al. Inhibitory effect of 2'-hydroxycinnamaldehyde on nitric oxide production through inhibition of NF-κB activation in RAW 264.7 cells. *Biochem Pharmacol.* (2005) 69:791–9. doi: 10.1016/j.bcp.2004.11.013

Singh G, Maurya S, Delampasona MP, Catalan CAN. A comparison of chemical, antioxidant and antimicrobial studies of cinnamon leaf and bark volatile oils, oleoresins and their constituents. *Food Chem. Toxicol.* (2007) 45:1650–61. doi: 10.1016/j.fct.2007.02.031

Kwon HK, Jeon WK, Hwang JS, Lee CG, So JS, Park JA, et al. Cinnamon extract suppresses tumor progression by modulating angiogenesis and the effector function of $CD8^+$ T cells. *Cancer Lett.* (2009) 278:174–82. doi: 10.1016/j.canlet.2009.01.015

Lv C, Yuan X, Zeng HW, Liu RH, Zhang WD. Protective effect of cinnamaldehyde against glutamate-induced oxidative stress and apoptosis in PC12 cells. *Eur J Pharmacol.* (2017) 815:487–94. doi: 10.1016/j.ejphar.2017.09.009

Sedighi M, Nazari A, Faghihi M, Rafieian-Kopaei M, Karimi A, Moghimian M, et al. Protective effects of cinnamon bark extract against ischemia-reperfusion injury and arrhythmias in rat. *Phytother. Res.* (2018) doi: 10.1002/ptr.6127. [Epub ahead of print].

Zhao LX, Jiang BC, Wu XB, Cao DL, Gao YJ. Ligustilide attenuates inflammatory pain via inhibition of NFκB-mediated chemokines production in spina astrocytes. *Eur J Neurosci.* (2014) 39:1391–402. doi: 10.1111/ejn.12502

Qian B, Li F, Zhao LX, Dong YL, Gao YJ, Zhang ZJ. Ligustilide ameliorates inflammatory pain and inhibits TLR4 upregulation in spinal astrocytes

Chen YJ, Huang XB, Li,. Z. X., Yin LL, Chen WQ, Li L. Tenuigenin protects cultured hippocampal neurons against methylglyoxal-induced neurotoxicity. *Eur. J. Pharmacol.* (2010) 645:1–8. doi: 10.1016/j.ejphar.2010.06.034

Chen Y, Huang X, Chen W, Wang N, Li L. Tenuigenin promotes proliferation and differentiation of hippocampal neural stem cells. *Neurochem Res.* (2012) 37:771–7. doi: 10.1007/s11064-011-0671-3

Wang, L.i M, Cao Y, Wang J, Zhang H, Zhou X, et al. Tenuigenin inhibits LPS-induced inflammatory responses in microglia via activating the Nrf2-mediated HO-1 signaling pathway. *Eur J Pharmacol.* (2017) 809:196– 202. doi: 10.1016/j.ejphar.2017.05.004

Tsai TY, Wu SN, Liu YC, Wu AZ, Tsai YC. Inhibitory action of L-type Ca2+ current by paeoniflorin, a major constituent of peony root, in NG108-15 neuronal cells. *Eur J Pharmacol.* (2005) 523:16–24. doi: 10.1016/j.ejphar.2005.08.042

Lee KK, Omiya Y, Yuzurihara M, Kase Y, Kobayashi H. Antispasmodic effect of shakuyakukanzoto extract on experimental muscle cramps in vivo: role of the active constituents of Glycyrrhizae radix. *J Ethnopharmacol.* (2013) 145:286–93. doi: 10.1016/j.jep.2012.11.005

Wang Z, Shen L, Li X, Shu X, Shan B, Zhang L, et al. Pain-relieving effect of a compound isolated from white peony root oral liquid on acute radiation-induced esophagitis. *Mol Med Rep.* (2013) 7:1950–4. doi: 10.3892/mmr.2013.1427

Seiwa C, Yamamoto M, Tanaka K, Fukutake M, Ueki T, Takeda S, et al. Restoration of FcRgamma/Fyn signaling repairs central nervous system demyelination. *J Neurosci Res.* (2007) 85:954–66. doi: 10.1002/jnr.21196

Sato N, Seiwa C, Uruse M, Yamamoto M, Tanaka K, Kawakita T, et al. Administration of chinpi, a component of the herbal medicine ninjin-youei-to, reverses age-induced demyelination. *Evid Based Complement Alternat Med.* (2011) 2011:617438. doi: 10.1093/ecam/neq001

Roohbakhsh A, Parhiz H, Soltani F, Rezaee R, Iranshahi M. Neuropharmacological properties and pharmacokinetics of the citrus flavonoids hesperidin and hesperetin–a mini-review. *Life Sci.* (2014) 113:1–6. doi: 10.1016/j.lfs.2014.07.029

Justin Thenmozhi A, William Raja TR, Manivasagam T, Janakiraman U, Essa MM. Hesperidin ameliorates cognitive dysfunction, osidative stress and apoptosis against aluminium chloride induced rat model of Alzheimer's disease. *Nutr Neurosci.* (2017) 20:360–8. doi: 10.1080/1028415X.2016.1144846

Yamauchi T, Kamon J, Waki H, Terauchi Y, Kubota N, Hara K, et al. The fat-derived hormone adiponectin reverses insulin resistance associated with both lipoatrophy and obesity. *Nat Med.* (2001) 7:941–936. doi: 10.1038/90984

Kadowaki T, Yamauchi T, Kubota N, Hara K, Ueki K, Tobe K. Adiponectin and adiponectin receptors in insulin resistance, diabetes, and the metabolic syndrome. *J Clin Invest.* (2006) 116:1784–92. doi: 10.1172/JCI29126

Na D, Liu FN, Miao ZF, Du ZM, Xu HM. Astragalus extract inhibits destruction of gastric cancer cells to mesothelial cells by anti-apoptosis. *World J Gastroenterol.* (2009) 15:570–7. doi: 10.3748/wjg.15.570

Xu A, Wang H, Hoo RL, Sweeney G, Vanhoutte PM, Wang Y, et al. Selective elevation of adiponectin production by the natural compounds derived from a medicinal herb alleviates insulin resistance and glucose intolerance in obese mice. *Endocrinology.* (2009) 150:625–33. doi: 10.1210/en.2008-0999

Hosseinzadeh H, Nassiri-Asl M. Pharmacological Effects of Glycyrrhiza spp. and Its Bioactive Constituents: Update and Review. *Phytother Res.* (2015) 29:1868–86. doi: 10.1002/ptr.5487

Dastagir G, Rizvi MA. Glycyrrhiza glabra L. *(Liquorice) Pak J Pharm Sci.* (2016) 29:1727–33.

Moon PD, Jeong HJ, Kim HM. Effects of schizandrin on the expression of thymic stromal lymphopoietin in human mast cell line HMC-1. *Life Sci.* (2012) 91:384–8. doi: 10.1016/j.lfs.2012.08.009

Kim YJ, Yoo SR, Chae CK, Jung UJ, Choi MS. Omija fruit extract improves endurance and energy metabolism by upregulating PGC-1α expression in the skeletal muscle of exercised rats. *J Med Food.* (2014) 17:28–35. doi: 10.1089/jmf.2013.3071

Araki R, Hiraki Y, Nishida S, Inatomi Y, Yabe T. Gomisin N ameliorates lipopolysaccharide-induced depressive-like behaviors by attenuating inflammation in the hypothalamic paraventricular nucleus and central nucleus of the amygdala in mice. *J Pharmacol Sci.* (2016) 132:138–44. doi: 10.1016/j.jphs.2016.09.004

Lee JY, Kim KY, Shin KY, Won BY, Jung HY, Suh YH. Effects of BT-11 on memory in healthy humans. *Neurosci Lett.* (2009) 454:111–4. doi: 10.1016/j.neulet.2009.03.024

Shin KY, Lee JY, Won BY, Jung HY, Chang KA, Koppula S, et al. BT-11 is effective for enhancing cognitive functions in the elderly humans. *Neurosci Lett.* (2009) 465:157–9. doi: 10.1016/j.neulet.2009. 08.033

Hsiao PJ, Lin KS, Chiu CC, Chen HW, Huang JS, Kao SY, et al. Use of traditional Chinese medicine (Ren Shen Yang Rong Tang) against microinflammation in hemodialysis patients: An open-label trial. *Complement Ther Med.* (2015) 23:363–71. doi: 10.1016/j.ctim.2015.03.002

Cyong J-C, Ki SM, Iijima K, Kobayashi T, Furuya M. Clinical and pharmacological studies on liver diseases treated with Kampo herbal medicine. *Am J Chin Med.* (2000) 28:351–60. doi: 10.1142/S0192415X00000416

Kaibori M, Ishizaki M, Matsui K, Kwon M, Imai R, Watanabe S, et al. Sorafenib alone versus a combination of sorafenib and ninjin'yoeito for the treatment of patients with advanced hepatocellular carcinoma: a retrospective study and pharmacological study in rats. *J Trad Med.* (2013) 30:221–8. doi: 10.11339/jtm.30.221

Xu Y, Chen Y, Li P, Wang XS. Ren Shen Yangrong Tang for fatigue in cancer survivors: A phase I/II open-label study. *J Altern Complement Med.* (2015) 21:281–7. doi: 10.1089/acm.2014.0211

3

Combined Use of Ninjin'yoeito Improves Subjective Fatigue Caused by Lenalidomide in Patients with Multiple Myeloma: A Retrospective Study

Tomoki Ito, Akiko Konishi, Yukie Tsubokura, Yoshiko Azuma, Masaaki Hotta, Hideaki Yoshimura, Takahisa Nakanishi, Shinya Fujita, Aya Nakaya, Atsushi Satake, Kazuyoshi Ishii and Shosaku Nomura*

First Department of Internal Medicine, Kansai Medical University, Hirakata, Japan

***Correspondence:**
Tomoki Ito
itot@hirakata.kmu.ac.jp

Lenalidomide is an immunomodulating derivative of thalidomide, which shows anti-tumor activity against myeloma cells with immunomodulation including augmentation of T-cell and natural killer cell function. Continuous treatment with this agent shows better survival benefit in patients with multiple myeloma and combined lenalidomide with dexamethasone (LEN-DEX) is a standard treatment regimen. However, fatigue is a frequent symptom resulting from lenalidomide administration. This side-effect therefore reduces quality of life for elderly patients and, furthermore, is a reason for treatment discontinuation. Unfortunately, appropriate preventive countermeasures against lenalidomide-related fatigue have not been established. Ninjin'yoeito is a traditional Chinese medicine made from the extracts of 12 herbal plants, which positively affects immunity and inflammation. It is used to treat fatigue, decreased appetite, anemia, and general malaise associated with malignant tumors and chemotherapy. We have previously reported that ninjin'yoeito significantly improved patients' subjective fatigue symptoms treated with melphalan-prednisone for multiple myeloma. In the present study, we assessed the benefits of ninjin'yoeito as a supplementary treatment for patients with myeloma, and its effect on lenalidomide treatment regime compliance. We retrospectively analyzed 36 cases of newly diagnosed or relapsed/refractory multiple myeloma. The study included patients receiving LEN-DEX with onset of general fatigue after lenalidomide administration (13 and 23 patients with or without ninjin'yoeito, respectively). Frequency of subjective fatigue was significantly decreased in patients administered ninjin'yoeito, compared to those treated with LEN-DEX alone (92.3 and 47.8 % of patients with and without ninjin'yoeito, respectively; $p = 0.008$). In addition, combined use of ninjin'yoeito and LEN-DEX showed a trend toward reduced rates of treatment discontinuation (7.7 % and 34.8 % of patients with and without ninjin'yoeito, respectively; $p = 0.076$). Our results suggest that ninjin'yoeito is an effective method for treating subjective fatigue caused by lenalidomide and may have the potential to extend lenalidomide treatment duration.

Keywords: Chinese medicine, lenalidomide, multiple myeloma, fatigue, ninjin'yoeito

INTRODUCTION

Lenalidomide (LEN) is an immunomodulating derivative of thalidomide and classified as immunomodulatory drug (IMiD) that has both direct tumoricidal and immunomodulatory effects in multiple myeloma (MM). LEN displays immunopotentiating activity, including augmentation of T and natural killer cell function (1–7).

LEN with dexamethasone (LEN-DEX) is a backbone regimen for MM. At present, the standard of care for patients with newly diagnosed or relapsed/refractory MM is to administer LEN combined with proteasome inhibitors or antibody-drugs. In addition, continuous treatment of LEN until progression diseases results in better survival benefit in MM patients (8–10).

Despite the benefits of LEN, general fatigue is sometimes an adverse event during its administration in clinical practice. In a randomized phase 3 trial consisting of newly diagnosed MM patients, grade 3 or 4 fatigue was observed in 7 to 9 % of the patients administered LEN-DEX as a first line treatment (9). Similarly, grade 3 or 4 fatigue has been reported for 6.5 % of relapsed or refractory MM patients (11). Furthermore, 47 % of patients receiving LEN maintenance therapy after autologous stem-cell transplantation experience fatigue to some extent (8). In clinical practice, LEN dosage is often reduced or treatment discontinued as a result of patients experiencing fatigue in addition to dysgeusia, anemia, and gastrointestinal symptoms. Unfortunately, at present there is no effective countermeasure against these adverse events.

Ninjin'yoeito (NYT) is a traditional Chinese medicine made from the extracts of 12 herbal plants, which has known beneficial effects on immunity and inflammation (12, 13). Components of NYT is listed in STORK (http://mpdb.nibiohn.go.jp/stork/). NYT has been used to treat fatigue, anorexia, anemia, and coldness of hands and feet. Notably, NYT not only has a supportive effect against MM with treatment of melphalan, but also relieves subjective symptoms, such as fatigue and pain (14). Although its mechanism of action is still largely unknown, NYT is therefore expected to improve quality of life for MM patients. In the present study, we focused on these activities and assessed whether combination of NYT is useful against the LEN-related subjective fatigue. Furthermore, we investigated whether discontinuation of LEN can be improved by combination use of NYT.

TABLE 1 | Patient base line characteristics.

	Lenalidomide + NYT ($n = 13$)	Lenalidomide alone ($n = 23$)	*p*-value
Age, median (range), years	72 (53-85)	67 (45-79)	$p = 0.213$
Sex, male/female, %	38.5 / 61.5	47.8% / 52.2%	$p = 0.731$
ECOG PS score, *n* (%)			
0	5 (38.5)	11 (47.8)	$p = 0.847$
1	5 (38.5)	8 (34.8)	
2	3 (23.1)	4 (17.4)	
ISS stage, *n* (%)			
I	4 (31.0)	6 (26.1)	$p = 0.765$
II	6 (46.2)	9 (39.1)	
III	3 (23.1)	8 (34.8)	
No. of prior therapies, *n* (%)			
0	2 (15.4)	7 (30.4)	$p = 0.589$
1	5 (38.5)	8 (34.8)	
≧2	6 (46.2)	8 (34.8)	
M protein subtype, *n* (%)			
IgG	7 (53.8)	14 (60.9)	$p = 0.898$
IgA	3 (23.1)	4 (17.4)	
BJP	3 (23.1)	5 (21.7)	
Doses of LEN, mean ± SD	14.2 ± 3.4 mg	14.6 ± 4.5 mg	$p = 0.804$
Severity of fatigue, *n* (%)*			
Grade 1	8 (61.5)	17 (73.9)	$p = 0.797$
Grade 2	4 (31.0)	5 (21.7)	
Grade 3	1 (7.7)	2 (8.7)	

ECOG, Eastern Cooperative Oncology Group; PS, Performance Status; ISS, International staging system; BJP, Bence Jones protein.
**Severity of fatigue was graded after 1 cycle-treatment of LEN-DEX and before administration of NYT.*
P-value regarding "age" was calculated by unpaired t-test with Welch's correction. P-value regarding "sex" was calculated by a two-sided Fisher's exact-test. P-value regarding "PS score," "ISS stage," "prior therapies," "M protein subtype," "doses of LEN," and "Severity of fatigue" were calculated by a Chi-square test.

PATIENTS AND METHODS

Patients and Treatment

We retrospectively analyzed 36 cases of newly diagnosed or relapsed/refractory receiving LEN-DEX with ($n = 13$) or without ($n = 23$) NYT between January 2011 and December 2017, who experienced general fatigue as a result of LEN-DEX treatment (**Table 1**). Patients received either oral lenalidomide 5–25 mg per day (depending on the judgment of a doctor in charge) on days 1–21 of each 28-day cycle. All patients received 20–40 mg oral dexamethasone on days 1, 8, 15, and 22 of each 28-day cycle (for 4 cycles) until disease progression. After 1 cycle-treatment of LEN-DEX, the severity of fatigue was graded using the National Cancer Institute Common Terminology Criteria for Adverse Events (NCI CTCAE) version 4.0 (code 10016256, grade 1-3) by clinical interview. We started oral administration of NYT (Kracie Pharma, Ltd) at a dose of 5.0 g/day when patients complained of grade 1 or more fatigue after LEN-DEX treatment according to the patients' requests, while continued LEN-DEX alone if the patients did not want NYT. Patient base line characteristics are shown in **Table 1**. We assessed the effectiveness of NYT for the severity or grade of subjective fatigue by clinical interview after every treatment cycle and we collected the data of discontinuation of LEN-DEX up to 6 months after administration. LEN-DEX were discontinued in total 9 patients. In these cases, severity or grade of fatigue was evaluated at the last cycle of LEN-DEX administration.

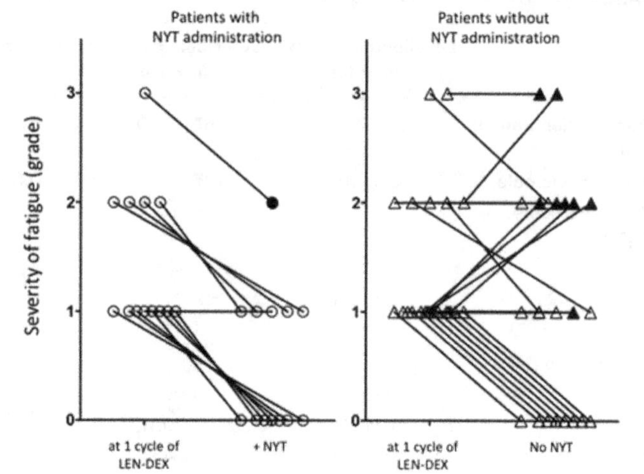

FIGURE 1 | Change of fatigue grade in patients treated with or without NYT. After 1 cycle-treatment of LEN-DEX, the severity of fatigue was graded, and then NYT was administered according to the patients' requests. When the patients did not want NYT, LEN-DEX alone were continued. Assessment of the effectiveness of NYT for the severity of subjective fatigue and LEN-DEX discontinuation up to 6 months. ○, Patients with NYT administration; Δ, Patients without NYT administration; ● and ▲, show LEN-DEX-discontinued patients within 6 months. For these 9 discontinued patients, severity of fatigue was evaluated at the last cycle of LEN-DEX administration.

This study was carried out in accordance with the recommendations of the International Conference on Harmonization guidelines for Good Clinical Practice with written informed consent from all subjects. All subjects gave written informed consent in accordance with the Declaration of Helsinki. The protocol was approved by the Institutional Review Board of Kansai Medical University.

Statistical Analysis

The data from 2 groups (LEN-DEX with and without NYT) were compared by 2-way Contingency Table Analysis using a Fisher's exact test. For the background of patient profile, *p*-value regarding "age" and "sex" were calculated by unpaired *t*-test with Welch's correction and two-sided Fisher's exact test, respectively. *P*-value regarding "PS score", "ISS stage," "prior therapies," "M protein subtype," "doses of LEN," and "Severity of fatigue" were calculated by a Chi-square test. A value of $p < 0.05$ was considered statistically significant. Data analysis was carried out with the software GraphPad Prism.

RESULTS

NYT was administered to 13 of the 36 patients with onset of general fatigue after 1 cycle of lenalidomide administration. Severity of fatigue in patients was shown in **Figure 1** and **Table 1**. For 12 patients (92.3 %), the grade of fatigue was reduced by the use of NYT in conjunction with LEN-DEX (**Figure 1** and **Table 2**). Of the 23 patients who continued LEN-DEX without NYT, 11 (47.8 %) had decrease in fatigue; however, the remaining 12 saw no improvement (5 had increased grade in fatigue during treatment) (**Figure 1**). Hence, NYT resulted in a significant increase in frequency of lower fatigue grade following its administration ($p = 0.008$).

TABLE 2 | Frequency of reduced grade of fatigue during treatment.

	Improvement of grade in fatigue	No improvement in fatigue	*p*-value
LEN-DEX + NYT ($n = 13$)	12	1	$p = 0.008$
LEN-DEX alone ($n = 23$)	11	12	

The data from 2 groups were analyzed by 2-way Contingency Table Analysis with the use of a one-sided Fisher's exact test.

TABLE 3 | Continuation of LEN-DEX treatment.

	Continuation of LEN-DEX	Discontinuation of LEN-DEX	*p*-value
LEN-DEX + NYT ($n = 13$)	12	1	$p = 0.076$
LEN-DEX alone ($n = 23$)	15	8	

The data from 2 groups were analyzed by 2-way Contingency Table Analysis with the use of a one-sided Fisher's exact test.

In addition, 12 of the 13 patients (92.3 %) administered NYT were able to continue LEN-DEX at least for the 6 months (**Figure 1** and **Table 3**). Of the 23 patients who did not receive NYT, 8 (34.8 %) failed to continue LEN-DEX. Hence, combined use of NYT and lenalidomide had a tendency toward suppressing LEN-DEX treatment discontinuation (7.7 and 34.8 % of patients with and without NYT, respectively, were unable to continue LEN-DEX treatment; $p = 0.076$).

DISCUSSION

MM remains an incurable disease with a severe prognosis; it is therefore necessary to aim for long-term disease control by specific and effective drugs. It was demonstrated that continuous therapy prolongs progression-free survival until first and second relapse and overall survival (15). Currently, lenalidomide is the main drug prescribed for continuous and maintenance therapy (16). After stem-cell transplantation, lenalidomide maintenance significantly prolonged not only progression-free survival, but also overall survival (8, 10). Therefore, avoiding dose reduction or treatment discontinuation due to intolerance and side-effects is important for extending patient survival and improving quality of life. The most common adverse events associated with lenalidomide include hematologic events, such as neutropenia, anemia, and thrombocytopenia; gastrointestinal disorders, such as nausea, vomiting, constipation, and diarrhea; and other side-effects, such as infections, and skin rashes. General disorders, such as fatigue and pyrexia are also significant adverse events (8, 9), which cause difficulty in continuing lenalidomide maintaining treatment regimens in clinical practice. However, there is no effective means for treating these general and subjective symptoms, with the exception of dose reduction or treatment discontinuation.

Previously, we found that NYT had the potential to repress general fatigue caused by melphalan (14). The present study suggests that NYT may also be useful for improving the symptoms of subjective fatigue caused by lenalidomide in patients with MM. A possible mechanism of NYT to relieve the fatigue caused by chemotherapy could be an effect of *Schisandra* as components of NYT. *Schisandra* has been shown to possess anti-athletic fatigue activity in mice (17) and improve endurance and energy metabolism in exercised rats (18). *Schisandra* has a potential to upregulate peroxisome proliferator-activated receptor-gamma coactivator (PGC)-1alpha in skeletal muscle, which is a key regulator of energy metabolism (18). Further studies are needed to clarify the detailed mechanisms involved in the anti-fatigue properties of NYT.

Supplementing lenalidomide administration with NYT could result in increased treatment durations and hence increase life expectancy. The limitations of our report are the retrospective analysis and a small number of patients derived from the setting of everyday clinical practice including several biases. In addition to this, there is a possibility that the effect we observed are attributed to the placebo effect. Additional research examining clinical outcomes using NYT need to be studied in the future.

AUTHOR CONTRIBUTIONS

TI planned, designed and wrote the paper. AK, YT, YA, MH, HY, TN, SF, AN, AS, KI, and SN contributed to acquisition and collection of patients' data. All authors read and approved the final manuscript.

FUNDING

This study was supported in part by a grant (17K09963 to T.I.) from the Ministry of Education, Science and Culture of Japan.

REFERENCES

Gandhi AK, Kang J, Capone L, Parton A, Wu L, Zhang LH, et al. Dexamethasone synergizes with lenalidomide to inhibit multiple myeloma tumor growth, but reduces lenalidomide-induced immunomodulation of T and NK cell function. *Curr Cancer Drug Targets* (2010) 10:155–67. doi: 10.2174/156800910791054239

Davies FE, Raje N, Hideshima T, Lentzsch S, Young G, Tai YT, et al. Thalidomide and immunomodulatory derivatives augment natural killer cell cytotoxicity in multiple myeloma. *Blood* (2001) 98:210–6. doi: 10.1182/blood.V98.1.210

Mitsiades N, Mitsiades CS, Poulaki V, Chauhan D, Richardson PG, Hideshima T, et al. Apoptotic signaling induced by immunomodulatory thalidomide analogs in human multiple myeloma cells: therapeutic implications. *Blood* (2002) 99:4525–30. doi: 10.1182/blood.V99.12.4525

Schafer PH, Gandhi AK, Loveland MA, Chen RS, Man HW, Schnetkamp PP, et al. Enhancement of cytokine production and AP-1 transcriptional activity in T cells by thalidomide-related immunomodulatory drugs. *J Pharmacol Exp Ther.* (2003) 305:1222–32. doi: 10.1124/jpet.102.048496

Wu L, Adams M, Carter T, Chen R, Muller G, Stirling D, et al. lenalidomide enhances natural killer cell and monocyte-mediated antibody-dependent cellular cytotoxicity of rituximab-treated CD20+ tumor cells. *Clin Cancer Res.* (2008) 14:4650–7. doi: 10.1158/1078-0432.CCR-07-4405

Benson DM Jr, Bakan CE, Mishra A, Hofmeister CC, Efebera Y, Becknell B, et al. The PD-1/PD-L1 axis modulates the natural killer cell versus multiple myeloma effect: a therapeutic target for CT-011, a novel monoclonal anti-PD-1 antibody. *Blood* (2010) 116:2286–94. doi: 10.1182/blood-2010-02-271874

Reddy N, Hernandez-Ilizaliturri FJ, Deeb G, Roth M, Vaughn M, Knight J, et al. Immunomodulatory drugs stimulate natural killer-cell function, alter cytokine production by dendritic cells, and inhibit angiogenesis enhancing the anti-tumour activity of rituximab *in vivo*. *Br J Haematol.* (2008) 140:36–45. doi: 10.1111/j.1365-2141.2007.06841.x

Attal M. Lauwers-Cances V, Marit G, Caillot D, Moreau P, Facon T, et al. Lenalidomide maintenance after stem-cell transplantation for multiple myeloma. *N Engl J Med.* (2012) 366:1782–91. doi: 10.1056/NEJMoa1114138

Benboubker L, Dimopoulos MA, Dispenzieri A, Catalano J, Belch AR, Cavo M, et al. Lenalidomide and dexamethasone in transplant- ineligible patients with myeloma. *N Engl J Med.* (2014) 371:906–17. doi: 10.1056/NEJMoa1402551

McCarthy PL, Owzar K, Hofmeister CC, Hurd DD, Hassoun H, Richardson PG et al. Lenalidomide after stem-cell transplantation for multiple myeloma. *N Engl J Med.* (2012) 366:1770–81. doi: 10.1056/NEJMoa1114083

Dimopoulos MA, Chen C, Spencer A, Niesvizky R, Attal M, Stadtmauer EA, et al. Long-term follow-up on overall survival from the MM-009 and MM-010 phase III trials of lenalidomide plus dexamethasone in patients with relapsed or refractory multiple myeloma. *Leukemia* (2009) 23:2147–52. doi: 10.1038/leu.2009.147

Yonekura K, Kawakita T, Saito Y, Suzuki A, Nomoto K. Augmentation of host resistance to Listeria monocytogenes infection by a traditional Chinese medicine, ren-shen-yang-rong-tang (Japanese name: ninjin'yoeito). *Immunopharmacol Immunotoxicol.* (1992) 14:165–90. doi: 10.3109/08923979209009218

Tanaka K, Sawamura S. Therapeutic effect of a traditional Chinese medicine, ren-shen-yang-rong-tang (Japanese name: Ninjin'yoeito) on nitric oxide-mediated lung injury in a mouse infected with murine cytomegalovirus. *Int Immunopharmacol.* (2006) 6:678–85. doi: 10.1016/j.intimp.2005.10.011

Nomura S, Ishii K, Fujita Y, Azuma Y, Hotta M, Yoshimura Y, et al. Immunotherapeutic effects of ninjin'yoeito on patients with multiple myeloma. *Curr. Trends Immunol.* (2014) 15:19–27.

Palumbo A, Gay F, Cavallo F, Di Raimondo F, Larocca A, Hardan I, et al. Continuous therapy versus fixed duration of therapy in patients with newly diagnosed multiple myeloma. *J Clin Oncol.* (2015) 33:3459–66. doi: 10.1200/JCO.2014.60.2466

Palumbo A, Hajek R, Delforge M, Krop Petrucciff M, Petrucci MT, Catalano J, et al. Continuous lenalidomide treatment for newly diagnosed multiple myeloma. *N Engl J Med.* (2012) 366:1759–69. doi: 10.1056/NEJMoa1112704

Cao S, Shang H, Wu W, Du J, Putheti R. Evaluation of anti-athletic fatigue activity of Schizandra chinensis aqueous extracts in mice *Afr J Pharm Pharmacol.* (2009) 3:593–7.

Kim YJ, Yoo SR, Chae CK, Jung UJ, Choi MS. Omija fruit extract improves endurance and energy metabolism by upregulating PGC-1α expression in the skeletal muscle of exercised rats. *J Med Food* (2014) 17:28–35. doi: 10.1089/jmf.2013.3071

4

Mesenchymal Stem Cell Therapy for Aging Frailty

Ivonne Hernandez Schulman[1,2], Wayne Balkan[1] and Joshua M. Hare[1]*

[1] *Interdisciplinary Stem Cell Institute, University of Miami Miller School of Medicine, Miami, FL, United States,* [2] *Katz Family Division of Nephrology and Hypertension, University of Miami Miller School of Medicine, Miami, FL, United States*

***Correspondence:**
Ivonne Hernandez Schulman
ischulman@med.miami.edu

Chronic diseases and degenerative conditions are strongly linked with the geriatric syndrome of frailty and account for a disproportionate percentage of the health care budget. Frailty increases the risk of falls, hospitalization, institutionalization, disability, and death. By definition, frailty syndrome is characterized by declines in lean body mass, strength, endurance, balance, gait speed, activity and energy levels, and organ physiologic reserve. Collectively, these changes lead to the loss of homeostasis and capability to withstand stressors and resulting vulnerabilities. There is a strong link between frailty, inflammation, and the impaired ability to repair tissue injury due to decreases in endogenous stem cell production. Although exercise and nutritional supplementation provide benefit to frail patients, there are currently no specific therapies for frailty. Bone marrow-derived allogeneic mesenchymal stem cells (MSCs) provide therapeutic benefits in heart failure patients irrespective of age. MSCs contribute to cellular repair and tissue regeneration through their multilineage differentiation capacity, immunomodulatory, and anti-inflammatory effects, homing and migratory capacity to injury sites, and stimulatory effect on endogenous tissue progenitors. The advantages of using MSCs as a therapeutic strategy include standardization of isolation and culture expansion techniques and safety in allogeneic transplantation. Based on this evidence, we performed a randomized, double-blinded, dose-finding study in elderly, frail individuals and showed that intravenously delivered allogeneic MSCs are safe and produce significant improvements in physical performance measures and inflammatory biomarkers. We thus propose that frailty can be treated and the link between frailty and chronic inflammation offers a potential therapeutic target, addressable by cell therapy.

Keywords: cell transplantation, regenerative medicine, inflammation, immunosenescence, geriatrics

DEFINITION AND EPIDEMIOLOGY OF FRAILTY

Frailty has been clinically defined as "a state of increased vulnerability resulting from aging-associated decline in reserve and function across multiple organ systems such that the ability to cope with everyday or acute stressors is compromised" (1). Central to this geriatric medical syndrome is the notion that it has multiple causes and contributors that lead to the characteristic decreases in strength, endurance, activity, energy levels, and physiologic function, which increase the susceptibility to dependency and death (2, 3). Of note, although frailty is not characterized as a disability, it does increase the risk of disability in affected individuals (3–5). Moreover, there is a close link between a patient's health and frailty (6, 7). These patients tend to show a greater risk of frailty when there are other comorbidities affecting their physical and psychological well-being, such as cardiovascular disease, diabetes, high blood pressure, cancer, or cognitive impairment (8). The main clinical presentations of frailty are falls, which are a result of impaired balance, gait, and awareness, fluctuating disability with independent and dependent days, and other non-specific signs and symptoms, such as unexplained weight loss, infections, and extreme fatigue.

Several instruments have been developed to assess frailty. These can be categorized as the unidimensional or phenotypic model, based on the physical or biological dimension, and multidimensional or cumulative deficit models, centered on the links between the physical, psychological, and social realms, all of which have been well validated (1, 8). The unidimensional or phenotypic model was first operationally defined by Fried et al. (9) and was used to develop the Cardiovascular Health Study (CHS) Index, commonly referred to as the "Physical Frailty Phenotype" (10). Using this model, frailty is defined as having three out of five phenotypic criteria indicating "compromised energetics": weak grip strength, low energy levels or self-reported exhaustion, slow gait speed, low physical activity (low energy expenditure), and/or unintentional weight loss (9). On the other hand, the Canadian Study of Health and Aging (CSHA) frailty index was developed using the cumulative deficit model (11, 12). The CSHA frailty index measures several age-associated health deficits (13), and is computed by counting the number of health deficits and dividing this number by the total number of health questions tested (12), with a score of 1 being the maximum index and indicating the poorest prognosis. Indeed, an index >0.7 is associated with a high risk of mortality (14). This index has been simplified for use in the outpatient clinic setting as the CSHA "clinical frailty scale" (15). This 7-point rapid screening tool, consisting of 7 variables ranging from fit to complete functional dependence, highly correlates with the frailty index. The maximum in this scale is a score of 7, indicating "severe frailty" (16).

A number of other instruments to assess frailty have been developed and validated, including the "FRAIL (Fatigue, Resistance, Ambulation, Illnesses, Loss of weight)" frailty scale by the International Academy of Nutrition and Aging (17), the "Study of Osteoporotic Fractures (SOF)" frailty scale (18), the "Frailty Instrument for Primary Care of the Survey of Health, the Aging and Retirement in Europe (SHARE-FI)" scale (19), and the "Groningen Frailty Indicator" (20). The FRAIL and SOF, for example, predict new disability at 3 and 9 years of follow up and the FRAIL predicts 9-year mortality in an African American population (21). A multidimensional instrument based on a "structural questionnaire" is the "Tilburg Frailty Indicator" (TFI) (22). This instrument is made up of 10 questions on determinants of frailty that include demographics and other lifestyle questions, as well as, 15 frailty elements arranged according to physical, psychological, and social aspects. The total score of the TFI ranges from 0 to 15, with frailty ascertained if the total score is 5 or greater.

In view of the aging population worldwide, there is a growing medical and scientific interest in the accurate diagnosis and treatment of frailty. Despite multinational efforts to reach an agreement on the definition of frailty and how to assess it with a simple and easily accessible tool, no consensus has been reached, as evidenced by the various definitions and multiple assessment tools being currently used in the literature. However, an agreement has been reached broadly defining frailty as a clinical syndrome characterized by increased vulnerability to stressors that leads to functional impairments and adverse health outcomes (2). This definition is considered to be useful in primary care assessments. Moreover, these functional impairments and health outcomes may be preventable or treatable by pharmacologic or non-pharmacologic interventions.

With regards to the prevalence of frailty in community dwelling individuals over the age of 65 in the United States, it was estimated at 7–12% using the frailty criteria validated in the CHS (10). Moreover, frailty prevalence increased with age from 3.9 to 25% in the 65–74 and over 85 age groups, respectively. Frailty prevalence was also found to be greater in women than men (8 vs. 5%). Ethnic differences in frailty prevalence were noted, with black Americans more likely to be frail than white Americans (13 vs. 6%) and Mexican Americans similar to Caucasians 7.8% (23), based on the Hispanic Established Populations Epidemiologic Studies of the Elderly. Compared to frailty, pre-frailty has a much greater prevalence, ranging between 35 and 50% in adults aged 65 or older. Pre-frailty is considered to be present in patients exhibiting one or two of the phenotypic criteria described in CHS and is reportedly more common in women than in men, just like frailty (9). There is also an association between pre-frailty and lower educational level and socio-economic status (24, 25). Despite the higher accumulation of deficits in women than in men of the same age, men exhibit a higher risk of mortality even though this accumulation is associated with mortality in both genders (26–28). Importantly, comorbidities, especially cardiovascular, pulmonary, musculoskeletal, neurologic, and psychiatric, are more prevalent in pre-frail compared to non-frail persons (24, 25, 29).

FRAILTY AND CARDIOVASCULAR PERFORMANCE

The prevalence of cardiovascular disease (CVD) increases substantially in individuals 65 years of age and over, and especially in individuals aged 80 and over (30). Not surprisingly, increased CVD prevalence is linked with increased prevalence and incidence of frailty, as shown in a meta-analysis of 54,250 elderly patients without frailty at baseline (31).

The aging cardiovascular system has some very specific phenotypic alterations (9, 30, 32). These include aortic stiffness due to increased collagen and decreased elastin, endothelial dysfunction, left ventricular hypertrophy, and a diminution in exercise induced increase in ejection fraction. These characteristic abnormalities are hypothesized to contribute to specific symptoms of the frailty syndrome and to increase the morbidity and mortality from CVD in elderly individuals (7, 10, 30). Several studies document the increased risk for mortality in frail elderly patients with cardiovascular events such as non-ST-segment elevation myocardial infarction (NSTEMI) (3, 7). Frail individuals have increased disease burden and therefore more prolonged recuperation vs. a non-frail subject (2, 8, 10). There are additional associations between frailty and other cardiovascular diagnoses including angina, myocardial infarction, hypertension, heart failure with reduced ejection (HFrEF), heart failure with preserved ejection fraction (HFpEF), and stroke (10, 30). Gait speed is one symptom of frailty that is linked with increased cardiovascular events and mortality, specifically in ST elevation myocardial infarction patients (33, 34). Importantly, frailty presents a major challenge to the ability of CVD patients to undergo surgery and other medical interventions successfully, thus affecting outcomes (30).

ROLE OF INFLAMMATION IN AGING AND FRAILTY

"Inflammaging" is a term that has been used to depict the particular molecular and cellular inter-related events that promote the process of aging (35). With aging, there is a continuous accumulation of damaged macromolecules and cells, generation of toxic metabolites and microbial byproducts, and development of cellular senescence and immunosenescence (36, 37). Not only does inflammaging accelerate the aging process, it is linked with and accelerates the diseases associated with aging, including cardiovascular diseases, cognitive, and neurologic impairments, cancer, and degenerative joint disease. Importantly, the increased susceptibility to disease and death is a result of these molecular inflammation-related changes in physiological systems. As such, measuring the molecules or biomarkers that mediate inflammation has become a useful tool to assess the aging process (37). For instance, there is evidence that circulating levels of pro-inflammatory cytokines increase during aging. High levels of TNF-α, interleukin-6 (IL-6), and C-reactive protein (CRP), even in elderly populations considered healthy, are independent predictors of mortality (38). This same inflammatory response underlies the tissue damage linked to various age-related chronic diseases (39). Indeed, a multitude of studies have now reliably demonstrated that chronically high levels of pro-inflammatory biomarkers do predict risk of morbidity and mortality in the elderly population (37).

Frailty involves aging-related decreases in organ physiologic reserve, leading to impaired ability to withstand stressors and resulting in increased vulnerability to disease. Frail patients manifest disturbances in the hematologic and inflammatory systems, which seem to be at the core of this geriatric syndrome (37, 40). For instance, frail patients have elevated levels of fibrinogen, IL-6, factor VIII, D-dimer, and CRP compared to non-frail patients (32, 41). Studies also report reduced hemoglobin, high leukocytes, elevated TNF-α, and low vitamin D as biomarkers of frailty. Importantly, the inflammatory cytokine IL-6 strongly correlates with the frailty phenotype and with unfavorable health outcomes (32, 42–44). Of note, among frail subjects, women exhibit higher concentrations of inflammatory and coagulation factors than men (41).

CRP is an example of one biomarker that has a higher concentration in women experiencing symptoms of frailty. Differential white blood cell counts, on the other hand, similarly predict frailty risk in men and women. Although there is still insufficient data to show which markers specifically affect men or women, dysregulated inflammation is a considerable key physiological marker in correlation with the frailty syndrome in both genders. It is of interest to note that the strong correlation between frailty and inflammatory and hematologic biomarkers is remarkably similar to the strong correlation between CVD and these same biomarkers, supporting the notion that frailty and CVD are clinically interrelated (37). Importantly, frail individuals also have characteristic declines in cardiovascular reserve, as described above, which may in turn contribute to the symptoms of the syndrome.

Substantial evidence has shown that chronic inflammation underlies the syndrome of aging frailty, leading to impairments in mobility and gait, sarcopenia, osteopenia, and decreased strength. High levels of circulating IL-6 correlate with the development of mobility disability (45) and high levels of IL-6 and TNF-α, either alone or together, are linked with decreased muscle mass and strength, increasing the susceptibility to sarcopenia (46, 47). Moreover, high levels of IL-6 and CRP are independently associated with decreases in physical performance and strength in the elderly (48, 49). The Women's Health and Aging Study (WHAS) demonstrated that elevated IL-6 levels in older women were associated with a greater decline in the ability to walk and a greater risk of acquiring physical disabilities (50). The MacArthur Studies of Successful Aging also found an association between decreased walking speed and grip strength and elevated levels of IL-6 and CRP (51). With regards to all-cause mortality predictors, elevated systemic IL-6 levels correlate strongly with various causes of death, as well as, with mortality in the near future (52, 53). A strong correlation is also present between CRP and early mortality and TNF-α and mortality among the elderly (54, 55). Since these inflammatory biomarkers are not specifically indicative of a particular disease or cause of mortality, these increases in systemic inflammation are thought to reflect a fundamental aspect of the aging process (37).

Chronic inflammation also causes remodeling of the immune system, which diminishes immune responses and contributes to increased mortality in subjects over 60 years of age with frailty (32, 42–44). Immunologic remodeling, in turn, is an important pathophysiologic contributor to frailty in older humans (56, 57). This functional impairment in cell-mediated and humoral immunity in frailty is well documented (58–60) and leads to an increased vulnerability to infectious diseases (40). However, the level of inflammation that affects individuals with frailty is "low-grade," for example, TNF-α levels range between 1.5 and 1.68 pg/ml (61). In this regard, it has been proposed that the chronicity of the inflammation causes more harm than the absolute level at any given time (62). This elevation in systemic TNF-α levels increases intracellular TNF-α in B cells, which causes a shift in B cell subsets producing an increased percentage of exhausted B cells and decreased switch memory B cells, thereby impairing B cell function (63, 64). In aging and frailty, T cell activity is also impaired, and can be assessed by a decrease in the ratio of CD4:CD8 cells (65). Together, these processes promote an immune cell refractory state where both T and B cell responses to *de novo* antigens and vaccines are diminished (66).

As there is no cure for aging or frailty, the therapeutic strategy is on developing approaches to lessen or at least regulate the effects of chronic inflammation on aging, with the goal to promote a healthier aging process. It is believed that frailty can ultimately be prevented or attenuated, and the link between frailty and inflammation offers a potential therapeutic target.

ENDOGENOUS STEM CELLS IN FRAILTY

An individual's endogenous stem cell production and function decreases with age and this decrease likely contributes to reduced ability to regenerate and repair organs and tissues (67–69). For instance, there is evidence that as mesenchymal stem cells (MSCs) undergo senescence, their multilineage differentiation and homing capacity and immunomodulatory and wound healing properties gradually disappear (69, 70). These aging-related declines may be due to intrinsic stem cell aging, for example there is evidence that aging induces a "quiescence-to-senescence switch" (71) in stem cells, and aging-related changes in extracellular matrix components and the stem cell niches in tissues (68, 72, 73). Collectively, these aging-related changes reduce stem cell self-renewal, maintenance and regenerative potential. With regard to frailty, altered and dysfunctional stem cell niches have been implicated in frailty syndrome (74, 75). As such, it has been proposed that a regenerative medicine therapeutic approach has the potential to improve or reverse the signs and symptoms of frailty (32, 70), as further discussed below.

MESENCHYMAL STEM CELLS AS A THERAPEUTIC STRATEGY FOR FRAILTY

Medical advances and a more health aware society have contributed to a longer living population. However, as the population ages, the growing number of frail elderly patients will continue to increase the demand for healthcare services. Therefore, novel medical therapies for frailty are under investigation to address this unmet need amongst the elderly population. Although certain diets, especially the Mediterranean diet (76, 77), nutritional supplements (78), hormonal supplements (79), and exercise regimes (80, 81) have been shown independently or in combination (82) to improve the signs and symptoms of frailty (8), there is currently no specific medical therapy available to prevent or treat the frailty syndrome.

There are specific features of the frailty syndrome that support a potential role of MSCs to ameliorate or improve frailty. MSCs are drawn to sites of injury, where they act to reduce inflammation and promote cellular repair (83). Notably, MSCs improve cardiovascular outcomes in patients with acute myocardial infarction (84), as well as, ischemic (85) and non-ischemic cardiomyopathy (86), reduce TNF-α and CRP levels, and are safe in patients irrespective of age (83, 87). The strong association between frailty and CVD and the growing database documenting safety and potential favorable effects of cell-based therapy in CVD provide justification for the assessment of potential benefits of cell therapy in subjects with frailty (88, 89; **Table 1**, **Figure 1**).

TABLE 1 | The potential effects of mesenchymal stem cells (MSCs) on frailty phenotypes.

Frailty phenotypes	Therapeutic MSC effects	Postulated mechanisms of action
Unintentional weight loss	↓ Chronic inflammation	↓ Inflammation, ↓ Onset of sarcopenia, ↓ TNF-α, ↓ IL-6, ↓ CRP, ↓IL-1ß, ↑ IL-10, ↑ TGF-ß
Low energy levels or exhaustion	↑ Pulmonary function, ↓ Chronic inflammation	↑ Endothelial function, ↓ Biomarkers of inflammation
Weak grip strength	↑ Physical performance	↑ Endogenous stem cell function
Slow gait speed	↑ 6-min walk distance	↑ Endothelial function, ↑ Cardiac performance, ↑Skeletal muscle performance
Low physical activity	↓ Chronic inflammation, ↑ Quality of life	↓ TNF-α, ↓ IL-6, ↓ CRP, ↓IL-1ß, ↑ IL-10, ↑ TGF-ß

Anti-inflammatory and Immunomodulatory Effects of Mesenchymal Stem Cells

MSCs can evade and modulate the host's immune system to prolong their therapeutic effects without being detected and eliminated. The absence of major histocompatibility complex (MHC)/human leukocyte antigen (HLA) class II and associated costimulatory molecules and low levels of MHC/HLA class I molecules expressed by MSCs (88, 89) enables them to evade detection by the host immune system. This absence of class II molecules provides the basis for allogeneic MSC therapy, although allogeneic MSCs may eventually induce an immune reaction due to their mismatched MHC-1 molecules, which can be recognized by the host CD8+ T-cells (90).

MSCs influence the host immune system in numerous ways. They reduce both B- and T-lymphocyte proliferation in a paracrine manner (secretion of factors) and by direct cell-cell contact (91, 92). MSCs reduce the expression of proinflammatory cytokines, including, TNF-α, interleukin (IL)-1β, IL-6, and CRP [see (93–95) for review; **Figure 1**]. The paracrine effects of MSCs are produced in response to either secretion of a wide array of individual factors, such as growth factors and cytokines, or via exosomes, small extracellular vesicles that contain proteins, peptides and microRNAs (miRNAs).

Factors secreted by MSCs include transforming growth factor (TGF)-β, hepatocyte growth factor (HGF) and interleukins, among many others [see (93) for review]. Many of these factors interact to produce an immunomodulatory effect (96). Furthermore, the effect of a specific factor may be modulated by the microenvironment (93). Perhaps the most well studied factor secreted by MSCs is TGF-ß. MSCs produce TGF-ß in response to IL-4 receptor mediated activation of the STAT6 pathway (97). TGF-ß inhibits the proliferation of CD4+ and CD8+ T-cells and the secretion of T helper1 (Th1) cells while increasing T-regulatory cells (Treg). Another factor secreted by MSCs, IL-10, is an anti-inflammatory and immunoregulatory cytokine also

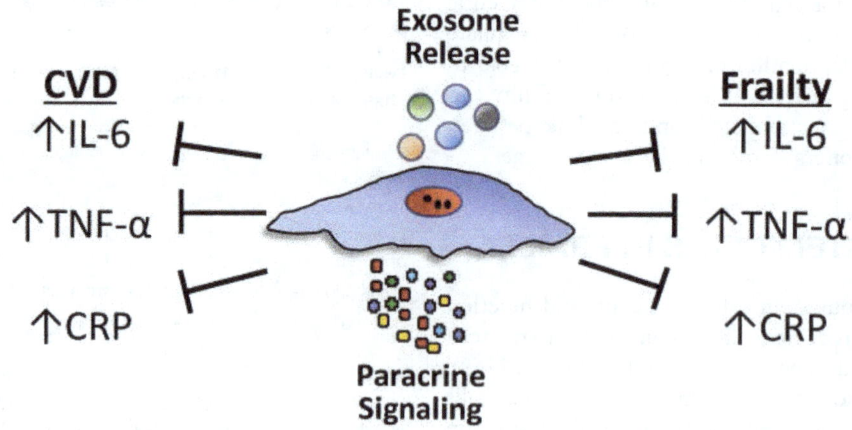

FIGURE 1 | Circulating levels of proinflammatory cytokines, particularly TNF-α, interleukin-6 (IL-6), and C-reactive protein (CRP), increase during aging and are independent predictors of mortality in frail patients. These same pro-inflammatory cytokines are elevated and underlie the tissue damage linked to various age-related chronic diseases, particularly cardiovascular diseases (CVD). Mesenchymal stem cells (MSCs) reduce the expression of proinflammatory cytokines, including TNF-α, IL-6, and CRP, in both CVD and frailty syndrome through paracrine effects or via exosomes. Paracrine effects involve the secretion of a multitude of individual growth factors and cytokines. Exosomes are small extracellular vesicles that contain proteins, peptides and microRNAs (miRNAs).

expressed by a variety of immune cells. MSC expression of IL-10 requires direct interaction with T-cells (98). IL-10 inhibits the ability of macrophages to produce pro-inflammatory cytokines. However, recent evidence suggests that increased production of IL-10 by cardiac macrophages promotes diastolic dysfunction (99). This result emphasizes that the effect of a specific factor, whether secreted by MSCs or another cell type, is dependent on context and it is the combination and interaction of secreted (and resident) factors that enable MSCs to modulate the host immune system.

MSCs also affect the immune system through their release of exosomes. Exosomes are 40–100 nm extracellular vesicles that can be isolated from MSC-conditioned media. *Ex vivo* studies demonstrate that MSC-derived exosomes reduce secretion of pro-inflammatory cytokines (IL-1ß, TNF-α) and increase production of TGF-ß by PBMCs, but don't affect PBMC proliferation (100). Administration of MSCs (101, 102) or MSC-derived exosomes (103) reduces the immune response in two mouse models of autoimmune disease, Type 1 diabetes mellitus and uveoretinitis. These results and those from many other studies, suggest that MSC-derived exosomes represent an alternative to stem cell therapy.

Exosomes are secreted by many cell types, including cells of the immune system. A recent study by Ipson et al. isolated exosomes from 7 frail and 7 robust individuals who suffered from similar chronic diseases. Eight exosome-derived miRNAs were identified that were differentially expressed in these two populations and are found at higher levels in frail individuals (104). While the sample size was small, this result suggests that exosome miRNA profiles may represent biomarkers for frailty. Perhaps isolating and administering MSC-derived exosomes containing miRNAs that can counteract these "frailty-specific" miRNAs, will provide a therapeutic option for treating frailty.

Not only do MSCs affect the host's immune system, but the host immune system also modulates the activity of MSCs (105–107). Exposure to interferon (IFN)-γ generally enhances the immunosuppressive action of MSCs while simultaneously increasing their HLA class I and II cell surface marker expression (94). However, low concentrations of both IFN-γ and TNF-α, can cause MSCs to become pro-inflammatory (94, 95). Furthermore, host-derived pro-inflammatory cytokines can impair the capability of MSCs to differentiate into bone, fat, and cartilage lineages [see (94)]. However, even after MSCs have differentiated into chondrocytes, they can exert immunosuppressive effects (108, 109).

MSCs are not all equal. Recent studies suggest that the tissue from which an MSC originates influences its immunomodulatory properties. Kim et al. compared the immunosuppressive properties of MSCs isolated from periodontal ligament, umbilical cord, and adipose tissue and determined that while they all similarly inhibited the proliferation and activation of PBMCs, UC-MSCs and to a lesser extent Ad-MSCs, secreted higher levels of immunosuppressive cytokines in response to IFN-γ (110). Furthermore, MSCs obtained from aged individuals possess reduced immunomodulatory properties compared to those from the young (111, 112). The tissue microenvironment into which MSCs migrate/are injected into also influences their immunosuppressive properties. MSCs located within an inflammatory microenvironment can suppress cytotoxic T cells (96, 113), induce T regulatory cells (114, 115), and stimulate macrophage polarization (116) (transition from an M1 to an M2 phenotype) thereby promoting an anti-inflammatory milieu. Furthermore, a recent study demonstrated that MSCs exert antibacterial effects (117) indicating that MSCs possess an immune function independent of the host's immune system.

Results of Phase I and II Clinical Trials of MSCs for Frailty

Currently, there is no specifically approved treatment for frail patients and therefore no established standard of care. The ultimate goal of a therapeutic strategy for frailty is to lengthen the healthy lifespan and restore or maintain cognitive and physical functionality of patients. We conducted a phase I and a phase II clinical trial, CRATUS (NCT02065245), investigating the safety (primary outcome) and efficacy (secondary outcome) of an intravenous infusion of allogeneic bone marrow-derived MSCs as a novel therapy for treating patients experiencing mild to moderate frailty (56, 57, 75). Efficacy outcomes included physical performance, quality of life, and systemic inflammation.

The phase I trial was a non-randomized, dose-escalation study in which 15 patients diagnosed with frailty, based on the CSHA clinical frailty scale, received allogeneic MSCs by intravenous infusion at doses of 20, 100, or 200 million MSCs (5 patients per group). All of the doses were administered as an 80 mL infusion at a speed of 2 mL/min, for a total infusion time of 40 min. Incidence of any treatment-emergent serious adverse events (TE-SAEs) at 1 month post-infusion was the primary outcome. Physical function measurements and circulating inflammatory biomarkers, measured at 3 and 6 months post-infusion, were the secondary outcomes. No TE-SAEs were reported with any of the doses at 1-month post-infusion and no clinically significant donor-specific immune reactions occurred during the first 6 months post-infusion. The six-min walk distance significantly increased at 3 and 6 months and circulating TNF-α levels significantly decreased at 6 months in all treatment groups. The best improvement in all efficacy outcomes was observed with the 100-million dose, except in the case of TNF-α, which showed a significant improvement with both the 100- and 200-million doses. The physical component of the SF-36 quality of life assessment also showed significant improvements in the 100-million dose group at all time points relative to baseline. This study indicated that allogeneic infusion of MSCs is safe and immunologically tolerated in aging frailty patients.

The phase II trial was a randomized, double-blinded, dose-finding study of intravenous allogeneic MSCs at doses of 100- or 200-million compared to placebo in 30 frailty patients (mean age 75.5 ± 7.3) (57). The primary outcome was safety, namely incidence of TE-SAEs at 1-month post-infusion. The secondary outcomes were physical performance measures, patient-reported quality outcomes, and immune markers of frailty, measured at 6 months post-infusion. There were no therapy-related TE-SAEs reported at 1-month post-infusion. Physical performance improved to a greater extent in the 100-million dose group and measures of immunologic parameters improved in both the 100-million and 200-million dose groups. The 6-min walk test, short physical performance exam, and forced expiratory volume in 1 s improved significantly in the 100-million dose group but not in the 200-million dose or placebo groups. Moreover, there was improvement noted in the female sexual quality of life questionnaire and decreases in serum TNF-α levels in the 100-million dose group. B cell intracellular TNF-α improved significantly in both the 100-million and 200-million dose groups compared to placebo. Early and late activated T-cells were decreased as well by MSC infusion compared to placebo. Although there were no safety concerns with the 200-million dose, there was no added benefit observed with this higher dose compared to the 100-million dose. In summary, intravenous allogeneic MSCs were found to be safe in individuals with aging frailty and produced significant benefits in measures of physical performance as well inflammatory biomarkers, which are important therapeutic outcomes in the frailty syndrome.

Allogeneic therapy was used in these studies because it offers "off-the-shelf" availability and a consistency to the cell product (118). These properties are extremely important as autologous cells may have deficiencies in function due to the underlying disease process, co-morbidities, lifestyle, concomitant medications, and/or patient age (119–121). Despite reports that allogeneic MSCs may be immunologically cleared more rapidly than autologous cells after differentiation (122), due to immunogenicity, this immunologic clearance might be beneficial in reducing any long-term risks of cell engraftment (123). Given the excellent safety profile and promising therapeutic efficacy demonstrated in these early phase trials (**Table 1**), studies with repeat dosing and longer follow up time (CRATUS; NCT02065245), as well as, a larger phase IIb (NCT03169231) clinical trial are ongoing to establish the efficacy of MSCs in the frailty syndrome.

AUTHOR CONTRIBUTIONS

IS drafted and edited the manuscript. WB wrote a section, edited the manuscript for scientific content, and made the figure. JH edited the manuscript for scientific content.

FUNDING

JH and IS are supported by the National Institute of Health (NIH) grants, UM1 HL113460, 1R01 HL134558-01, 1R01 HL137355-01, as well as by the Starr and Soffer Family Foundations.

REFERENCES

Chen X, Mao G, Leng SX. Frailty syndrome: an overview. *Clin Int Aging* (2014) 9:433–41. doi: 10.2147/CIA.S45300

Morley JE, Vellas B, van Kan GA, Anker SD, Bauer JM, Bernabei R, et al. Frailty consensus: a call to action. *J Am Med Dir Assoc.* (2013) 14:392–7. doi: 10.1016/j.jamda.2013.03.022

Ekerstad N, Swahn E, Janzon M, Alfredsson J, Lofmark R, Lindenberger M, et al. Frailty is independently associated with 1-year mortality for elderly patients with non-ST-segment elevation myocardial infarction. *Eur J Prev Cardiol.* (2014) 21:1216–24. doi: 10.1177/2047487313490257

Ebrahimi Z, Wilhelmson K, Eklund K, Moore CD, Jakobsson A. Health despite frailty: exploring influences on frail older adults' experiences of health. *Geriatr Nurs.* (2013) 34:289–94. doi: 10.1016/j.gerinurse.2013.04.008

Koller K, Rockwood K. Frailty in older adults: implications for end-of-life care. *Cleve Clin J Med.* (2013) 80:168–74. doi: 10.3949/ccjm.80a.12100

Jylha M, Guralnik JM, Balfour J, Fried LP. Walking difficulty, walking speed, and age as predictors of self-rated health: the women's health and aging study. *J Gerontol A Biol Sci Med Sci.* (2001) 56:M609–17. doi: 10.1093/gerona/56.10.M609

Newman AB, Gottdiener JS, McBurnie MA, Hirsch CH, Kop WJ, Tracy R, et al. Associations of subclinical cardiovascular disease with frailty. *J Gerontol A Biol Sci Med Sci.* (2001) 56:M158–66. doi: 10.1093/gerona/56.3.M158

Sacha J, Sacha M, Sobon J, Borysiuk Z, Feusette P. Is it time to begin a public campaign concerning frailty and pre-frailty? a review article. *Front Physiol.* (2017) 8:484. doi: 10.3389/fphys.2017.00484

Fried LP, Tangen CM, Walston J, Newman AB, Hirsch C, Gottdiener J, et al. Frailty in older adults: evidence for a phenotype. *J Gerontol A Biol Sci Med Sci.* (2001) 56:M146–56. doi: 10.1093/gerona/56.3.M146

Fried LP, Kronmal RA, Newman AB, Bild DE, Mittelmark MB, Polak JF, et al. Risk factors for 5-year mortality in older adults: the Cardiovascular Health Study. *JAMA* (1998) 279:585–92.

Rockwood K, Mitnitski A. Frailty in relation to the accumulation of deficits. *J Gerontol A Biol Sci Med Sci.* (2007) 62:722–7. doi: 10.1093/gerona/62. 7.722

Clegg A, Young J, Iliffe S, Rikkert MO, Rockwood K. Frailty in elderly people. *Lancet* (2013) 381:752–62. doi: 10.1016/S0140-6736(12)62 167-9

Rockwood K, Blodgett JM, Theou O, Sun MH, Feridooni HA, Mitnitski A, et al. A Frailty index based on deficit accumulation quantifies mortality risk in humans and in mice. *Sci Rep.* (2017) 7:43068. doi: 10.1038/srep 43068

Rockwood K, Mitnitski A. Limits to deficit accumulation in elderly people. *Mech Ageing Dev.* (2006) 127:494–6. doi: 10.1016/j.mad.2006.01.002

Ritt M, Ritt JI, Sieber CC, Gassmann KG. Comparing the predictive accuracy of frailty, comorbidity, and disability for mortality: a 1-year follow-up in patients hospitalized in geriatric wards. *Clin Interv Aging* (2017) 12:293–304. doi: 10.2147/CIA.S124342

Rockwood K, Song X, MacKnight C, Bergman H, Hogan DB, McDowell I, et al. A global clinical measure of fitness and frailty in elderly people. *CMAJ* (2005) 173:489–95. doi: 10.1503/cmaj.050051

Morley JE, Malmstrom TK, Miller DK. A simple frailty questionnaire (FRAIL) predicts outcomes in middle aged african americans. *J Nutr Health Aging* (2012) 16:601–8. doi: 10.1007/s12603-012-0084-2

Ensrud KE, Ewing SK, Cawthon PM, Fink HA, Taylor BC, Cauley JA, et al. A Comparison of frailty indexes for the prediction of falls, disability, fractures and mortality in older men. *J Am Geriatr Soc.* (2009) 57:492–8. doi: 10.1111/j.1532-5415.2009.02137.x

Romero-Ortuno R, Walsh CD, Lawlor BA, Kenny RA. A Frailty Instrument for primary care: findings from the Survey of Health, Ageing and Retirement in Europe (SHARE). *BMC Geriatrics* (2010) 10:57. doi: 10.1186/1471-2318-10-57

Drubbel I, Bleijenberg N, Kranenburg G, Eijkemans RJC, Schuurmans MJ, de Wit NJ, et al. Identifying frailty: do the frailty index and groningen frailty indicator cover different clinical perspectives? A cross- sectional study. *BMC Family Pract.* (2013) 14:64. doi: 10.1186/1471-229 6-14-64

Malmstrom TK, Miller DK, Morley JE. A comparison of four frailty models. *J Am Geriatr Soc.* (2014) 62:721–6. doi: 10.1111/jgs. 12735

Gobbens RJ, van Assen MA, Luijkx KG, Wijnen-Sponselee MT, Schols JM. The Tilburg frailty indicator: psychometric properties. *J Am Med Direct Assoc.* (2010) 11:344–55. doi: 10.1016/j.jamda.2009. 11.003

Ottenbacher KJ, Graham JE, Snih SA, Raji M, Samper-Ternent R, Ostir GV, et al. Becoming frail: findings from the hispanic established populations epidemiologic study of the elderly. *Am J Public Health* (2009) 99:673–9. doi: 10.2105/AJPH.2008.143958

Raji MA, Al Snih S, Ostir GV, Markides KS, Ottenbacher KJ. Cognitive status and future risk of frailty in older Mexican Americans. *J Gerontol A Biol Sci Med Sci.* (2010) 65:1228–34. doi: 10.1093/gerona/glq121

Danon-Hersch N, Rodondi N, Spagnoli J, Santos-Eggimann B. Prefrailty and chronic morbidity in the youngest old: an insight from the Lausanne cohort Lc65+. *J Am Geriatr Soc.* (2012) 60:1687–94. doi: 10.1111/j.1532-5415.2012.04113.x

Mitnitski AB, Mogilner AJ, MacKnight C, Rockwood K. The mortality rate as a function of accumulated deficits in a frailty index. *Mech Ageing Dev.* (2002) 123:1457–60. doi: 10.1016/S0047-6374(02)00082-9

Mitnitski AB, Mogilner AJ, MacKnight C, Rockwood K. The accumulation of deficits with age and possible invariants of aging. *Sci. World J.* (2002) 2:1816–22. doi: 10.1100/tsw.2002.861

Puts MT, Lips P, Deeg DJ. Sex differences in the risk of frailty for mortality independent of disability and chronic diseases. *J Am Geriatr Soc.* (2005) 53:40–7. doi: 10.1111/j.1532-5415.2005.53008.x

Fernandez-Garrido J, Ruiz-Ros V, Buigues C, Navarro-Martinez R, Cauli O. Clinical features of prefrail older individuals and emerging peripheral biomarkers: a systematic review. *Arch Gerontol Geriatr.* (2014) 59:7–17. doi: 10.1016/j.archger.2014.02.008

Paneni F, Diaz Canestro C, Libby P, Luscher TF, Camici GG. The aging cardiovascular system: understanding it at the cellular and clinical levels. *J Am Coll Cardiol.* (2017) 69:1952–67. doi: 10.1016/j.jacc.2017.01.064

Afilalo J, Karunananthan S, Eisenberg MJ, Alexander KP, Bergman H. Role of frailty in patients with cardiovascular disease. *Am J Cardiol.* (2009) 103:1616–21. doi: 10.1016/j.amjcard.2009.01.375

Kanapuru B, Ershler WB. Inflammation, coagulation, and the pathway to frailty. *Am J Med.* (2009) 122:605–13. doi: 10.1016/j.amjmed.2009.01.030

Bouillon K, Batty GD, Hamer M, Sabia S, Shipley MJ, Britton A, et al. Cardiovascular disease risk scores in identifying future frailty: the Whitehall II prospective cohort study. *Heart* (2013) 99:737–42. doi: 10.1136/heartjnl-2012-302922

Matsuzawa Y, Konishi M, Akiyama E, Suzuki H, Nakayama N, Kiyokuni M, et al. Association between gait speed as a measure of frailty and risk of cardiovascular events after myocardial infarction. *J Am Coll Cardiol.* (2013) 61:1964–72. doi: 10.1016/j.jacc.2013.02.020

Franceschi C, Bonafe M, Valensin S, Olivieri F, De Luca M, Ottaviani E, et al. Inflamm-aging. An evolutionary perspective on immunosenescence. *Ann N Y Acad Sci.* (2000) 908:244–54. doi: 10.1111/j.1749-6632.2000.tb06651.x

Franceschi C, Campisi J. Chronic inflammation (inflammaging) and its potential contribution to age-associated diseases. *J Gerontol A Biol Sci Med Sci.* (2014) 69(Suppl. 1):S4–9. doi: 10.1093/gerona/glu057

Gonzalez R, Woynarowski D, Geffner L. Stem cells targeting inflammation as potential anti-aging strategies and therapies. *Cell Tissue Transpl Ther.* (2015) 7:1–8. doi: 10.4137/CTTT.S19477

Bruunsgaard H, Pedersen BK. Age-related inflammatory cytokines and disease. *Immunol Allergy Clin North Am.* (2003) 23:15–39. doi: 10.1016/S0889-8561(02)00056-5

Licastro F, Candore G, Lio D, Porcellini E, Colonna-Romano G, Franceschi C, et al. Innate immunity and inflammation in ageing: a key for understanding age-related diseases. *Immun Ageing* (2005) 2:8. doi: 10.1186/1742-4933-2-8

Mitnitski A, Collerton J, Martin-Ruiz C, Jagger C, von Zglinicki T, Rockwood K, et al. Age-related frailty and its association with biological markers of ageing. *BMC Med.* (2015) 13:161. doi: 10.1186/s12916-015-0400-x

Gale CR, Baylis D, Cooper C, Sayer AA. Inflammatory markers and incident frailty in men and women: the English Longitudinal Study of Ageing. *Age* (2013) 35:2493–501. doi: 10.1007/s11357-013-9528-9

Ershler WB, Keller ET. Age-associated increased interleukin-6 gene expression, late-life diseases, and frailty. *Annu Rev Med.* (2000) 51:245–70. doi: 10.1146/annurev.med.51.1.245

de Gonzalo-Calvo D, Neitzert K, Fernandez M, Vega-Naredo I, Caballero B, Garcia-Macia M, et al. Differential inflammatory responses in aging and disease: TNF-alpha and IL-6 as possible biomarkers. *Free Radic Biol Med.* (2010) 49:733–7. doi: 10.1016/j.freeradbiomed.2010.05.019

Bruunsgaard H, Andersen-Ranberg K, Hjelmborg J, Pedersen BK, Jeune B. Elevated levels of tumor necrosis factor alpha and mortality in centenarians. *Am J Med.* (2003) 115:278–83. doi: 10.1016/S0002-9343(03)00329-2

Ferrucci L, Harris TB, Guralnik JM, Tracy RP, Corti MC, Cohen HJ, et al. Serum IL-6 level and the development of disability in older persons. *J Am Geriatr Soc.* (1999) 47:639–46.

Visser M, Pahor M, Taaffe DR, Goodpaster BH, Simonsick EM, Newman AB, et al. Relationship of interleukin-6 and tumor necrosis factor-alpha with muscle mass and muscle strength in elderly men and women: the

Health ABC Study. *J Gerontol A Biol Sci Med Sci.* (2002) 57:M326–32. doi: 10.1093/gerona/57.5.M326

Schaap LA, Pluijm SM, Deeg DJ, Harris TB, Kritchevsky SB, Newman AB, et al. Higher inflammatory marker levels in older persons: associations with 5-year change in muscle mass and muscle strength. *J Gerontol A Biol Sci Med Sci.* (2009) 64:1183–9. doi: 10.1093/gerona/glp097

Cesari M, Penninx BW, Pahor M, Lauretani F, Corsi AM, Rhys Williams G, et al. Inflammatory markers and physical performance in older persons: the InCHIANTI study. *J Gerontol A Biol Sci Med Sci.* (2004) 59:242–8. doi: 10.1093/gerona/59.3.M242

Barbieri M, Ferrucci L, Ragno E, Corsi A, Bandinelli S, Bonafe M, et al. Chronic inflammation and the effect of IGF-I on muscle strength and power in older persons. *Am J Physiol Endocrinol Metab.* (2003) 284:E481–7. doi: 10.1152/ajpendo.00319.2002

Ferrucci L, Penninx BW, Volpato S, Harris TB, Bandeen-Roche K, Balfour J, et al. Change in muscle strength explains accelerated decline of physical function in older women with high interleukin-6 serum levels. *J Am Geriatr Soc.* (2002) 50:1947–54. doi: 10.1046/j.1532-5415.2002.50605.x

Taaffe DR, Harris TB, Ferrucci L, Rowe J, Seeman TE. Cross-sectional and prospective relationships of interleukin-6 and C-reactive protein with physical performance in elderly persons: MacArthur studies of successful aging. *J Gerontol A Biol Sci Med Sci.* (2000) 55:M709–15. doi: 10.1093/gerona/55.12.M709

Newman AB, Sachs MC, Arnold AM, Fried LP, Kronmal R, Cushman M, et al. Total and cause-specific mortality in the cardiovascular health study. *J Gerontol A Biol Sci Med Sci.* (2009) 64:1251–61. doi: 10.1093/gerona/glp127

Walston JD, Matteini AM, Nievergelt C, Lange LA, Fallin DM, Barzilai N, et al. Inflammation and stress-related candidate genes, plasma interleukin-6 levels, and longevity in older adults. *Exp Gerontol.* (2009) 44:350–5. doi: 10.1016/j.exger.2009.02.004

Jenny NS, Yanez ND, Psaty BM, Kuller LH, Hirsch CH, Tracy RP. Inflammation biomarkers and near-term death in older men. *Am J Epidemiol.* (2007) 165:684–95. doi: 10.1093/aje/kwk057

Harris TB, Ferrucci L, Tracy RP, Corti MC, Wacholder S, Ettinger WH Jr, et al. Associations of elevated interleukin-6 and C-reactive protein levels with mortality in the elderly. *Am J Med.* (1999) 106:506–12.

Golpanian S, DiFede DL, Khan A, Schulman IH, Landin AM, Tompkins BA, et al. Allogeneic human mesenchymal stem cell infusions for aging frailty. *J Gerontol Ser A Biolog Sci Med Sci.* (2017) 72:1505–12. doi: 10.1093/gerona/glx056

Tompkins BA, DiFede DL, Khan A, Landin AM, Schulman IH, Pujol MV, et al. Allogeneic mesenchymal stem cells ameliorate aging frailty: a phase II randomized, double-blinded, placebo controlled clinical trial. *J Gerontol Ser A Biol Sci Med Sci.* (2017) 72:1513–22. doi: 10.1093/gerona/glx137

Ghatreh-Samani M, Esmaeili N, Soleimani M, Asadi-Samani M, Ghatreh-Samani K, Shirzad H. Oxidative stress and age-related changes in T cells: is thalassemia a model of accelerated immune system aging? *Cent Eur J Immunol.* (2016) 41:116–24. doi: 10.5114/ceji.2015.56973

Pinti M, Appay V, Campisi J, Frasca D, Fulop T, Sauce D, et al. Aging of the immune system: focus on inflammation and vaccination. *Eur J Immunol.* (2016) 46:2286–301. doi: 10.1002/eji.201546178

Qin L, Jing X, Qiu Z, Cao W, Jiao Y, Routy JP, et al. Aging of immune system: Immune signature from peripheral blood lymphocyte subsets in 1068 healthy adults. *Aging* (2016) 8:848–59. doi: 10.18632/aging.100894

Hubbard RE, O'Mahony MS, Savva GM, Calver BL, Woodhouse KW. Inflammation and frailty measures in older people. *J Cell Mol Med.* (2009) 13:3103–9. doi: 10.1111/j.1582-4934.2009.00733.x

De Martinis M, Franceschi C, Monti D, Ginaldi L. Inflammation markers predicting frailty and mortality in the elderly. *Exp Mol Pathol.* (2006) 80:219– 27. doi: 10.1016/j.yexmp.2005.11.004

Frasca D, Blomberg BB. Inflammaging decreases adaptive and innate immune responses in mice and humans. *Biogerontology* (2016) 17:7–19. doi: 10.1007/s10522-015-9578-8

Frasca D, Diaz A, Romero M, Landin AM, Blomberg BB. Age effects on B cells and humoral immunity in humans. *Ageing Res Rev.* (2011) 10:330–5. doi: 10.1016/j.arr.2010.08.004

Strindhall J, Skog M, Ernerudh J, Bengner M, Lofgren S, Matussek A, et al. The inverted CD4/CD8 ratio and associated parameters in 66-year- old individuals: the Swedish HEXA immune study. *Age* (2013) 35:985–91. doi: 10.1007/s11357-012-9400-3

Frasca D, Diaz A, Romero M, Landin AM, Phillips M, Lechner SC, et al. Intrinsic defects in B cell response to seasonal influenza vaccination in elderly humans. *Vaccine* (2010) 28:8077–84. doi: 10.1016/j.vaccine.2010.10.023

Zhuo Y, Li SH, Chen MS, Wu J, Kinkaid HY, Fazel S, et al. Aging impairs the angiogenic response to ischemic injury and the activity of implanted cells: combined consequences for cell therapy in older recipients. *J Thorac Cardiovasc Surg.* (2010) 139:1286–94.e1–2. doi: 10.1016/j.jtcvs.2009. 08.052

Jones DL, Rando TA. Emerging models and paradigms for stem cell ageing. *Nat Cell Biol.* (2011) 13:506–12. doi: 10.1038/ncb05 11-506

Yu KR, Kang KS. Aging-related genes in mesenchymal stem cells: a mini-review. *Gerontology* (2013) 59:557–63. doi: 10.1159/0003 53857

Raggi C, Berardi AC. Mesenchymal stem cells, aging and regenerative medicine. *Muscles Ligaments Tendons J.* (2012) 2:239–42.

Sousa-Victor P, Gutarra S, Garcia-Prat L, Rodriguez-Ubreva J, Ortet L, Ruiz-Bonilla V, et al. Geriatric muscle stem cells switch reversible quiescence into senescence. *Nature* (2014) 506:316–21. doi: 10.1038/nature 13013

Geissler S, Textor M, Schmidt-Bleek K, Klein O, Thiele M, Ellinghaus A, et al. In serum veritas-in serum sanitas? Cell non-autonomous aging compromises differentiation and survival of mesenchymal stromal cells via the oxidative stress pathway. *Cell Death Dis.* (2013) 4:e970. doi: 10.1038/cddis.2013.501

Ballard VL. Stem cells for heart failure in the aging heart. *Heart Fail Rev.* (2010) 15:447–56. doi: 10.1007/s10741-010-9160-z

Lopez-Otin C, Blasco MA, Partridge L, Serrano M, Kroemer G. The hallmarks of aging. *Cell* (2013) 153:1194–217. doi: 10.1016/j.cell.2013. 05.039

Golpanian S, DiFede DL, Pujol MV, Lowery MH, Levis-Dusseau S, Goldstein BJ, et al. Rationale and design of the allogeneiC human mesenchymal stem cells (hMSC) in patients with aging fRAilTy via intravenoUS delivery (CRATUS) study: a phase I/II, randomized, blinded and placebo controlled trial to evaluate the safety and potential efficacy of allogeneic human mesenchymal stem cell infusion in patients with aging frailty. *Oncotarget* (2016) 7:11899–912. doi: 10.18632/oncotarget.7727

Voelker R. The mediterranean diet's fight against frailty. *JAMA* (2018) 319:1971–2. doi: 10.1001/jama.2018.3653

Kojima G, Avgerinou C, Iliffe S, Walters K. Adherence to mediterranean diet reduces incident frailty risk: systematic review and meta-analysis. *J Am Geriatr Soc.* (2018) 66:783-8. doi: 10.1111/jgs.15251

Kim CO, Lee KR. Preventive effect of protein-energy supplementation on the functional decline of frail older adults with low socioeconomic status: a community-based randomized controlled study. *J Gerontol A Biol Sci Med Sci.* (2013) 68:309–16. doi: 10.1093/gerona/gls167

O'Connell MD, Wu FC. Androgen effects on skeletal muscle: implications for the development and management of frailty. *Asian J Androl.* (2014) 16:203–12. doi: 10.4103/1008-682X.122581

Cadore EL, Moneo AB, Mensat MM, Munoz AR, Casas-Herrero A, Rodriguez-Manas L, et al. Positive effects of resistance training in frail elderly patients with dementia after long-term physical restraint. *Age* (2014) 36:801–11. doi: 10.1007/s11357-013-9599-7

Cadore EL, Rodriguez-Manas L, Sinclair A, Izquierdo M. Effects of different exercise interventions on risk of falls, gait ability, and balance in physically frail older adults: a systematic review. *Rejuvenation Res.* (2013) 16:105–14. doi: 10.1089/rej.2012.1397

Artaza-Artabe I, Saez-Lopez P, Sanchez-Hernandez N, Fernandez-Gutierrez N, Malafarina V. The relationship between nutrition and frailty: effects of protein intake, nutritional supplementation, vitamin D and exercise on muscle metabolism in the elderly. A systematic review. *Maturitas* (2016) 93:89–99. doi: 10.1016/j.maturitas.2016.04.009

Bagno L, Hatzistergos KE, Balkan W, Hare JM. Mesenchymal stem cell-based therapy for cardiovascular disease: progress and challenges. *Mol Ther.* (2018) 26:1610–23. doi: 10.1016/j.ymthe.2018.05.009

Hare JM, Traverse JH, Henry TD, Dib N, Strumpf RK, Schulman SP, et al. A randomized, double-blind, placebo-controlled, dose-escalation study of intravenous adult human mesenchymal stem cells (prochymal) after acute myocardial infarction. *J Am Coll Cardiol.* (2009) 54:2277–86. doi: 10.1016/j.jacc.2009.06.055

Hare JM, Fishman JE, Gerstenblith G, Difede Velazquez DL, Zambrano JP, Suncion VY, et al. Comparison of allogeneic vs autologous bone marrow-derived mesenchymal stem cells delivered by transendocardial injection in patients with ischemic cardiomyopathy: the POSEIDON randomized trial. *JAMA* (2012) 308:2369–79. doi: 10.1001/jama.2012.25321

Hare JM, DiFede DL, Rieger AC, Florea V, Landin AM, El-Khorazaty J, et al. Randomized comparison of allogeneic versus autologous mesenchymal stem cells for nonischemic dilated cardiomyopathy: POSEIDON-DCM trial. *J Am Coll Cardiol.* (2017) 69:526–37. doi: 10.1016/j.jacc.2016.11.009

Golpanian S, El-Khorazaty J, Mendizabal A, DiFede DL, Suncion VY, Karantalis V, et al. Effect of aging on human mesenchymal stem cell therapy in ischemic cardiomyopathy patients. *J Am Coll Cardiol.* (2015) 65:125–32. doi: 10.1016/j.jacc.2014.10.040.

Jacobs SA, Roobrouck VD, Verfaillie CM, Van Gool SW. Immunological characteristics of human mesenchymal stem cells and multipotent adult progenitor cells. *Immunol Cell Biol.* (2013) 91:32–9. doi: 10.1038/icb.2012.64

Ryan JM, Barry FP, Murphy JM, Mahon BP. Mesenchymal stem cells avoid allogeneic rejection. *J Inflamm.* (2005) 2:8. doi: 10.1186/1476-9255-2-8

Berglund AK, Fortier LA, Antczak DF, Schnabel LV. Immunoprivileged no more: measuring the immunogenicity of allogeneic adult mesenchymal stem cells. *Stem Cell Res Ther.* (2017) 8:288. doi: 10.1186/s13287-017-0742-8

Munoz-Fernandez R, Prados A, Leno-Duran E, Blazquez A, Garcia- Fernandez JR, Ortiz-Ferron G, et al. Human decidual stromal cells secrete C-X-C motif chemokine 13, express B cell-activating factor and rescue B lymphocytes from apoptosis: distinctive characteristics of follicular dendritic cells. *Hum Reprod.* (2012) 27:2775–84. doi: 10.1093/humrep/des198

Castro-Manrreza ME, Mayani H, Monroy-Garcia A, Flores-Figueroa E, Chavez-Rueda K, Legorreta-Haquet V, et al. Human mesenchymal stromal cells from adult and neonatal sources: a comparative *in vitro* analysis of their immunosuppressive properties against T cells. *Stem Cells Dev.* (2014) 23:1217–32. doi: 10.1089/scd.2013.0363

Fontaine MJ, Shih H, Schafer R, Pittenger MF. Unraveling the mesenchymal stromal cells' paracrine immunomodulatory effects. *Transfus Med Rev.* (2016) 30:37–43. doi: 10.1016/j.tmrv.2015.11.004

Najar M, Krayem M, Merimi M, Burny A, Meuleman N, Bron D, et al. Insights into inflammatory priming of mesenchymal stromal cells: functional biological impacts. *Inflamm Res.* (2018) 67:467–77. doi: 10.1007/s00011-018-1131-1

Shi Y, Wang Y, Li Q, Liu K, Hou J, Shao C, et al. Immunoregulatory mechanisms of mesenchymal stem and stromal cells in inflammatory diseases. *Nat Rev Nephrol.* (2018) 14:493–507. doi: 10.1038/s41581-018-0023-5

Di Nicola M, Carlo-Stella C, Magni M, Milanesi M, Longoni PD, Matteucci P, et al. Human bone marrow stromal cells suppress T-lymphocyte proliferation induced by cellular or nonspecific mitogenic stimuli. *Blood* (2002) 99:3838–43. doi: 10.1182/blood.V99.10.3838

Takeda K, Tanaka T, Shi W, Matsumoto M, Minami M, Kashiwamura S, et al. Essential role of Stat6 in IL-4 signalling. *Nature* (1996) 380:627–30. doi: 10.1038/380627a0

Nasef A, Chapel A, Christelle M, Bouchet S, Lopez M, Mathieu N, et al. Identification of IL-10 and TGF-beta transcripts involved in the inhibition of T-lymphocyte proliferation during cell contact with human mesenchymal stem cells. *Gene Exp.* (2007) 13:217–26. DOI: doi: 10.3727/000000006780666957

Hulsmans M, Sager HB, Roh JD, Valero-Munoz M, Houstis NE, Iwamoto Y, et al. Cardiac macrophages promote diastolic dysfunction. *J Exp Med.* (2018) 215:423–40. doi: 10.1084/jem.20171274

Chen W, Huang Y, Han J, Yu L, Li Y, Lu Z, et al. Immunomodulatory effects of mesenchymal stromal cells-derived exosome. *Immunol Res.* (2016) 64:831–40. doi: 10.1007/s12026-016-8798-6

Kota DJ, Wiggins LL, Yoon N, Lee RH. TSG-6 produced by hMSCs delays the onset of autoimmune diabetes by suppressing Th1 development and enhancing tolerogenicity. *Diabetes* (2013) 62:2048–58. doi: 10.2337/db12-0931

Ko JH, Lee HJ, Jeong HJ, Kim MK, Wee WR, Yoon SO, et al. Mesenchymal stem/stromal cells precondition lung monocytes/macrophages to produce tolerance against allo- and autoimmunity in the eye. *Proc Natl Acad Sci USA.* (2016) 113:158–63. doi: 10.1073/pnas.15229 05113

Shigemoto-Kuroda T, Oh JY, Kim DK, Jeong HJ, Park SY, Lee HJ, et al. MSC-derived extracellular vesicles attenuate immune responses in two autoimmune murine models: type 1 diabetes and uveoretinitis. *Stem Cell Rep.* (2017) 8:1214–25. doi: 10.1016/j.stemcr.2017.04.008

Ipson BR, Fletcher MB, Espinoza SE, Fisher AL. Identifying exosome- derived MicroRNAs as candidate biomarkers of frailty. *J Frailty Aging* (2018) 7:100–3. doi: 10.14283/jfa.2017.45

Chen K, Wang D, Du WT, Han ZB, Ren H, Chi Y, et al. Human umbilical cord mesenchymal stem cells hUC-MSCs exert immunosuppressive activities through a PGE2-dependent mechanism. *Clin Immunol.* (2010) 135:448–58. doi: 10.1016/j.clim.2010.01.015

Krampera M, Cosmi L, Angeli R, Pasini A, Liotta F, Andreini A, et al. Role for interferon-gamma in the immunomodulatory activity of human bone marrow mesenchymal stem cells. *Stem Cells* (2006) 24:386–98. doi: 10.1634/stemcells.2005-0008

Bortolotti F, Ruozi G, Falcione A, Doimo S, Dal Ferro M, Lesizza P, et al. *In vivo* functional selection identifies cardiotrophin-1 as a cardiac engraftment factor for mesenchymal stromal cells. *Circulation* (2017) 136:1509–24. doi: 10.1161/CIRCULATIONAHA.117.029003

Du WJ, Reppel L, Leger L, Schenowitz C, Huselstein C, Bensoussan D, et al. Mesenchymal stem cells derived from human bone marrow and adipose tissue maintain their immunosuppressive properties after chondrogenic differentiation: role of HLA-G. *Stem Cells Dev.* (2016) 25:1454–69. doi: 10.1089/scd.2016.0022

Lee HJ, Kang KS, Kang SY, Kim HS, Park SJ, Lee SY, et al. Immunologic properties of differentiated and undifferentiated mesenchymal stem cells derived from umbilical cord blood. *J Vet Sci.* (2016) 17:289–97. doi: 10.4142/jvs.2016.17.3.289

Kim JH, Jo CH, Kim HR, Hwang YI. Comparison of immunological characteristics of mesenchymal stem cells from the periodontal ligament, umbilical cord, and adipose tissue. *Stem Cells Int.* (2018) 2018:8429042. doi: 10.1155/2018/8429042

Wu LW, Wang YL, Christensen JM, Khalifian S, Schneeberger S, Raimondi G, et al. Donor age negatively affects the immunoregulatory properties of both adipose and bone marrow derived mesenchymal stem cells. *Trans Immunol.* (2014) 30:122–7. doi: 10.1016/j.trim.2014. 03.001

Kizilay Mancini O, Shum-Tim D, Stochaj U, Correa JA, Colmegna I. Age, atherosclerosis and type 2 diabetes reduce human mesenchymal stromal cell-mediated T-cell suppression. *Stem Cell Res Ther.* (2015) 6:140. doi: 10.1186/s13287-015-0127-9

Maggini J, Mirkin G, Bognanni I, Holmberg J, Piazzon IM, Nepomnaschy I, et al. Mouse bone marrow-derived mesenchymal stromal cells turn activated macrophages into a regulatory-like profile. *PLoS ONE* (2010) 5:e9252. doi: 10.1371/journal.pone.0009252

Li H, Wang L, Pang Y, Jiang Z, Liu Z, Xiao H, et al. In patients with chronic aplastic anemia, bone marrow-derived MSCs regulate the Treg/Th17 balance by influencing the Notch/RBP- J/FOXP3/RORgammat pathway. *Sci Rep.* (2017) 7:42488. doi: 10.1038/srep 42488

Lee HJ, Kim SN, Jeon MS, Yi T, Song SU. ICOSL expression in human bone marrow-derived mesenchymal stem cells promotes induction of regulatory T cells. *Sci Rep.* (2017) 7:44486. doi: 10.1038/srep 44486

Melief SM, Schrama E, Brugman MH, Tiemessen MM, Hoogduijn MJ, Fibbe WE, et al. Multipotent stromal cells induce human regulatory T cells through a novel pathway involving skewing of monocytes toward anti- inflammatory macrophages. *Stem Cells* (2013) 31:1980–91. doi: 10.1002/ste m.1432

Alcayaga-Miranda F, Cuenca J, Khoury M. Antimicrobial activity of mesenchymal stem cells: current status and new perspectives of antimicrobial peptide-based therapies. *Front Immunol.* (2017) 8:339. doi: 10.3389/fimmu.2017.00339

Boyle AJ, McNiece IK, Hare JM. Mesenchymal stem cell therapy for cardiac repair. *Methods Mol Biol.* (2010) 660:65–84. doi: 10.1007/978-1-60761-705-1_5

Kissel CK, Lehmann R, Assmus B, Aicher A, Honold J, Fischer- Rasokat U, et al. Selective functional exhaustion of hematopoietic progenitor cells in the bone marrow of patients with postinfarction heart failure. *J Am Coll Cardiol.* (2007) 49:2341–9. doi: 10.1016/j.jacc.2007. 01.095

Kovacic JC, Moreno P, Hachinski V, Nabel EG, Fuster V. Cellular senescence, vascular disease, and aging: part 1 of a 2-part review. *Circulation* (2011) 123:1650–60. doi: 10.1161/CIRCULATIONAHA.110.0 07021

Heiss C, Keymel S, Niesler U, Ziemann J, Kelm M, Kalka C. Impaired progenitor cell activity in age-related endothelial dysfunction. *J Am Coll Cardiol.* (2005) 45:1441–8. doi: 10.1016/j.jacc.2004. 12.074

Huang XP, Sun Z, Miyagi Y, McDonald Kinkaid H, Zhang L, Weisel RD, et al. Differentiation of allogeneic mesenchymal stem cells induces immunogenicity and limits their long-term benefits for myocardial repair. *Circulation* (2010) 122:2419–29. doi: 10.1161/CIRCULATIONAHA.110.9 55971 von Bahr L, Batsis I, Moll G, Hagg M, Szakos A, Sundberg B, et al. Analysis of tissues following mesenchymal stromal cell therapy in humans indicates limited long-term engraftment and no ectopic tissue formation. *Stem Cells* (2012) 30:1575–8. doi: 10.1002/stem.1118

5

A Clinical Study of Ninjin'yoeito with Regard to Frailty

Naoya Sakisaka[1]*, Kazuo Mitani[2], Sadahiro Sempuku[3], Tamaki Imai[4], Yoshinori Takemoto[5], Hiroaki Shimomura[6] and Takahisa Ushiroyama[7]

[1] Sakisaka Clinic, Osaka, Japan, [2] Mitani Family Clinic, Osaka, Japan, [3] Sempuku Clinic, Osaka, Japan, [4] Imai Clinic, Osaka, Japan, [5] Takemoto Clinic, Nara, Japan, [6] Shimomura Clinic of Internal Medicine, Osaka, Japan, [7] Osaka Medical College Health Science Clinic, Osaka, Japan

****Correspondence:***
Naoya Sakisaka
naoyas@bca.bai.ne.jp

Frailty in older people is strongly associated with poor nutrition, which is particularly important in the present-day superaging society. This study initially investigated a number of cases of frailty where there was a speedy recovery after administration of a dual deficiency of qi and blood preparation, ninjin'yoeito (NYT), formulated for frail patients who suffer from kiketuryokyo status. Based on these observations, a more extensive investigation involving a greater number of cases was completed. The findings of the effects of NYT on frailty are reported here.

Keywords: ninjin'yoeito, frailty, sarcopenia, kampo, elder

INTRODUCTION

As Japan's population rapidly ages, the problems of "poor nutrition" and "nutritional deficiency" in a superaging society have grown in importance. Frailty in elderly people is strongly associated with poor nutrition, and it can cause sarcopenia, which manifests in a decrease in muscle mass (1). To resolve such issues, the Ministry of Health, Labor, and Welfare announced that starting in 2018 it will implement nationwide "Frailty" countermeasures (2).

Those who work in health care for the elderly understand that people shift between frail and healthy conditions, so appropriate interventions should be made as necessary. When treating frailty through nutritional therapy, the active intake of protein, vitamin D, vitamin E, vitamin C, and so on has been recommended (3). As for exercise therapy, strength training at a slightly intense level, two to three times a week, in addition to aerobic exercise, such as walking, is recommended (4). However, there has been little research on the use of medication to treat frailty and sarcopenia.

In a previous study, the author administered a dual deficiency of qi and blood preparation, NYT, to patients affected by frailty and who were suffering from *kiketuryokyo*, and found that in a number of cases, the patients recovered quickly from a state of frailty to a healthy condition (5). On the basis of the findings of the previous study, we carried out a cohort study that examined the effects of NYT on frailty. These findings are reported here.

STUDY SUBJECTS

The subjects were chosen from six medical facilities that participated in this research study from April 2016 to March 2018. They were elderly patients who were over the age of 65 and could walk without assistance, and who had at least one of the following symptoms: decreased strength after illness, malaise, hypophagia, night sweats, cold hands and feet, or anemia. The exclusion criteria included the following: (1) patients who had taken *Kampo* (i.e., Chinese medicine) or crude drugs within the 2 weeks before the commencement of the study; (2) obese patients with a body mass index (BMI) of over 25; and (3) patients whose physician in charge deemed their involvement in the study to be unsuitable. Furthermore, a group of patients whose background matched the study's criteria was set up as the control group.

METHOD

NYT group: Kracie Ninjin'yoeito Granule Extract, which contains 7.5 g of ninjin'yoeito, was given over two to three administrations throughout the day, delivered orally before or during meals. Right and left grip strength, weight, BMI, muscle mass, body fat percentage, lean body mass, muscle quality score, estimated bone mass, body age, and thigh circumference were measured at 0, 8, 16, and 24 weeks. All variables, except grip strength and thigh circumference, were measured using a body composition meter RD-903 or RD-501 (Tanita Corporation, Tokyo, Japan). Statcel 3 software (OMS Publishing Inc., Saitama, Japan) was used as the statistical analysis software.

Control group: No placebos were administered as the group was observed and continued with their conventional treatment. The same items as the NYT group were measured. The envelope method was used as a method of grouping.

This study has been screened by an ethical committee that included the presence of a lawyer and third parties (Medical Corporation Sakisaka Clinic Ethical Committee, approval number: 160201).

RESULTS

NYT group: 64 patients (male/female = 18/46), average age 78.5 ± 6.5 years.

Control group: 49 patients (male/female = 17/32), average age 76.0 ± 6.3 years (**Table 1**).

Because the missing value was 8 weeks' data and 16 weeks' data, it was compared at 0 and 24 weeks.

TABLE 1 | Patient background.

	Ninjin'yoeito Group ($n = 64$)	Control group ($n = 49$)	*P*-value
Age, years	78.5 ± 6.5	76.0 ± 6.3	*
Sex (Male/Female)	18/46	17/32	n.s.
Height, cm	153.1 ± 9.1	156.3 ± 8.2	n.s.
Right-hand grip strength, kg	18.0 ± 5.7	22.1 ± 7.2	**
Left-hand grip strength, kg	16.9 ± 5.9	21.5 ± 7.5	**
Weight, kg	50.7 ± 9.7	53.7 ± 8.8	n.s.
BMI, kg/m^2	21.5 ± 2.9	22.0 ± 2.8	n.s.
Body fat percentage, %	26.8 ± 9.4	25.3 ± 9.2	n.s.
Muscle mass, kg	34.1 ± 7.1	37.9 ± 6.5	*
Muscle quality score, points	41.8 ± 17.0	42.6 ± 16.0	n.s.
Estimated bone mass, kg	2.0 ± 0.5	2.2 ± 0.4	*
Body age, years	69.7 ± 7.5	66.1 ± 8.1	*
Thigh circumference, cm	42.5 ± 5.7	42.1 ± 4.9	n.s.
Lean body mass, kg	36.8 ± 6.4	40.2 ± 7.1	*

The comparisons between groups for variables, other than sex, were carried out using Welch's t-test. The comparison between groups for sex was carried out using the chi-square test. Both sides were tested at $p < 0.05$ (*), $p < 0.01$ (**).

Grip Strength

For the right-hand grip strength, the NYT group had significantly improved ($p < 0.01$). There was no change in the control group. With regard to the amount of change before and after administration, when the two groups were compared, a significant improvement was seen in the NYT group ($p < 0.01$) (**Figure 1**).

For the left-hand grip strength, the NYT group had significantly improved ($p < 0.01$), whereas the control group had significantly deteriorated ($p < 0.05$). With regard to the amount of change before and after administration, when the two groups were compared, a significant improvement was seen in the NYT group ($p < 0.001$) (**Figure 2**).

Weight and BMI

For weight and BMI, there were no changes in the NYT group or the control group (data not shown).

Muscle Mass

There was no change in the NYT group, but in the control group, muscle mass had significantly deteriorated ($p < 0.05$). With regard to the amount of change before and after administration, there was no difference between the groups when they were compared (data not shown).

Body Fat Percentage

For body fat percentage, there were no changes in the NYT group or the control group (data not shown).

Lean Body Mass

For lean body mass, there were no changes in the NYT group or the control group (data not shown).

Muscle Quality Score

No changes were observed in the NYT group, but in the control group, the muscle quality score had significantly deteriorated ($p < 0.05$). With regard to the amount of change before and after administration, when the two groups were compared, a significant difference was observed ($p < 0.05$) (**Figure 3**).

Estimated Bone Mass

For estimated bone mass, there were no changes in the NYT group or the control group (data not shown).

Body Age

There were no changes in the NYT group, but the body age had significantly deteriorated in the control group ($p < 0.05$). With regard to the amount of change

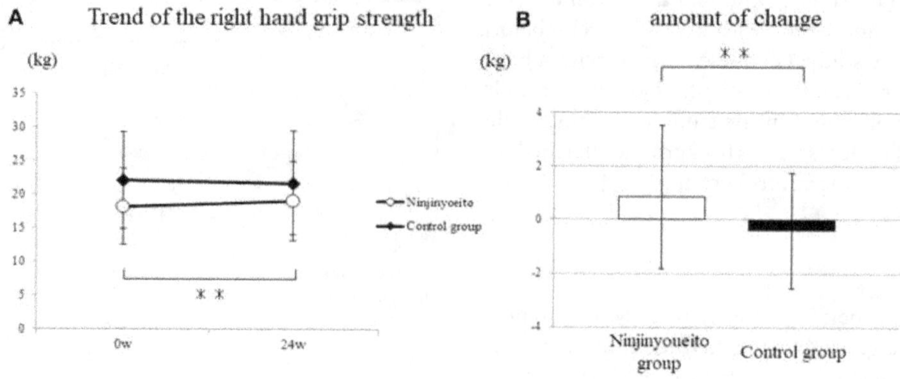

	0w	24w	P-value
Ninjinyoeito group	18.2±5.7	19.0±5.8	**
Control group	22.1±7.2	21.7±7.7	n.s.

	Amount of changes	P-value
Ninjinyoeito group	0.80±2.67	**
Control group	-0.43±2.16	

*p<0.05: Paired t-test in each group. **p<0.01:Welch's t test. control group vs Ninjinyoeito group. mean ± SD.

FIGURE 1 | Change in right-hand grip strength between both groups. The grip strength of the groups was compared using the paired *t*-test. The amount of change of each group was compared using Welch's *t*-test. Both sides were tested at $p < 0.05$ (*), $p < 0.01$ (**). Ninjin'yoeito group: 61 cases; control group: 49 cases. A significant improvement was seen in the ninjin'yoeito group. There were no changes in the control group. With regard to the amount of change before and after administration, when both groups were compared, the ninjin'yoeito group showed significant improvement.

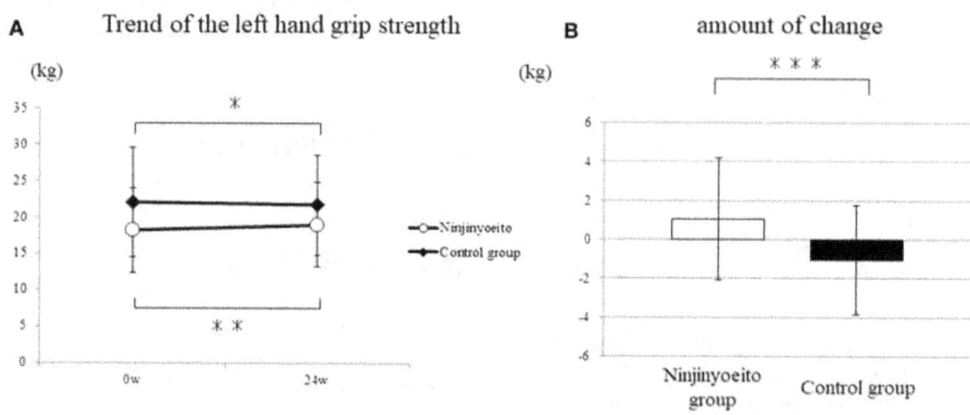

	0w	24w	p-value
Ninjinyoeito group	17.9±5.8	19.0±5.8	**
Control group	21.5±7.5	20.5±6.9	*

	Amount of changes	p-value
Ninjinyoeito group	1.10±3.15	***
Control group	-1.03±2.82	

Paired t-test in each group. ***p<0.001:Welch's t test. control group vs Ninjinyoeito group. mean ± SD.

FIGURE 2 | Change in left-hand grip strength between both groups. The grip strength of the groups was compared using the paired t-test. The amount of change of each group was compared using Welch's *t*-test. Both sides were tested at $p < 0.05$ (*), $p < 0.01$ (**), $p < 0.001$ (***). Ninjin'yoeito group: 61 cases; control group: 49 cases. A significant improvement was seen in the ninjin'yoeito group. Left-hand grip strength had significantly deteriorated in the control group. With regard to the amount of change before and after administration, when both groups were compared, the ninjin'yoeito group showed significant improvement.

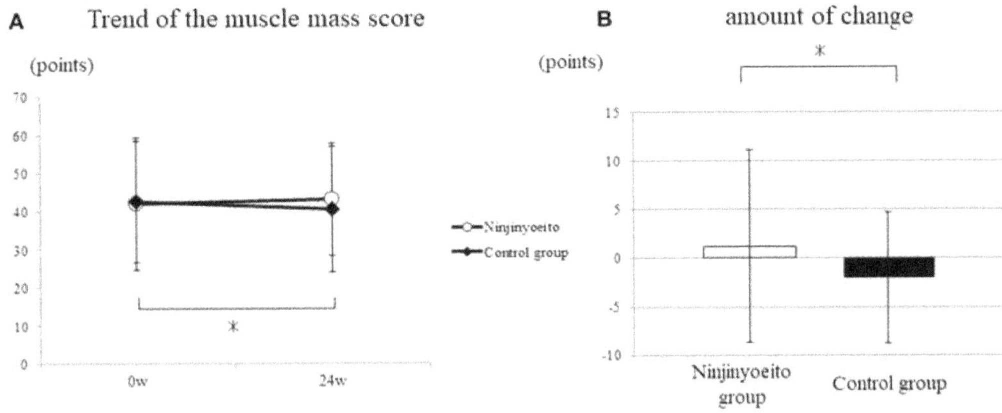

	0w	24w	p-value
Ninjinyoeito group	41.9±17.3	43.2±14.9	n.s.
Control group	42.6±16.0	40.6±16.5	*

	Amount of changes	p-value
Ninjinyoeito group	1.20±9.95	*
Control group	-2.04±6.71	

*p<0.05: Paired t-test in each group. *p<0.05:Welch's t test. control group vs Ninjinyoeito group. mean ± SD.

FIGURE 3 | Change in the muscle quality score between both groups. The muscle quality scores of each group were compared using the paired t-test. The amount of change of each group was compared using Welch's *t*-test. Both sides were tested, and $p < 0.05$ was set as the level of significance. Ninjin'yoeito group: 61 cases; control group: 49 cases. No changes were observed in the ninjin'yoeito group, but in the control group, muscle quality scores had significantly deteriorated. With regard to the amount of change before and after administration, when both groups were compared, the ninjin'yoeito group showed significant improvement.

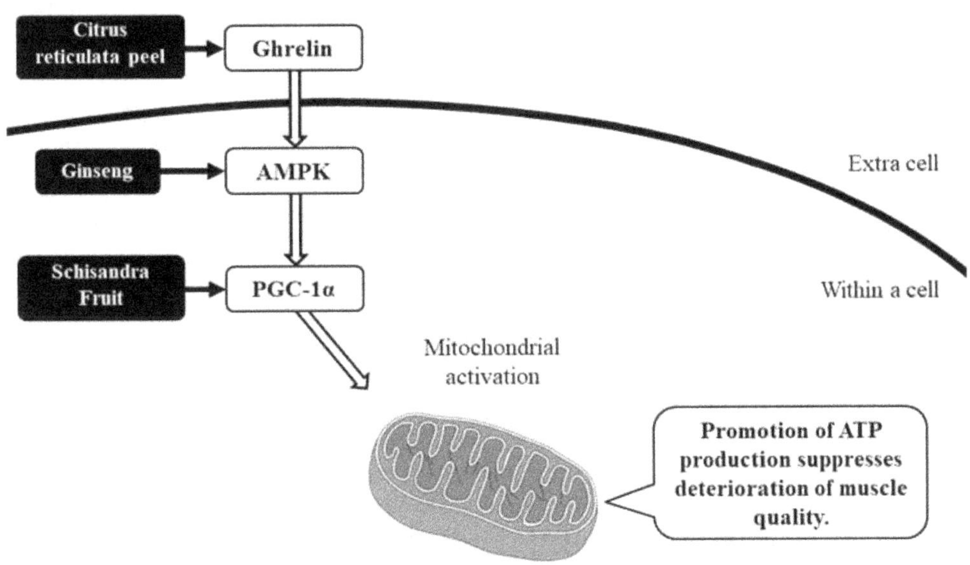

FIGURE 4 | Estimated mechanism of the action of ninjin'yoeito against muscle weakness. We can surmise that citrus reticulata peel promotes ghrelin production, ginseng activates AMPK, and Schisandra fruit induces the expression of *PGC-1α* in the skeletal muscle, which activates muscle mitochondria and increases energy production efficiency.

before and after administration, there was no difference between the groups when they were compared (data not shown).

Thigh Circumference

For thigh circumference, there were no changes in the NYT group or the control group (data not shown).

DISCUSSION

Not only does frailty lead to a noticeable decline in activity of daily living (6), but it also causes an increase in the number of people requiring nursing care (7), becoming a significant burden for families and society. It should thus not be treated as a personal issue, but as a societal problem.

Frailty can be classified into three different types: physical frailty, mental and psychological frailty, and social frailty (8). Physical frailty mainly takes the form of sarcopenia. People with mental and psychological frailty display signs of depression and mild cognitive decline. Furthermore, social frailty is demonstrated by those in isolated environments, such as those who live alone or shut themselves up in their room. It is important to note that these three types of frailty are not independent of one another, as they influence each other and are reversible. Health care and nursing care professionals who often examine frail patients should help them to return to a healthy state by accurately assessing their frailty, and providing them with meal and exercise guidance, as well as medication as needed.

While routinely examining many frail patients, the author noticed that *kiketuryokyo* was at the root of the condition. So, when the patients were administered NYT, which is a typical *kiketsu* complementary agent, several of them experienced dramatic improvements in the level of frailty. Moreover, these patients' depressive symptoms also improved considerably. Therefore, these results show that NYT can be effective in treating mental and psychological frailty (5). The results of the cohort study found that the administration of NYT improved the patients' grip strength in their right and left hands, and they were able to maintain their muscle quality.

There are many unanswered questions concerning the effect of NYT on muscles, but from the basic research reported thus far we can surmise that citrus reticulata peel promotes ghrelin production (9), ginseng activates activated protein kinase (AMPK) (10), and Schisandra fruit induces the expression of *PGC-1α* in skeletal muscle (11), which in turn activates muscle mitochondria and increases energy production efficiency (**Figure 4**). It is thought that NYT, which includes these crude drugs, has great potential to act as a form of "frailty treatment" in the future.

CONCLUSIONS

This study, which included more than 100 patients, suggests that NYT improves grip strength in both hands and maintains muscle quality. Therefore, NYT, a dual deficiency of qi and blood preparation, may be effective in treating physical frailty; however, there is a need to further study the effectiveness by increasing the number of cases further.

AUTHOR CONTRIBUTIONS

NS analyzed the data and wrote this report. KM, SS, TI, YT, HS, and TU provided the patient data.

REFERENCES

Xue QL, Bandeen-Roche K, Varadhan R, Zhou J, Fried LP. Initial manifestations of frailty criteria and the development of frailty phenotype in the Women's Health and Aging Study II. *J Gerontol A Biol Sci Med Sci.* (2008) 63:984–90.

Ministry of Health, Labour and Welfare. *Annual Health, Labour and Welfare Report.* (2016).

Bartali B, Frongillo EA, Bandinelli S, Lauretani F, Semba RD, Fried LP, et al. Low nutrient intake is an essential component of frailty in older persons. *J Gerontol A Biol Sci Med Sci.* (2006) 61:589–93. doi: 10.1093/gerona/61.6.589

Bonnefoy M, Cornu C, Norman S, Boutitie F, Bugnard F, Rahmani A, et al. The effects of exercise and protein-energy supplements on body composition and muscle function in frail elderly individuals: a long-term controlled randomized study. *Br J Nutr.* (2003) 89:731–9. doi: 10.1079/BJN2003836

Sakisaka A. Frailty and ninjin'yoeito. *Phil Kampo.* (2017) 64:17–9.

Murata S, Otao H, Murata J, Horie J. Relationship between the 10-second chair-stand test for the frail elderly (Frail CS-10) and activities of daily living (ADL). *Rigakuryoho Kagaku* (2011) 26:101–4. doi: 10.1589/rika.26.101

Kanzaki K. *Frailty and Geriatric syndrome. Frailty: The Most Important Task and Prevention Strategy in Super Aging Society.* 1st ed. Tokyo: Ishiyaku Publishers, Inc (2014). p. 23–30.

Arai H. Implication of frailty in elderly care. *Japanese J Geriatr.* (2014) 51:497–501.

Takeda K. Rikkunshito increases acyl ghrelin secretion by 5-HT2 receptor antagonism and improves anorexia caused by cisplatin. *Rec Prog Kampo Med Obstetr Gynecol.* (2008) 25:19–26.

Park MW, Ha J, Chung SH. 20 (S)-ginsenoside Rg3 enhances glucose stimulated insulin secretion and activates AMPK. *Biol Pharm Bull.* (2008) 31:748–51. doi: 10.1248/bpb.31.748

Kim YJ, Yoo SR, Chae CK, Jung UJ, Choi MS. Omija fruit extract improves endurance and energy metabolism by upregulating PGC-1 α expression in the skeletal muscle of exercised rats. *J Med Food.* (2014) 17:28–35. doi: 10.1089/jmf.201 3.3071

6

Kampo Medicines for Frailty in Locomotor Disease

Hajime Nakae[1,2]*, *Yuko Hiroshima*[2] *and Miwa Hebiguchi*[2]

[1] Department of Emergency and Critical Care Medicine, Akita University Graduate School of Medicine, Akita, Japan, [2] Department of Traditional Japanese Medicine, Akita University Hospital, Akita, Japan

***Correspondence:**
Hajime Nakae
nakaeh@doc.med.akita-u.ac.jp

Frailty is a syndrome that includes broad problems of senility and consists of three domains: physical, psychological, and social. Kampo medicine is used for intervention in cases of hypofunction in a mental or physical state. Kampo treatment, using Hojin formulations such as Hachimijiogan and Gosyajinkigan, is useful in patients with "jinkyo," or kidney hypofunction. Ketsu includes both blood and its metabolic products that circulate throughout the body. Oketsu is a disturbance of ketsu and is considered to be a microcirculation disorder. Anti-oketsu formulations, such as Keishibukuryogan and Jidabokuippo, are useful in the treatment of trauma patients who are experiencing swelling and pain. "Ki" is the universal energy that exists in the world. Hoki formulations, such as Rikkunshito and Hochuekkito, are useful in patients with poor appetites for reinforcing vital energy. Juzentaihoto and Ninjinyoeito are useful in patients with hypofunction of ki and ketsu, which are accompanying symptoms of coldness or cutaneous dryness. Thus, Kampo medicines can be used as a superior approach for the management of frailty.

Keywords: traditional Japanese medicine, sarcopenia, locomotive syndrome, hypofunctional constitution, trauma, Gosyajinkigan, Jidabokuippo

INTRODUCTION

Recently, sarcopenia, frailty, and locomotive syndrome have become known as disorders that are mainly caused by aging (1). These disorders have been considered in the context of a long life expectancy and illustrate the importance of promoting preventive care in Japan where the aging society progress (2, 3).

Here, we provide an outline regarding prevention and intervention for frailty in locomotor disease using Kampo medicine.

FRAILTY AND SARCOPENIA

Since physiological residual function decreases in a senile state, it becomes difficult to endure a higher level of stress, thereby resulting in frailty. Notably, frailty is considered to be a state that is easy to enter into, in the context of a bionomics disorder, and may require nursing care.

Sarcopenia is a syndrome that is characterized by progressive and generalized loss of skeletal muscle mass and strength, with a risk of adverse outcomes such as physical disability, poor quality of life, and death (4). Further, frailty includes both physical and mental problems, such as cognitive dysfunction or depression, and social problems, including economic hardship (5). Thus, frailty is a problem that is widely indicative of a senile state, consisting of these three domains. Frailty is defined as a clinical syndrome in which three or more of the following criteria are present: unintentional weight loss (10 lbs. in the previous year), self-reported exhaustion, weakness (grip strength), slow walking speed, and low physical activity (6). Among these criteria, weakness and slowness are also indicative of sarcopenia, suggesting that sarcopenia is a central element of a physical frailty (7).

INTERVENTION AND PREVENTION OF FRAILTY

For intervention and prevention of frailty, exercise therapy and nutrition care for sarcopenia is critical. Elderly people cannot perform exercise therapy because of weakening physical strength and a variety of physical symptoms. Pain control plays a key role in locomotor disease. However, elderly people cannot often utilize nonsteroidal anti-inflammatory drugs (NSAIDs) because of gastrointestinal (GI) disorder or renal dysfunction. Furthermore, it may be difficult to tolerate Western medicines, due to the side effects of anticonvulsant or opioid drugs.

In such cases, Kampo medicines may be useful to raise of physical strength and improve appetite (**Figure 1**).

TREATMENT WITH KAMPO MEDICINE FOR THE LOCOMOTOR DISEASE

Frailty is a state between disability and robust health. If appropriate intervention is performed against frailty, it is possible for frail patients to return to a healthy state (8). This concept is similar to "mibyo," or presymptomatic disease, in Kampo medicine. Mibyo is a state between illness and health, which can require treatment to prevent diseases from worsening and spreading to other parts of the body. Western medicine has no tests and, hence, no treatments available for people who have minor symptoms; however, Kampo recognizes even the slightest of these abnormalities, and takes action against them. In short, intervention by Kampo preparations and lifestyle guidance can change the body, such that it does not become ill, thereby preserving the health of the individual.

Frailty includes mental problems. In Kampo medicine, since ki, the universal energy that exists in the world, is considered to be a basic element of life, it is thought to support all mental, as well as physical, functions and bodily structures. This concept is referred to as the "relation of mind and body." Therefore, there are similarities between the philosophy of Kampo medicine and frailty, such that mind and body are regarded as inseparable.

Kampo medicine intervenes in cases of hypofunction in a mental or physical state, in a manner that is known as hypofunctional constitution. Notably, when elderly people with coldness suffer from reduced lower limb and bladder function, Kampo treatment is well applied. These symptoms are diagnosed as "jinkyo," kidney hypofunction. Hojin formulations for jinkyo, such as Rokumigan (RG), Hachimijiogan (HJG), and Gosyajinkigan (GJG), are used. HJG consists of Rehmannia Root, Cornus Fruit, Dioscorea Rhizome, Alisma Rhizome, Hoelen, Moutan Bark, Cinnamon Bark, and Aconite Tuber. It is applied in cases of nephritis, diabetes, impotence, sciatica, lumbago, bladder catarrh, prostatic hypertrophy, and hypertension, among others. Kawago has studied whether HJG can improve quality of life in Japanese patients with peripheral arterial disease (PAD). In the patients with the intermittent claudication caused

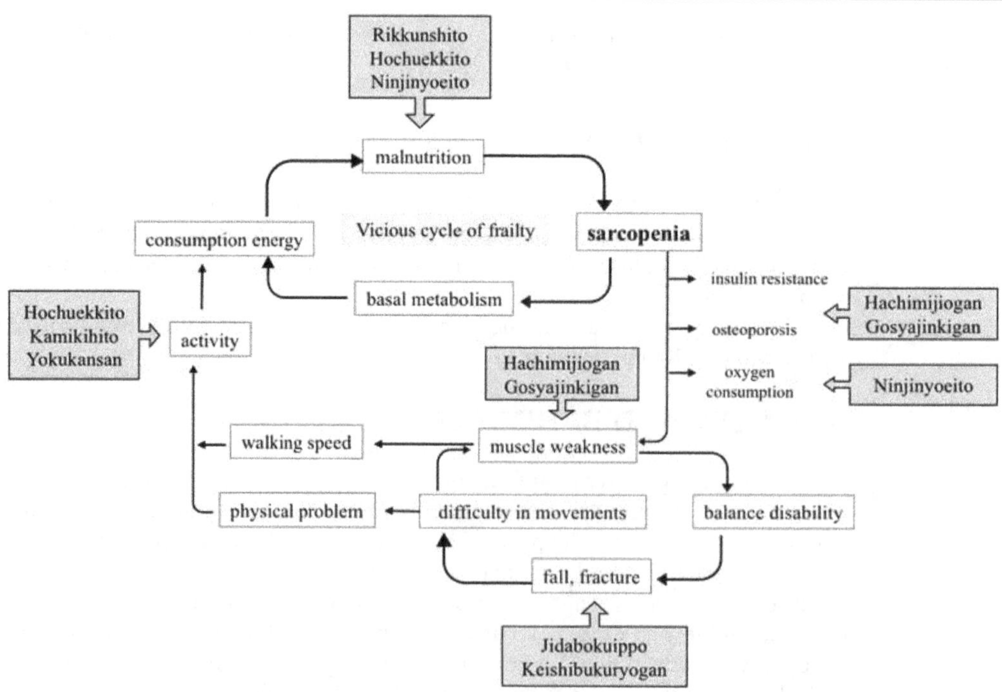

FIGURE 1 | Approach to frailty treatment, using Kampo medicines.

TABLE 1 | Vasodilatory activities in Hojin formulations ((9), revised).

	Pharmacological action	Rokumigan	Hachimijiogan	Gosyajinkigan
Vascular endothelial cell	Nitric oxide synthesis	+	+	+
	Prostaglandin I_2 synthesis	−	−	−
Vascular smooth muscle cell	Calcium channel inhibitor	+	+	+
	Protein kinase C inhibitor	+	+	+
	Beta receptor agonist	−	+	+

by PAD, it was suggested that HJG administration might improve quality of life (10). GJG is a prescription that adds Achyranthes Root and Plantago Seed to HJG. It is applied in cases of lumbago, coldness of the lower part of the body, micturition abnormalities (diuresis, urinary frequency, night urination), visual impairment (cataracts, blurred vision), hearing impairment (hearing loss, tinnitus), and edematous tendency. GJG is typically used for numbness in the lower limbs. In terms of pain relief effects, central analgesia has been observed through the stimulation of the κ opioid receptor, whereas peripheral analgesia has been observed through increased nitric oxide-production (11, 12). In a mouse model of neuropathic pain, analgesia has been reported through suppression of TNF—α expression from activated microglia (13). In a clinical setting, it was reported that GJG contributed to the suppression of peripheral neuropathy with the FOLFOX therapy for colorectal cancer (14). However, GJG did not prevent oxaliplatin-associated peripheral neuropathy in a multicenter randomized phase III trial (15). There remains controversy regarding whether GJG prevents chemotherapy-induced peripheral neuropathy in patients undergoing neurotoxic chemotherapy (9). Watanabe investigated whether GJG reduces the onset of diabetic complications (16). After 5 years of observation, 116 patients underwent analysis. Deterioration of the ankle reflex was suppressed in the GJG group. In addition, glycated hemoglobin and fasting plasma glucose were reduced in the GJG group. Kishida showed that GJG suppressed sarcopenia via the IGF-1/insulin pathway, maintained the expression of mitochondrial-related transcription factors, and suppressed TNF-α in senescence-accelerated mice (17). These results indicate that GJG is a promising candidate for relief from sarcopenia. Satoh reported that decreased pharmacological aging was observed in a single medical preparation, and that multicomponent composition medicines, such as Hojin formulations, showed an anti-aging effect (18). Interestingly, the vascular relaxant effect differs among three preparations (RG, HJG, and GJG; **Tables 1, 2**). Thus, GJG improves disuse atrophy through analgesia and prevents frailty. Herbal formulations containing Rehmannia Root as major ingredient are known as Rehmannia drug group. Since the Rehmannia drug group does not include licorice, there is no risk of pseudoaldosteronism. Nevertheless, Rehmannia Root might cause a GI disorder. When GI disorder develops, the administration of the Rehmannia drug group should be avoided before a meal; rather, it should be taken after a meal. Another option is the use of Rehmannia Root together with Anchusan (AS); this combination is used in patients with hypofunctional constitution and abdominal pain, as well as heartburn, nausea, vomiting, epigastric discomfort, and malaise. Aconite Tuber is also added to improve "ki," which gradually decreases through aging. Aconite Tuber provides antioxidant activity, analgesia, and an increased vascular flow (19, 20). Small amounts of Aconite Tuber can be used for arthralgia and somatic pain with coldness in elderly patients (21). Even in a kidney hypofunction state (jinkyo), when the clockwise circulation of ki is disturbed or a GI disorder is caused by Rehmannia Root, the Keishito (KT) group should be used instead. KT is used in patients who exhibit signs such as hypofunction, poor digestion, and exhaustion. KT consists of five herbs; Cinnamon Bark, Peony Root, Jujube Fruit, Ginger Rhizome, and Glycyrrhiza Root. Each formulation in KT group has a modified admixture based on the combination of the five KT herbs. Keishikajutsubuto (KKJBT) is a prescription that includes additional Atractyloids Lanceae Rhizome and Aconite Tuber, in combination with KT. It is applied in cases of coldness or to manage symptoms that become worse in cold (22). Kakkonkajutsubuto (KTKJBT) is a prescription that includes additional Atractyloids Lanceae Rhizome and Aconite Tuber, in combination with Kakkonto. It is applied in cases of pain and stiffness of the upper body (23).

TABLE 2 | Behaviors in Hojin formulations ((9), revised).

Pharmacological action	Clinical effect
Calcium channel inhibitor	Anti-atherogenic effect
Beta receptor agonist	Improvement of urinary disturbance
Protein kinase C inhibitor	Improvement of coldness in legs
Anticoagulant and antithrombogenic activities	Improvement of numbness in legs
Superoxide dismutase mimicking activity	
Lipid metabolism regulation	
Glycometabolism regulation	
Diuretic activity	
Improvement of kidney function	

"Ketsu" means red liquid. Ketsu includes both blood and its metabolic products that circulate throughout the body supplying nutrients to cells under the high-level control of ki. "Sui" means colorless liquids, bodily fluid or water. Sui includes all bodily fluids other than ketsu. Ki is represented by the nervous system, ketsu immunological function, and sui the various hormonal secretions that affect metabolism according to the theory of ki, ketsu, and sui. Swelling and pain caused by trauma is regarded as "oketsu." Oketsu is a disturbance of ketsu and is considered

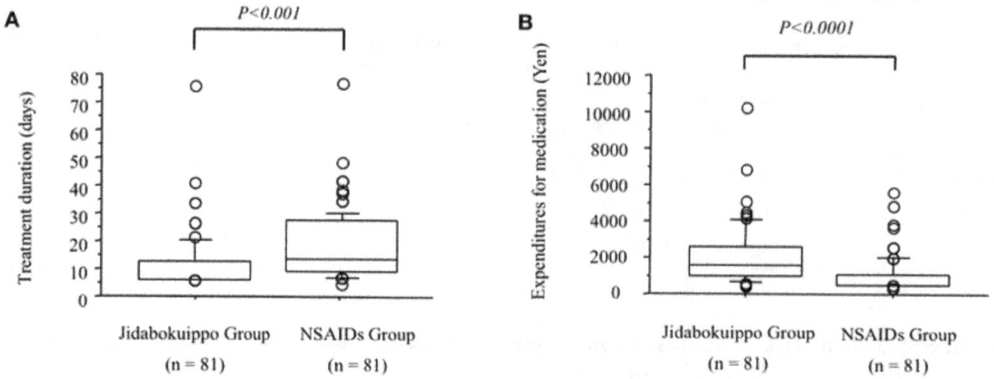

FIGURE 2 | Comparison of treatment durations and expenditures for medication between the jidabokuippo (JDI) and the non-steroidal anti-inflammatory drugs (NSAIDs) groups ((24) revised). **(A)**. Median treatment duration is significantly lower in the JDI group than in the NSAIDs group ($P < 0.001$). **(B)** Median expenditures for medication are significantly lower in the JDI group than in the NSAIDs group ($P < 0.0001$).

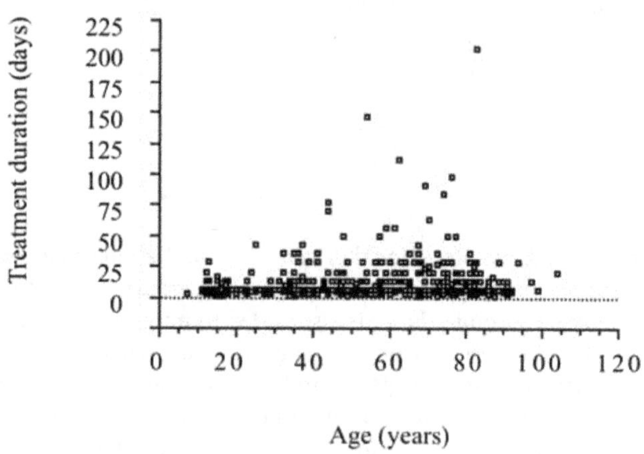

FIGURE 3 | Relationship between ages and treatment durations ((25) revised). A significant correlation is observed between the parameters. ($n = 643$, $r = 0.150$, $P < 0.0005$).

to be a microcirculation disorder. Keishibukuryogan (KBG), Jidabokuippo (JDI), and Tsudosan (TS) are used to treat oketsu. Kampo formulations exhibit antioxidant activity that is thought to be associated with swelling reduction (26, 27). We compared the efficacies of JDI and NSAIDs in patients with rib fracture by analyzing the treatment duration (24). Our results suggested, that compared with NSAIDs, JDI could shorten the duration of treatment and may provide a promising analgesic agent, from a medical economic viewpoint (**Figure 2**). It is unclear whether JDI effectively shortens the healing period or whether NSAIDs effectively delay healing. In either case, our results prove the non-inferiority of JDI to NSAIDs. We have used JDI for the treatment of various traumas, including multiple injuries, as well as simple bruise and sprain (28, 29). In our previous study, the efficacy rate was 91.6% in 643 patients with trauma who underwent JDI treatment (25). The necessary treatment period became longer with age (**Figure 3**). This may reflect the fact that wound healing increases with aging. Early intervention for pain control caused by trauma is necessary for elderly people, for the purpose of frailty prevention.

Even in a case of locomotor disease, when a patient complains of poor appetite, which is caused due to deficiency of ki, Hoki formulations for reinforcing vital energy, such as Rikkunshito (RT) and Hochuekkito (HET), should be used initially. Juzentaihoto (JTT) and Ninjinyoeito (NYT) are used for concomitant hypofunction of ki and ketsu, along with the accompanying symptoms of coldness or cutaneous dryness. NYT demonstrates hematopoietic activity and is effective for osteoporosis management (30). Frailty and apathy negatively affect the progression of Alzheimer's disease (31, 32). Ohsawa reported that NYT was effective for anorexia of aging in Alzheimer's disease (33).

Needless to say, Kampo medicines are not magical panaceas for frailty with locomotor disease. In order to engage in these problems, cooperation among various types of professions is required.

CONCLUSION

Pain control, as well as nutritional and mental management, are important for cases of frailty with locomotor disease. Since Kampo formulations are composed of multiple crude drugs, a single prescription can address several symptoms simultaneously. Thus, Kampo medicines can be used as a superior approach for the treatment of frailty.

AUTHOR CONTRIBUTIONS

HN conceived the original idea, and developed it in collaboration with YH and MH. HN wrote the first draft of the article. All authors contributed to revisions.

REFERENCES

Nakamura K. A "super-aged" society and the "locomotive syndrome". *J Orthop Sci.* (2008) **13**:1–2. doi: 10.1007/s00776-007-1202-6

Nakamura K, Ogata T. Locomotive syndrome: definition and management. *Clinic Rev Bone Miner Metab.* (2016) **14**:56–67. doi: 10.1007/s12018-016-9208-2

Akahane M, Maeyashiki A, Tanaka Y, Imamura T. The impact of musculoskeletal diseases on the presence of locomotive syndrome. *Mod Rheumatol.* (2018) **12**:1–16. doi: 10.1080/14397595.2018.1452173

Cruz-Jentoft AJ, Baeyens JP, Bauer JM, Boirie Y, Cederholm T, Landi F, et al. Sarcopenia: European consensus on definition and diagnosis: report of the European working group on sarcopenia in older people. *Age Ageing* (2010) **39**:412–23. doi: 10.1093/ageing/afq034

Ouchi Y, Arai H. *Statements for Frailty from the Japan Geriatric Society*. (2014). Available online at: https://www.jpn-geriat-soc.or.jp/info/topics/pdf/20140513_01_01.pdf

Fried LP, Tangen CM, Walston J, Newman AB, Hirsch C, Gottdiener J, et al. Frailty in older adults: evidence for a phenotype. *J Gerontol A Biol Sci Med Sci.* (2001) **56**:M146–56. doi: 10.1093/gerona/56.3.M146

Xue QL, Bandeen-Roche K, Varadhan R, Zhou J, Fried LP. Initial manifestations of frailty criteria and the development of frailty phenotype in the Women's Health and Aging Study II. *J Gerontol A. Biol Sci Med Sci.* (2008) **63**:984–90. doi: 10.1093/gerona/63.9.984

Kuzuya M. Impact of sarcopenia and frailty on elderly health. *Jpn J Geriat.* (2009) **46**:279–85.

Kuriyama A, Endo K. Goshajinkigan for prevention of chemotherapy-induced peripheral neuropathy: a systematic review and meta-analysis. *Support Care Cancer* (2018) **26**:1051–59. doi: 10.1007/s00520-017-4028-6

Kawago K, Shindo S, Inoue H, Akasaka J, Motohashi S, Urabe G, et al. The effect of Hachimi-Jio-Gan (Ba-Wei-Di-Huang-Wan) on the quality of life in patients with peripheral arterial disease: a prospective study using Kampo medicine. *Ann Vasc Dis.* (2016) **9**:289–94. doi: 10.3400/avd.oa.15-00133

Suzuki Y, Goto K, Ishige A, Komatsu Y, Kamei J. Antinociceptive effect of Gosha-jinki-gan, a Kampo medicine, in streptozotocin-induced diabetic mice. *Jpn J Pharmacol.* (1999) **79**:169–75.

Suzuki Y, Goto K, Ishige A, Komatsu Y, Kamei J.. Antinociceptive mechanism of Gosha-jinki-gan in streptozotocin-induced diabetic animals: role of nitric oxide in the periphery. *Jpn J Pharmacol.* (1999) **79**:387–91. doi: 10.1254/jjp.79.387

Nakanishi M, Nakae A, Kishida Y, Baba K, Sakashita N, Shibata M, et al. Gosha-jinki-Gan (GJG) ameliorates allodynia in chronic constriction injury-model mice via suppression of TNF-α expression in the spinal cord. *Mol Pain.* (2016) **12**:1–6. doi: 10.1177/1744806916656382

Kono T, Hata T, Morita S, Munemoto Y, Matsui T, Kojima H, et al. Goshajinkigan oxaliplatin neurotoxicity evaluation (GONE): a phase 2, multicenter, randomized, double-blind, placebo-controlled trial of goshajinkigan to prevent oxaliplatin-induced neuropathy. *Cancer Chemother Pharmacol.* (2013) **72**:1283–90. doi: 10.1007/s00280-013-2306-7

Oki E, Emi Y, Kojima H, Higashijima J, Kato T, Miyake Y, et al. Preventive effect of Goshajinkigan on peripheral neurotoxicity of FOLFOX therapy (GENIUS trial): a placebo-controlled, double-blind, randomized phase III study. *Int J Clin Oncol.* (2015) **20**:767–75. doi: 10.1007/s10147-015-0784-9

Watanabe K, Shimada A, Miyaki K, Hirakata A, Matsuoka K, Omae K, et al. Long-term effects of goshajinkigan in prevention of diabetic complications: a randomized open-labeled clinical trial. *Evid Based Complement Alternat Med.* (2014) **2014**:128726. doi: 10.1155/2014/128726

Kishida Y, Kagawa S, Arimitsu J, Nakanishi M, Sakashita N, Otsuka S., et al. Go-sha-jinki-Gan (GJG), a traditional Japanese herbal medicine, protects against sarcopenia in senescence-accelerated mice. *Phytomedicine* (2015) **22**:16–22. doi: 10.1016/j.phymed.2014.11.005

Satoh H, Nishida S, Tsuchida K. Kampo pharmacology: modulation by Hojin formulations of age-dependent vasodilatation and the dependence of diseases. *Nihon Yakurigaku Zasshi.* (2016) **147**:144–7. doi: 10.1254/fpj.147.144

Nakae H. Clinical evaluation of the finger tissue blood volume during shuchi-bushi powder administration. *Kampo Med.* (2008) **59**:809–12. doi: 10.3937/kampomed.59.809

Nakae H. Clinical evaluation of oxidative stress after taking powdered processed Aconite Tuber. *Kampo Med.* (2010) **61**:15–8. doi: 10.3937/kampomed.61.15

Nakae, H. Efficacy of powdered processed Aconite Tuber in patients with arthralgia and somatic pain. *Jpn J Occup Traumatol.* (2010) **58**:150–4.

Hamaguchi S, Komatsuzaki M, Kitajima T, Egawa H. A retrospective study assessing Kampo medicine for the treatment of lower extremity symptoms caused by lumber spinal diseases. *Kampo Med.* (2017) **68**:366–71. doi: 10.3937/kampomed.68.366

Nakae H, Hebiguchi M, Horikawa A, Kodama H. Efficacy of Kakkonkajutsubuto in patients with scapulohumeral periarthritis. *Pers Med Univers.* (2014) **2**:30–5.

Nakae H, Yokoi A, Kodama H, Horikawa A. Comparison of the effects on rib fracture between the traditional Japanese medicine Jidabokuippo and nonsteroidal anti-Inflammatory drugs: a randomized controlled trial. *Evid Based Complement Alternat Med.* (2012) **2012**:837958. doi: 10.1155/2012/837958

Nakae H, Hebiguchi M, Hiroshima Y, Okuyama M, Igarashi T. Jidabokuippo use in patients with trauma. *Kampo Newest Ther.* (2016) **25**:245–51.

Nakae, H. Clinical evaluation of oxidative stress after taking jidabokuippo. *Kampo Med.* (2010) **61**:847–52. doi: 10.3937/kampomed.61.847

Nakae H. Determination of the total antioxidant capacity for comparing different types of suspensions of Kampo extract. *Int J Integrative Med.* (2011) **3**:62–6.

Nakae H, Hebiguchi M, Okuyama M. Jidabokuippo use in patients with fractures of the extremities. *Pers Med Univers.* (2015) **4**:66–9. doi: 10.1016/j.pmu.2014.10.002

Nakae H, Okuyama M, Igarashi T. Traumatic lateral abdominal wall hematoma treated with Kampo medicines. *Traditional Kampo Med.* (2015) **2**:102–4. doi: 10.1002/tkm2.1022

Fujii Y, Imamura M, Han M, Hashino S, Zhu X, Kobayashi H, et al. Recipient-mediated effect of a traditional Chinese herbal medicine, ren-shen- yang-rong-tang (Japanese name: ninjin-youei-to), on hematopoietic recovery following lethal irradiation and syngeneic bone marrow transplantation. *Int J Immunopharmacol.* (1994) **16**:615–22. doi: 10.1016/0192-0561(94)90134-1

Spalletta G, Long JD, Robinson RG, Trequattrini A, Pizzoli S, Caltagirone C, et al. Longitudinal neuropsychiatric predictors of death in Alzheimer's disease. *J Alzheimers Dis.* (2015) **48**:627–36. doi: 10.3233/JAD-150391

Kojima G, Liljas A, Iliffe S, Walters K. Prevalence of frailty in mild to moderate Alzheimer's disease: a systematic review and meta-analysis. *Curr Alzheimer Res.* (2017) **14**:1256–63. doi: 10.2174/1567205014666170417104236

Ohsawa M, Tanaka Y, Ehara Y, Makita S, Onaka K. A Possibility of simultaneous treatment with the multicomponent drug, Ninjin'yoeito, for anorexia, apathy, and cognitive dysfunction in frail Alzheimer's disease patients: an open-label pilot study. *J Alzheimer Dis Rep.* (2017) **1**:229–35. doi: 10.3233/ADR-170026

7

Frailty and *Caenorhabditis elegans* as a Benchtop Animal Model for Screening Drugs Including Natural Herbs

*Katsuyoshi Matsunami**

Department of Pharmacognosy, Graduate School of Biomedical and Health Sciences, Hiroshima University, Hiroshima, Japan

***Correspondence:**
Katsuyoshi Matsunami
matunami@hiroshima-u.ac.jp

Caenorhabditis elegans has been used in research for years to clarify the genetic cascades and molecular mechanisms of aging, longevity, and health span. Health span is closely related to frailty; however, frailty has a different concept and is evaluated using various parameters in humans, such as Fried's Frailty Criteria. The *C. elegans* model has several advantages when performing a chemical screen to identify drug candidates. Several mouse models of frailty were recently developed, including a homozygous *IL-10* knockout. These mouse models are useful for understanding human frailty; however, they are not appropriate for primary drug screening because they require large spaces, expensive cost, and time consuming assessments. Therefore, a combination of these models may be a promising tool for discovering drugs and understanding the mechanisms of frailty. In addition, natural products, and herbs are attractive sources of novel drugs with pharmacological activity and low toxicity, in fact, over 60% of currently-available drugs are estimated to be related to natural compounds. In this review, the possibility of identifying natural agents (i.e., herb extracts and compounds) that could improve frailty are proposed, and the advantages and limitations of these models are also discussed.

Keywords: frailty, *Caenorhabditis elegans*, drug screening, natural herbs, model animal

INTRODUCTION

Frailty is a complex geriatric syndrome that is associated with increased vulnerability and a reduced physiological reserve that could lead to adverse health outcomes such as an increased risk of falls, dependency, disability, hospitalization, and mortality (1, 2). Shimada et al. performed a population-based survey to ascertain the prevalence of frailty in 5104 older (≥65 years; mean age: 71 years) Japanese adults (3). The authors showed that the rate of frailty increased with age and the overall prevalence of frailty was 11.3% (5.6, 7.2, 16, and 34.9% in the 65–69, 70–74, 75–79, and ≥80 age groups, respectively) (3). The global prevalence of physical frailty assessed using Fried's criteria was summarized by Choi et al. (4). The authors included data from the USA, Europe, and Asia and found that the prevalence of frailty and prefrailty varied between 4.9 and 27.3%, and 34.6 and 50.9%, respectively (4).

The global population is aging rapidly. In 2015, ~8.5% of the global population (7.3 billion) was aged ≥65. The number of older individuals is continuing to increase and is estimated to reach 12.0% (equivalent to 1 billion people) of the global population by 2030, and 16.7% (9.4 billion) by 2050. This increase in population is mainly due to low fertility and increased life expectancy (5).

Frailty is associated with multisystem impairments and chronic disease risk factors including cognitive impairment, diabetes, osteoporosis, chronic cardiovascular disease, kidney disease, malnutrition, chronic inflammation, and sarcopenia (2, 6, 7). These risk factors are related to the quality of life of older people and eventual mortality (2, 8–10). Therefore, given the emergent trend in global aging, interventions against frailty are a major concern (11).

FRAILTY CRITERIA IN HUMANS

Clinical frailty criteria were first introduced in cardiovascular health studies and included unintentional weight loss, self-reported fatigue or feelings of unusual tiredness or weakness, low activity levels (based on the frequency and duration of physical activity), slow walking times, and low grip strength (based on body mass index). These criteria were used to define frailty as either non-frail, prefrail, or frail (Fried Frailty Index) (10). In addition, the Clinical Global Impression of Change in Physical Frailty (CGIC-PF) (12); the Fatigue, Resistance, Ambulation, Illnesses, and Loss of Weight questionnaire (FRAIL scale) (13); the Canadian Study of Health and Aging (CSHA) clinical frailty scale (14); and the Gerontopole Frailty Screening Tool (GFST) (15) are also used to assess frailty.

Frailty is considered to be a dynamic process of accelerated aging in the absence of disability (16); however, it is difficult to understand the molecular and genetic mechanisms of human aging and frailty due to the ethical problem, genetic diversity, and lifestyle variability of the older human population.

MAMMALIAN MODELS OF FRAILTY

Several mouse models and their assessment tools were recently developed and provided an invaluable opportunity to conduct research into the mechanisms of frailty, the interventions to ameliorate frailty, and the effects of frailty on adverse outcomes using validated models (17–24).

Parks et al. were the first to attempt to establish a mouse frailty scale, which contained 31 parameters including activity levels, hemodynamics, body composition, and serum analysis. The authors found that frailer older mice showed the greatest myocyte hypertrophy and the worst peak contraction (17). However, this assessment had its limitations, as the experimental equipment used is uncommon for most laboratories. Whitehead et al. were the next to report an animal frailty index that contained visually-inspected and non-invasive assessment parameters (18). Liu and Graber et al. reported another mouse frailty index that used an activity wheel, a rotarod, and an inverted-cling grip device and resembled the Fried Frailty Test used in humans (19).These criteria provide a platform for validated preclinical animal models and have been implemented for a wide range of applications (25).

Graber et al. evaluated the effects of physical interventions in old mice using the mouse frailty index established by themselves (19). The authors found that voluntary aerobic exercise significantly improved the frailty score in C57BL/6 mouse (26). The effects of dietary and pharmaceutical interventions on frailty were also investigated using the criteria developed by Whitehead (18), and these treatments significantly reduced the mouse frailty index in DBA/2J and C57BL/6J mouse (27).

In addition, a rat frailty index was also recently developed (28, 29). Miller et al. selected criterion tests and configured appropriate cutoff points and indices to identify frailty in aged Fischer F344 rats. This model adapted existing clinical and preclinical indices, including grip strength, endurance, walking speed, and physical activity, that were used in human and mouse frailty indices. Yorke et al. also independently developed a rat frailty index for aged Fischer F344 rats using 27 criteria (29).

Animal models, such as transgenic and gene knockout mice, continue to be useful tools for preclinical studies in various diseases. Walston et al. reported a frail mouse model (i.e., IL-$10^{tm/tm}$) and characterized the physical and biological features to be similar to those seen in human frailty (30, 31). Mice carrying a homozygous targeted mutation of the *IL-10* gene (IL-$10^{tm/tm}$) were first generated by Kuhn et al. (32). This mouse was developed as a model of colitis but was found to exhibit a frail phenotype that was characterized by inflammation, reduced muscle strength, and a reduced health span. Aged IL-$10^{tm/tm}$ mice showed stiffer vasculature, which was in accordance with the increased COX-2 activity and thromboxane A2 receptor activation (33). In addition, ATP synthesis and the free energy released from ATP hydrolysis in skeletal muscle was reduced in this frail mouse model, which provides some mechanistic insight into skeletal muscle weakness in mouse and human frailty (33). Higher glucose level may be a risk factor for frailty in older human adults (34), and frail and prefrail older adults present lower estimated resting metabolic rate (eRMR) than non-frail adults, together with lower expired volume (Ve) and oxygen consumption (VO_2) values that were partially compensated by an respiratory frequency (RF) increase (35).

Westbrook et al. investigated the older IL-$10^{tm/tm}$ mice concerning on metabolic parameters shown in older humans, i.e., glucose metabolism, oxygen consumption (VO_2), respiratory quotient (RQ), spontaneous locomotor activity, body composition, and plasma adipokine levels. Interestingly, VO_2, fat mass, plasma adiponectin, and leptin were decreased with age in IL 10 $^{tm/tm}$ mice compared to controls, although insulin sensitivity, glucose homeostasis, locomotor activity, and RQ were not significantly altered. These findings suggest that frailty of this mouse model may be caused by reduction of fat mass, hormonal secretion and energy metabolism (36). Deepa et al. reported a new mouse model of frailty, Sod1KO mouse lacking the antioxidant enzyme Cu/Zn superoxide dismutase (24). The Sod1KO mice exhibited some features of human frailty including weight loss, weakness, low physical activity levels, exhaustion, increased inflammation, and sarcopenia. Dietary restriction in the Sod1KO mouse prevented the progression of frailty (24).

Thus, mouse frailty indices and normal and genetically-modified mouse models are important research tools that allow us to understand the biological mechanisms of frailty and evaluate novel interventions to ameliorate frailty. However, drug screening in mammalian models is expensive, time-consuming, requires large amount of drug candidates, and is relatively low throughput for many laboratories, although mammalian models are the most reliable and important platforms for preclinical studies.

CAENORHABDITIS ELEGANS: A BENCHTOP ANIMAL MODEL FOR INITIAL DRUG SCREENING

Non-mammalian model organisms are attractive options for discovering antifrailty drugs. Among the various well-known model organisms (i.e., *Danio rerio* (zebrafish), *Drosophila melanogaster* (fruit fly), and the nematode, *C. elegans*), *C. elegans* is the most studied animal in the field of aging, lifespan, and health span (37). It was first introduced to the field of basic biology in 1963 and has been used in a variety of studies assessing development (38), cell death (39), RNA interference (RNAi) (40), and aging (41). In fact, the genetic basis of aging has first recognized in *C. elegans* via the discovery of *age-1*, *daf-2*, and *daf-16* mutants (42–44). The lifespan was doubled by mutations in the *age-1* (PI3K, phosphoinositide 3-kinase) or *daf-2* (InR, insulin/IGF-1 receptor) genes, and reduced in the *daf-16* (FOXO transcription factor) mutant. Following this pioneering discovery, many researchers have used this model to focus on the genetic analysis and exploration of chemical interventions for longevity.

The pioneering research using *C. elegans* revealed that numerous pathways, including insulin/insulin-like growth factor-1 signaling, target of rapamycin signaling, AMP-activated protein kinase, sirtuins, mitochondrial stress-signaling pathways, and caloric restriction (45), were conserved in different organisms (e.g., *C. elegans*, *D. melanogaster*, and *Mus musculus*), and several chemicals have been investigated as potential candidates for extending life-span (41, 46, 47) (**Figure 1**).

C. elegans have many desirable features for drug discovery, such as their ease of maintenance in the laboratory, their transparent bodies for anatomical observation, their high genetic homology (60–80%) to humans, the publication of the complete genome sequence (48–50), conserved biological molecular responses, essentially no ethical problems, their high fertility rates (~250 eggs/worm within several days), and the availability of molecular biology tools (i.e., transgenic, gene knockouts, and RNAi knockdowns) (37). In addition, their short lifespan (~3 weeks) and small size are favorable for the screening of antiaging drugs due to the reduced experimental costs and their capacity for high throughput (51) (**Table 1**).

Frailty is defined as a condition of decreased physiological reserves by multisystem dysregulation and increased vulnerability to stressors (2). Similarly, aging is defined as the decreased adaptability to internal and external stress and increased vulnerability to disease and mortality by an accumulation of deficits derived from the progressive structural and functional decline of proteins, cellular organelles, tissues, and organs (52, 53). Both of these definitions have a lot in common, although the phrases are different.

Moreover, many age-associated features described in mammals, including neuromuscular degeneration, weakness

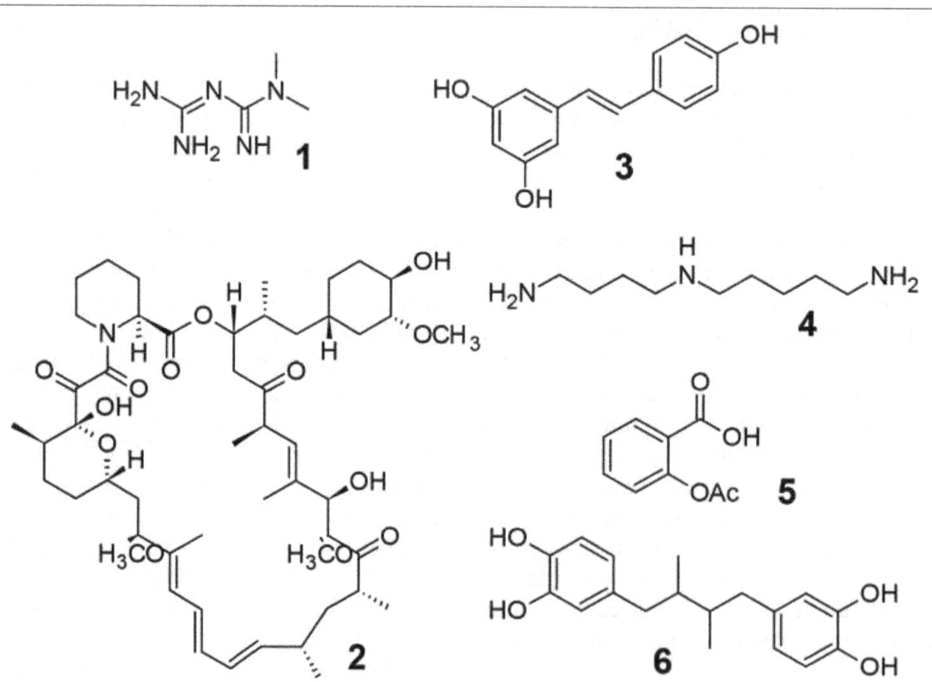

FIGURE 1 | Aging modulating compounds. 1; Metformin (biguanide antiglycemic agent, AMPK activation), 2; Rapamycin (immune suppressing agent, mTOR inhibitor), 3; Resveratrol (polyphenol, sirtuin activator), 4; Spermidine (polyamine, induction of autophagy), 5; Aspirin (COX inhibitor, antithrombosis, antioxidant), 6; Masoprocol (catechol, antioxidant, antiinflammation).

TABLE 1 | Feature of *C. elegans*.

- Multicellular animal
- Small size (~1 mm in length)
- Short life cycle (~3 days)
- High progeny production (~250 offspring in ~3 days)
- Conservation of cellular processes and genes

(Homologs have been identified for 60–80% of human genes)

- ADMET characteristics
- Low husbandry and animal costs
- Simple and high-throughput screening assays
- Availability of mutant and transgenic strains

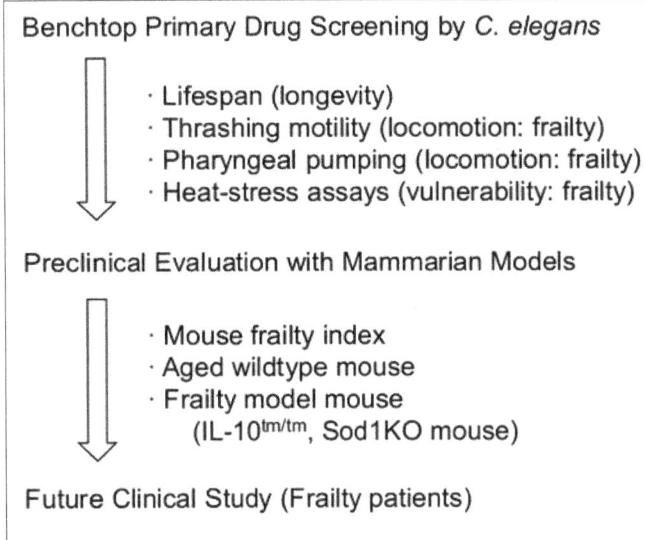

SCHEME 1 | Plausible work flow for anti-frailty agents.

to stressors, elevated infection levels, decreased physiological activity, and increased mortality, are also observed in *C. elegans* models (54).

Aging in *C. elegans* is also characterized by a severe loss of muscle mass and function (sarcopenia) (55), which gradually interferes with movement and the ingestion of food. Muscle mitochondrial energy dysregulation (56–58) and an accumulation of oxidative damage and aggregates in muscle cells are also likely to be related to muscle dysfunction in aged *C. elegans* (59, 60).

Several research papers have recently documented the relationship between lifespan, health span, and frailty in *C. elegans*. Newell et al. reported that mutants of age-related pathway genes in *C. elegans* showed that long-lived mutants displayed prolonged midlife movement and did not prolong the frailty period assessed by locomotor decline (56, 61); however, Bansal et al. previously reported controversial results showing that some long-lived mutants increased the proportion of the frailty period rather than health span (62).

When considering an improvement in quality of life, the health span-to-gerospan ratio is much more important than lifespan extension alone (62). Therefore, interventions focusing on the health span along with lifespan of the aging population are favorable.

Aging is characterized by muscular dysfunction as observed in sarcopenia and frailty. These two phenotypes are substantially overlapped with each other, and many of the adverse outcomes of frailty are probably mediated by sarcopenia (63–65).

In aged *C. elegans*, a gross decline in general behaviors (i.e., locomotion and feeding) is correlated with degeneration of muscle structure and contractile function (55). Loss of muscle mass is the major cause of aging-related functional decline, sarcopenia, and frailty. Several factors are correlated with sarcopenia including contraction-related cellular injury, oxidative stress, endocrine changes, and a reduced regenerative potential. In addition, both functional and structural decline in the pharynx during aging is significantly delayed in mutants with reduced muscle contraction rates that affect the initiation and progression of sarcopenia during aging (55, 60).

In addition, *C. elegans* containing a transgenic strain of human amyloid beta 1–42 (Aβ) under a neuron-specific promoter, as an Alzheimer's disease model, showed eight-fold slower locomotion than wildtype worms. This model seems consistent with the frailty seen in Alzheimer's patients (66–68). Tan et al. found a high prevalence of frailty in Parkinson's disease recently (69). The transgenic *C. elegans* of human α-synuclein gene as a Parkinson's disease model has been used for the demonstration of a natural product, squalamine, for the reduction of α-synuclein aggregation and muscle paralysis (70).

Sonowal et al. recently showed that small molecules, indole and derivatives, e.g., indole-3-carboxaldehyde and indole acetic acid, from commensal microbiota could extend the health span (i.e., the non-frailty period) of *C. elegans*. These compounds were also effective in *D. melanogaster* and *M. musculus*, therefore these compounds may become potential drug candidates to extend the health span and reduce frailty in humans (71). In this research, a lifespan assay (to measure longevity), two locomotion assays related to sarcopenia (e.g., a thrashing motility assay and a pharyngeal pumping assay), and a heat-stress assay (to measure vulnerability) were performed in *C. elegans*. These assays are popular, reliable, and well-studied so far as the *C. elegans* health span assay (72).

CONCLUSION

According to the 2016 review by Newman and Cragg, natural products continue to be an important source of clinical trial drugs and drug candidates; for example, ~65% of small-molecule drugs approved from 1981 to 2014 were directly or indirectly related to natural compounds (73). Among the various natural resources (i.e., plants, microbials, and marine organisms), plants have a long history of medicinal use that goes back to the ancient records of Mesopotamia, which chronicled their use in the treatment of various diseases. The total number of higher plants species in the world is estimated to be around 250,000; however, many of these remain to be characterized phytochemically. Thus, natural products and herbs are still attractive sources of novel drugs with pharmacological activity and low toxicity (74).

The *C. elegans* model is advantageous when performing a chemical screen to identify drug candidates to increase the health span. Among the various health span assays, longevity, thrashing motility, pharyngeal pumping, and heat stress assays are preferable as they have already been successfully utilized for the discovery of candidate compounds (71).

Wildtype and genetically-modified mouse models are useful for estimating efficacy on human frailty; however, they have several disadvantages for primary drug screening because of their scale, cost, and labor intensiveness. Therefore, the combination of these models may provide a promising workflow to discover drugs and understand the mechanism of frailty (**Scheme 1**).

AUTHOR CONTRIBUTIONS

The author confirms being the sole contributor of this work and has approved it for publication.

ACKNOWLEDGMENTS

This work was supported by JSPS KAKENHI grant number JP 17K08336.

REFERENCES

Walston J, Fried LP. Frailty and the older man. *Med Clin North Am.* (1999) 83:1173–94. doi: 10.1016/S0025-712570157-7

Fried LP, Ferrucci L, Darer J, Williamson JD, Anderson G. Untangling the concepts of disability, frailty, and comorbidity: implications for improved targeting and care. *J Gerontol A Biol Sci Med Sci.* (2004) 59:255–63. doi: 10.1093/gerona/59.3.M255

Shimada H, Makizako H, Doi T, Yoshida D, Tsutsumimoto K, Anan Y, et al. Combined prevalence of frailty and mild cognitive impairment in a population of elderly Japanese people. *J Am Med Dir Assoc.* (2013) 14:518–24. doi: 10.1016/j.jamda.2013.03.010

Choi J, Ahn A, Kim S, Won CW. Global prevalence of physical frailty by Fried's criteria in community-dwelling elderly with national population-based surveys. *J Am Med Dir Assoc.* (2015) 16:548–50. doi: 10.1016/j.jamda.2015.02.004

Wan H, Daniel G, Paul K. *U.S. Census Bureau, International Population Reports, P95/16-1, An Aging World: 2015.* Washington, DC: U.S. Government Publishing Office (2016).

Walston J, McBurnie MA, Newman A, Tracy RP, Kop WJ, Hirsch CH, et al. Frailty and activation of the inflammation and coagulation systems with and without clinical comorbidities: results from the Cardiovascular Health Study. *Arch Intern Med.* (2002) 162:2333–41. doi: 10.1001/archinte.162.20.2333

Sánchez GS, Garcia PC, Salva A, Sanchez AR, Granados GV, Cuadros MJ, et al. Frailty in community-dwelling older adults: association with adverse outcomes. *Clin Interv Aging* (2017) 12:1003–11. doi: 10.2147/CIA. S139860

Fulop T, Larbi A, Witkowski JM, McElhaney J, Loeb M. Mitnitski A, et al. Aging, frailty and age-related diseases. *Biogerontology* (2010) 11:547–63. doi: 10.1007/s10522-010-9287-2

Shamliyan T, Talley KM, Ramakrishnan R, Kane RL. Association of frailty with survival: a systematic literature review. *Ageing Res Rev.* (2013) 12:719–36. doi: 10.1016/j.arr.2012.03.001

Fried LP, Tangen CM, Walston J, Newman AB, Hirsch C, Gottdiener J, et al. Frailty in older adults: evidence for a phenotype. *J Gerontol A Biol Sci Med Sci.* (2001) 56:M146–57. doi: 10.1093/gerona/56.3.M146

Fried LP. Interventions for human frailty: physical activity as a model. *Cold Spring Harb Perspect Med.* (2016) 6:a025916. doi: 10.1101/cshperspect.a025916

Studenski S, Hayes RP, Leibowitz RQ, Bode R, Lavery L, Walston J, et al. Clinical global impression of change in physical frailty: development of a measure based on clinical judgment. *J Am Geriatr Soc.* (2004) 52:1560–6. doi: 10.1111/j.1532-5415.2004.52423.x

Morley JE, Malmstrom TK, Miller DK. A simple frailty questionnaire (FRAIL) predicts outcomes in middle aged African Americans. *J Nutr Health Aging* (2012) 16:601–8.

Rockwood K, Song X, MacKnight C, Bergman H, Hogan DB, McDowell I, et al. A global clinical measure of fitness and frailty in elderly people. *Can Med Ass J.* (2005) 173:489–95. doi: 10.1503/cmaj. 050051

Subra J, Gillette GS, Cesari M, Oustric S, Vellas B. The integration of frailty into clinical practice: preliminary results from the Gerontopole. *J Nutr Health Aging* (2012) 16:714–20. doi: 10.1007/s12603-012-0391-7

Landi F, Calvani R, Cesari M, Tosato M, Martone AM, Bernabei R, et al. Sarcopenia as the biological substrate of physical frailty. *Clin Geriatr Med.* (2015) 31:367–74. doi: 10.1016/j.cger.2015.04.005

Parks RJ, Fares E, MacDonald JK, Ernst MC, Sinal CJ, Rockwood K, et al. A procedure for creating a frailty index based on deficit accumulation in aging mice. *J Gerontol A Biol Sci Med Sci.* (2012) 67:217–27. doi: 10.1093/gerona/glr193

Whitehead JC, Hildebrand BA, Sun M, Rockwood MR, Rose RA, Rockwood K, et al. A clinical frailty index in aging mice: comparisons with frailty index data in humans. *J Gerontol A Biol Sci Med Sci.* (2014) 69:621–32. doi: 10.1093/gerona/glt136

Liu H, Graber TG, Ferguson-Stegall L, Thompson LV. Clinically relevant frailty index for mice. *J Gerontol A Biol Sci Med Sci.* (2014) 69:1485–91. doi: 10.1093/gerona/glt188

Howlett SE. Assessment of frailty in animal models. *Interdiscip Top Gerontol Geriatr.* (2015) 41:15–25. doi: 10.1159/000381131

Kane AE, Huizer PA, Mach J, Mitchell SJ, de Cabo R, Le Couteur DG, et al. A comparison of two mouse frailty assessment tools. *J Gerontol A Biol Sci Med Sci.* (2017) 72:904–9. doi: 10.1093/gerona/glx009

Seldeen KL, Pang M, Troen BR. Mouse models of frailty: an emerging field. *Curr Osteoporos Rep.* (2015) 13:280–6. doi: 10.1007/s11914-015-0283-y

Kane AE, Hilmer SN, Mach J, Mitchell SJ, de Cabo R, Howlett SE. Animal models of frailty: current applications in clinical research. *Clin Interv Aging* (2016) 11:1519–29. doi: 10.2147/CIA.S105714

Deepa SS, Bhaskaran S, Espinoza S, Brooks SV, McArdle A, Jackson MJ, et al. A new mouse model of frailty: the Cu/Zn superoxide dismutase knockout mouse. *Geroscience* (2017) 39:187–98. doi: 10.1007/s11357-017-9975-9

Kane AE, Ayaz O, Ghimire A, Feridooni HA, Howlett SE. Implementation of the mouse frailty index. *Can J Physiol Pharmacol.* (2017) 95:1149–55. doi: 10.1139/cjpp-2017-0025

Graber TG, Ferguson-Stegall L, Liu H, Thompson LV. Voluntary aerobic exercise reverses frailty in old mice. *J Gerontol A Biol Sci Med Sci.* (2015) 70:1045–58. doi: 10.1093/gerona/glu163

Kane AE, Hilmer SN, Boyer D, Gavin K, Nines D, Howlett SE, et al. Impact of longevity interventions on a validated mouse clinical frailty index. *J Gerontol A Biol Sci Med Sci.* (2016) 71:333–9. doi: 10.1093/gerona/glu315

Miller MG, Thangthaeng N, Shukitt-Hale BA. Clinically relevant frailty index for aging rats. *J Gerontol A Biol Sci Med Sci.* (2017) 72:892–6. doi: 10.1093/gerona/glw338

Yorke A, Kane AE, Hancock Friesen CL, Howlett SE, O'Blenes S. Development of a rat clinical frailty index. *J Gerontol A Biol Sci Med Sci.* (2017) 72:897–903. doi: 10.1093/gerona/glw339

Walston J, Fedarko N, Yang H, Leng S, Beamer B, Espinoza S, et al. The physical and biological characterization of a frail mouse model. *J Gerontol A Biol Sci Med Sci.* (2008) 63:391–8. doi: 10.1093/gerona/63.4.391

Ko F, Yu Q, Xue QL, Yao W, Brayton C, Yang H, et al. Inflammation and mortality in a frail mouse model. *Age* (2012) 34:705–15. doi: 10.1007/s11357-011-9269-6

Kuhn R, Lohler J, Rennick D, Rajewsky K, Muller W. Interleukin- 10-deficient mice develop chronic enterocolitis. *Cell* (1993) 75:263–74. doi: 10.1016/0092-867480068-P

Akki A, Yang H, Gupta A, Chacko VP, Yano T, Leppo MK, et al. Skeletal muscle ATP kinetics are impaired in frail mice. *Age* (2014) 36:21–30. doi: 10.1007/s11357-013-9540-0

Zaslavsky O, Walker RL, Crane PK, Gray SL, Larson EB. Glucose levels and risk of frailty. *J Gerontol A Biol Sci Med Sci.* (2016) 71:1223–9. doi: 10.1093/gerona/glw024

Pedro A, Luis R, Pedro MSJ, Teresa FR, Sergio SR, Miguel FS. Energetics of aging and frailty: the FRADEA Study. *J Gerontol A Biol Sci Med Sci.* (2016) 71:787–96. doi: 10.1093/gerona/glv182

Westbrook RM, Yang HL, Langdon JM, Roy CN, Kim JA, Choudhury PP, et al. Aged interleukin-10tm1Cgn chronically inflamed mice have substantially reduced fat mass, metabolic rate, and adipokines. *PLoS ONE* (2017) 12:e0186811. doi: 10.1371/journal.pone.0186811

Strange K. Drug discovery in fish, flies, and worms. *ILAR J.* (2016) 57:133–43. doi: 10.1093/ilar/ilw034

Vuong-Brender TT, Yang X, Labouesse M. *C. elegans* embryonic morphogenesis. *Curr Top Dev Biol.* (2016) 116:597–616. doi: 10.1016/bs.ctdb.2015.11.012

Malin JZ, Shaham S. Cell death in *C. elegans* development. *Curr Top Dev Biol.* (2015) 114:1–42. doi: 10.1016/bs.ctdb.2015.07.018

Ohkumo T, Masutani C, Eki T, Hanaoka F. Use of RNAi in *C. elegans*. *Methods Mol Biol.* (2008) 442:129–37. doi: 10.1007/978-1-59745-191-8_10

Lapierre LR, Hansen M. Lessons from *C. elegans*: signaling pathways for longevity. *Trends Endocrinol Metab.* (2012) 23:637–44. doi: 10.1016/j.tem.2012.07.007

Klass MR. A method for the isolation of longevity mutants in the nematode *Caenorhabditis elegans* and initial results. *Mech Ageing Dev.* (1983) 22:279–86. doi: 10.1016/0047-637490082-9

Friedman DB, Johnson TE. A mutation in the age-1 gene in *Caenorhabditis elegans* lengthens life and reduces hermaphrodite fertility. *Genetics* (1988) 118:75–86.

Kenyon C, Chang J, Gensch E, Rudner A, Tabtiang R. A *C. elegans* mutant that lives twice as long as wild type. *Nature* (1993) 366:461–4. doi: 10.1038/366461a0

Bitto A, Wang AM, Bennett CF, Kaeberlein M. Biochemical genetic pathways that modulate aging in multiple species. *Cold Spring Harb Perspect Med.* (2015) 5:a025114. doi: 10.1101/cshperspect.a025114

Kumar S, Lombard DB. Finding Ponce de Leon's pill: challenges in screening for anti-aging molecules. *F1000Res* (2016) 5:406. doi: 10.12688/f1000research.7821.1

Pan H, Finkel T. Key proteins and pathways that regulate lifespan. *J Biol Chem.* (2017) 292:6452–60. doi: 10.1074/jbc.R116.771915

The *C. elegans* Sequencing Consortium. Genome sequence of the nematode *C. elegans*: a platform for investigating biology. *Science* (1998) 282:2012–8. doi: 10.1126/science.282.5396.2012

Kaletta T, Hengartner MO. Finding function in novel targets: *C. elegans* as a model organism. *Nat Rev Drug Discov.* (2006) 5:387–98. doi: 10.1038/nrd2031

Markaki M, Tavernarakis N. Modeling human diseases in *Caenorhabditis elegans*. *Biotechnol J.* (2010) 5:1261–76. doi: 10.1002/biot.201000183

Rangaraju S, Solis GM, Petrascheck M. High-throughput small-molecule screening in *Caenorhabditis elegans*. *Methods Mol Biol.* (2015) 1263:139–55. doi: 10.1007/978-1-4939-2269-7_11

Holliday R. Developmental and cell biology series. In: Barlow PW, Bray D, Green D, Kirk DL, editors . *Understanding Aging*. Vol. 30. Cambridge, NY: Cambridge University Press (1995). p. 41–66.

Neal SF. The biology of aging and frailty. *Clin Geriatr Med.* (2011) 27:27–37. doi: 10.1016/j.cger.2010.08.006

Torgovnick A, Schiavi A, Maglioni S, Ventura N. Healthy aging: what can we learn from *Caenorhabditis elegans*? *Z Gerontol Geriatr.* (2013) 46:623–8. doi: 10.1007/s00391-013-0533-5

Glenn CF, Chow DK, David L, Cooke CA, Gami MS, Iser WB, et al. Behavioral deficits during early stages of aging in *Caenorhabditis elegans* result from locomotory deficits possibly linked to muscle frailty. *J Gerontol A Biol Sci Med Sci.* (2004) 59:1251–60. doi: 10.1093/gerona/59. 12.1251

Newell SBL, Cypser JR, Kechris K, Kitzenberg DA, Tedesco PM, Johnson TE. Movement decline across lifespan of *Caenorhabditis elegans* mutants in the insulin/insulin-like signaling pathway. *Aging Cell* (2018) 17:e12704. doi: 10.1111/acel.12704

Sebastian D, Palacin M, Zorzano A. Mitochondrial dynamics: coupling mitochondrial fitness with healthy aging. *Trends Mol Med.* (2017) 23:201–15. doi: 10.1016/j.molmed.2017.01.003

Gaffney CJ, Shephard F, Chu J, Baillie DL, Rose A, Constantin TD, et al. Degenerin channel activation causes caspase-mediated protein degradation and mitochondrial dysfunction in adult *C. elegans* muscle. *J Cachexia Sarcopenia Muscle* (2016) 7:181–92. doi: 10.1002/jcsm.12040

Ayyadevara S, Balasubramaniam M, Suri P, Mackintosh SG, Tackett AJ, Sullivan DH, et al. Proteins that accumulate with age in human skeletal-muscle aggregates contribute to declines in muscle mass and function in *Caenorhabditis elegans*. *Aging (Albany NY)* (2016) 8:3486–97. doi: 10.18632/aging.101141

Chow DK, Glenn CF, Johnston JL, Goldberg IG, Wolkow CA. Sarcopenia in the *Caenorhabditis elegans* pharynx correlates with muscle contraction rate over lifespan. *Exp Gerontol.* (2006) 41:252–60. doi: 10.1016/j.exger.2005.12.004

Herndon LA, Schmeissner PJ, Dudaronek JM, Brown PA, Listner KM, Sakano Y, et al. Stochastic and genetic factors influence tissue-specific decline in ageing *C. elegans*. *Nature* (2002) 419:808–14. doi: 10.1038/nature01135

Bansal A, Zhu LJ, Yen K, Tissenbaum HA. Uncoupling lifespan and healthspan in *Caenorhabditis elegans* longevity mutants. *Proc Natl Acad Sci USA.* (2015) 112:E277–86. doi: 10.1073/pnas.1412192112

Cederholm T. Overlaps between frailty and sarcopenia definitions. *Nestle Nutr Inst Workshop Ser.* (2015) 83:65–9. doi: 10.1159/000382063

Bernabei R, Martone AM, Vetrano DL, Calvani R, Landi F, Marzetti E. Frailty, physical frailty, sarcopenia: a new conceptual model. *Stud Health Technol Inform.* (2014) 203:78–84. doi: 10.3233/978-1-61499-425-1-78

Keevil VL, Romero OR. Ageing well: a review of sarcopenia and frailty. *Proc Nutr Soc.* (2015) 74:337–47. doi: 10.1017/S0029665115002037

Machino K, Link CD, Wang S, Murakami H, Murakami S. A semi- automated motion-tracking analysis of locomotion speed in the *C. elegans* transgenics overexpressing beta-amyloid in neurons. *Front Genet.* (2014) 5:202. doi: 10.3389/fgene.2014.00202

Koch G, Belli L, Giudice TL, Lorenzo FD, Sancesario GM, Sorge R, et al. Frailty among Alzheimer's disease patients. *CNS Neurol Disord Drug Targets* (2013) 12:507–11. doi: 10.2174/1871527311312040010

Kulmala J, Nykänen I, Mänty M, Hartikainen S. Association between frailty and dementia: a population-based study. *Gerontology* (2014) 60:16–21. doi: 10.1159/000353859

Perni M, Galvagnion C, Maltsev A, Meisl G, Müller MB, Challa PK, et al. A natural product inhibits the initiation of α-synuclein aggregation and suppresses its toxicity. *Proc Natl Acad Sci USA.* (2017) 114:E1009–17. doi: 10.1073/pnas.1610586114

Tan AH, Hew YC, Lim SY, Ramli NM, Kamaruzzaman SB, Tan MP, et al. Altered body composition, sarcopenia, frailty, and their clinico- biological correlates, in Parkinson's disease. *Parkinsonism Relat Disord.* (2018). doi: 10.1016/j.parkreldis.2018.06.020. [Epub ahead of print].

Sonowal R, Swimm A, Sahoo A, Luo L, Matsunaga Y, Wu Z, et al. Indoles from commensal bacteria extend healthspan. *Proc Natl Acad Sci USA.* (2017) 114:E7506–15. doi: 10.1073/pnas.1706464114

Keith SA, Amrit FR, Ratnappan R, Ghazi A. The *C. elegans* healthspan and stress-resistance assay toolkit. *Methods* (2014) 68:476–86. doi: 10.1016/j.ymeth.2014.04.003

Newman DJ, Cragg GM. Natural products as sources of new drugs from 1981 to 2014. *J Nat Prod* (2016) 79:629–61. doi: 10.1021/acs.jnatprod.5b01055

Matsunami K. Current topics: natural products chemistry of global tropical and subtropical plants. *Chem Pharm Bull.* (2018) 66:467–8. doi: 10.1248/cpb.c18-ctf6605

8

Clinical Practice Guidelines and Evidence for the Efficacy of Traditional Japanese Herbal Medicine (Kampo) in Treating Geriatric Patients

Shin Takayama, Ryutaro Arita, Akiko Kikuchi, Minoru Ohsawa, Soichiro Kaneko and Tadashi Ishii*

Department of Education and Support for Regional Medicine, Department of Kampo Medicine, Tohoku University Hospital, Sendai, Japan

***Correspondence:**
Shin Takayama
takayama@med.tohoku.ac.jp

Frailty is defined as a state of increased vulnerability to poor resolution of homeostasis following stress, which increases the risk of adverse outcomes such as falls, delirium, and disability in the elderly. Recently in Japan, clinical practice guidelines (CPG) have recommended kampo treatment. We conducted a search for reports on Japanese CPG and kampo medicine in the treatment of symptoms in the elderly. The search was performed using the databases PubMed, Ichushi Web, J-Stage, Japan Medical Publishers Association, Medical Information Network Distribution Service, and CPG containing kampo products in Japan; reports from January 1st, 2012 to October 31st, 2017 were reviewed. Over the past 5 years, nine CPGs have recommended kampo treatment based on the evidence for improvement in skin symptoms, cough, gastro-intestinal dysfunction, urinary dysfunction, and dementia. Treatments with kampo medicine are performed depending on the coexistence of manifestations based on the original kampo concept, i.e., cognitive dysfunction and dementia with sarcopenia showing urinary disorder. Each kampo formula includes multiple crude drugs that have several pharmacological functions; these drugs include alkaloids, glycosides, and polysaccharides. Thus, kampo formula has an effect on multiple organs and coordinates the relationship between the brain, endocrine system, immune system, and skeletal muscles. Kampo treatment can be considered as supporting holistic medicine in elderly individuals with frailty.

Keywords: review, herbal medicine, kampo medicine, guidelines, geriatrics, elderly

INTRODUCTION

Frailty is defined as a state of increased vulnerability to poor resolution of homeostasis following stress, which increases the risk of adverse outcomes such as falls, delirium, and disability in the elderly (1–3). Frailty involves disorders in multiple inter-related physiological systems, including the brain, the endocrine system, the immune system, and the skeletal muscle, resulting in weight loss, exhaustion, low energy expenditure, slow gait speed, and weak grip strength (4). The left side of **Figure 1** shows an overview of the hypothesized molecular, physiological, and clinical pathways involved in the pathogenesis of frailty (5). In addition to exercise intervention combined with nutrition, multifunctional pharmacological agents are probably required for preventing frailty.

In the super aged society in Japan, the percentage of the elderly population (aged over 65 years) is expected to exceed 30% in 2025 and reach 39.9% in 2060 (6). Frailty is one of the reasons for need of nursing care in the elderly, thus the medical, social, and economical correspondence has been a research focus. Traditional Japanese medicine (kampo) has been applied for the treatment of comorbid symptoms or disorder for the past 1500 years. Kampo medicine includes multiple crude drugs that have several pharmacological functions including alkaloids, glycoside, and polysaccharide (7). Thus, kampo medicine has an effect on multiple organs and coordinates the relationship between the brain, endocrine system, immune system, skeletal muscles, and the patients' emotional condition. The right side of the **Figure 1** shows the kampo concept for frailty. We believe that concomitant use with western medicine and kampo medicine can contribute to management of patients with frailty. Evidence based on clinical studies has grown in the past two decades; and recently, in Japan, clinical practice guidelines (CPG) for symptoms in the elderly gave some recommendations for use of kampo medicine.

In this report, we review CPG regarding kampo and the evidence of the efficacy of kampo medicine in the treatment of the elderly. We also discuss the characteristics of the kampo concept.

MATERIALS AND METHODS

Literature Search

We conducted data base searches for Japanese CPG and kampo medicine for the symptoms in elderlies in PubMed, Ichushi Web, J-Stage, Japan Medical Publishers Association, Medical Information Network Distribution Service, and Clinical Practice Guideline Containing Kampo products. The search was restricted to CPGs published between January 1st 2012 to October 31st 2017. We used the following search strategy: 1. CPG; 2. Kampo medicine; 3. Herbal medicine; 4. #1–3 in Japanese; 5. #1 OR #2 AND #3 OR; and 6. #4 OR #5.

Selection Criteria

We included research articles published in English or Japanese that were related to CPG using kampo medicine. CPGs that mentioned the recommendation strength with quality of evidence and studies that included elderly subjects were selected. Physical therapy, massage therapy, acupuncture, and acupuncture-related techniques were excluded.

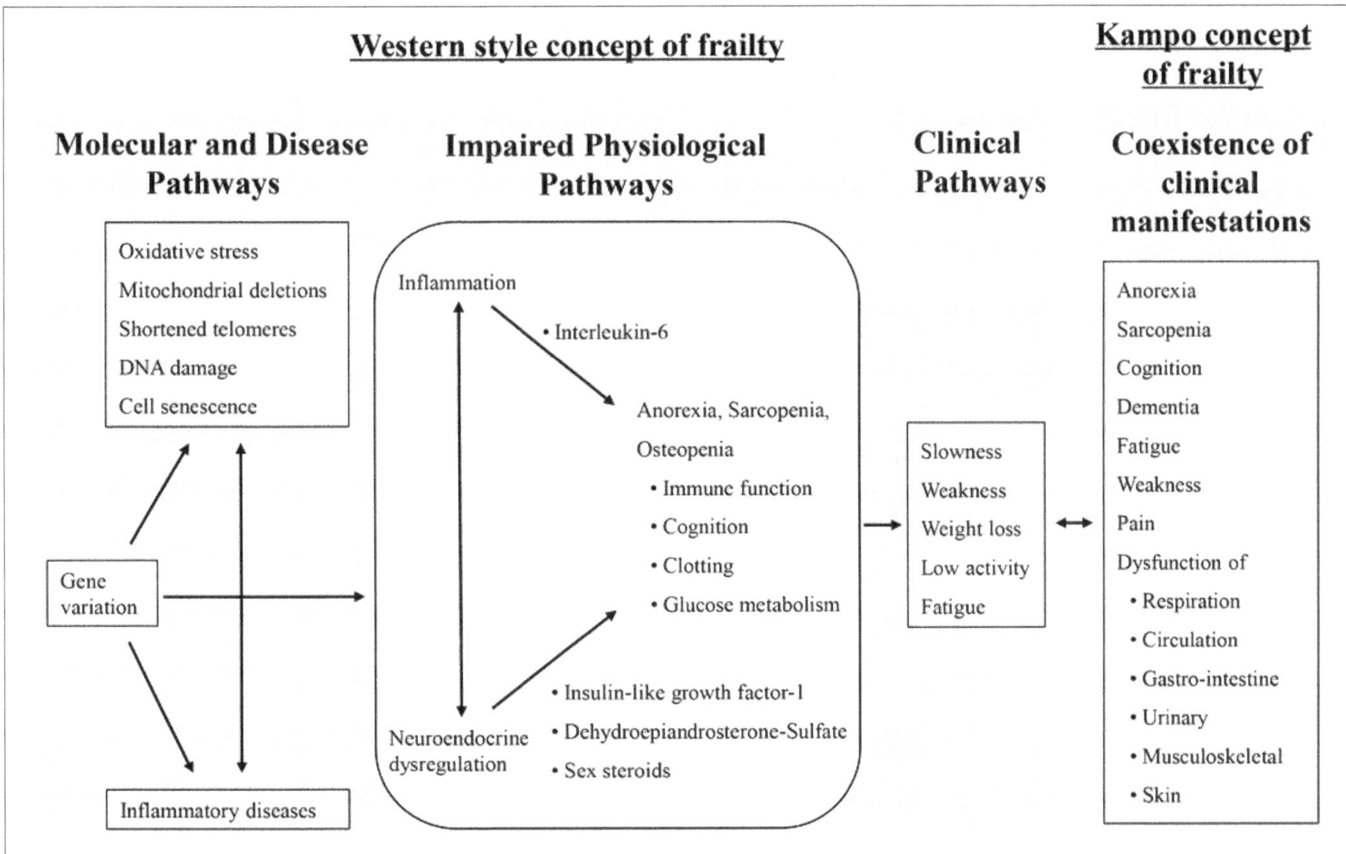

FIGURE 1 | An overview of the hypothesized molecular, physiological, and clinical pathways involved in frailty and the kampo concept of frailty [adapted from (2, 5)].

Data Extraction

Eligible articles were categorized by two independent researchers (ST and SK). Specifically, information from the articles or CPGs was extracted and tabulated, and eligible CPG were classified according to the name of CPG, symptoms or diseases, clinical question, mention about quality of evidence, and recommendation strength.

RESULTS

General Aspects

The review process flowchart is shown in **Figure 2**; and the eligible PCGs are shown in **Table 1**. Over the past 5 years, the following eligible nine CPGs have given some recommendations for kampo treatment based on the evidence for skin symptoms, allergy, cough, gastro-intestinal dysfunction, urinary dysfunction, and dementia: Clinical Practice Guideline for the Pruritus cutaneus universalis (8), Practical Guideline for the Management of Allergic Rhinitis in Japan (9), The Japanese Respiratory Society guidelines for management of cough (10), Evidence-based Clinical Practice Guidelines for GERD (11), Evidence-based Clinical Practice Guidelines for Functional Dyspepsia (12), Evidence-based Clinical Practice Guidelines for Irritable Bowel Syndrome (13), Evidence-based clinical practice guidelines for chronic constipation (14), Clinical guidelines for overactive bladder syndrome (15), and Practice Guideline for Dementia (16).

Randomized Clinical Trial Involving Elderly Patients With Each Symptom Introduced in the Clinical Practice Guidelines

Skin Symptoms

CPG for pruritus gave some recommendations (permission) for pruritus or dry skin based on some RCTs. Five RCTs for skin symptom were selected in the CPG focused on the elderly. Ohkawara et al. reported the efficacy and safety of orengedokuto or goshajinkigan for the symptom in senile pruritus (17). Orengedokuto (Huang-Lian-Jie-Du-Tang) (18) or goshajinkigan (Niu-Che-Shen-Qi-Wan) (18) improved the subjective and objective symptom with no significant difference in the efficacy and safety as compared to Clemastine Fumarate that is potent and selective histamine H1 receptor antagonist. Iida et al. reported the efficacy of tokiinshi (Dang-Gui-Yin-Zi) (18) for moisture holding ability evaluated with a measurement device for the water content of the skin corneum in patients with senile pruritus (19). Tokiinshi significantly improved dry skin compared with no treatment. Ishioka et al. reported the efficacy of hachimijiogan (Ba-Wei-Di-Huang-Wan) (18) for the subjective symptom in patients with senile pruritus (20). Hachimijiogan improved the subjective symptom with no significant difference in efficacy compared to Ketotifen Fumarate that is selective histamine H1 receptor antagonist. In addition, Ishioka reported no significant difference in efficacy between hachimijiogan and rokumigan (Liu-Wei-Wan) (18) for treatment of subjective symptom in patients with senile pruritus (21). Ohkuma et al. reported that orengedokuto with tokiinshi, orengedokuto alone, or tokiinshi alone significantly improved the itchy symptom with no significant difference in efficacy compared with anti-histamine (22).

Allergy Symptoms

CPG for nasal allergy recommended use of kampo medicine for perennial nasal allergy with a referred RCT. Baba et al. reported the efficacy and safety of shoseiryuto (Xiao-Qing-Long-Tang) (18) for perennial allergic rhinitis in a double-blind RCT including elderly subjects (23). The shoseiryuto group showed more moderate to high improvement than that of the placebo

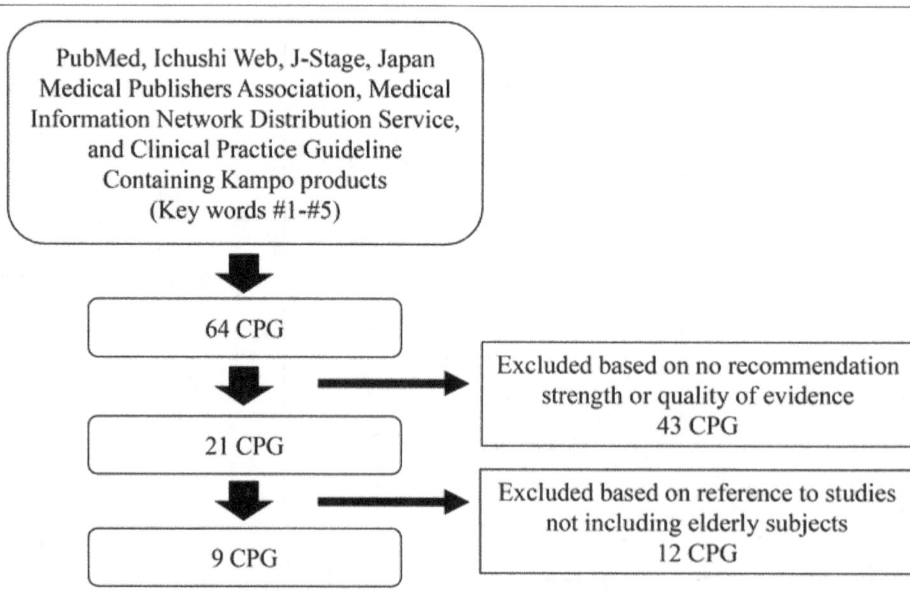

FIGURE 2 | Flowchart of the review process. CPG, clinical practice guideline.

TABLE 1 | Overview of CPGs included in the study.

Clinical practice guideline	Clinical question	Symptom	Kampo medicine	Evidence (number of RCT including elderly subjects)	Recommendation	Publication year	Reference
Clinical Practice Guideline for the Pruritus cutaneus universalis	Is kampo medicine effective for pruritus?	Skin pruritus, Senile pruritus	tokiinshi, orengedokuto, goshajinkigan, hachimijiogan, rokumigan	At least one RCT (5)	Permit	2012	(7)
Practical Guideline for the Management of Allergic Rhinitis in Japan	What are the indications for effective kampo medicine treatment in patients with allergic rhinitis?	Allergic Rhinitis	shoseiryuto	Double-blind RCT (1)	Recommend	2015	(8)
The Japanese Respiratory Society guidelines for management of cough	What is a non-specific therapeutic agent for dry cough?	Dry cough	bakumondoto	At least one RCT (1)	Recommend	2012	(9)
	What is a non-specific therapeutic agent for moist cough?	Moist cough	shoseiryuto	At least one RCT (1)	Recommend		
Evidence-based Clinical Practice Guidelines for GERD 2015 (2nd Edition)	Identification of drug with additional gastro-intestinal regulation effect of or kampo medicine combined with proton pump inhibitor.	GERD (addition to PPI, refractory to PPI)	rikkunshito	Low quality of evidence (1)	Low recommendation	2015	(10)
Evidence-based Clinical Practice Guidelines for Functional Dyspepsia	Is kampo medicine effective for Functional Dyspepsia?	Functional Dyspepsia	rikkunshito, (hangekobokuto)	High quality of evidence (2)	Low recommendation	2014	(11)
Evidence-based Clinical Practice Guidelines for Irritable Bowel Syndrome	Is kampo medicine effective for Irritable Bowel Syndrome?	Irritable Bowel Syndrome	keishikashakuyakuto	Low quality of evidence (1)	Low recommendation	2014	(12)
Evidence-based clinical practice guidelines for chronic constipation 2017	Is kampo medicine effective for chronic constipation?	Chronic constipation	daiokanzoto, daikenchuto	Low quality of evidence (2)	Low recommendation	2017	(13)
Clinical guidelines for overactive bladder syndrome		Overactive bladder	goshajinkigan	Small scale RCT (1)	Recommend	2015	(14)
Practice Guideline for Dementia 2017	Patient indications for effective non-medication or medication for agitation.	Agitation	yokukansan	Low (1)	Suggest	2017	(15)
	Patient indications for effective non-medication or medication for hallucinations and delusions.	Hallucinations, delusions	yokukansan	Low (0)	Suggest		
	How do you identify correspondence to dysphagia (including prevention for pneumonia)?	Correspondence to dysphagia (including prevention for pneumonia)	hangekobokuto	Very low (1)	Suggest		
	How do you respond in case of edema? (side effect)	Edema	yokukansan	Low (0)	Suggest		
	Is there treatment for behavioral and psychological symptoms of dementia, and for the sleep behavior disorder associated with Lewy body disease, and the rem period?	Behavioral and psychological symptoms of dementia and the sleep behavior disorder symptom of patients with Lewy body disease	yokukansan	Low (0)	Suggest		

group, with statistical significance. Mild side effects were detected in both groups with no significant group-wise difference.

Cough Symptoms

CPG for cough recommended use of kampo medicine for cough in the elderly with two referred RCTs focused on the elderly. Irifune et al. reported the efficacy of bakumondoto (Mai-Men-Dong-Tang) (18) for post-infectious prolonged cough in elderly patients (24). As compared to procaterol hydrochloride, bakumondoto with procaterol hydrochloride was more effective in treating post-infectious prolonged cough. Mukaida et al. reported the efficacy of bakumondoto for cough in elderly patients diagnosed with chronic obstructive pulmonary disease (25). Additional bakumondoto treatment was more effective than regular medication in suppressing the severity of cough.

Gastro-Intestinal Symptoms

CPG for Gastro Esophageal Reflux Disease (GERD), Functional Dyspepsia (FD), Irritable Bowel Syndrome (IBS), and chronic constipation gave weak recommendation for use of kampo medicine for these conditions with referred RCT. In a double-blind RCT including elderly patients, Tominaga et al. reported the efficacy of rikkunshito (Liu-Jun-Zi-Tang) (18) for patients with GERD who were refractory to treatment with proton-pump inhibitor (PPI) (26). Rikkunshito combined with PPI significantly decreased the frequency scale of the GERD symptoms' score, similar to the decrease seen on treatment with a double dose of PPI. Subgroup analysis showed that the patients of male sex or low body mass index showed more improvement compared with the other subgroups.

Harasawa et al. reported that the regular dose of rikkunshito significantly improved dysmotility-like dyspepsia than the low dose of rikkunshito in a double-blind RCT including elderly subjects (27). Arai et al. reported that there was a significant improvement in dyspeptic symptoms in patients treated with either rikkunshito or domperidone that is peripheral D2-like receptor antagonist, based on the Gastrointestinal Symptom Rating Scale score (28). The improvements of reflux and indigestion symptoms in patients treated with rikkunshito showed good correlations with the increased levels of acylated ghrelin.

Sasaki et al. reported the efficacy and safety of keishikasyakuyakuto (Gui-Zhi-Jia-Shao-Yao-Tang) (18) for functional abdominal pain of irritable bowel syndrome in a double-blind RCT including elderly subjects (29). Abdominal pain in irritable bowel syndrome with diarrhea significantly decreased after keishikasyakuyakuto administration, and the effect was superior to that of a placebo. Adverse effects of keishikasyakuyakuto were not significantly different from the placebo, suggesting the safety of keishikasyakuyakuto.

Miyoshi et al. reported the efficacy and safety of daiokanzoto (Da-Huang-Gan-Cao-Tang) (18) for constipation in a double-blind RCT including elderly subjects (30). Daiokanzoto was significantly effective for constipation compared to the placebo. There were no significant differences in safety between daiokanzoto and the placebo.

Horiuchi et al. reported the effect of daikenchuto (Da-Jian-Zhong-Tang) (18) in patients with chronic constipation in an RCT including elderly subjects (31). The addition of daikenchuto to sennoside resulted in significant improvement in bloating and abdominal pain and significant decrease in the gas volume score.

Urinary Symptoms

CPG for overactive bladder syndrome gave weak recommendation for use of kampo medicine with a referred RCT (32). In an RCT including elderly patients, Nishizawa et al. reported the efficacy of goshajinkigan for patients with over active bladder compared with propiverine hydrochloride. During the 1-year observation period, propiverine hydrochloride significantly improved the symptom of over active bladder in the first month, however, goshajinkigan significantly improved the symptom of over active bladder after 2 months. The incidence of adverse event related to treatment with goshajinkigan was lower than that with propiverine hydrochloride.

Dementia and Related Symptoms

CPG for dementia and related symptom gave weak recommendation for use of kampo medicine with two referred RCTs. Mizukami et al. reported the effectiveness and safety of yokukansan (Yi-Gan-San) (18) for the treatment of behavioral and psychological symptoms of dementia (BPSD) in patients with dementia associated with Alzheimer's disease or Lewy bodies (33). The mean total of the Neuropsychiatric Inventory score used to evaluate BPSD were significantly improved by the additional yokukansan administration. Subscale analysis showed significant improvements in delusions, hallucinations, agitation/aggression, depression, anxiety, and irritability/lability. There were no serious adverse reactions. Iwasaki et al. examined the effect of hangekobokuto (Ban-Xia-Hou-Pu-Tang) (18) on swallowing reflex among the elderly (34). Compared to the placebo, hangekobokuto significantly improved time from the water injection to the onset of swallowing. Furthermore, substance P in the saliva of patients administered with hangekobokuto significantly increased. Based on the result, Iwasaki et al. reported that treatment with hangekobokuto reduced the risk of pneumonia and pneumonia-related mortality in elderly patients with dementia in an RCT with 12-month patients' follow-up (35).

Adverse Effects

Adverse effects were not searched by the above steps. Additional hand searching for adverse effects showed that four CPG indicated the side effect of kampo medicine and introduce caution for using kampo medicine.

Guidelines for the management of hypertension 2014 (36) introduces the side effect of kampo medicine, western medicinal drugs, or health supplement that includes Glycyrrhiza. Glycyrrhiza includes glycyrrhizin which has potential to induce pseudo aldosteronism. If increase of blood pressure and/or hypokalemia are confirmed, withdrawing of suspicious products should be considered. In case it is difficult to stop use of the products, aldosterone antagonist can be prescribed.

Clinical Practice Guideline for the Management of Upper Tract Urothelial Carcinoma (37) introduces the side effect of crude drugs including aristolochic acid. Some studies indicated that aristolochic acid was associated with nephropathy, uropathy, or urothelial cancer. In Japan, crude drugs approved by the Ministry of Health, Labor and Welfare do not include aristolochic acid, but patients can use imported drugs.

Consensus statement for the diagnosis and treatment of drug-induced lung injuries (38) introduced the side effect of kampo medicine, especially shosaikoto (Xiao-Chai-Hu-Tang) (18), which can induce interstitial pneumonia in rare cases. The prevalence of shosaikoto-induced interstitial pneumonia is reported as under 0.1%, however, national survey reported the mortality rate of 10 in 100 cases of interstitial pneumonia induced by shosaikoto. If drug-induced interstitial pneumonia is expected, use of the suspected drug should be discontinued.

The guideline Japanese Society of Laboratory Medicine 2015 (39) introduced drug-induced edema, hypertension, and liver dysfunction. Comments for edema and hypertension induced by Glycyrrhiza were similar with prior comments in Guidelines for the management of hypertension 2014. Kampo medicine is one of the drugs that induce liver injury or hepatitis, therefore side effect correspondence is considered important.

DISCUSSION

Interpretation of Results

Nine CPG gave some recommendations for total 13 kampo medicines in treatment of the symptom in the elderly. Each kampo medicine includes multiple crude drugs which have several pharmacological functions; thus, kampo medicine affects multiple organs and coordinates the interrelation between the brain, endocrine system, immune system, and skeletal muscle in elderly patients.

Characteristics of Kampo Medicine Introduced in CPGs

Table 2 show the over view of 13 kampo medicines introduced in CPG, its indications and components referred from STORK (40), and its characteristics in kampo theory. Kampo medicine have multiple effect on organs result in improving symptom.

Orengedokuto, tokiinshi, goshajinkigan, hachimijiogan, and rokumigan were recommended in patients with skin symptom. In the kampo concept, orengedokuto is used to improve inflammation in skin and other organs and improve irritation. Therefore, it should be used in patients with reddish skin and worsening itchy symptom with irritation. Goshajinkigan, hachimijiogan, and rokumigan were categorized in similar kampo medicine. They have been used for dry skin, urinary disorder, and sarcopenia. These kampo medicine include crude drugs to moisturize the skin, strengthen the muscles, promote microcirculation, and control urination. Additional effects include the following: for tokiinshi, suppressing itchiness, for goshajinkigan, warming the body and improving edema and lumber pain, for hachimijiogan, controlling cold and hot feeling and improving edema, and for rokumigan, controlling hot feeling and improving edema. These kampo medicines can be selected depending on not only the skin condition but also cold/hot sensation and water balance. Kishida et al. reported that goshajinkigan suppressed sarcopenia via the IGF-1/insulin pathway, maintained the expression of mitochondrial-related transcription factors, and suppressed TNF-α in SAMP8 mice, indicating that goshajinkigan is a promising candidate for relief from sarcopenia (41). CPG and results from the study suggested that goshajinkigan can be applied for skin symptom with additional expected effect on sarcopenia.

Shoseiryuto was selected for use in patients with allergic rhinitis and cough. Bakumondoto was selected for use in patients with cough. These kampo medicines have opposite effects on water imbalance in the upper respiratory tract. Shoseiryuto can improve the occurrence of excess water in thin secretion, thus it is applied in cases with allergic rhinitis and cough with thin secretion. Shoseiryuto decreased the number of T-helper (Th) 2 cells and the level of interleukin-4. The Th1 cells were not altered (42). Since shoseiryuto does not affect the histamine H1 receptors, there are fewer side-effects such as sedation and drowsiness. On the other hand, bakumondoto can moisturize and improve the dryness and sensitivity of the upper respiratory tract epithelium. Thus, it is applied in case of dry cough without secretion after respiratory infection. Ophiopogonis Radix, another herb in bakumondoto, has anti-inflammatory activity; and its active components include ruscogenin and ophiopogonin D.

Rikkunshito was recommended for patients with PPI-refractory GEARD and FD. It supplies vital energy to the digestive organs and promotes peristalsis from the stomach to the intestine. Thus, this kampo medicine is more suitable for patients with fatigue, anorexia, and gastric hypomotility resulting in weight loss. A recent study reported that rikkunshito increased plasma ghrelin levels in humans and mice (43) and restored the decreased plasma ghrelin levels induced by serotonin release in rats.

Keishikashakuyakuto was recommended for irritable bowel syndrome. It can be applied for both diarrhea, constipation, and mix-type IBS. It can control contraction and expansion of the intestine, resulting in pain relief and control of the stool condition.

Daiokanzoto and daikenchuto were recommended for constipation. Daiokanzoto is applied for constipation in patients whose vital energy is sufficient; whereas, daikenchuto is applied for constipation in patients with low vital energy, and characteristics of low body weight and abdominal distention, because it includes the crude drug, ginseng, which can supply energy to the digestive function. Daikenchuto treats abdominal symptoms via enhancing the secretions of motilin (44), substance P (45), calcitonin gene-related peptide, and adrenomedullin (46, 47), and activating the transient receptor potential of the vanilloid receptor complex (48).

Yokukansan was recommended for patients with BPSD. It has been used for irritation and sleep disorder of children since ancient times. Recently, it has been applied for the symptom in

TABLE 2 | Over view of 13 kampo medicines introduced in CPG, its indications and components referred from STORK (40), and its characteristics in kampo theory.

		Kampo medicine												
		orengedok uto	**goshajinki gan**	**tokiinshi**	**hachimiji ogan**	**rokumigan**	**shoseiryuto**	**bakumond oto**	**rikkunsh ito**	**keishikashaku yakuto**	**daiokanz oto**	**daikench uto**	**yokukan san**	**hangekobo kuto**
Clinical manifestation of frailty according to the traditional concept	Anorexia							O	O			O	O	
	Sarcopenia		O		O	O								
	Cognition		O		O	O								
	Dementia	O											O	
	Fatigue								O					O
	Weakness		O		O	O			O					
	Pain		O		O					O		O		
	Dysfunction of Respiration						O	O						O
	Circulation		O	O	O	O								
	Gastro-intestine							O	O	O	O	O		O
	Urinary		O		O	O								
	Musculoskeletal		O		O	O								
	Skin	O	O	O	O	O								
Indications		The relief of the following symptoms of those patients who have ruddy face with comparatively strong constitution, a touch of hot flushes, and a tendency to irritability: nose bleeding, hypertension, insomnia, neurosis, gastritis, alcoholic hangover, climacteric disturbance and automatic imbalance syndrome peculiar to women resembling climacteric disturbance, dizziness, palpitation, eczema or dermatitis and pruritus cutaneous	The relief of the following symptoms of those patients with decreased urine volume or polyuria sometimes having dry mouth who are easily fatigued and easily feel cold in the extremities: Leg pain, low back pain, numbness, blurred vision in old patients, pruritus, dysuria, frequent urination and edema	The relief of the following symptoms of those patients with oversensitivity to cold: Chronic eczema (with little exudation) and itching	The relief of the following symptoms of those patients with severe fatigue or malaise, decreased urinary output or increased urinary frequency, dry mouth, and alternate cold and hot feeling in the extremities: Nephritis, diabetes mellitus, impotence, sciatica, low back pain, beriberi, cystorrhea, prostatic hypertrophy and hypertension	The relief of the following symptoms of those patients with decreased urine volume or polyuria sometimes having dry mouth who are easily fatigued: Dysuria, frequent urination, edema and pruritus	Watery sputum, watery nasal discharge, nasal obstruction, sneezing, stridor, coughing, lacrimation in the following diseases: Bronchitis, bronchial asthma, rhinitis, allergic rhinitis, allergic conjunctivitis, and common cold	The relief of the following symptoms: Coughing with a hard, obstructive sputum, bronchitis, and bronchial asthma	The relief of the following symptoms of those patients with weak stomach, loss of appetite and full stomach pit, and those who are easily fatigued, anemic and likely to have cold limbs: Gastritis, gastric atony, gastroptosis, maldigestion, anorexia, gastric pain, vomiting	The relief of the following symptoms of those patients with abdominal distension: Tenesmus alvi and abdominal pain	Constipation	The relief of abdominal cold feeling and pain accompanied by abdominal flatulence	The relief of the following symptoms of those patients with delicate constitution and nervousness: Neurosis, insomnia, night cry in children, and peevishness in children	The relief of the following symptoms of those patients who have depressed feelings and a feeling of foreign body in the throat and oesophagus and who sometimes have palpitation, dizziness, nausea, etc.: Anxiety neurosis, nervous gastritis, hyperemesis gravidarum, coughing, hoarseness, nervous oesophageal stricture, and insomnia

(Continued)

TABLE 2 | Continued

	Kampo medicine												
	orengedokuto	**goshajinkigan**	**tokiinshi**	**hachimijiogan**	**rokumigan**	**shoseiryuto**	**bakumondoto**	**rikkunshito**	**keishikashakuyakuto**	**daiokanzoto**	**daikenchuto**	**yokukansan**	**hangekobokuto**
Components of kampo medicine	JP Scutellaria Root	JP Rehmannia Root	JP Japanese Angelica Root	JP Rehmannia Root	JP Rehmannia Root	JP Pinellia Tuber	JP Ophiopogon Tuber	JP Atractylodes Lancea Rhizome	JP Peony Root	JP Rhubarb	JP Processed Ginger	JP Atractylodes Lancea Rhizome	JP Pinellia Tuber
	JP Coptis Rhizome	JP Achyranthes Root	JP Rehmannia Root	JP Cornus Fruit	JP Cornus Fruit	JP Processed Ginger	JP Brown Rice	JP Ginseng	JP Cinnamon Bark	JP Glycyrrhiza	JP Ginseng	JP Poria Sclerotium	JP Poria Sclerotium
	JP Gardenia Fruit	JP Cornus Fruit	JP Tribulus Fruit	JP Dioscorea Rhizome	JP Dioscorea Rhizome	JP Glycyrrhiza	JP Pinellia Tuber	JP Pinellia Tuber	JP Jujube		JP Zanthoxylum Fruit	JP Cnidium Rhizome	JP Magnolia Bark
	JP Phellodendron Bark	JP Dioscorea Rhizome	JP Peony Root	JP Alisma Rhizome	JP Alisma Rhizome	JP Cinnamon Bark	JP Jujube	JP Poria Sclerotium	JP Glycyrrhiz		JP Koi	JP Uncaria Hook	JP Perilla Herb
		JP Plantago Seed	JP Cnidium Rhizome	JP Poria Sclerotium	JP Poria Sclerotium	JP Schisandra Fruit	JP Glycyrrhiza	JP Jujube	JP Ginger			JP Japanese Angelica Root	JP Ginger
		JP Alisma Tuber	JP Saposhnikovia Root and Rhizome	P Moutan Bark	JP Moutan Bark	JP Asiasarum Root	JP Ginseng	JP Citrus Unshiu Peel				JP Bupleurum Root	
		JP Poria Sclerotium	JP Polygonum Root	JP Cinnamon Bark		JP Peony Root		JP Glycyrrhiza				JP Glycyrrhiza	
		JP Moutan Bark	JP Astragalus Root	JP Powdered Processed Aconite Root		JP Ephedra Herb		JP Ginger					
		JP Cinnamon Bark	JP Schizonepeta Spike										
		JP Powdered Processed Aconite Root	JP Glycyrrhiza										

JP, The Japanese Pharmacopoeia.

elderly patients. With regard to the characteristics of yokukansan, it does not induce extrapyramidal symptoms, however, it controls the concentration of serotonin in the synaptic cleft via partial agonist action on the serotonin 1A receptor (49), downregulates expression of the serotonin 2A receptor (50), inhibits the release of glutamate resulting in a decreased concentration of glutamate at synaptic clefts in the brain, and promotes glutamate uptake by astrocytes (51–53).

Hangekobokuto was recommended for use in patients with dysphagia. It has been used for pharyngeal discomfort since ancient times. It can soothe sensation in the pharynx and improve swallowing and cough reflex. It is reported that hangekobokuto modulates cerebral levels of 5-hydroxytryptamine, noradrenaline, and dopamine in mice (54).

There are some advantages in kampo treatment. As a super-aging society, the increased cost of medical insurance is a serious problem in Japan. The medical cost of kampo medicine is relatively lower than that of western medicine. This treatment can improve the target symptoms and contribute to holistic control of whole-body conditions, as mentioned above. Furthermore, kampo medicine has been applied for disease prevention and maintenance of quality of life since ancient times. Kampo medicine may contribute to health in elderly individuals. Based on these aspects, both CPG and research regarding kampo medicine for geriatric patients should be continued. The clinical application of kampo medicine has been performed depending on the patients' clinical history and physical sign. In this review, we demonstrated the present status of CPG involving kampo medicine for geriatrics. Clinical and basic research studies are currently on going. In future, more information on evidence-based detailed application will become available.

Limitation

A limitation of this review is that the target subjects of the RCT referenced in the CPG do not necessarily correspond to elderly patients. The articles cited in ref. (16–19, 22, 23) were limited in their study of elderly subjects. However, the articles cited in ref. (20, 21, 25–33) included elderly subjects as a portion of the study population. The number of RCTs with only elderly subjects was very small; thus, we included studies with elderly subjects as a portion of the study population. Despite this limitation, this review demonstrated the use of Japanese CPG and kampo medicine in the treatment of symptoms in elderly patients.

CONCLUSION

Japanese CPG gave some recommendation for use of kampo medicine for symptoms in the elderly. In the CPG, evidence related to kampo medicine for several symptoms is provided, and each kampo medicine includes multiple crude drugs that have multiple pharmacological functions. Thus, the treatment can be considered as holistic medicine which can lead to support of elderly patients with frailty.

AUTHOR CONTRIBUTIONS

ST designed the study, confirmed the CPG and articles, and wrote the manuscript. SK proof read the CPG and the manuscript. AK, MO, RA, and TI gave advice for the study design and manuscript.

ACKNOWLEDGMENTS

This study was supported by our university's administration fund.

REFERENCES

Fried LP, Tangen CM, Walston J, Newman AB, Hirsch C, Gottdiener J, et al. Frailty in older adults: evidence for a phenotype. *J Gerontol A Biol Sci Med Sci.* (2001) 56:M146–56.

Walston J, Hadley EC, Ferrucci L, Guralnik JM, Newman AB, Studenski SA, et al. Research agenda for frailty in older adults: toward a better understanding of physiology and etiology: summary from the American Geriatrics Society/ National Institute on Aging Research Conference on Frailty in Older Adults. *J Am Geriatr Soc.* (2006) 54:991–1001. doi: 10.1111/j.1532-5415.2006.00745.x

Eeles EM, White SV, O'Mahony SM, Bayer AJ, Hubbard RE. The impact of frailty and delirium on mortality in older inpatients. *Age Ageing* (2012) 41:412–6. doi: 10.1093/ageing/afs021

Clegg A, Young J, Iliffe S, Rikkert MO, Rockwood K. Frailty in older people. *Lancet* (2013) 381:752–62. doi: 10.1016/S0140-6736(12)62167-9

Hazzard WR, Blass JP, Halter JB, Ouslander JG, Tinetti ME. (eds). *Principles of Geriatric Medicine and Gerontology.* 5th ed. New York, NY: McGraw-Hill (2003). p. 1487–502.

Arai H, Ouchi Y, Toba K, Endo T, Shimokado K, Tsubota K, et al. Japan as the front-runner of super-aged societies: perspectives from medicine and medical care in Japan. *Geriatr Gerontol Int.* (2015) 15:673–87. doi: 10.1111/ggi.12450

Satoh H. Pharmacological characteristics of Kampo medicine as a mixture of constituents and ingredients. *J Integr Med.* (2013) 11:11–6. doi: 10.3736/jintegrmed2013003

Satoh T, Yokozeki H, Katayama I, Murota H, Tokura Y, Boku N, et al. Clinical Practice Guideline for the Pruritus cutaneus universalis [in Japanese]. *Jpn J Dermatol.* (2012) 122:267–80.

Okubo K, Kurono Y, Ichimura K, Enomoto T, Okamoto Y, Kawauchi H, et al. *Practical Guideline for the Management of Allergic Rhinitis in Japan.* Life Science Press [in Japanese] (2015).

Kohno S, Okada K, Kadota J, Shioya T, Tanaka H, Tokuyama K, et al. *The Japanese Respiratory Society Guidelines for Management of Cough.* Medical Revew Co., Ltd. [in Japanese] (2012).

Kinoshita Y, Iwakiri K, Ashida K, Iwakiri R, Oshima T, Ohara S, et al. *Evidence-Based Clinical Practice Guidelines for GERD 2015.* 2nd ed. Nankodo Press [in Japanese] (2015).

Miwa H, Kusano M, Arisawa T, Oshima T, Kato T, Joh T, et al. *Evidence- based Clinical Practice Guidelines for Functional Dyspepsia.* Nankodo Press [in Japanese] (2014).

Fukudo S, Kaneko H, Akiho H, Inamori M, Endo Y, Okumura T, et al. *Evidence-based Clinical Practice Guidelines for Irritable Bowel Syndrome.* Nankodo Press [in Japanese] (2014).

Miwa H, Torii A, Maeda K, Akiho H, Araki Y, Iijima H, et al. *Evidence-based Clinical Practice Guidelines for Chronic Constipation 2017.* Nankodo Press [in Japanese] (2017).

Takeda M, Yokoyama O, Goto M, Homma Y, Asakura H, Yamanishi T, et al. *Clinical Guidelines for Overactive Bladder Syndrome.* 2nd ed. RichHill Medical Inc. [in Japanese] (2015).

Nakashima K, Tomimoto H, Aiba I, Akishita M, Kurita S, Iijima S, et al. *Practice Guideline for Dementia 2017.* Igaku-Shoin Ltd. [in Japanese] (2017).

Ohkawara A, Furuya K, Kurisu Y, Asada Y, Higashida T, Takeda K, et al. Experience with Orengedokuto (TJ-15) and Goshajinkigan (TJ-107) for the treatment of senile pruritus [in Japanese]. *Nishinihon Hifuka* (1991) 53:1234–41.

Appendix - Composition and Indications of 148 Ethical Prescriptions. KAIM (The Journal of Kampo, Acupuncture, and Integrative Medicine) Special Edition - Current Kampo Medicine | November 2006, http://www.kaim.us/special_TOC.html)

Toshihiro I, Chiak N, Hiroyuki S. The effects of Toki-Inshi and a bath preparation containing licorice extract on patients with Senile Pruritus [in Japanese]. *Kampo Med.* (1996) 47:35–41.

Ishioka T, Aoi R. Comparative evaluation of hachimijiogan and ketotifen fumarate on senile pruritus [in Japanese]. *Shinyaku Rinsho* (1992) 41:2603–8.

Ishioka T. Comparative evaluation of Rokumigan and Hachimi- jiohgan on senile pruritus [in Japanese]. *Ther Res.* (1995) 16:1497–504.

Ohkuma M. Treatment of pruritus by Chinese drugs [in Japanese]. *J Med Pharm Soc WAKAN YAKU* (1993)10:126–30.

Baba S, Takasaka T, Inamura N, Sato M, Suzuki S, Endo S, et al. Double-blind clinical trial of Sho-seiryu-to (TJ-19) for perennial nasal allergy [in Japanese]. *Pract Otol.* (1995) 88:389–405.

Irifune K, Hamada H, Ito R, Katayama H, Watanabe A, Kato A, et al. Antitussive effect of bakumondoto a fixed kampo medicine (six herbal components) for treatment of post-infectious prolonged cough: controlled clinical pilot study with 19 patients. *Phytomedicine* (2011) 18:630–3. doi: 10.1016/j.phymed.2011.02.017

Mukaida K, Hattori N, Kondo K, Morita N, Murakami I, Haruta Y, et al. A pilot study of the multiherb Kampo medicine bakumondoto for cough in patients with chronic obstructive pulmonary disease. *Phytomedicine* (2011) 18:625–9. doi: 10.1016/j.phymed.2010.11.006

Tominaga K, Iwakiri R, Fujimoto K, Fujiwara Y, Tanaka M, Shimoyama, et al. Rikkunshito improves symptoms in PPI-refractory GERD patients: a prospective, randomized, multicenter trial in Japan. *J Gastroenterol.* (2012) 47:284–92. doi: 10.1007/s00535-011-0488-5

Harasawa S, Miyoshi A, Miwa T, Masamune O, Matsuo Y, Mori H, et al. Double-blind multicenter post-marketing clinical trial of TJ-43 TSUMURA Rikkunshi-to for the treatment of dysmotility-like dyspepsia [in Japanese]. *Igaku Ayumi* (1998) 187:207–29.

Arai M, Matsumura T, Tsuchiya N, Sadakane C, Inami R, Suzuki T, et al. Rikkunshito improves the symptoms in patients with functional dyspepsia, accompanied by an increase in the level of plasma ghrelin. *Hepatogastroenterology* (2012) 59:62-6. doi: 10.5754/hge11246

Sasaki D, Uehara A, Hiwatashi N, Sekiguchi T, Nakahara A, Nakai Y, et al. Clinical efficacy of keishikashakuyakuto in patients with irritable bowel syndrome: a multicenter collaborative randomized controlled study [in Japanese]. *Rinsho Kenkyu* (1998)75:1136–52.

Miyoshi A, Masamune O, Fukutomi H, Mori H, Miwa T, Kojima K, et al. The clinical effects of TSUMURA Dai-Kanzo-To extract granules for ethical use (TJ-84) on constipation using double blind test [in Japanese]. *Gastroenterology* (1994) 18:299–312.

Horiuchi A, Nakayama Y, Tanaka N. Effect of traditional Japanese medicine, daikenchuto (TJ-100) in patients with chronic constipation. *Gastroenterol Res.* (2010) 3:151–5. doi: 10.4021/gr219w

Nishizawa Y, Nishizawa Y, Yoshioka F, Amakata Y, Nosaka S, Fushiki S, et al. Efficacy and safety of Chinese traditional medicine, Niu-Che-Shwn-Qi-Wan (Japanese name: goshajinki-gan) versus propiverine hydrochloride on health-related quality of life in patients with overactive bladder in prospective randomized comparative study [in Japanese]. *Kampo New Ther.* (2007) 16:131–42.

Mizukami K, Asada T, Kinoshita T, Tanaka K, Sonohara K, Nakai R, et al. Randomized cross-over study of a traditional Japanese medicine (kampo), yokukansan, in the treatment of the behavioural and psychological symptoms of dementia. *Int J Neuropsychopharmacol.* (2009) 12:191–9. doi: 10.1017/S146114570800970X

Iwasaki K, Cyong JC, Kitada S, Niu K, Ohrui T, Okitsu R, et al. A traditional Chinese herbal medicine, banxia houpo tang, improves cough reflex of patients with aspiration pneumonia. *J Am Geriatr Soc.* (2002) 50:1751–2.

Iwasaki K, Kato S, Monma Y, Niu K, Ohrui T, Okitsu R, et al. A pilot study of banxia houpu tang, a traditional Chinese medicine, for reducing pneumonia risk in older adults with dementia. *J Am Geriatr Soc.* (2007) 55:2035–40. doi: 10.1111/j.1532-5415.2007.0 1448.x

Shimamoto K, Ando K, Ishimitsu T, Ito S, Ito M, Ito H, et al. *Guidelines for the Management of Hypertension 2014.* Life Science Publishing Co. Ltd. [in Japanese] (2014).

Oya M, Ichikawa T, Nishiyama H, Jinzaki M, Kamai T, Kawauchi A, et al. *Clinical Practice Guideline for the Management of Upper Tract Urothelial Carcinoma.* Medical Review Co., Ltd. [in Japanese] (2014).

Azuma A, Kanazawa M, Kameda H, Kusumoto M, Kubo K, Tsuruma A, et al. *Consensus Statement for the Diagnosis and Treatment of Drug-Induced Lung Injuries* Medical Review Co. Ltd., [in Japanese] (2012).

Iinuma Y, Izuhara K, Koshiba T, Tanaka M, Higashida S, Toyama K, et al. *Japanese Society of Laboratory Medicine Guideline 2015.* Uchudo Yagi Bookstore Co. Ltd., [in Japanese] (2015).

Department of Pharmacognosy, Phytochemistry and Narcotics (DPPN), National Institute of Health Sciences (NIHS) of Japan and National Institutes of Biomedical Innovation, Health and Nutrition (NIBIOHN). Standards of Reporting Kampo Products (STORK). http://mpdb.nibiohn.go.jp/stork/.

Kishida Y, Kagawa S, Arimitsu J, Nakanishi M, Sakashita N, Otsuka S, et al. Go-sha-jinki-Gan (GJG), a traditional Japanese herbal medicine, protects against sarcopenia in senescence-accelerated mice. *Phytomedicine* (2015) 22:16–22. doi: 10.1016/j.phymed.2014. 11.005

Ko E, Rho S, Cho C, Choi H, Ko S, Lee Y, et al. So-Cheong-Ryong-Tang, tradititional Korean medicine, suppresses Th2 lineage development. *Biol Pharm Bull* (2004) 27:739–43. doi: 10.1248/bpb.27.739

Matsumura T, Arai M, Yonemitsu Y, Maruoka D, Tanaka T, Suzuki T, et al. The traditional Japanese medicine Rikkunshito increases the plasma level of ghrelin in humans and mice. *J Gastroenterol.* (2010) 45:300–7. doi: 10.1007/s00535-009-0166-z

Nagano T, Itoh H, Takeyama M. Effect of Dai-kenchu-to on levels of 3 brain- gut peptides (motilin, gastrin and somatostatin) in human plasma. *Biol Pharm Bull.* (1999) 22:1131–3.

Kono T, Koseki T, Chiba S, Ebisawa Y, Chisato N, Iwamoto J, et al. Colonic vascular conductance increased by Daikenchuto via calcitonin gene-related peptide and receptoractivity modifying protein 1. *J Surg Res.* (2008) 150:78–84. doi: 10.1016/j.jss.2008.02.057

Kono T, Kaneko A, Hira Y, Suzuki T, Chisato N, Ohtake N, et al. Anticolitis and -adhesion effects of Daikenchuto via endogenous adrenomedullin enhancement in Crohn's disease mouse model. *J Crohns Colitis* (2010) 4:161– 70. doi: 10.1016/j.crohns.2009.09.006

Kono T, Omiya Y, Hira Y, Kaneko A, Chiba S, Suzuki T, et al. Daikenchuto (TU-100) ameliorates colon microvascular dysfunction via endogenous adrenomedullin in Crohn's disease rat model. *J Gastroenterol.* (2011) 46:1187– 96. doi: 10.1007/s00535-011-0438-2

Kikuchi D, Shibata C, Imoto H, Naitoh T, Miura K, Unno M. Intragastric Dai-Kenchu-To, a Japanese herbal medicine, stimulates colonic motility via transient receptor potential cation channel subfamily V member 1 in dogs. *Tohoku J Exp Med.* (2013) 230:197–204. doi: 10.1620/tjem. 230.197

Terawaki K, Ikarashi Y, Sekiguchi K, Nakai Y, Kase Y. Partial agonistic effect of yokukansan on human recombinant serotonin 1A receptors expressed in the membranes of Chinese hamster ovary cells. *J Ethnopharmacol.* (2010) 127:306–12. doi: 10.1016/j.jep.2009.11.003

Egashira N, Iwasaki K, Ishibashi A, Hayakawa K, Okuno R, Abe M, et al. Repeated administration of Yokukansan inhibits DOI-induced head-twitch response and decreases expression of 5-hydroxytryptamine (5-HT) 2A receptors in the prefrontal cortex. Prog. Neuropsychopharmacol. *Biol Psychiatry* (2008) 32:1516–20. doi: 10.1016/j.pnpbp.2008. 05.010

Takeda A, Itoh H, Tamano H, Yuzurihara M, Oku N. Suppressive effect of Yokukansan on excessive release of glutamate and aspartate in the hippocampus of zinc-deficient rats. *Nutr Neurosci.* (2008) 11:41–6. doi: 10.1179/147683008X301414

Takeda A, Tamano H, Itoh H, Oku N. Attenuation of abnormal glutamate release in zinc deficiency by zinc and Yokukansan. *Neurochem Int.* (2008) 53:230–5. doi: 10.1016/j.neuint.2008. 07.009

Kawakami Z, Ikarashi Y, Kase Y. Glycyrrhizin and its metabolite 18 beta-glycyrrhetinic acid in glycyrrhiza, a constituent herb of yokukansan, ameliorate thiamine deficiency-induced dysfunction of glutamate transport in cultured rat cortical astrocytes. *Eur J Pharmacol.* (2010) 626:154–8. doi: 10.1016/j.ejphar.2009.09.046

Kaneko A, Cho S, Hirai K, Okabe T, Iwasaki K, Nanba Y, et al. Hange-koboku-to, a Kampo medicine, modulates cerebral levels of 5-HT (5-hydroxytryptamine), NA (noradrenaline) and DA (dopamine) in mice. *Phytother Res.* (2005) 19:491–5. doi: 10.1002/ptr. 1669

9

Semen Cassiae Extract Improves Glucose Metabolism by Promoting GIUT4 Translocation in the Skeletal Muscle of Diabetic Rats

Meiling Zhang[1,2†], Xin Li[3†], Hangfei Liang[3], Huqiang Cai[3], Xueling Hu[3], Yu Bian[3], Lei Dong[3], Lili Ding[3], Libo Wang[4], Bo Yu[1,2], Yan Zhang[3] and Yao Zhang[1,2*]*

[1] *Key Laboratory of Myocardial Ischemia Mechanism and Treatment, Ministry of Education, Harbin Medical University, Harbin, China,* [2] *Department of Cardiology, The Second Affiliated Hospital of Harbin Medical University, Harbin, China,* [3] *State Province Key Laboratories of Biomedicine – Pharmaceutics of China, Key Laboratory of Cardiovascular Medicine Research, Ministry of Education, Department of Pharmacology, College of Pharmacy, Harbin Medical University, Harbin, China,* [4] *Department of Medicinal Chemistry and Natural Medicine Chemistry, College of Pharmacy, Harbin Medical University, Harbin, China*

***Correspondence:**
Yao Zhang
yaozhang_grace@163.com
Yan Zhang
zhangyan@ems.hrbmu.edu.cn

† *These authors have contributed equally to this work.*

Diabetes mellitus is a clinical syndrome characterised by hyperglycaemia; its complications lead to disability and even death. Semen Cassiae is a traditional Chinese medicine, which has anti-hypertensive, anti-hyperlipidaemia, anti-oxidation, and anti-ageing properties. Our study was designed to evaluate the action of total anthraquinones of Semen Cassiae extract (SCE) on the improvement of glucose metabolism in diabetic rats and to elucidate the underlying mechanism. First, we evaluated the effect of SCE on normal rats. Next, we observed the effect of SCE using a rat model of diabetes, which was established by feeding rats with high-energy diet for 4 weeks and a single intraperitoneal injection of streptozotocin (STZ; 30 mg/kg) 3 weeks after starting the high-energy diet. Rats in different SCE groups (administered 54, 108, and 324 mg/kg/day of SCE) and metformin group (162 mg/kg/day, positive control drug) were treated with the corresponding drugs 1 week before starting high-energy diet and treatment continued for 5 weeks; meanwhile, rats in the control group were administered the same volume of sodium carboxymethyl cellulose solution (vehicle solution). One week after STZ injection, fasting blood glucose (FBG), oral glucose tolerance (OGT), fasting serum insulin (FSI) and serum lipids were quantified. Finally, the expression of proteins in the phosphatidylinositol-3-kinase (PI3K)–Akt–AS160–glucose transporter isoform 4 (GLUT4) signalling pathway was detected by western blotting. The data indicated that the levels of FBG and serum lipids were significantly lowered, and OGT and FSI were markedly increased in diabetic rats treated with SCE (108 mg/kg/day); however, SCE did not cause hypoglycaemia in normal rats. The molecular mechanisms were explored in the skeletal muscle. SCE markedly restored the decreased translocation of GLUT4 in diabetic rats. Moreover, the protein expressions of phosphorylated-AS160 (Thr642), phosphorylated-Akt (Ser473) and PI3K were significantly increased after SCE treatment in the skeletal muscle. These results indicate that SCE exerts an anti-hyperglycaemic effect by promoting GLUT4 translocation through the activation of the PI3K–Akt–AS160 signalling pathway. Our findings suggest that treatment with SCE, containing anthraquinones, could be an effective approach to enhance diabetes therapy.

Keywords: diabetes, Semen Cassiae, anthraquinones, anti-hyperglycaemia, PI3K–Akt–AS160–GLUT4 pathway

INTRODUCTION

Diabetes mellitus has become a global public health problem. In 2015, the total number of adults worldwide suffering from DM was 415 million and every 6 s a person died from DM (5 million deaths); this includes 109.6 million people in the People's Republic of China (ranking first in the number of diabetes patients). By 2040, 642 million adults will have diabetes and the number in China will be 150 million (International Diabetes Federation, 2015). A persistently high level of BG can lead to serious complications, including damage to the hearts, blood vessels, kidneys, eyes, and nerves. DM and its complications impose an enormous burden on medical costs. This is an urgent problem for medical scientists all over the world, including China. In recent years, many clinical trials have confirmed that the positive interventions during the early period of DM to improve glucose tolerance and FBG could effectively postpone and reduce the development from prediabetes into type 2 DM (Knowler et al., 2002; DeFronzo and Abdul-Ghani, 2011; Perreault et al., 2012).

Traditional Chinese medicine is a treasure of China and an important part of traditional medicine in the world. It has a history of more than 5,000 years. DM was first recorded in *Huang Di Nei Jing*, the earliest traditional Chinese medicine records during the Warring States period to the Western Han Dynasty at more than 2,000 years ago; it was recorded as the symptom of polyuria, polydipsia, polyphagia, and weight loss and defined as "Xiao Ke Zheng" for the first time in China (Zhang, 2007; Sun, 2011). Herbs used in traditional Chinese medicine and their extracts have been reported to effectively prevent and treat DM (Liu et al., 2013, 2016; Lan and Zhu, 2015; Zhang Y. et al., 2016). Their anti-diabetic effects are multi-dimensional (Xiong et al., 1997; Li and Liu, 2010; Li et al., 2012). The combination of traditional Chinese medicine and western medicine in treating DM began in 1990s (Vray and Attali, 1995) and has become significantly popular in China (Huyen et al., 2012; Lian et al., 2015; Hu and Meng, 2017).

Semen Cassiae, called Jue Ming Zi in China, is the seed of *Cassia obtusifolia* L. or *Cassia tora* L. of the Leguminosae family initially recorded in *Shennong Bencao Jing* (Huang, 1982; Chinese Pharmocopoeia Committee, 2009). It is locally used as a variety of roasted tea. Semen Cassiae is currently used for its anti-pyretic, eyesight-improving, bowel-relaxing, anti-hypertensive, and anti-hyperlipidaemic effects (Li et al., 2003; Cheng et al., 2005; Zhang et al., 2006; Wang, 2010). It has been reported that Semen Cassiae contains anthraquinones, as the main active components, naphtopyrones, glycosides, amino acids, trace elements, polysaccharides, and other ingredients (Chunjuan et al., 2015). Fu et al. (2014) and Kim et al. (2014) found that the anthraquinones of Semen Cassiae could improve diabetic nephropathy and myocardial ischaemia and reperfusion injury in rats with DM induced by high-fat diet combined with STZ. Nevertheless, the preventive effect and underlying mechanism of SCE on DM have not yet been investigated.

The current study aimed to evaluate whether the alcohol extract (total anthraquinones) from Semen Cassiae has an anti-hyperglycaemic effect in rats with DM and to explore the possible underlying mechanisms.

Abbreviations: AUC, area under curve; BG, blood glucose; DM, diabetes mellitus; FBG, fasting blood glucose; FSI, fasting serum insulin; GSV, GLUT4 storage vesicle; HDL-C, high-density lipoprotein cholesterol; LDL-C, low-density lipoprotein cholesterol; mTOR, mammalian target of rapamycin; OGT, oral glucose tolerance; SCE, Semen Cassiae extract; SCE-L, low-dose Semen Cassiae extract; SCE-H, high-dose Semen Cassiae extract; SCE-M, middle-dose Semen Cassiae extract; STZ, streptozotocin; TC, total cholesterol; TGs, triglycerides.

MATERIALS AND METHODS

Plant Material

For extract preparation, parched Semen Cassiae was purchased from Beijing Tongrentang (Tongrentang, Beijing, China) and authenticated by a pharmacognosy expert, Prof. Guoyu Li at Harbin University of Commerce. The plant materials of Semen Cassiae we used in this study were the seed of *C. obtusifolia* L. of the Leguminosae family. A voucher specimen (article number: 20160119) was deposited at the College of Pharmacy, Harbin Medical University, China.

Extraction of Total Anthraquinones From Semen Cassiae

Dry Semen Cassiae (2 kg) was soaked in 50% ethanol (Lin, 2001; Liu W.M. et al., 2009; Lu and Yuan, 2010) for 12 h at a 1:7 ratio. Then it was extracted twice under heating reflux for 2 h each time. The extract was filtered and concentrated by using a rotavapor (R-300, BUCHI, Switzerland), and then lyophilised. The powder of SCE was sealed and stored in a dark at room temperature.

Determination of Total Anthraquinones Content

Preparation of the Sample Solution

Semen Cassiae extract powder (0.5 g) was hydrolysed with 10% HCl (30 mL) for 20 min under ultrasonication (KQ-100VDE, Kun Shan Ultrasonic Instruments, Co., Ltd., China), and then mixed with chloroform (30 mL). The mixture was refluxed under heating for 1 h and extracted by chloroform until the chloroform layer became colourless. The combined chloroform extract was concentrated by decompression. Then, the extract was dissolved in 1% $Mg(CH_3COO)_2$ solution (50 mL), and 1 mL of the solution was diluted 100 times for detection by UV-VIS spectrophotometry (UV2550, Daojin, Japan) (Kang et al., 2011; Wang, 2013).

Preparation of Analytical Standards

Emodin was used as the calibration sample (Xi'an Nat Biotechnique, Co., Ltd., Xi'an, China). After accurately weighing and dissolving 1.3 mg of emodin in 1% $Mg(CH_3COO)_2$ solution, the volume was made up to 10 mL to obtain the stock solution. With 1% $Mg(CH_3COO)_2$ solution as control, the absorbance of the stock solution was scanned in the range of 400–800 nm, and the results showed that emodin maximally absorbed at 513 nm. Accurately measured 0.4, 0.6, 0.8, 1.0, 1.2, and 1.4 mL of this stock solution was added into 1% $Mg(CH_3COO)_2$ solution and the volumes were made up to 10 mL to obtain standard samples. The absorbance of different concentrations of emodin was measured at 513 nm and the standard curve was plotted. The content of total anthraquinones in SCE was calculated by interpolating with the standard curve.

Diabetes Mellitus Animal Model

Animals

Male Sprague-Dawley rats (180 ± 20 g body weight) of SPF grade were purchased from Liaoning Longevity Biotechnology, Co., Ltd. (Liaoning, China). The rats were housed at controlled temperature (23 ± 2°C) and relative humidity (50–60%) and a 12 h light/dark cycle. All experimental procedures were approved by the ethics committee of the Second Affiliated Hospital of Harbin Medical University (approbation number: KY2016-226).

Dosage Design of SCE

The adult dose of Semen Cassiae recommended by the pharmacopoeia of the People's Republic of China is 9–15 g per day (Chinese Pharmocopoeia Committee, 2009), and we chose a dosage of 11 g/day Semen Cassiae for the study.

As described in Section "Total Anthraquinone Content in SCE," the content of total anthraquinones in Semen Cassiae was 6.8%. Considering the average human body weight as 70 kg, the dosage of SCE (total anthraquinones) for humans is: 11 g (weight of the original medicine of Semen Cassiae) × 6.8% (total anthraquinones content in SCE)/70 kg (average human body weight)/day = 10.69 mg/kg/day. According to the evaluation of the auxiliary hypoglycaemic function of registered health foods recommended by the China National Food and Drug Administration (China Healthy Food and Cosmetic Product Department, China State Food and Drug Administration Bureau, 2012), three doses of SCE should be tested as follows:

(1) low-dose SCE: five folds of the SCE dose for humans = 5 × 10.69 mg/kg/day (the dose of SCE for humans) = 53.45 mg/kg/day ≈ 54 mg/kg/day;
(2) middle-dose SCE: 10 folds of the SCE dose for humans = 10 × 10.69 mg/kg/day (the dose of SCE for humans) ≈ 108 mg/kg/day;
(3) high-dose SCE: 30 folds of the SCE dose for humans = 30 × 10.69 mg/kg/day (the dose of SCE for humans) ≈ 324 mg/kg/day.

Diabetic Rat Model

The diabetic rat model was established using a high-energy diet for 4 weeks and combined with low-dose STZ (30 mg/kg, Sigma, United States). The high-energy diet (Beijing Hua Fukang Biotechnology, Co., Ltd., Beijing, China) included lard (10.0%), sucrose (15.0%), egg yolk powder (15.0%), casein (5.0%), cholesterol (1.2%), sodium cholate (0.2%), calcium bicarbonate (0.6%), mineral meal (0.4%), and normal diet (52.6%).

Experimental Designing and Sampling

To evaluate the hypoglycaemic effect of SCE on normal rats, FBG of 20 male healthy Sprague-Dawley rats was quantified by a glucometer (ACCU-CHEK® Active, Roche, Ireland), and then the rats were randomly divided into a control group and an SCE treatment group according to FBG with 10 rats in each group. Rats in the SCE treatment group were administered SCE at a dose of 324 mg/kg/day (SCE was dissolved in 0.5% sodium carboxymethyl cellulose solution), and the same volume (10 mL/kg) of 0.5% sodium carboxymethyl cellulose solution was administered to rats in the control group by gavage once a day for 30 days. Then, FBG levels were measured in blood samples obtained from the tip of the tail after fasting the rats for 12 h with free access to water.

To evaluate the hypoglycaemic effect of SCE on diabetic rats, FBG and BG levels after 0.5, 1 and 2 h of the administration of 2 g/kg glucose (Tianjin Xinzheng, Co., Ltd., Tianjin, China) of 80 male healthy Sprague-Dawley rats were determined after fasting for 12 h. Based on FBG and BG levels 0.5 h after glucose administration, the rats were divided into the following six groups: control group (control, n = 10), DM group (n = 14), metformin (Alphapharm, Pty, Ltd., Australia) group (MET, 162 mg/kg/day, n = 14), SCE-L group (54 mg/kg/day, n = 14), SCE-M group (108 mg/kg/day, n = 14), and SCE-H group (324 mg/kg/day, n = 14). Rats were fed the normal diet (Beijing Keao Xieli Feed, Co., Ltd., Beijing, China) for the first week of the experiment. From the second week onwards, high-energy diet was provided to rats in the DM, SCE and MET treatment groups for 4 weeks; rats in the control group were fed the normal diet. At 3 weeks, rats in all groups, except the control group, were administered STZ as a single intraperitoneal injection at a dose of 30 mg/kg. During the experimental period, SCE and MET were administered daily to the respective treatment groups by gavage. The control and DM groups were administered the same volume of vehicle solution.

Fasting Blood Glucose, Fasting Serum Insulin, Oral Glucose Tolerance, Area Under Curve of Glucose, and Serum Lipid Determination

One day before the experiment was completed, all rats were fasted for 12 h, and the blood samples were withdrawn from the tip of the tail to test the level of FBG. Further, rats of the treatment groups were treated with SCE or metformin, and rats in the control and DM groups were administered the same volume of vehicle solution. After 15 min, 2 g/kg of glucose was administered to the rats, and the level of BG was measured at 0.5, 1, and 2 h after glucose administration. The AUC of glucose was calculated using the following formula:

$$AUC_{glucose} = (0hBG + 0.5hBG) \times 0.5/2 + (2hBG + 0.5hBG) \times 1.5/2.$$

At the end of the experiment, the blood samples were withdrawn from the abdominal aorta after fasting for 12 h and serum samples were separated to test FSI using a rat insulin ELISA Kit (Cusabio Biotech, Co., Wuhan, China); serum levels of TC, TG, LDL-C and HDL-C were also measured by using corresponding commercially available assay kits (Sichuan Mike Biological Polytron Technologies, Inc., Chengdu, China).

Western Blot Analysis

About 30 mg of skeletal muscle isolated from each rat was homogenised in a lysis buffer (P00138, Beyotime, Jiangsu, China) containing 1% protease inhibitor (P1005, Beyotime) and 10% phosphatase inhibitor (4906845001, Roche, United States) solution (for phosphorylated proteins) to obtain total proteins. The Membrane and Cytosol Protein Extraction Kit (P0033, Beyotime) was used to obtain membrane proteins from about 40 mg of skeletal muscle from each rat. Western blot analyses were performed using a standard blotting protocol, as described previously (Zhang Y. et al., 2016). Protein concentration was determined using the BCA protein assay kit (P0010S, Beyotime) by spectrophotometry (BioTek, United States). Total proteins (80 μg) and membrane proteins (100 μg) were separated by 10 or 8% SDS-PAGE and 8% *Bis–Tris* gel electrophoresis (Solarbio, China), respectively, and transferred onto nitrocellulose membranes (Invitrogen, United States). After blocking with 5% free-fat milk (BD Biosciences, United States) for 2 h at room temperature, membranes were incubated with the primary antibodies against AS160 (2670S, 1:1000, Cell Signaling Technology, Boston, MA, United States), phosphorylated-AS160 (Thr642, 4288S, 1:1000, Cell Signaling Technology), glucose transporter isoform 4 (GLUT4) (ab654, 1:1000, Abcam, Cambridge, United Kingdom), Akt (ab8805, 1:1000, Abcam), phosphorylated-Akt (Ser473, 4051S, 1:1000, Cell Signaling Technology), phosphatidylinositol-3-kinase (PI3K; 3821S, 1:1000, Cell Signaling Technology) and GAPDH (TA-08, 1:2000, ZSGB-BIO, Beijing, China) with gentle agitation at 4°C overnight and then incubated with secondary antibodies (1:10000, LICOR, United States) for 1 h at room temperature. Protein levels were quantified using the Odyssey software (LICOR) by densitometry. To normalise the data, expression levels of target proteins are presented as fold changes relative to GAPDH.

Statistical Analysis

Data are presented as the mean ± SD. One-way ANOVA was performed for multiple comparisons analysis and two-sided Student's *t*-test was used to compare differences between two groups by GraphPad Prism 5.0. $P < 0.05$ was considered to indicate a statistical significance.

RESULTS

Total Anthraquinone Content in SCE

The standard curve was plotted with concentration as the abscissa and absorbance as the ordinate. The linear equation was $Y = 21.324C + 0.024$ ($R^2 = 0.9992$) with a relative standard deviation of 0.38%. The results showed that the emodin had a good linearity relationship with the absorbance in the range of 0.0052–0.0182 mg/mL. The weight of the extract obtained from 2 kg of Semen Cassiae after extraction with 50% ethanol was 334.4 g; the extraction efficiency was 16.72%. Total anthraquinones content in SCE was 6.8% (**Table 1**).

Hypoglycaemic Effect of SCE

Fasting blood glucose levels in SCE-treated rats (5.3 ± 0.4 mmol/L) did not statistically differ from those in control rats (5.3 ± 0.6 mmol/L), indicating that SCE has no hypoglycaemic effect on normal rats (**Table 2**).

However, FBG levels in rats in the DM group were significantly higher than those in control rats ($^{**}P < 0.01$ vs. control group). The AUC of glucose in DM model rats was significantly higher than those in control rats ($^{**}P < 0.01$ vs. control group), indicating that OGT of DM model rats was obviously attenuated (**Table 3**). Meanwhile, FSI levels in DM model rats were lower than those in control rats ($^{*}P < 0.05$ vs. control group) and insulin resistance index (IRI) in DM model rats was higher than that in control rats ($^{*}P < 0.05$ vs. control group) (**Table 4**). The above results showed that the rat model of DM was established successfully.

As shown in **Table 3**, FBG levels in rats treated with SCE (108 mg/kg/day) were significantly lower than those in DM

TABLE 1 | Determination of total anthraquinone content in Semen Cassiae.

Sample	Total anthraquinone	Extractionrate (accounting for medicinal herbs)
Extract of Semen Cassiae by 50% ethanol	6.8%	16.72%

TABLE 2 | Effect of SCE on fasting blood glucose in normal rats (x̄ ± SD).

Groups	*n*	Dose (mg/kg)	Fasting blood glucose (mmol/L)	
			Before treatment	After treatment
Control	9	–	4.72 ± 0.37	5.33 ± 0.63
SCE	10	324	4.87 ± 0.58	5.30 ± 0.36

Control: rats were fed with normal diet; SCE: rats were fed with normal diet and treated with SCE (Semen Cassiae extract). SCE group showed no significant difference compared with control group (P > 0.05).

TABLE 3 | Effect of SCE on fasting blood glucose and glucose tolerance in diabetic rats ($\bar{x} \pm$ SD, n = 8).

Groups	Dose (mg/kg/day)	Blood glucose (mmol/L)				AUC (mmol/L·h)
		FBG	0.5 h	1 h	2 h	
Control	–	5.19 ± 0.27	7.54 ± 0.53	8.44 ± 0.65	5.99 ± 0.44	13.33 ± 0.72
DM	–	20.20 ± 3.28**	30.40 ± 3.68**	29.85 ± 5.74**	29.10 ± 2.06**	57.28 ± 4.30**
MET	162	10.89 ± 2.35##	21.37 ± 5.65##	20.31 ± 5.65##	16.00 ± 8.07##	36.09 ± 11.12##
SCE-L	54	16.89 ± 2.77	29.99 ± 2.79	31.85 ± 1.33	28.14 ± 4.15	55.31 ± 4.48
SCE-M	108	11.14 ± 6.64##	23.48 ± 5.78##	29.93 ± 4.18	23.06 ± 5.08#	43.56 ± 9.80##
SCE-H	324	16.23 ± 2.91	29.49 ± 2.35	32.33 ± 1.27	26.70 ± 2.06	53.57 ± 3.09

*Control: rats were fed with normal diet. DM: diabetes mellitus, rats were fed with high-energy diet and treated with STZ. MET (metformin): DM + MET. SCE (Semen Cassiae extract): DM + SCE. L: low-dose, M: middle-dose, and H: high-dose. *P < 0.05, **P < 0.01 vs. control group, #P < 0.05 and ##P < 0.01 vs. DM group.*

TABLE 4 | Effect of SCE on fasting serum insulin level and insulin resistance in diabetic rats ($\bar{x} \pm$ SD, n = 8).

Groups	Dose (mg/kg/day)	FSI (mIU/L)	IRI
Control	–	16.36 ± 2.42	3.77 ± 0.57
DM	–	13.32 ± 2.51*	11.65 ± 0.78**
MET	162	16.81 ± 5.60	7.76 ± 1.48##
SCE-L	54	13.91 ± 4.98	10.34 ± 3.43
SCE-M	108	18.67 ± 4.79#	8.28 ± 3.22#
SCE-H	324	17.89 ± 3.07#	12.73 ± 2.33

*Control: rats were fed with normal diet. DM: diabetes mellitus, rats were fed with high-energy diet and treated with STZ. MET (metformin): DM + MET. SCE (Semen Cassiae extract): DM + SCE. L: low-dose, M: middle-dose, and H: high-dose. *P < 0.05, **P < 0.01 vs. control group, #P < 0.05 and ##P < 0.01 vs. DM group.*

model rats ($^{\#\#}P$ < 0.01 vs. DM group); moreover, the AUC of glucose was significantly lower in SCE-treated rats than in DM model rats ($^{\#\#}P$ < 0.01 vs. DM group). Furthermore, as shown in **Table 4**, SCE treatment (108 mg/kg/day) significantly increased FSI levels ($^{\#}P$ < 0.05 vs. DM group) and decreased IRI ($^{\#}P$ < 0.05 vs. DM group). These data indicate that SCE (108 mg/kg/day) lowers FBG and IRI, thereby enhancing OGT and FSI.

Signalling Mechanisms Responsible for the Anti-diabetic Properties of SCE in Diabetic Rats

SCE Promotes Glucose Uptake by Transporting GLUT4 to the Sarcolemma in Skeletal Muscle

After determining the hypoglycaemic efficacy of SCE, we investigated the underlying mechanism. Skeletal muscle is the major site of glucose uptake in the body (Yang, 2014). On the one hand, the skeletal muscle can store glucose as glycogen, and on the other hand, it can oxidise glucose to produce energy after glucose transfer (by glucose transporters). The major glucose transporter that mediates this uptake is GLUT4 (gene name, SLC2A4) (Huang and Czech, 2007). Therefore, we examined whether SCE could influence GLUT4 membrane trafficking. **Figures 1A,B** indicates that the protein expression of membrane GLUT4 and cytoplasm GLUT4 in the skeletal muscle of DM model rat was significantly lower than that of control rats (membrane GLUT4: $^{***}P$ < 0.001 vs. control group; cytoplasm GLUT4: $^{**}P$ < 0.01 vs. control group). Membrane GLUT4 expression in rats treated with SCE (108 mg/kg/day) was higher than that in DM model rats ($^{\#\#}P$ < 0.01 vs. DM group, **Figure 1A**); however, the difference in the level of cytoplasm GLUT4 was not statistically significant (**Figure 1B**). This indicates that SCE (108 mg/kg/day) could promote glucose uptake by transporting GLUT4 to the sarcolemma in skeletal muscle.

SCE Regulates the Transport of GLUT4 to the Sarcolemma by Activating the PI3K–Akt–AS160 Signalling Pathway

In the absence of insulin stimulation, GLUT4 is stored in GLUT4 storage vesicles (GSVs). Under insulin stimulation, insulin binds to its receptor and triggers a cascade of reactions, resulting in the movement of GSVs to the cell membrane, where vesicle membranes fuse with the cell membrane, and GLUT4 is transported to the cell membrane (Zorzano et al., 1996). AS160 (Akt substrate of 160 kDa) is a substrate protein of the protein kinase Akt. Under normal conditions, its Rab-GTPase-activating protein (Rab-GAP) domain adheres to the Rab protein present on GSVs. GTPase is active at this time, and it hydrolyses GTP to GDP. Rab combines to GDP and maintains an inactive status. This makes GSVs stay in the cytoplasm. When the Akt phosphorylation site in AS160 is phosphorylated by p-Akt, Rab-GTPase is inactivated, GTP is not hydrolysed to GDP, Rab combines to GTP and maintains an active status and GSVs move to the cell membrane and transport GLUT4 to the cell membrane (Sano et al., 2003). Therefore, Akt and its downstream AS160 play an important role in GLUT4 translocation.

To explore why SCE could promote GLUT4 translocation to the membrane of skeletal muscle, we determined whether SCE could influence both AS160 and Akt proteins. As shown in **Figure 2**, the protein expression of p-AS160 and t-AS160 (total AS160) was significantly lower in DM model rats than that in control rats (p-AS160: $^{**}P$ < 0.01; t-AS160: $^{*}P$ < 0.05 vs. control group). In contrast, levels of p-AS160 and t-AS160 expression in the SCE (108 mg/kg/day) treatment group were significantly higher than those in the DM group ($^{\#\#}P$ < 0.01 vs. DM group). Similarly, the protein expression level of p-Akt and t-Akt in the DM group was significantly lower than that in the control group ($^{*}P$ < 0.05 vs. control group, **Figure 3**), and levels of p-Akt and t-Akt expression were significantly higher in the SCE

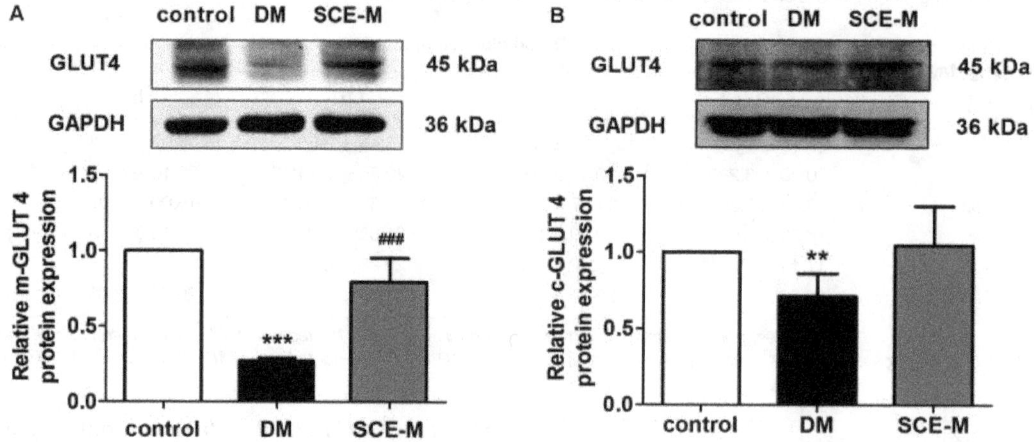

FIGURE 1 | Effect of SCE on GLUT4 expression in skeletal muscle of diabetic rats. Relative protein levels of glucose transporter isoform 4 (GLUT4) in the **(A)** plasma membrane and **(B)** cytoplasm measured by western blot analysis in the control, diabetes mellitus (DM) and middle-dose of SCE-M groups (n = 4). $^{**}P < 0.01$, $^{***}P < 0.001$ vs. control group and $^{\#\#\#}P < 0.001$ vs. DM group; mean ± SD.

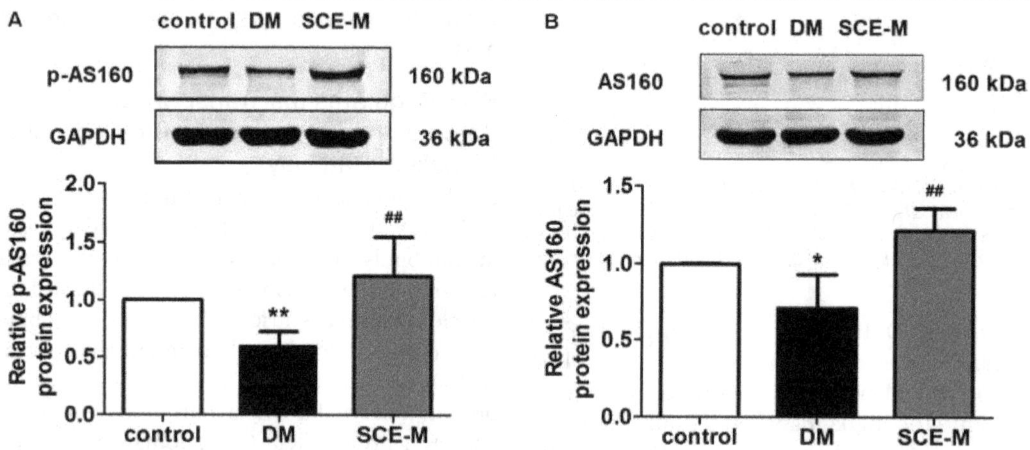

FIGURE 2 | Effect of SCE on AS160 expression in skeletal muscle of diabetic rats. **(A)** Relative protein levels of the phosphorylated form of AS160 (phosphorylated at Thr642). **(B)** Total protein levels of AS160 in the control, DM and SCE-M groups (n = 4). $^{*}P < 0.05$, $^{**}P < 0.01$ vs. control group and $^{\#\#}P < 0.01$ vs. DM group; mean ± SD.

(108 mg/kg/day) treatment group than in the DM group (p-Akt: $^{\#\#}P < 0.01$; t-Akt: $^{\#}P < 0.05$ vs. DM group, **Figure 3**).

Phosphatidylinositol-3-kinase activates Akt through the actions of two intermediate protein kinases, phosphosinsositide-dependent kinase 1 and Rictor/mTOR (Vanhaesebroeck and Alessi, 2000; Sarbassov et al., 2005). Thus, we evaluated the action of SCE on PI3K expression in diabetic rats. The protein expression of PI3K (**Figure 4**), upstream of Akt, was decreased in the DM group ($^{*}P < 0.05$ vs. control group), but significantly increased in the SCE (108 mg/kg/day) treatment group ($^{\#\#}P < 0.01$ vs. DM group). These data indicate that SCE could promote GLUT4 translocation by activating the PI3K–Akt–AS160 signalling pathway.

Hypolipidaemic Effect of SCE in Diabetic Rats

As shown in **Table 5**, levels of TC, TG, and LDL-C were all significantly higher and the level of HDL-C was significantly lower in the DM group than those in the control group ($^{**}P < 0.01$ vs. control group). These results indicate that diabetes-induced dysfunction in lipid metabolism was successfully induced in rats. Levels of TC and LDL-C were significantly lower and the level of HDL-C was higher in rats treated with SCE (108 mg/kg/day) than those in DM model rats ($^{\#\#}P < 0.01$ or $^{\#}P < 0.05$ vs. DM group). However, there was no difference in the level of TG between the DM and SCE treatment groups.

DISCUSSION

In the present study, we found that SCE containing anthraquinones is effective in lowering BG in diabetic rats and promoting glucose uptake by inducing the translocation of GLUT4 in skeletal muscle through the activation of the

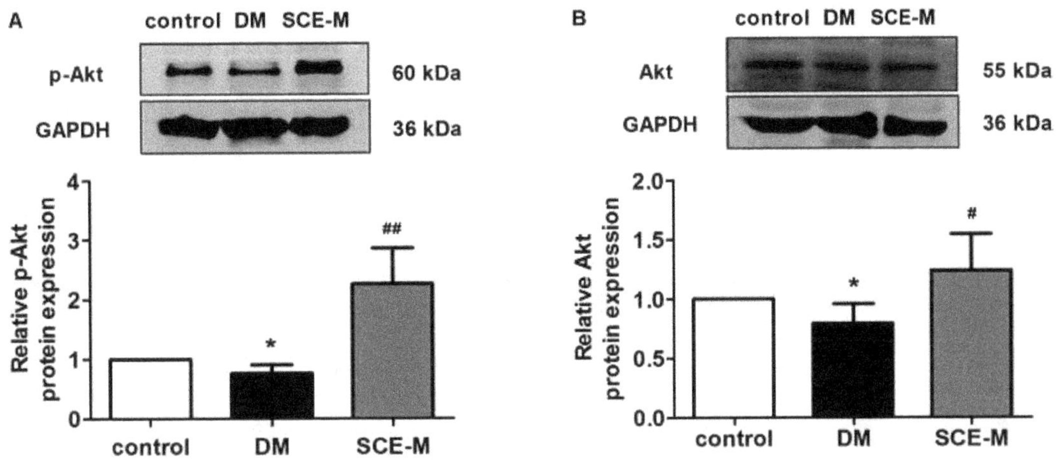

FIGURE 3 | Western blot analysis of Akt protein levels. **(A)** Relative protein levels of the phosphorylated form of Akt (phosphorylated at Ser473). **(B)** Total protein levels of Akt in the control, DM and SCE-M groups (n = 4). *P < 0.05 vs. control group, #P < 0.05 and ##P < 0.01 vs. DM group; mean ± SD.

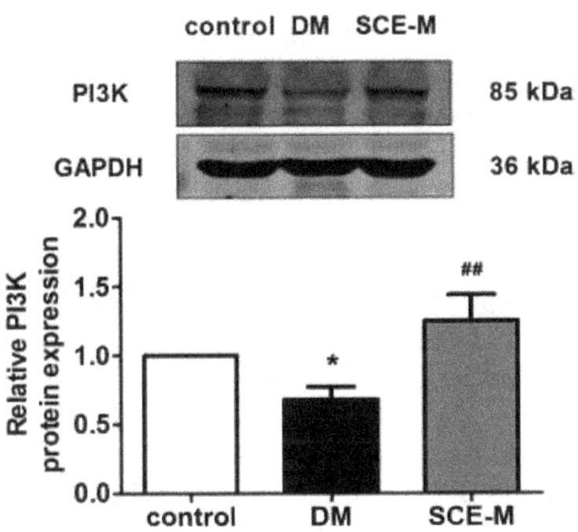

FIGURE 4 | Western blot analysis of phosphatidylinositol-3-kinase (PI3K) protein levels. Relative protein levels of the PI3K in the control, DM and SCE-M groups (n = 4). *P < 0.05 vs. control group, #P < 0.05 and ##P < 0.01 vs. DM group; mean ± SD.

PI3K–Akt–AS160 signalling pathway. This may be the possible mechanism for anti-hyperglycaemic effect of SCE (**Figure 5**).

Type 2 DM is a metabolic disease characterised by hyperglycaemia and reduced insulin secretion either because of pancreatic β cell dysfunction or decreased insulin sensitivity (Skelly, 2006). Up to 95% of all diagnosed cases of DM in adults are of type 2 DM. Therefore, it is important to find better strategies for the treatment and prevention of type 2 DM. To achieve this goal, an appropriate experimental model is considered as an important tool for understanding the pathogenesis of type 2 DM and the effects of therapeutic agents. High-energy diet combined with STZ induces type 2 DM in rats, which simulates the human pathogenesis, and is suitable for the testing of anti-diabetic compounds (Reed et al., 2000). Zhang M. et al. (2008) demonstrated that high-energy diet combined with multiple low doses of STZ (30 mg/kg) can be used to develop a stable animal model of type 2 DM. In this study, hyperglycaemia was induced by feeding the rats with high-energy diet for 4 weeks and a single low dose of STZ (30 mg/kg) injection at the end of the third week. Rats with the FBG ≥ 7.8 mmol/L or BG level ≥ 11. mmol/L after 2 h in the OGT test were considered diabetic (American Diabetes Association, 2012). As shown in **Tables 3–5**, levels of FBG, 2-h BG, AUC of glucose, IRI, TC, TG, and LDL-C in diabetic rats were significantly increased, and FSI and HDL-C were significantly decreased, indicating that DM model rats developed glycolipid metabolism disorder and insulin resistance. Thus, the model of type 2 DM in this study was established successfully.

Drugs used in traditional Chinese medicine have shown excellent efficacy and safety in the clinical treatment of DM (Zhang Y. et al., 2008; Kianbakht et al., 2013). Semen Cassiae, a well-known traditional Chinese medicine, has been used to treat for hyperlipidaemia, DM, acute liver injury, inflammation, photophobia, hypertension, headache, dizziness, and Alzheimer's disease (Dong et al., 2017). Management methods for agents used as both food and Chinese herbal medicines were promulgated by the (Ministry of Commerce of the People's Republic of China, 2014), and included 101 substances as both food and medicine, including Semen Cassiae (Ministry of Commerce of the People's Republic of China, 2014). As food, Semen Cassiae is commonly drunk as a type of roasted tea infusion for improving health in human daily life. Therefore, SCE is generally used as medicine.

To ensure the quality of research on traditional Chinese medicine, Semen Cassiae used in this study was identified by a pharmacognosy expert and they were the seeds of *C. obtusifolia* L. of the Leguminosae family. A variety of ingredients have been isolated from Semen Cassiae, and anthraquinones are considered the primary active constituents (Yang et al., 2015). Numerous studies have confirmed that the effect of alcohol extraction process used in our study is obviously better than that of water extraction process in terms of total anthraquinone extraction efficiency (Liu W.M. et al., 2009; Lu and Yuan, 2010). UV–VIS spectrophotometry is a simple, sensitive and

TABLE 5 | Effect of SCE on blood lipid levels in diabetic rats ($\bar{x} \pm SD$, $n = 8$).

Groups	Dose (mg/kg/day)	TC (mmol/L)	TG (mmol/L)	HDL-C (mmol/L)	LDL-C (mmol/L)
Control	–	1.33 ± 0.13	3.12 ± 0.06	0.26 ± 0.02	0.09 ± 0.02
DM	–	2.65 ± 0.35**	3.54 ± 0.26**	0.15 ± 0.02**	0.25 ± 0.07**
MET	162	2.12 ± 0.57	3.96 ± 0.56	0.29 ± 0.05##	0.25 ± 0.05
SCE-L	54	1.70 ± 0.34##	3.46 ± 0.22	0.22 ± 0.04##	0.20 ± 0.07
SCE-M	108	1.81 ± 0.26##	3.41 ± 0.16	0.20 ± 0.03#	0.14 ± 0.04##
SCE-H	324	1.82 ± 0.18#	3.51 ± 0.12	0.19 ± 0.02	0.19 ± 0.04

Control: rats were fed with normal diet. DM: diabetes mellitus, rats were fed with high-energy diet and treated with STZ. MET (metformin): DM + MET. SCE (Semen Cassiae extract): DM + SCE. L: low-dose, M: middle-dose, and H: high-dose. $^{*}P < 0.05$, $^{**}P < 0.01$ *vs. control group,* $^{\#}P < 0.05$ *and* $^{\#\#}P < 0.01$ *vs. DM group.*

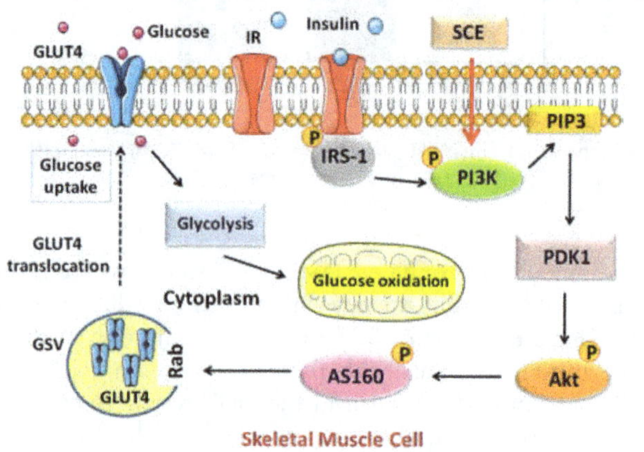

FIGURE 5 | Schematic diagram of the pathway activated by SCE in skeletal muscle that regulates GLUT4 translocation to the cell membrane. GLUT4, glucose transporter isoform 4; IR, insulin receptor; IRS, insulin receptor substrate; PI3K, phosphatidylinositol-3-kinase; PIP3, phosphatidylinositol (PI)-3, 4, 5-tiphosphate; PDK1, phosphosinsositide-dependent kinase 1; Akt, protein kinase Akt or protein kinase B (PKB); AS160, Akt substrate of 160 kDa; GSV, GLUT4 storage vesicle; SCE, Semen Cassiae extract.

reproducible method to quantify the content of anthraquinones in SCE (Kang et al., 2011; Wang, 2013). Our experimental data also support this, and the content of total anthraquinones extracted from Semen Cassiae was 6.8% with the extraction rate as 16.72% (**Table 1**).

Because mechanisms of compounds in the treatment of DM are very complex, the study of single Chinese medicines has become a trend to study the target and mechanism of drug action (Zhang X.N. et al., 2016). The study of Semen Cassiae in the treatment of DM and its complications is still in its initial stage. Our data (**Table 2**) showed that the administration of SCE at 324 mg/kg/day for 30 days does not affect FBG level in normal rats. Most notably, we discovered that SCE effectively lowers BG and increases insulin sensitivity in diabetic rats. It decreased levels of FBG, 2-h BG, AUC of glucose, IRI, TC and LDL-C, and increased the levels of FSI and HDL-C (**Tables 3–5**).

Skeletal muscle is the major site of postprandial insulin-dependent glucose uptake (Yang, 2014). Insulin resistance in skeletal muscle occurs much earlier before the development of β cell dysfunction and overt hyperglycaemia (DeFronzo and Tripathy, 2009). Therefore, we explored the potential mechanisms for the observed effects of SCE in skeletal muscle.

Glucose transporters (GLUTs) play an important role in regulating BG levels. GLUT4 is the most important insulin-sensitive glucose transporter protein in skeletal muscle. It is mainly localised in intracellular GSVs, and is translocated to the plasma membrane due to various stimuli to promote postprandial glucose uptake into muscle cells (Yang, 2014; Ueda-Wakagi et al., 2015). In the present study, we found that the membrane and cytoplasm GLUT4 levels in DM model rats were significantly lower than that those in control rats, and SCE (108 mg/kg/day) treatment increased the levels of membrane-bound GLUT4. Therefore, our results reveal a potential mechanism for the efficacy of SCE (108 mg/kg/day) in enhancing glucose uptake by promoting GLUT4 translocation to the cell membrane in skeletal muscle cells.

In skeletal muscle, the translocation of GLUT4 and the promotion of glucose uptake are regulated by insulin (Ueda-Wakagi et al., 2015). In the insulin pathway, the binding of insulin activates the tyrosine kinase of its receptor, which phosphorylates insulin receptor substrate-1 and activates the p85 regulatory subunit of PI3K. Activated PI3K induces the phosphorylation of downstream Akt and AS160 to regulate GLUT4 translocation. In diabetic rats, the PI3K–Akt–AS160 signalling pathway was inhibited and SCE (108 mg/kg/day) restored the activation of this signalling pathway. Therefore, SCE (108 mg/kg/day) could lower BG by regulating the PI3K–Akt–AS160–GLUT4 axis.

Previous studies have revealed that ethanol and aqueous extracts of Semen Cassiae significantly decreased the serum levels of TC, TG, and LDL-C; however, the level of HDL-C is increased (Li et al., 2002; Patil et al., 2004; Zhang et al., 2006; Wang et al., 2014). Our results show that SCE (108 mg/kg/day) significantly reduces levels of TC and LDL-C, and increases levels of HDL-C, but the levels of TG did not change compared with those in DM model rats. Our results on TG-lowering effects of SCE are different from those reported previously probably because the hypolipidaemic effect of SCE in a hyperlipidaemia model is different from that in a DM model with glucose and lipid metabolism disorder or because it may take a longer time to lower TG levels (Kim et al., 2014).

For many years, metformin has been the gold standard in the treatment of type 2 DM; therefore, we chose metformin as the positive control drug. In this experiment, metformin clearly demonstrated its hypoglycaemic effect. As shown in **Table 3**, levels of FBG, BG at 0.5, 1 and 2 h, and AUC of glucose were significantly reduced in the MET group ($^{\#\#}P < 0.01$ vs.

DM group). However, there was no difference between the MET group and the DM group in levels of FSI and lipids. It makes sense, because the BG-lowering mechanism of metformin is generally attributed to decreased hepatic gluconeogenesis, delayed intestinal glucose absorption and increased glucose utilisation by the intestine, particularly anaerobic glucose metabolism (Bailey et al., 2008). This is also the reason why metformin is typically taken before meals. Therefore, Semen Cassiae is superior to metformin in regulating the level of blood lipids in type 2 DM.

The present study verifies the pharmacological effects of SCE (108 mg/kg/day), especially its effects on promoting the translocation of GLUT4 and lowing BG by promoting GLUT4 translocation through the activation of the PI3K–Akt–AS160 signalling pathway in rats with DM induced by high-energy diet and low-dose STZ. Moreover, SCE (108 mg/kg/day) exerts an anti-hyperlipidaemic effect. These are beneficial to delay the progression from prediabetes to DM. Therefore, treatment with SCE could be an effective approach to prevent the development of DM and to assist the treatment of DM. Furthermore, the PI3K signalling pathway is also commonly activated in cancer. mTOR is a major node in the pathway; approximately 50% of solid tumours are associated with the activation of the PI3K–Akt–mTOR pathway (Liu P. et al., 2009). Khan et al. (2016) found that hyperglycaemia is common in patients treated with PI3K–Akt–mTOR inhibitors; the agents targeting this pathway are associated with hyperglycaemia due to their interaction with the insulin–glucose regulatory axis. Recently, it was reported that NLRC3 is an inhibitory sensor of the PI3K–mTOR pathway in cancer (Karki et al., 2016); however, the relationship between NLRC3 and PI3K–Akt–AS160–GLUT4, NLRC3 and PI3K–Akt–mTOR signalling pathway in DM is not known. Moreover, it is not clear whether SCE can influence NLRC3 in diabetes. Besides, to deduce the exact mechanism of the anti-hyperglycaemic effects of SCE, further studies on the inhibition of the activity of GSK-3, which inhibits glycogen synthesis (MacAulay and Woodgett, 2008; Khan et al., 2017) and glucose absorption, are needed to explain the regulation of glucose homeostasis by SCE.

Numerous western medicines are derived from plants, such as artemisinin. As early as 1,578, 1,892 traditional Chinese medicines were described in *Compendium of Materia Medica* (*Bencao Gangmu*) (Cui and Li, 2006). Studies on these traditional Chinese medicines can help us discover additional drugs with high efficiencies and low toxicities. The experimental design of this study was based on a combination of ancient literature and records of traditional Chinese medicine and methods used in modern medical research. This study aims to establish standards for the quality control of plant materials and analyse active ingredients in herb formulations. Such standardized and scientific research will increase the global reach of traditional Chinese medicine.

CONCLUSION

This study reveals that SCE, containing anthraquinones as the main components, prevents hyperglycaemia by promoting GLUT4 translocation through the activation of the PI3K–Akt–AS160 signalling pathway. Thus, SCE treatment could be effectively used to postpone the development of DM and to assist the treatment of DM.

AUTHOR CONTRIBUTIONS

YnZ and YoZ contributed conception and design of the study. MZ, XL, and BY organized the database. MZ and XL performed the statistical analysis and wrote the first draft of the manuscript. LW performed the extraction and content determination of Semen Cassiae extract. HL and HC performed the animal experiments. XH and YB performed the fasting serum insulin and serum lipids detection. MZ, HL, and LeD performed the western blot analysis. HL, HC, XH, YB, LeD, and LiD performed the FBG and BG level detection. All authors contributed to manuscript revision, read and approved the submitted version.

FUNDING

This study was supported by the National Natural Science Foundation of China (Grant Nos. 81770255 and 81503070), the Natural Science Fund Project of Heilongjiang Province of China (Grant No. H201314), Harbin Medical University Innovation Fund Foundation Research Project (Grant No. 2017JCZX56), and the Project of Central Guidance for the Development of Local Science and Technology (Grant No. ZY16A07).

ACKNOWLEDGMENTS

We would like to thank Science and Technology Park of Harbin Medical University for providing the laboratory. We are also thankful for the supports from the Department of Pharmacology of Harbin Medical University.

REFERENCES

American Diabetes Association (2012). Standards of medical care in diabetes–2012. *Diabetes Care* 35(Suppl. 1), S11–S63. doi: 10.2337/dc12-s011

Bailey, C. J., Wilcock, C., and Scarpello, J. H. (2008). Metformin and the intestine. *Diabetologia* 51, 1552–1553. doi: 10.1007/s00125-008-1053-5

Cheng, L. L., Sun, M., and Tu, L. (2005). Antibacterial activity of semen cassiae extract on plant pathogenic bacteria. *J. Sichuan Univ. Sci. Eng.* 18, 53–55.

China Healthy Food and Cosmetic Product Department, China State Food and Drug Administration Bureau (2012). *Methodology for Evaluating the Assistant Anti-hyperglycaemic Function, No. 107 File.* Beijing: China Food and Drug Administration.

Chinese Pharmocopoeia Committee (2009). *Pharmacopoeia of the People's Republic of China.* Beijing: Chemical Industry Press, 34.

Chunjuan, Y., Shuhong, W., Xiaowei, G., Jiahui, S., Lu, L., and Lijun, W. (2015). Simultaneous determination of seven anthraquinones in rat plasma by Ultra High Performance Liquid Chromatography-tandem Mass

Spectrometry and pharmacokinetic study after oral administration of Semen Cassiae extract. *J. Ethnopharmacol.* 169, 305–313. doi: 10.1016/j.jep.2015.04.008

Cui, S., and Li, S. O. A. (2006). *Compendium of Materia Medica (Bencao Gangmu).* Beijing: Foreign Languages Press.

DeFronzo, R. A., and Abdul-Ghani, M. (2011). Type 2 diabetes can be prevented with early pharmacological intervention. *Diabetes Care* 34(Suppl. 2), S202–S209. doi: 10.2337/dc11-s221

DeFronzo, R. A., and Tripathy, D. (2009). Skeletal muscle insulin resistance is the primary defect in type 2 diabetes. *Diabetes Care* 32(Suppl. 2), S157–S163. doi: 10.2337/dc09-S302

Dong, X., Fu, J., Yin, X., Yang, C., Zhang, X., Wang, W., et al. (2017). Cassiae semen: a review of its phytochemistry and pharmacology (Review). *Mol. Med. Rep.* 16, 2331–2346. doi: 10.3892/mmr.2017.6880

Fu, F., Tian, F., Zhou, H., Lv, W., Tie, R., Ji, L., et al. (2014). Semen cassiae attenuates myocardial ischemia and reperfusion injury in high-fat diet streptozotocin-induced type 2 diabetic rats. *Am. J. Chin. Med.* 42, 95–108. doi: 10.1142/S0192415X14500062

Hu, J., and Meng, Q. (2017). Knowledge map analysis of Chinese medicine treatment of type 2 diabetes based on CiteSpace. *Chin. J. Trad. Chin. Med. Pharm.* 32, 4102–4106.

Huang, J. (1982). *Shennong Bencao Jing*, 1st Edn. Beijng: Chinese Ancient Books Publishing House.

Huang, S., and Czech, M. P. (2007). The GLUT4 glucose transporter. *Cell Metab.* 5, 237–252. doi: 10.1016/j.cmet.2007.03.006

Huyen, V. T., Phan, D. V., Thang, P., Ky, P. T., Hoa, N. K., and Ostenson, C. G. (2012). Antidiabetic effects of add-on gynostemma pentaphyllum extract therapy with sulfonylureas in type 2 diabetic patients. *Evid. Based Complement. Alternat. Med.* 2012, 452313. doi: 10.1155/2012/452313

International Diabetes Federation (2015). *IDF Diabetes ATLAS-*, 7th Edn. Belgium: Karakas Print, 13.

Kang, J., Qu, L. B., Wu, Y. J., and Zeng, J. W. (2011). Determination of total anthraquinone in Semen Cassiae by spectrophotometry. *Tradit. Chin. Med. Res.* 24, 35–37.

Karki, R., Man, S. M., Malireddi, R. K., Kesavardhana, S., Zhu, Q., Burton, A. R., et al. (2016). NLRC3 is an inhibitory sensor of PI3K-mTOR pathways in cancer. *Nature.* doi: 10.1038/nature20597 [Epub ahead of print].

Khan, I., Tantray, M. A., Alam, M. S., and Hamid, H. (2017). Natural and synthetic bioactive inhibitors of glycogen synthase kinase. *Eur. J. Med. Chem.* 125, 464–477. doi: 10.1016/j.ejmech.2016.09.058

Khan, K. H., Wong, M., Rihawi, K., Bodla, S., Morganstein, D., Banerji, U., et al. (2016). Hyperglycemia and Phosphatidylinositol 3-Kinase/Protein Kinase B/Mammalian Target of Rapamycin (PI3K/AKT/mTOR) Inhibitors in Phase I Trials: Incidence, Predictive Factors, and Management. *Oncologist* 21, 855–860. doi: 10.1634/theoncologist.2015-0248

Kianbakht, S., Khalighi-Sigaroodi, F., and Dabaghian, F. H. (2013). Improved glycemic control in patients with advanced type 2 diabetes mellitus taking Urtica dioica leaf extract: a randomized double-blind placebo-controlled clinical trial. *Clin. Lab.* 59, 1071–1076.

Kim, Y. S., Jung, D. H., Sohn, E., Lee, Y. M., Kim, C. S., and Kim, J. S. (2014). Extract of Cassiae semen attenuates diabetic nephropathy via inhibition of advanced glycation end products accumulation in streptozotocin-induced diabetic rats. *Phytomedicine* 21, 734–739. doi: 10.1016/j.phymed.2013.11.002

Knowler, W. C., Barrett-Connor, E., Fowler, S. E., Hamman, R. F., Lachin, J. M., Walker, E. A., et al. (2002). Reduction in the incidence of type 2 diabetes with lifestyle intervention or metformin. *N. Engl. J. Med.* 346, 393–403. doi: 10.1056/NEJMoa012512

Lan, J. Q., and Zhu, C. J. (2015). Recent advances in pharmacological intervention for prediabetes. *Yao Xue Xue Bao* 50, 1565–1572.

Li, C. H., Li, X. E., and Guo, B. J. (2002). The effects of Cassia seed extracts on reducing blood lipid. *J. South Chin. Norm. Univ.* 98, 29–32.

Li, J., and Liu, D. (2010). Effect of salvia Miltiorrhiza on antioxidant function in streptozotocin-induced diabetic Rats. *Progress in Veterinary Medicine* 31, 30–33.

Li, X. E., Guo, B. J., and Zeng, Z. (2003). Experimental study on the antihypertensive effect of proein, oligosaccharide and anthraquinone glycosides in the Semen Cassiae. *Chin. Tradit. Herb. Drugs* 34, 842–842.

Li, Y., Pi, X., Liu, C., Gong, Y., and Li, Z. (2012). The mechanism of hypoglycemic effect of lily polysaccharide in vitro. *Lishizhen Med. Mater. Medica Res.* 23, 1964–1966.

Lian, F., Tian, J., Chen, X., Li, Z., Piao, C., Guo, J., et al. (2015). The efficacy and safety of Chinese herbal medicine Jinlida as add-on medication in type 2 diabetes patients ineffectively managed by metformin monotherapy: a double-blind, randomized, placebo-controlled, multicenter trial. *PLoS One* 10:e0130550. doi: 10.1371/journal.pone.0130550

Lin, J. (2001). The technology of extracting semen cassiae from Jueming jiangzhi powder. *Tradit. Chin. Drug Res. Clin. Pharmacol.* 12, 115–117.

Liu, P., Cheng, H., Roberts, T. M., and Zhao, J. J. (2009). Targeting the phosphoinositide 3-kinase pathway in cancer. *Nat. Rev. Drug Discov.* 8, 627–644. doi: 10.1038/nrd2926

Liu, S. Z., Deng, Y. X., Chen, B., Zhang, X. J., Shi, Q. Z., and Qiu, X. M. (2013). Antihyperglycemic effect of the traditional Chinese scutellaria-coptis herb couple and its main components in streptozotocin-induced diabetic rats. *J. Ethnopharmacol.* 145, 490–498. doi: 10.1016/j.jep.2012.11.017

Liu, W. M., Jiang, B., Zeng, Y. E., Chen, R. D., and Lin, P. J. (2009). Study on effect of water and alcohol extracting process on Anthraquinone content in Semen cassiae. *Lishizhen Med. Mater. Medica Res.* 20, 2270–2271.

Liu, Y., Li, X., Xie, C., Luo, X., Bao, Y., Wu, B., et al. (2016). Prevention effects and possible molecular mechanism of mulberry leaf extract and its formulation on rats with insulin-insensitivity. *PLoS One* 11:e0152728. doi: 10.1371/journal.pone.0152728

Lu, S. W., and Yuan, H. (2010). Selection of optimum extraction process for semen cassiae with orthogonal design. *J. Shandong Med. Coll.* 32, 105–108.

MacAulay, K., and Woodgett, J. R. (2008). Targeting glycogen synthase kinase-3 (GSK-3) in the treatment of Type 2 diabetes. *Expert Opin. Ther. Targets* 12, 1265–1274. doi: 10.1517/14728222.12.10.1265

Ministry of Commerce of the People's Republic of China (2014). Both food and Chinese herbal medicine material catalogue management method according to tradition. *Beverage Ind.* 6:6.

Patil, U. K., Saraf, S., and Dixit, V. K. (2004). Hypolipidemic activity of seeds of Cassia tora Linn. *J. Ethnopharmacol.* 90, 249–252. doi: 10.1016/j.jep.2003.10.007

Perreault, L., Pan, Q., Mather, K. J., Watson, K. E., Hamman, R. F., and Kahn, S. E. (2012). Effect of regression from prediabetes to normal glucose regulation on long-term reduction in diabetes risk: results from the Diabetes Prevention Program Outcomes Study. *Lancet* 379, 2243–2251. doi: 10.1016/s0140-6736(12)60525-x

Reed, M. J., Meszaros, K., Entes, L. J., Claypool, M. D., Pinkett, J. G., Gadbois, T. M., et al. (2000). A new rat model of type 2 diabetes: the fat-fed, streptozotocin-treated rat. *Metabolism* 49, 1390–1394. doi: 10.1053/meta.2000.17721

Sano, H., Kane, S., Sano, E., Miinea, C. P., Asara, J. M., Lane, W. S., et al. (2003). Insulin-stimulated phosphorylation of a Rab GTPase-activating protein regulates GLUT4 translocation. *J. Biol. Chem.* 278, 14599–14602. doi: 10.1074/jbc.C300063200

Sarbassov, D. D., Guertin, D. A., Ali, S. M., and Sabatini, D. M. (2005). Phosphorylation and regulation of Akt/PKB by the rictor-mTOR complex. *Science* 307, 1098.

Skelly, A. H. (2006). Type 2 diabetes mellitus. *Nurs. Clin. North Am.* 41, 531–547. doi: 10.1016/j.cnur.2006.07.011

Sun, X. (2011). The understanding of diabetes in the Yellow Emperor's Medicine Classic. *GUANG MING ZHONG YI* 26, 1313–1314.

Ueda-Wakagi, M., Mukai, R., Fuse, N., Mizushina, Y., and Ashida, H. (2015). 3-O-Acyl-epicatechins Increase Glucose Uptake Activity and GLUT4 Translocation through Activation of PI3K Signaling in Skeletal Muscle Cells. *Int J Mol Sci* 16, 16288–16299. doi: 10.3390/ijms160716288

Vanhaesebroeck, B., and Alessi, D. R. (2000). The PI3K–PDK1 connection: more than just a road to PKB. *Biochem. J.* 346(Pt 3), 561–576.

Vray, M., and Attali, J. R. (1995). Randomized study of glibenclamide versus traditional Chinese treatment in type 2 diabetic patients. Chinese-French Scientific Committee for the Study of Diabetes. *Diabete Metab.* 21, 433–439.

Wang, C. P. (2010). Antioxidation effect of Cassiae Seed on lens of aged rats: an active site research. *J. Shanxi Coll. Tradit. Chin.* 11, 12–13.

Wang, Y. (2013). Determiantion of anthraquinones in Semen Cassia by UV Spectrophotometry. *Clinical Journal of Traditional Chinese Medicine* 25, 730–732.

Wang, Y. H., Gao, L., Zhou, W. J., and Yan-Miao, M. A. (2014). Effects of ethanol extraction from cassiae semen on serum IL-6 and TNF-α in Hyperlipidemia Rats. *Chin. J. Exp. Tradit. Med. Formul.* 20, 178–181. doi: 10.1016/j.jep.2015.04.008

Xiong, M. Q., Lin, A. Z., and Zhu, Z. Z. (1997). Effects of supplemented taohe chengqi decoction in treating insulin resistance in rats with non-insulin dependent diabetes mellitus. *Zhongguo Zhong Xi Yi Jie He Za Zhi* 17, 165–168. doi: 10.1016/B978-0-12-800101-1.00005-3

Yang, C., Wang, S., Guo, X., Sun, J., Liu, L., and Wu, L. (2015). Simultaneous determination of seven anthraquinones in rat plasma by ultra high performance liquid chromatography-tandem mass spectrometry and pharmacokinetic study after oral administration of Semen Cassiae extract. *J. Ethnopharmacol.* 169, 305–313. doi: 10.1016/j.jep.2015.04.008

Yang, J. (2014). Enhanced skeletal muscle for effective glucose homeostasis. *Prog. Mol. Biol. Transl. Sci.* 121, 133–163. doi: 10.1016/b978-0-12-800101-1.00005-3

Zhang, H. (2007). Recognize of diabetes in internal canon of medicine of the yellow emperor. *Chin. Arch. Tradit. Chin. Med.* 25, 1239–1241. doi: 10.1155/2008/704045

Zhang, J. X., Wan, L., Hu, Y.-J., Qu, Q.-L., and Shi, J. (2006). Study on the effective part of reducing blood lipid in semen cassiae. *Lishizhen Med. Mater. Medica Res.* 17, 904–905.

Zhang, M., Lv, X. Y., Li, J., Xu, Z. G., and Chen, L. (2008). The characterization of high-fat diet and multiple low-dose streptozotocin induced type 2 diabetes rat model. *Exp. Diabetes Res.* 2008:704045. doi: 10.1155/2008/704045 doi: 10.1038/srep34284

Zhang, X. N., Qin, S. L., and Wei, M. H. (2016). Study on the hypoglycemic effects of single Chinese herbs. *Cardiovasc. Disease J. Integr. Tradit. Chin. West. Med.* 4, 117–118. doi: 10.1210/jc.2007-2404

Zhang, Y., Li, X., Li, J., Zhang, Q., Chen, X., Liu, X., et al. (2016). The anti-hyperglycemic efficacy of a lipid-lowering drug Daming capsule and the underlying signaling mechanisms in a rat model of diabetes mellitus. *Sci. Rep.* 6:34284. doi: 10.1038/srep34284

Zhang, Y., Li, X., Zou, D., Liu, W., Yang, J., Zhu, N., et al. (2008). Treatment of type 2 diabetes and dyslipidemia with the natural plant alkaloid berberine. *J. Clin. Endocrinol. Metab.* 93, 2559–2565. doi: 10.1210/jc.2007-2404

Zorzano, A., Munoz, P., Camps, M., Mora, C., Testar, X., and Palacin, M. (1996). Insulin-induced redistribution of GLUT4 glucose carriers in the muscle fiber. In search of GLUT4 trafficking pathways. *Diabetes* 45(Suppl. 1), S70–S81.

10

The Modulatory Properties of Li-Ru-Kang Treatment on Hyperplasia of Mammary Glands Using an Integrated Approach

Shizhang Wei[1], Liqi Qian[2], Ming Niu[3], Honghong Liu[4], Yuxue Yang[1], Yingying Wang[1], Lu Zhang[1], Xuelin Zhou[1], Haotian Li[1], Ruilin Wang[2], Kun Li[1] and Yanling Zhao[1]**

[1] Department of Pharmacy, 302 Hospital of People's Liberation Army, Beijing, China, [2] Department of Traditional Chinese Medicine, First Affiliated Hospital of Chinese PLA General Hospital, Beijing, China, [3] China Military Institute of Chinese Medicine, 302 Hospital of People's Liberation Army, Beijing, China, [4] Department of Integrative Medical Center, 302 Hospital of People's Liberation Army, Beijing, China

***Correspondence:**
Ming Niu
nmbright@163.com
Yanling Zhao
zhaoyl2855@126.com

Background: Li-Ru-Kang (LRK) has been used in the treatment of hyperplasia of mammary glands (HMG) for several decades and can effectively improve clinical symptoms. This study aims to investigate the mechanism by which LRK intervenes in HMG based on an integrated approach that combines metabolomics and network pharmacology analyses.

Methods: The effects of LRK on HMG induced by estrogen-progesterone in rats were evaluated by analyzing the morphological and pathological characteristics of breast tissues. Moreover, UPLC-QTOF/MS was performed to explore specific metabolites potentially affecting the pathological process of HMG and the effects of LRK. Pathway analysis was conducted with a combination of metabolomics and network pharmacology analyses to illustrate the pathways and network of LRK-treated HMG.

Results: Li-Ru-Kang significantly improved the morphological and pathological characteristics of breast tissues. Metabolomics analyses showed that the therapeutic effect of LRK was mainly associated with the regulation of 10 metabolites, including *prostaglandin E2*, *phosphatidylcholine*, *leukotriene B4*, and *phosphatidylserine*. Pathway analysis indicated that the metabolites were related to arachidonic acid metabolism, glycerophospholipid metabolism and linoleic acid metabolism. Moreover, principal component analysis showed that the metabolites in the model group were clearly classified, whereas the metabolites in the LRK group were between those in the normal and model groups but closer to those in the normal group. This finding indicated that these metabolites may be responsible for the effects of LRK. The therapeutic effect of LRK on HMG was possibly related to the regulation of 10 specific metabolites. In addition, we further verified the expression of protein kinase C alpha (PKCα), a key target predicted by network pharmacology analysis, and showed that LRK could significantly improve the expression of PKCα.

Conclusion: Our study successfully explained the modulatory properties of LRK treatment on HMG using metabolomics and network pharmacology analyses.

This systematic method can provide methodological support for further understanding the complex mechanism underlying HMG and possible traditional Chinese medicine (TCM) active ingredients for the treatment of HMG.

Keywords: Li-Ru-Kang, hyperplasia of mammary glands, modulatory properties, metabolomics, network pharmacology

INTRODUCTION

Hyperplasia of mammary glands is one of the most common breast diseases in middle-aged women and accounts for more than 70% of all breast disease (Chen et al., 2015). HMG is easily overlooked because of its clinical characteristics until the generation of mammary carcinoma. (Zhang et al., 2012). The morbidity of HMG has increased due to increased work-related stress and competitive career pressures along with the fast pace of modern life (Li et al., 2017a). However, there is still not a sufficient understanding of the etiology of HMG, and pertinent therapeutic strategies are limited. Hormone or endocrine therapy is one of the most commonly used methods to mitigate the clinical symptoms of HMG. Nevertheless, the side effects also decrease the quality of life for patients who receive long-term treatment. Surgical treatment as a form of therapy is hardly accepted by most patients with recurring symptoms (Henry, 2014). Therefore, finding a more appropriate treatment with fewer side effects and more therapeutic advantages is the current goal standard for treating HMG.

Traditional Chinese medicine (TCM) has been practiced in China for thousands of years to treat acute and chronic diseases. Its application in the prevention and treatment of HMG has garnered increasing attention. To explore the mechanism of action and active substances of TCM, a variety of constructive technologies have been used over the past few decades, such as metabolomics, proteomics, genomic arrays and network pharmacology (Xu et al., 2017). However, few researchers fully integrate the aforementioned techniques.

Li-Ru-Kang is composed of *Curcumae radix*, *Prunellae spica*, *Pseudobulbus cremastrae Seu pleiones*, *Radix bupleuri*, *licorice*, *Polygonum multiflorum*, *Crassostrea gigas* and *Cornu cervi*, and has been used for the treatment of HMG for several decades as a cipher prescription based on the clinical experience of many medical experts. Clinical researches showed that the total effective rate of LRK in the treatment of HMG was 88.0%. Moreover, LRK showed obvious superiority in improving the patients' symptoms and abnormalities of gonadal hormone (Qian et al., 2007).

As a rapidly developing technology, metabolomics can discover the pathogenesis of diseases by detecting more than 1,000 molecules in various biological fluids, such as urine, saliva, and blood. This technology has been successfully applied to the diagnosis and identification of various diseases, such as coronary heart disease (Li et al., 2017c), early chronic kidney disease (Benito et al., 2018) and thyroid cancer (Navas-Carrillo et al., 2017). Metabolomics has also been widely applied in the field of TCM (Li et al., 2017b; Liu et al., 2017) and provides insight into the complex network mechanisms of HMG. In addition, network pharmacology has also been successfully applied to the study of TCM molecular mechanisms and can provide a deep understanding of the complex relationship between TCM components and diseases.

In this study, we elucidated the bioactive components, potential biomarkers and possible mechanisms of LRK in the treatment of HMG using metabolomics and network pharmacology.

MATERIALS AND METHODS

Water Extract of LRK Preparation

Curcumae radix, Prunellae spica, Pseudobulbus cremastrae Seu pleiones, Radix bupleuri, licorice, Polygonum multiflorum, Crassostrea gigas and *Cornu cervi* were purchased from He yanling, Co., Ltd. (Beijing, China). The origin and quality of the 8 herbs were identified according to the Chinese Pharmacopeia (2015 Edition). Water extract from LRK was prepared by extracting the mixture of the 8 herbs (at a ratio of 12: 12: 9: 10: 30: 10: 9: 6, respectively) twice with water for 1 h. The extract was then decanted, filtered and dried under reduced pressure. The final ratio of powder to raw herb was 9.2%.

Animals

Female Sprague-Dawley rats weighing 200 ± 5 g (license number: SCXK-(A) 2012-0004) were obtained from the laboratory animal center of Military Medical Science Academy of the PLA. All studies were performed in accordance with the Guiding Principles for the Care and Use of Laboratory Animals of China. The animals were housed in the same feeding environment (temperature: 25 ± 2°C; humidity: 50 ± 10%) and fed based on lighting conditions (12:12 h light: dark cycle) with a standard diet and water *ad libitum*. After acclimatization for 7 days, all animals were randomly divided into six groups (n = 6): a normal group (A), a model group (B), a tamoxifen-treated HMG group (C), a low dose LRK-treated HMG group (D), a medium dose LRK-treated HMG group (E) and a high dose LRK-treated HMG group (F). Rats in the B, C, D, E, and F groups were intramuscularly injected with estrogen (0.5 mg/kg/d) for 25 days, followed by progestogen (5 mg/kg/d) for another 5 days to induce the experimental HMG model (Wang et al., 2011). Rats in groups D, E, and F were given 0.6, 1.2 and 2.4 g/kg LRK orally for 30 days, respectively. Rats in groups A and B were treated with an equal volume of saline. Rats in group C were given oral tamoxifen (4 mg/kg/d) for 30 days. All animal studies were approved by the Ethical Committee of 302 Military Hospital of China.

Sample Preparation

After the last treatment, all rats were sacrificed. Blood samples were collected and centrifuged at 3000 × g for 10 min to obtain serum for mass spectrometry. The mammary samples were rapidly excised and fixed in 10% paraformaldehyde solution for histopathological analysis. Paraffin-embedded sections ranging from 4 to 5 μm in thickness were stained with haematoxylin-eosin (H & E). The stained sections were analyzed with a Nikon microscope (Nikon Instruments Corporation, Shanghai, China) and Image-Pro Plus 7200 software.

Sample Handling

Briefly, 200 μL of serum samples and 600 μL of methanol were mixed uniformly and allowed to stand for 20 min at 4°C. The samples were centrifuged at 12,000 rpm at 4°C for 10 min to obtain the supernatant and then filtered through a syringe filter (0.22 μm) to obtain the sample for injection.

Chromatography and Mass Spectrometry

Chromatography was carried out using an Agilent 1290 series UHPLC system. The sample injection volume was 4 μL, and all samples were detected at 4°C on a ZORBAX RRHD 300 SB-C18 column (2.1 mm × 100 mm, 1.8 μm; Agilent, United States). The mobile phases were composed of 0.1% formic acid in acetonitrile (solvent A) and 0.1% formic acid in water (solvent B), and the flow rate was 0.30 mL/min. The gradient was set as follows: the first minute: 95% A; 1.0 to 9.0 min: 95–60% A; 9.0 to 19.0 min: 60–10% A; 19.0 to 21.0 min: 10–0% A; and 21.0 to 25.0 min: 0% A. After injection of the 10 samples and the QC sample compounded with all samples, a blank was injected to guarantee the stability and repeatability of the UPLC-QTOF/MS systems.

Mass spectrometry was performed using an Agilent 6550 Q-TOF/MS instrument (Agilent Technologies, Santa Clara, CA, United States) with an electrospray ionization source (ESI) in both positive and negative ionization mode. The following electrospray source parameters were used: the electrospray capillary voltages were 3.0 kV (negative ionization mode) and 4.0 kV (positive ionization mode); the gas temperature was 200°C (negative ionization mode) and 225°C (positive ionization mode); the mass range ranged from m/z 80 to 1000; the gas flow was 11 L/min; the nebulizer was 35 pisg in negative ionization mode and 45 pisg in positive ionization mode; the sheath gas temperature was set to 350°C, and the sheath gas flow was 12 L/min; the nozzle voltage was 500 V in both negative and positive ionization modes.

Data Extraction and Multivariate Analysis

MassHunter Profinder software (Agilent, California, United States) was used to extract sample data for peak detection and alignment. Full scan mode was applied in the mass range of 80–1000 m/z. The initial and final retention times were set for data collection. The resultant data matrices were normalized using MetaboAnalyst 3.0[1] and then introduced to SIMCA-P 13.0 software (Umetrics, Umea, Sweden) for PCA and PLSDA analysis. PCA was used as an unsupervised pattern recognition approach to reduce the dimension of the UPLC-QTOF/MS data and disclose intrinsic clustering of samples. PLS-DA analysis was employed to maximize the differences in inter-class discrimination and minimize the differences in inter-class discrimination. The variables with VIP >1.5 and |p(corr)| ≥0.58 in the PLS-DA analysis were further evaluated with an independent sample *t*-test.

Biomarkers Identification and Pathway Enrichment Analysis

The significant variables ($p < 0.05$ in ANOVA) were selected as potential biomarkers for further pathway enrichment analysis. These biomarkers were identified by METLIN[2], and the identified compound names were resubmitted to MetaboAnalyst 3.0 to analyse their signaling pathways.

Identification of Drug Targets and Potential Metabolites and Network Construction

To systematically elucidate the complex relationships between potential metabolites and their associated targets, we conducted network analysis using network pharmacology. The ingredients with an oral bioavailability (OB) ≥30% and a drug-likeness (DL) >0.18 from *Radix bupleuri, licorice, Pseudobulbus cremastrae Seu pleiones, Prunellae spica, Polygonum multiflorum* and *Curcumae radix* were put into the TCMSP database[3], and their corresponding chemical components were also collected from the same database (Huang et al., 2017). The ingredients and corresponding targets of *Cornu cervi* and *Crassostrea gigas* were retrieved from the BATMAN-TCM database[4]. The protein targets of potential metabolites were collected from the MBROLE 2.0 database[5] (Lopez-Ibanez et al., 2016). Different protein ID types were converted to UniProt IDs. Then, the "metabolite-target-chemical components" interactive network was established by using protein–protein interaction (PPI) information. Cytoscape 2.8.3 (National Institute of General Medical Sciences, United States) was applied to visualize and analyse the network.

Immunohistochemistry

To evaluate the effect of LRK on the expression of PKCα in breast tissue of HMG rats, immunohistochemistry was performed as described previously (Chen et al., 2014). Breast tissue slides were incubated with anti- PKCα (Abcam, Cambridge, MA, United States) for 12 h at 4°C. After treatment with HRP-conjugated goat anti-mouse IgG and 50 μL of streptavidin-peroxidase solutions for 30 min at RT, the sections were stained with DAB and counterstained with hematoxylin. The positive areas showed the color of brown yellow.

Statistical Analysis

Data were expressed as the mean ± SE and analyzed with the SPSS 13.0 software program (Chicago, United States). The

[1] http://www.metaboanalyst.ca/

[2] http://metlin.scripps.edu/

[3] http://lsp.nwu.edu.cn/tcmsp.php

[4] http://bionet.ncpsb.org/batman-tcm/

[5] http://csbg.cnb.csic.es/mbrole2/

differences between the group means were calculated by ANOVA. $p < 0.05$ was considered statistically significant, and $p < 0.01$ was considered highly significant. The results of the three-dimensional matrix containing the peak index, sample name, and peak area were introduced into SIMCA-P 13.0 software for pattern recognition analysis of PCA and PLS-DA.

RESULTS

Therapeutic Effects of LRK on HMG

The average diameter and height of nipples (Left 2 and Right 2) were measured as indices of HMG. As shown in **Figure 1**, rats given estrogen and progesterone displayed remarkable increases in the average nipple diameter and height. The administration of LRK (2.4 and 1.2 g/kg) markedly decreased the average nipple diameter and height, respectively. Pathological studies provided direct evidence of protective effects of LRK on HMG. In **Figure 2**, the mammary tissues of the rats in the normal group exhibited normal morphological structures with no abnormal features. By contrast, the mammary tissues of the rats in the model group displayed more acinus and lobules, expanded mammary lumens, and hyperplastic ducts. Conversely, treatment with LRK (2.4 and 1.2 g/kg) ameliorated these morphological changes. These results preliminarily verified that 2.4 and 1.2 g/kg LRK significantly protected the mammary tissue in the rats with HMG induced by estrogen and progesterone.

Multivariate Statistical Analysis

Principal component analysis (PCA) and orthogonal partial least squares-discriminant analysis (OPLS-DA) are pattern recognition approaches frequently used to classify metabolic phenotypes and identify different metabolites to evaluate variation among complex data sets. Score plots revealed a direct image of observational clusters. A distinguished classification between the clustering of the normal and model groups and the normal and LRK groups was observed in both the positive (**Figure 3A**) and negative modes (**Figure 3B**). Further multivariate analysis was needed to explore which metabolites caused these differences.

Orthogonal partial least squares-discriminant analysis was used to identify potential biomarkers that were significantly changed between the normal, model and LRK groups. The parameters R^2X (cum), R^2Y (cum), and Q^2 (cum) were used to provide an estimate of how well the model fit the data. We further determined whether the metabolite fingerprints in the serum differed between the normal, model, and LRK groups by constructing an OPLS-DA model. A distinguished classification between the clustering of the normal, model, and LRK groups was observed in both the positive (**Figure 4**) and negative models (Supplementary Figure S1), suggesting a significant serum biochemical perturbation in the model and LRK groups. The R^2X (cum), R^2Y (cum), and Q^2 (cum) of OPLS-DA in our positive model were 0.506, 0.936, 0.79, respectively, using the data from the control and model groups and 0.304, 0.87, 0.748, respectively, using the data from the model and LRK groups. The R^2X (cum), R^2Y (cum), and Q^2 (cum) of OPLS-DA in our negative model were 0.261, 0.908, 0.768, respectively, using the data from the control and model groups and 0.233, 0.97, 0.806, respectively, using the data from the model and LRK groups. The corresponding parameter results indicated that models were of good quality and provided accurate predictions. Variables further away from the origin in the corresponding S-plots were thought to contribute more significantly were more thus responsible for the separation between the normal and model groups as well as the model and LRK groups in both the positive (**Figures 4B,E**) and negative ionization models (Supplementary Figure S1). These variables may therefore be regarded as

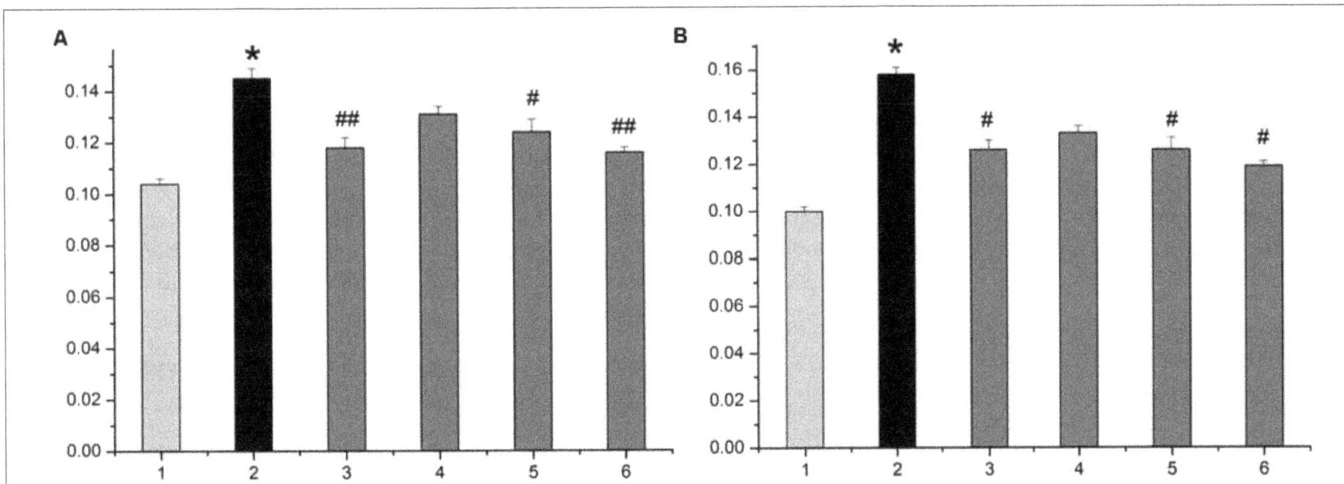

FIGURE 1 | The average diameter and height of nipples in the HMG rats. **(A)** The average diameter of nipples. **(B)** The average height of nipples. 1: normal group. 2: model group. 3: tamoxifen-treated HMG group (4 mg/kg). 4: low-dose LRK-treated HMG group (0.6 g/kg). 5: medium-dose LRK-treated HMG group (1.2 g/kg). 6: high-dose LRK-treated HMG group (2.4 g/kg). Data are expressed as the mean ± SE ($n = 6$). $^*p < 0.01$ compared with the normal group; $^{\#\#}p < 0.01$, $^{\#}p < 0.05$ compared with the model group.

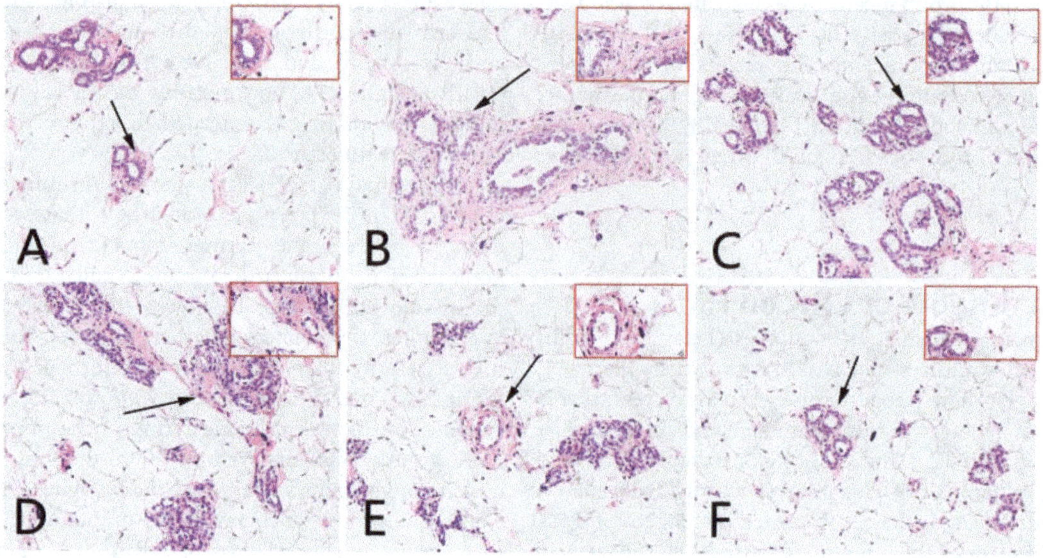

FIGURE 2 | Effects of LRK on the histopathology of mammary tissues using haematoxylin and eosin staining (200× and 400×). **(A)** Normal group. **(B)** Model group. **(C)** Tamoxifen-treated HMG group (4 mg/kg). **(D)** Low-dose LRK-treated HMG group (0.6 g/kg). **(E)** Medium-dose LRK-treated HMG group (1.2 g/kg). **(F)** High dose LRK-treated HMG group (2.4 g/kg). The magnified areas (×400) are marked with a black arrow in the pathological tissue figures (200×).

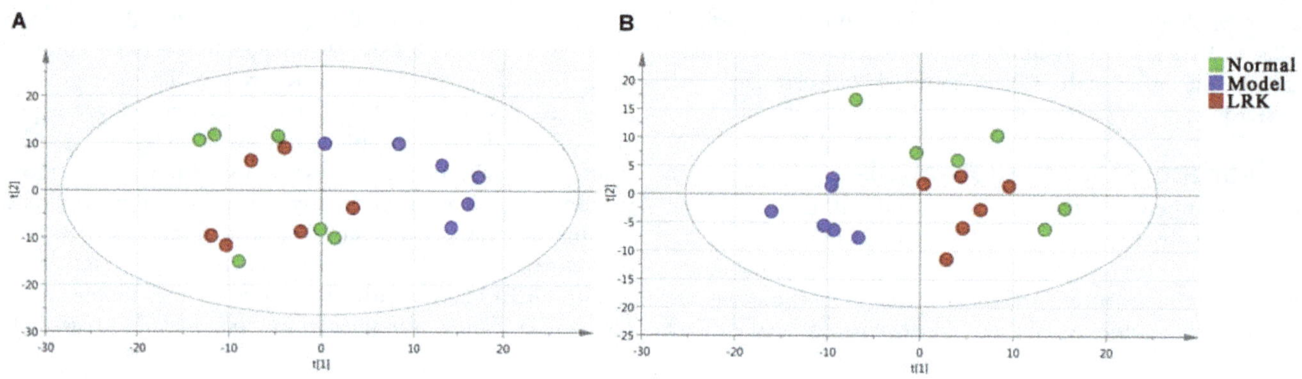

FIGURE 3 | Principal component analysis (PCA) score plot of the control, model and LRK (2.4 g/kg) groups. **(A)** ESI+ model. **(B)** ESI- model.

potential biomarkers. Permutation tests with 100 iterations were performed to validate the model. These tests compared the goodness of fit of the original model with the goodness of fit of randomly permuted models. As shown in **Figures 4C,F**, the validation plots indicated that the original models were valid.

Identification of Potential Metabolites in HMG Treatment

Among the 1986 signals detected in the control, model and 2.4 g/kg LRK groups, variables that significantly contributed to the clustering and discrimination were identified according to a threshold of VIP ≥1.5 and |p(corr)| ≥ 0.58. Those thresholds were obtained after OPLS-DA processing these variables. According to the VIP and |p(corr)|, 366 variables were selected from the control, model and 2.4 g/kg LRK groups as the candidates for fold-changes and ANOVA analyses. The candidates that significantly differed among the groups with fold change exceeding two were identified as candidate biomarkers for METLIN and Metaboanalyst identification. Ten potential biomarkers were summarized in **Table 1** with their corresponding formula, retention time, m/z, and differences by group.

Pathway Analysis of HMG Treatment

Herein, 10 potential metabolites were expressed at significant levels. Pathway analysis was performed in detail using Metaboanalyst. HMG-associated metabolites were responsible for metabolizing arachidonic acid, glycerophospholipid, linoleic acid, sphingolipid, alpha-linolenic acid, glycine, serine, threonine, arginine, proline, and purine (**Table 2** and **Figure 5**). The top three metabolic pathways were arachidonic acid, glycerophospholipid and linoleic acid.

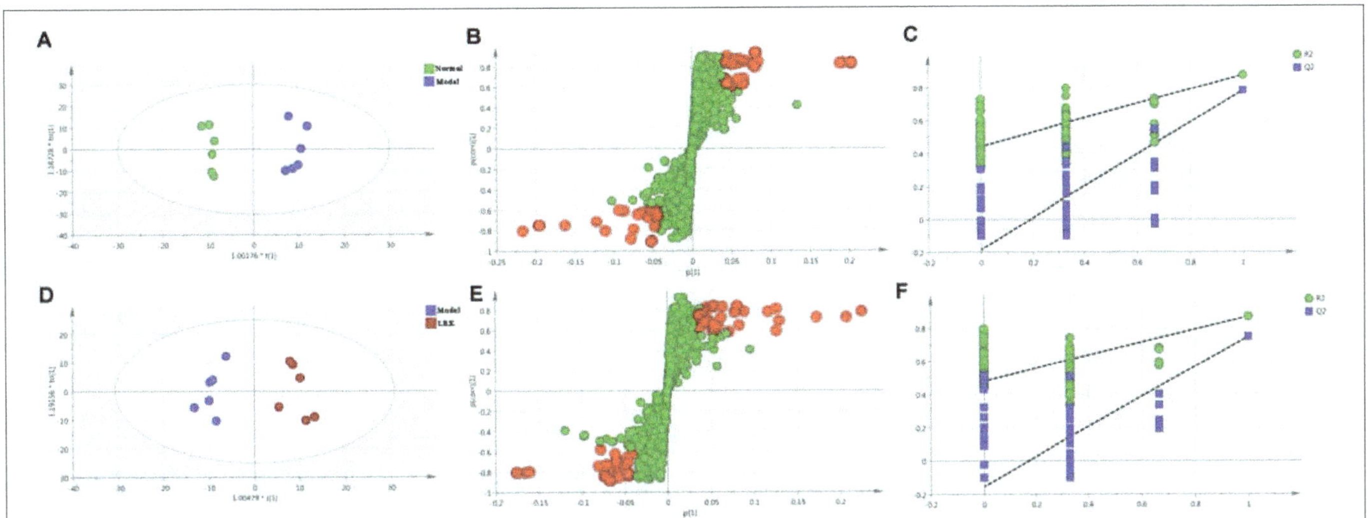

FIGURE 4 | The OPLS-DA score plots, S-plots and 100-permutation test generated from the OPLS-DA data of the normal, model and LRK groups in ESI+ mode. OPLS-DA score plots were the pair-wise comparisons between the normal and model groups **(A)** as well as between the model and LRK groups **(D)**. S-plots of the OPLS-DA model for the normal and model groups **(B)** as well as for the model and LRK groups **(E)**. The 100-permutation test of the OPLS-DA model was for the normal and model groups **(C)** as well as for the model and LRK groups **(F)**.

TABLE 1 | Identified metabolites of the serum from different groups.

No	Metabolites	Formula	R.T. (min)	Mass (m/z)	Ratio changes (significance)	
					Control/Model	LRK/Model
1	Sulfolithocholylglycine	$C_{26}H_{42}NO_7S$	7.36	536.2628	0.40^{**}	$0.45^{\#\#}$
2	Leukotriene B4	$C_{20}H_{32}O_4$	6.57	339.2557	0.23^{**}	$0.16^{\#\#}$
3	Phosphatidylcholine	$C_{10}H_{18}NO_8PR_2$	6.9	792.5771	1.36^{**}	$1.07^{\#}$
4	Ceramide	$C_{19}H_{36}NO_3R$	6.57	678.6891	3.10^{**}	$2.98^{\#\#}$
5	Prostaglandin E2	$C_{20}H_{32}O_5$	10.99	375.2233	3.50^{**}	$2.72^{\#\#}$
6	3-Hydroxypicolinic acid	$C_6H_5NO_3$	1.25	173.9994	0.68^{**}	$0.67^{\#\#}$
7	5-Amino-4-imidazole carboxylate	$C_4H_5N_3O_2$	1.06	162.006	3.88^{**}	$3.04^{\#\#}$
8	Phosphatidylserine	$C_8H_{12}NO_{10}PR_2$	6.96	854.5852	6.43^{**}	$3.23^{\#\#}$
9	Coenzyme Q9	$C_{54}H_{82}O_4$	6.95	829.5664	0.14^{**}	$0.58^{\#\#}$
10	Gamma-glutamyl-L-putrescine	$C_9H_{19}N_3O_3$	4.73	216.1361	0.20^{**}	$0.51^{\#\#}$

$^{**}P < 0.01$ compared with normal group; $^{\#\#}P < 0.01$, $^{\#}P < 0.05$ compared with model group.

"Potential Metabolite-Target-Component" Interactive Network and Analysis

To reveal the proteins targets and chemical components of LRK regulation, the "potential metabolite-target-component" interactive network was structured by combing the drug targets and the targets associated with potential metabolites. As shown in **Figure 6**, 445 drug targets, 170 targets associated with potential metabolites, and 3 potential metabolites, including phosphatidylserine (C02737), prostaglandin E2 (C00584) and phosphatidylcholine (C00157), participated in the "potential metabolite-target-component" interactive network (**Figure 6A**). Five drug targets, including *protein kinase C alpha type* (P17252), *prostaglandin E synthase* (O14684), *prostaglandin E2 receptor EP3 subtype* (P43115), *group IIE secretory phospholipase A2* (Q9NZK7) and *phospholipase B1* (Q6P1J6), directly regulated the 3 potential metabolites (**Figure 6B**). The 5 drug targets were directly regulated by multiple chemical components, including *beta-sitosterol, quercetin, p-coumaric acid* and *naringenin*, which were collected from 4 herbs, including *Curcumae radix, Prunellae spica, Radix bupleuri* and *Pseudobulbus cremastrae Seu pleiones* in LRK (**Figure 7**).

The Effect of LRK on the Expression of PKCα in Breast Tissue of HMG Rats

Analysis of the network pharmacology prediction results showed that the greatest number of chemical components directly connected to PKCα, suggesting that PKCα may play a more important role in the treatment of HMG by LRK. Therefore, to verify the authenticity of the network pharmacology prediction results, we evaluated the expression of PKCα in breast tissue by immunohistochemistry. The results indicated the expression of

TABLE 2 | Results of integrating enrichment analysis of biomarkers with MetaboAnalyst 3.0.

No	Pathway Name	Match Status	*p*	−log(p)	Impact
1	Arachidonic acid metabolism	3/62	0.0059386	0.0059386	0.0059386
2	Glycerophospholipid metabolism	2/39	0.023519	0.023519	0.023519
3	Linoleic acid metabolism	1/15	0.048758	0.089758	0.089758
4	Sphingolipid metabolism	1/25	0.14536	0.14536	0.14536
5	alpha-Linolenic acid metabolism	1/29	0.16669	0.16669	0.16669
6	Glycine, serine and threonine metabolism	1/48	0.26143	0.26143	0.26143
7	Arginine and proline metabolism	1/77	0.38685	0.94973	0.01185
8	Purine metabolism	1/92	0.44363	0.81278	0.0162

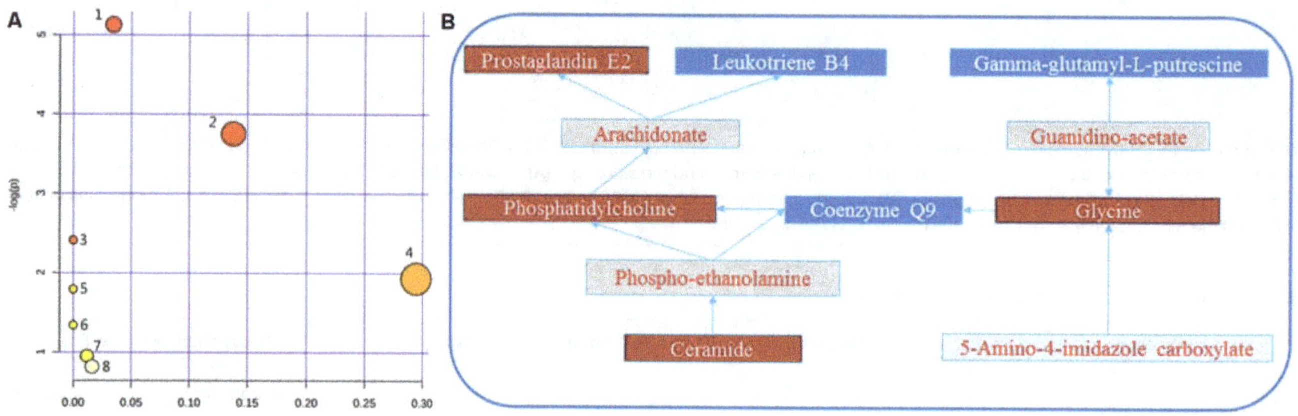

FIGURE 5 | (A) Metabolomic Pathway construction of the metabolic pathways involved in the effects of LRK on HMG. **(B)** Signaling networks associated with the differentially expressed metabolic pathways. 1: Arachidonic acid metabolism. 2: Glycerophospholipid metabolism. 3: Linoleic acid metabolism. 4: Sphingolipid metabolism. 5: alpha-linolenic acid metabolism. 6: Glycine, serine and threonine metabolism. 7: Arginine and proline metabolism. 8: Purine metabolism. The red solid box represents the peak area of the LRK/model >1. The blue solid box represents the peak area of LRK/model < 1.

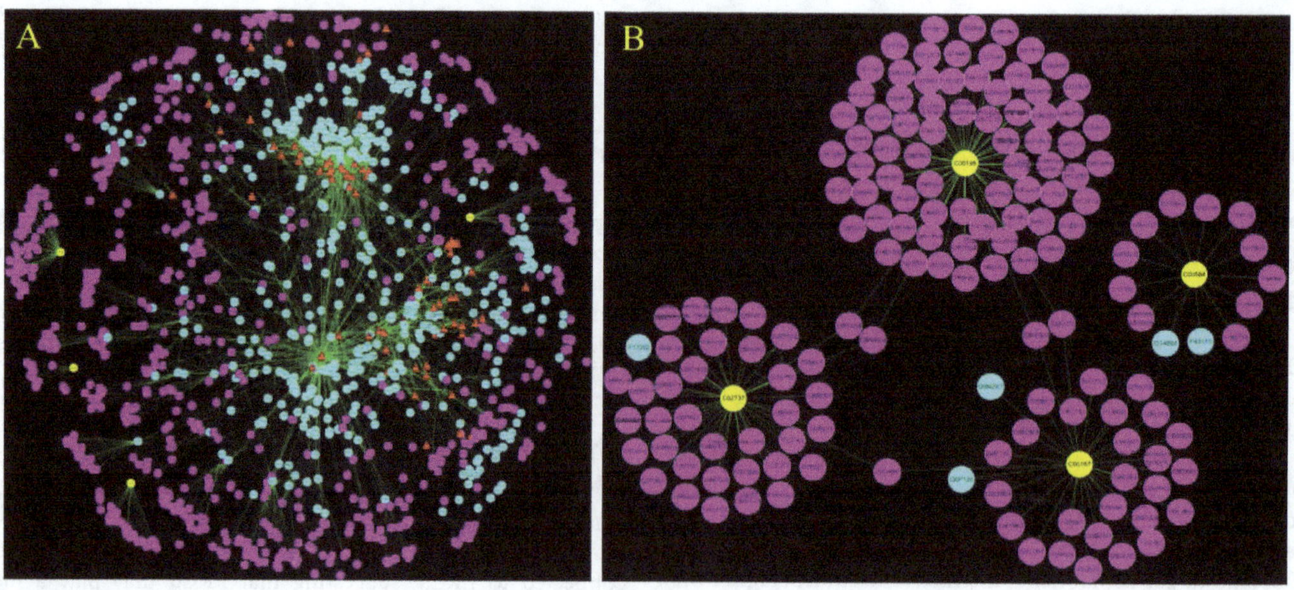

FIGURE 6 | The "potential metabolite-target-component" interactive network with all target information **(A)** and key target information **(B)** participating in the treatment of HMG by LRK. The red triangles represent active chemical constituents of LRK. The blue dots represent the protein targets of drugs. The yellow dots represent potential metabolites. The purple dots represent the targets associated with potential metabolites.

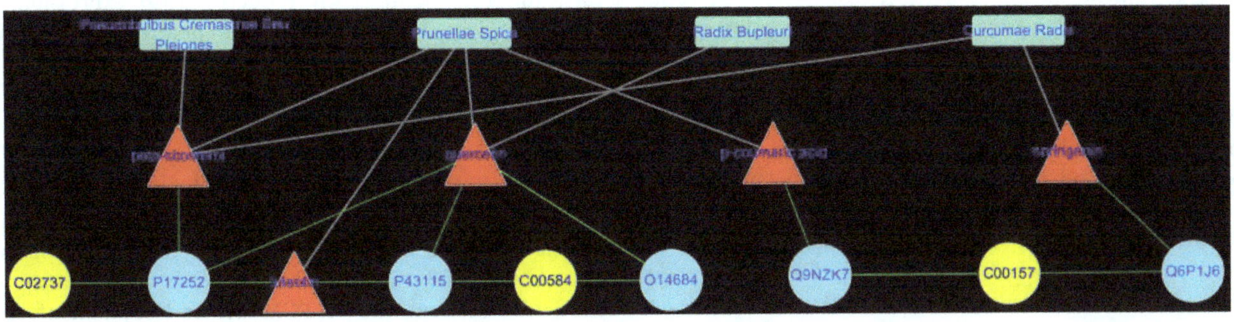

FIGURE 7 | The "potential metabolite-target-component-herb" interactive network participating in the treatment of HMG by LRK. The red triangles represent active chemical constituents of LRK. The blue dots represent the protein targets of herbs. The yellow dots represent the potential metabolites. The blue rectangles represent herbs.

PKCα was significantly increased in the breast tissues of rats in the model group, while the different doses of LRK significantly reduced the expression of PKCα (**Figure 8**).

DISCUSSION

The morbidity rate of HMG is increasing annually and continues to affect younger women (Zhang et al., 2008). HMG is classified in the "Rupi" category according to TCM theory (Fan et al., 2013). While network pharmacology and metabonomics have been applied to TCM research (Su et al., 2017; Wang et al., 2017), few studies have attempted to combine these two approaches. Metabolomics can analyze and detect small molecules in bodily fluids to determine which compounds have significant abnormalities and to uncover the mechanism of disease development. Network pharmacology can analyze the interaction of macromolecule targets corresponding to chemical components and diseases and reveal the molecular mechanisms of drug treatment. By combining metabolomics and network pharmacology, we were able to gain a deeper understanding of the molecular mechanisms underlying TCM treatment.

Li-Ru-Kang is made up of 8 kinds of herbs. It has been effective in treating HMG for decades. In this study, we combined metabonomics and network pharmacology analyses to evaluate the efficacy, active components and possible molecular mechanisms of LRK in the treatment of HMG. LRK significantly improved the morphological characteristics of nipples and reduced the pathological state of HMG in rats. Furthermore, we described the metabolomic feature profile and metabolite interaction network of LRK in treating HMG. LRK exhibited protective effects against HMG by reversing potential metabolites to normal levels. Ten metabolites were significantly regulated by LRK. Seven of these metabolites, including prostaglandin E2, leukotriene B4, phosphatidylcholine, coenzyme Q9, ceramide, gamma-glutamyl-L-putrescine and 5-amino-4-imidazole carboxylate, could interact in different ways. The results indicated that the occurrence and development of HMG were caused by changes in many aspects of physiologically and pathologically related molecules and that most of the changes in the body's molecules were interrelated. LRK regulated these

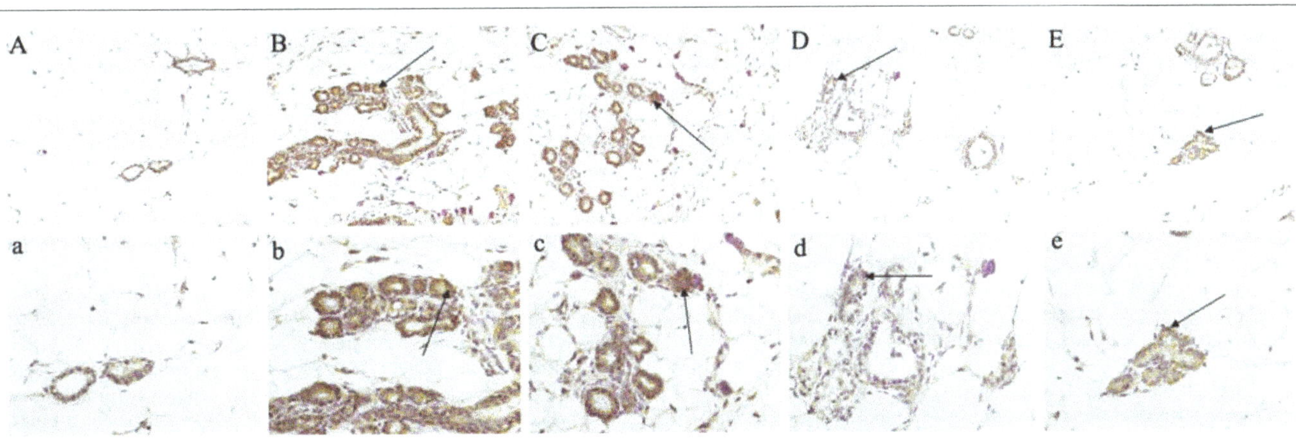

FIGURE 8 | Effects of LRK on the expression of PKCα in breast tissue of HMG rats using immunohistochemistry (200× and 400×). **(A)** (200**×**) and **a** (400**×**) : normal group. **(B)** (200**×**) and **b** (400**×**): model group. **(C)** (200**×**) and **c** (400**×**): low-dose LRK-treated HMG group (0.6 g/kg). **(D)** (200**×**) and **d** (400**×**): medium-dose LRK-treated HMG group (1.2 g/kg). **(E)** (200**×**) and **e** (400**×**): high dose LRK-treated HMG group (2.4 g/kg).

10 biomarkers to normalize their expression levels, indicating that LRK could be used to treat HMG via multiple pathways and multiple targets.

To obtain a deeper understanding of the LRK mechanism for treating HMG and the correlation between LRK chemical components and metabolites, we further combined the network pharmacology method to establish the "potential metabolite-target-component" interactive network. The results showed that four chemical components, *beta-sitosterol, quercetin, p-coumaric acid* and *naringenin*, which come from *Curcumae radix, Prunellae spica, Radix bupleuri* and *Pseudobulbus cremastrae Seu pleiones*, acted directly on multiple targets that are directly related to metabolites, including *prostaglandin E synthase, protein kinase C alpha type, prostaglandin E2 receptor EP3 subtype, group IIE secretory phospholipase A2* and *phospholipase B1*. The results suggested that multiple components in LRK played an important role in regulating the endogenous physical disturbance of the body, thus indicating the advantages of LRK in the clinical treatment of HMG. By investigating the pathogenesis of HMG, we found that inflammation and oxidative stress mechanisms played a key role in the development of HMG (Holloway et al., 2012). At the same time, some drugs act on HMG by exerting anti-inflammatory and antioxidant pharmacological effects (Das Gupta et al., 2015; Huang et al., 2017). Studies have shown that beta-sitosterol (Villasenor et al., 2002; Tan et al., 2008), quercetin (Kamaraj et al., 2007), p-coumaric acid (Ilavenil et al., 2016) and naringenin (Cavia-Saiz et al., 2010; Chen et al., 2013) in LRK have anti-inflammatory and antioxidant pharmacological activities. The network pharmacology results showed that PKCα was the target directly connected to the four chemical components. This target is also the most closely related target to inflammation and oxidative stress (Kopach et al., 2013; Andersson et al., 2016). Therefore, to verify the accuracy of the network pharmacology prediction results, we further examined the expression of PKCα in the breast tissues of HMG rats. The expression of PKCα was increased significantly in HMG rats, and LRK significantly reduced PKCα expression. These results suggested that the network pharmacology prediction results were credible. This experiment also demonstrated the significance of PKCα in the pathogenesis of HMG and LRK treatment.

This study systematically explored the molecular mechanism of LRK for the treatment of HMG by combining metabonomics and network pharmacology analyses. In addition, this innovative research method can provide new ideas for research on the molecular mechanisms of TCM in the treatment of complex diseases.

AUTHOR CONTRIBUTIONS

SW and LQ performed the experiments, analyzed the data, and wrote the manuscript. MN, HHL, YY, YW, LZ, XZ, and HTL collected and prepared samples. RW, KL, and YZ performed the analyses.

FUNDING

This work was financially supported by Project of the Project of Chinese Medicine Education Association (No. 2016SKT-M035), Chinese Medicine Education Association (No. 2016SKT-Z003) and Beijing Municipal Science & Technology Commission (No. Z171100001717013), and State Natural Science Foundation (No. 81573631).

REFERENCES

Andersson, A., Bluwstein, A., Kumar, N., Teloni, F., Traenkle, J., Baudis, M., et al. (2016). PKCalpha and HMGB1 antagonistically control hydrogen peroxide-induced poly-ADP-ribose formation. *Nucleic Acids Res.* 44, 7630–7645. doi: 10.1093/nar/gkw442

Benito, S., Sanchez-Ortega, A., Unceta, N., Jansen, J. J., Postma, G., Andrade, F., et al. (2018). Plasma biomarker discovery for early chronic kidney disease diagnosis based on chemometric approaches using LC-QTOF targeted metabolomics data. *J. Pharm. Biomed. Anal.* 149, 46–56. doi: 10.1016/j.jpba.2017.10.036

Cavia-Saiz, M., Busto, M. D., Pilar-Izquierdo, M. C., Ortega, N., Perez-Mateos, M., and Muniz, P. (2010). Antioxidant properties, radical scavenging activity and biomolecule protection capacity of flavonoid naringenin and its glycoside naringin: a comparative study. *J. Sci. Food Agric.* 90, 1238–1244. doi: 10.1002/jsfa.3959

Chen, T., Li, J., Chen, J., Song, H., and Yang, C. (2015). Anti-hyperplasia effects of *Rosa rugosa* polyphenols in rats with hyperplasia of mammary gland. *Environ. Toxicol. Pharmacol.* 39, 990–996. doi: 10.1016/j.etap.2015.02.014

Chen, Y., Nie, Y. C., Luo, Y. L., Lin, F., Zheng, Y. F., Cheng, G. H., et al. (2013). Protective effects of naringin against paraquat-induced acute lung injury and pulmonary fibrosis in mice. *Food Chem. Toxicol.* 58, 133–140. doi: 10.1016/j.fct.2013.04.024

Chen, Y. W., Tsai, M. Y., Pan, H. B., Tseng, H. H., Hung, Y. T., and Chou, C. P. (2014). Gadoxetic acid-enhanced MRI and sonoelastography: non-invasive assessments of chemoprevention of liver fibrosis in thioacetamide-induced rats with Sho-Saiko-To. *PLoS One* 9:e114756. doi: 10.1371/journal.pone.0114756

Das Gupta, S., So, J. Y., Wall, B., Wahler, J., Smolarek, A. K., Sae-Tan, S., et al. (2015). Tocopherols inhibit oxidative and nitrosative stress in estrogen-induced early mammary hyperplasia in ACI rats. *Mol. Carcinog.* 54, 916–925. doi: 10.1002/mc.22164

Fan, Y., Pei, X., Liu, Z., Xia, Z., Zhang, D., Song, A., et al. (2013). Effectiveness of external Sanjierupi Gao on mastalgia caused by mammary gland hyperplasia: a placebo controlled trial. *J. Tradit. Chin. Med.* 33, 603–607. doi: 10.1016/S0254-6272(14)60028-5

Henry, N. L. (2014). Endocrine therapy toxicity: management options. *Am. Soc. Clin. Oncol. Educ. Book* e25–e30. doi: 10.14694/EdBook_AM.2014.34.e25

Holloway, R. W., Bogachev, O., Bharadwaj, A. G., McCluskey, G. D., Majdalawieh, A. F., Zhang, L., et al. (2012). Stromal adipocyte enhancer-binding protein (AEBP1) promotes mammary epithelial cell hyperplasia via proinflammatory and hedgehog signaling. *J. Biol. Chem.* 287, 39171–39181. doi: 10.1074/jbc.M112.404293

Huang, J., Tang, H., Cao, S., He, Y., Feng, Y., Wang, K., et al. (2017). Molecular targets and associated potential pathways of Danlu capsules in hyperplasia of mammary glands based on systems pharmacology. *Evid. Based Complement. Alternat. Med.* 2017:1930598. doi: 10.1155/2017/1930598

Ilavenil, S., Kim da, H., Srigopalram, S., Arasu, M. V., Lee, K. D., Lee, J. C., et al. (2016). Potential application of p-coumaric acid on differentiation of C2C12 skeletal muscle and 3T3-L1 preadipocytes-an in vitro and in silico approach. *Molecules* 21:E997. doi: 10.3390/molecules21080997

Kamaraj, S., Vinodhkumar, R., Anandakumar, P., Jagan, S., Ramakrishnan, G., and Devaki, T. (2007). The effects of quercetin on antioxidant status and tumor markers in the lung and serum of mice treated with benzo(a)pyrene. *Biol. Pharm. Bull.* 30, 2268–2273. doi: 10.1248/bpb.30.2268

Kopach, O., Viatchenko-Karpinski, V., Atianjoh, F. E., Belan, P., Tao, Y. X., and Voitenko, N. (2013). PKCalpha is required for inflammation-induced trafficking of extrasynaptic AMPA receptors in tonically firing lamina II dorsal horn neurons during the maintenance of persistent inflammatory pain. *J. Pain* 14, 182–192. doi: 10.1016/j.jpain.2012.10.015

Li, X., Xin, P., Wang, C., Wang, Z., Wang, Q., and Kuang, H. (2017a). Mechanisms of traditional Chinese medicine in the treatment of mammary gland hyperplasia. *Am. J. Chin. Med.* 45, 443–458. doi: 10.1142/S0192415X 17500276

Li, X., Zhang, A., Sun, H., Liu, Z., Zhang, T., Qiu, S., et al. (2017b). Metabolic characterization and pathway analysis of berberine protects against prostate cancer. *Oncotarget* 8, 65022–65041. doi: 10.18632/oncotarget. 17531

Li, Y., Zhang, D., He, Y., Chen, C., Song, C., Zhao, Y., et al. (2017c). Investigation of novel metabolites potentially involved in the pathogenesis of coronary heart disease using a UHPLC-QTOF/MS-based metabolomics approach. *Sci. Rep.* 7:15357. doi: 10.1038/s41598-017-15737-3

Liu, P., Shang, E. X., Zhu, Y., Yu, J. G., Qian, D. W., and Duan, J. A. (2017). Comparative analysis of compatibility effects on invigorating blood circulation for cyperi rhizoma series of herb pairs using untargeted metabolomics. *Front. Pharmacol.* 8:677. doi: 10.3389/fphar.2017.00677

Lopez-Ibanez, J., Pazos, F., and Chagoyen, M. (2016). MBROLE 2.0-functional enrichment of chemical compounds. *Nucleic Acids Res.* 44, W201–W204. doi: 10.1093/nar/gkw253

Navas-Carrillo, D., Rodriguez, J. M., Montoro-Garcia, S., and Orenes-Pinero, E. (2017). High-resolution proteomics and metabolomics in thyroid cancer: deciphering novel biomarkers. *Crit. Rev. Clin. Lab. Sci.* 54, 446–457. doi: 10. 1080/10408363.2017.1394266

Qian, L. Q., Pei, X. H., Xu, Z. Y., and Wang, C. (2007). Clinical observation on treatment of hyperplasia of mammary gland by Lirukang Granule. *Chin. J. Integr. Med.* 13, 120–124. doi: 10.1007/s11655-007-0120-y

Su, G., Wang, H., Gao, Y., Chen, G., Pei, Y., and Bai, J. (2017). ^{1}H-NMR-based metabonomics of the protective effect of *Coptis chinensis* and berberine on cinnabar-induced hepatotoxicity and nephrotoxicity in rats. *Molecules* 22:1855. doi: 10.3390/molecules22111855

Tan, M. A., Takayama, H., Aimi, N., Kitajima, M., Franzblau, S. G., and Nonato, M. G. (2008). Antitubercular triterpenes and phytosterols from *Pandanus tectorius* Soland. var. *laevis*. *J. Nat. Med.* 62, 232–235. doi: 10.1007/s11418-007-0218-8

Villasenor, I. M., Angelada, J., Canlas, A. P., and Echegoyen, D. (2002). Bioactivity studies on beta-sitosterol and its glucoside. *Phytother. Res.* 16, 417–421. doi: 10.1002/ptr.910

Wang, L., Zhao, D., Di, L., Cheng, D., Zhou, X., Yang, X., et al. (2011). The anti-hyperplasia of mammary gland effect of *Thladiantha dubia* root ethanol extract in rats reduced by estrogen and progestogen. *J. Ethnopharmacol.* 134, 136–140. doi: 10.1016/j.jep.2010.11.071

Wang, N., Zhao, G., Zhang, Y., Wang, X., Zhao, L., Xu, P., et al. (2017). A network pharmacology approach to determine the active components and potential targets of *Curculigo orchioides* in the treatment of osteoporosis. *Med. Sci. Monit.* 23, 5113–5122. doi: 10.12659/MSM.904264

Xu, T., Pi, Z., Liu, S., Song, F., and Liu, Z. (2017). Chemical profiling combined with "omics" technologies (CP-Omics): a strategy to understand the compatibility mechanisms and simplify herb formulas in traditional Chinese medicines. *Phytochem. Anal.* 28, 381–391. doi: 10.1002/pca.2685

Zhang, G., Li, D., Guo, H., Ma, Y., Liao, R., Tan, B., et al. (2012). Modulation of expression of p16 and her2 in rat breast tissues of mammary hyperplasia model by external use of rupifang extract. *J. Tradit. Chin. Med.* 32, 651–656. doi: 10.1016/S0254-6272(13)60087-4

Zhang, L. J., Song, A. F., Wang, Z. H., and Lu, Y. (2008). Effects of the needling method for regulating kidney and smoothing liver on endocrine and immune functions in the patient with hyperplasia of mammary glands. *Zhongguo Zhen Jiu* 28, 648–652.

11

Antibacterial Activity and Mechanism of Action of Aspidinol Against Multi-Drug-Resistant Methicillin-Resistant *Staphylococcus aureus*

Xin Hua[1†], Qin Yang[1†], Wanjiang Zhang[1], Zhimin Dong[2], Shenye Yu[1], Stefan Schwarz[3] and Siguo Liu[1]*

[1] Division of Bacterial Diseases, State Key Laboratory of Veterinary Biotechnology, Harbin Veterinary Research Institute, Chinese Academy of Agricultural Sciences, Harbin, China, [2] Tianjin Animal Science and Veterinary Research Institute, Tianjin, China, [3] Institute of Microbiology and Epizootics, Department of Veterinary Medicine, Freie Universität Berlin, Berlin, Germany

***Correspondence:**
Siguo Liu
liusiguo@caas.cn

† These authors have contributed equally to this work.

This study aimed at investigating the antibacterial activity of aspidinol, an extract from *Dryopteris fragrans* (L.) Schott, against methicillin-resistant *Staphylococcus aureus* (MRSA). MRSA isolates were treated with aspidinol to determine the differential expression of genes and associated pathways following the drug treatment. Aspidinol displayed significant anti-MRSA activity, both *in vivo* (minimum inhibitory concentration = 2 μg/mL) and *in vitro*, and achieved an antibacterial effect comparable to that of vancomycin. In the lethal septicemic mouse study, a dose of 50 mg/kg of either aspidinol or vancomycin provided significant protection from mortality. In the non-lethal septicemic mouse study, aspidinol and vancomycin produced a significant reduction in mean bacterial load in murine organs, including the spleen, lung, and liver. After treatment with aspidinol, we found through RNA-seq and RT-PCR experiments that the inhibition of the formation of ribosomes was the primary *S. aureus* cell-killing mechanism, and the inhibition of amino acid synthesis and the reduction of virulence factors might play a secondary role.

Keywords: aspidinol, anti-MRSA activity, antimicrobial mechanism, RNA-seq, inhibit ribosomes synthesis

INTRODUCTION

Methicillin-resistant *Staphylococcus aureus* (MRSA) is the most common pathogen and is associated with high morbidity and mortality in both humans and animals (VanEperen and Segreti, 2016). MRSA causes nosocomial infections, pneumonia (Woods and Colice, 2014), sepsis (Taylor, 2013), and skin infections (Mihu et al., 2015). In January 2017, MRSA was officially ranked as one of the 12 deadliest drug-resistant bacteria by WHO (2017). Antibiotics are the most effective tool to combat infections due to pathogenic bacteria. While new antimicrobial agents are becoming increasingly difficult to develop, medicine is currently unable to keep pace with the emergence of resistant bacteria (Rennie, 2012). Therefore, it is imperative to develop new agents to fight resistant bacteria, especially MRSA.

Natural products are alternative tools in the fight against drug-resistant bacteria, and synthetic approaches are unable to replace natural products (Guzman et al., 2010; Vandal et al., 2015; Farah et al., 2016). Chinese herb *Dryopteris fragrans* (L.) Schott is a deciduous perennial herbaceous plant of *Dryopteris*, it is widely distributed in many countries and is mainly grown in northeast of China (Zhong et al., 2017). As a traditional Chinese herb medicine, *D. fragrans* was used to treat a variety of diseases, especially skin diseases such as psoriasis, rashes, dermatitis, and beriberi (Huang et al., 2014). Recently, there are also reports of the antibacterial (Gao et al., 2016), anti-tumor (Zhang et al., 2012), anti-inflammatory, and antifungal activity of its extracts (Huang et al., 2014; Peng et al., 2016). Aspidinol is a phloroglucinol derivative from the stem and leaf of traditional *D. fragrans* (Zhao et al., 2014; Gao et al., 2016). To date, the research on aspidinol has been rather limited; only one publication has reported that it has anti-cancer activity (Zhao et al., 2014).

In this study, aspidinol was found to be an effective anti-MRSA agent. We have verified that aspidinol efficiently cleared intracellular bacteria and exhibited excellent *in vivo* activity, which indicated its potential for application as an antibacterial agent to treat systemic MRSA infections. Building upon this seminal work, we investigated the anti-MRSA mechanism of aspidinol. RNA-seq demonstrated that aspidinol appears to interfere with multiple biological pathways in *S. aureus* and that this interference ultimately results in the killing of MRSA.

Herein, we report for the first time the validation process of the anti-MRSA activity of aspidinol and identify its mode of action. All of the findings strongly verified the potential therapeutic application of aspidinol as a novel antibacterial agent.

MATERIALS AND METHODS

Strains and Growth Conditions

The *S. aureus* strains ATCC 29213 and ATCC 33591 (MRSA) were obtained from the American Type Culture Collection. The clinical MSSA and MRSA isolates used in this study were provided by the First Affiliated Hospital of Harbin Medical University, Harbin, China. A complete list of bacterial strains used in this study can be found in **Supplementary Table S1**. All strains were maintained in Mueller-Hinton broth (MHB, Oxoid, Basingstoke, United Kingdom), frozen at −80°C until use, and cultured in MHB at 37°C under aerobic conditions.

Antimicrobial Agents

Aspidinol, vancomycin, and linezolid were purchased from Sigma-Aldrich (Bornem, Belgium). Aspidinol was stored in DMSO at −20°C. All antibiotics were dissolved in ultrapure water.

Minimum Inhibitory Concentration and Minimum Bactericidal Concentration

Broth microdilution was used to determine the minimum inhibitory concentration (MIC) according to CLSI standards M07-A9. The test medium used for most species was MHB, and the cell concentration was adjusted to approximately 5×10^5 cells/mL. After 20 h of incubation at 35 ± 2°C, the MIC was read as the lowest concentration of antibiotic that inhibited visible growth of the bacteria. The minimum bactericidal concentration (MBC) was defined as the lowest concentration of aspidinol to kill *S. aureus* ATCC 33591 cells. *S. aureus* ATCC 33591 cells from the MIC assays were resuspended in fresh media and plated onto Mueller-Hinton agar (MHA). After incubating for 24 h at 37°C, the colonies were enumerated. All experiments were performed with three replicates.

Time-Dependent Killing

An overnight culture of cells (*S. aureus* ATCC 33591) was diluted 1:5,000 in MHB and incubated at 37°C at 220 r.p.m. for 2 h after overnight culture. The bacteria cells were then treated with aspidinol, linezolid, or vancomycin at a concentration of 10 × MIC. One milliliter aliquots were removed at 2, 4, 6, 8, 12, 24, and 48 h, and 1 mL of MHB was added as a replacement. The suspension was centrifuged at 10,000 *g* for 1 min, and the pellet was resuspended in 100 mL of sterile PBS buffer. The diluted suspensions were plated onto MHA plates and incubated at 37°C overnight for CFU calculation. All experiments were performed with three replicates.

Cytotoxicity Assay

Macrophage cells (RAW264.7) were seeded at a density of 10,000 cells per well into a 96-well cell culture plate (NEST, Nest Biotech Co. Ltd, NJ, United States) and incubated overnight at 37°C in DMEM media containing 10% fetal bovine serum (FBS). Cells were then treated with aspidinol for 24 h at different concentrations ranging from 0 to 128 μg/mL. The treated cells were washed four times with PBS, and DMEM media containing the MTS assay reagent, 3-(4,5-dimethylthiazol-2-yl)-5-(3carboxymethoxyphenyl)-2-(4-sulfophenyl)-2H-tetrazolium) (Promega, Madison, WI, United States) was then added. After 4 h of incubation at 37°C, the absorbance was measured using an ELISA microplate reader (Molecular Devices, Sunnyvale, CA, United States). The percent cell viability of the aspidinol-treated cells was calculated.

Intracellular Infection Assay

After overnight incubation, macrophage cells (RAW 264.7) were infected with MRSA ATCC 33591 for 30 min at a multiplicity of infection (MOI) ratio of 100:1. The infected cells were then washed three times with DMEM medium containing 10 IU lysostaphin. Aspidinol (20 μg/mL), vancomycin (20 μg/mL), or linezolid (10 μg/mL) were added in complete DMEM medium containing 4 IU lysostaphin, which was then used to incubate the infected cells at 37°C (with 5% CO_2). After 24 h, the cells were washed three times with PBS and lysed with 0.1% Triton X-100 (Sigma-Aldrich). The cell lysates were plated onto MHA plates and incubated for 24 h at 37°C, followed by CFU determination.

Biofilm Assay

Staphylococcus aureus ATCC 33591 was cultured in tryptic soy broth containing 1% glucose. A biofilm formed after 24 h of incubation at 37°C. The medium was then removed, and the biofilm washed with PBS. The drugs at a concentration of 10 × MIC were added and incubated for an additional 24 h at 37°C. The 96-well plates were washed again, and the biofilms were stained with 0.1% (wt/vol) crystal violet. The 96-well plates were washed and air-dried, and finally, the biofilm mass was dissolved using 95% ethanol. A microplate reader (Bio-Tek Instruments, Inc., United States) was used to measure the intensity of crystal violet. The data were presented as the percent of biofilm mass reduction in the treated groups in relation to the control group.

Scanning Electron Microscopy

The method of biofilm formation was carried out as described above on a glass coverslip in 24-well plates. The formed biofilm was fixed with 2.5% glutaraldehyde in 0.1 M sodium cacodylate buffer (pH 7.2) at 4°C for 10 min and then washed three times with PBS. Next, the biofilm was fixed with 1% osmic acid at room temperature for 10 min. Gradual dehydration was then carried out with ethyl alcohol (60, 70, 80, 90, 95, and 100%), and tertiary butanol was used as a displacement liquid (60, 70, 80, 90, 95, and 100%). Finally, the samples were freeze-dried overnight. The specimens were then sputter coated with gold for observation using a JSM 7500 (JEOL, Tokyo, Japan).

Mouse Studies

Eight-week-old female BALB/c mice (Vital River, Beijing, China) were used in all of the mouse studies. The animal experiments were performed in accordance with the animal ethics guidelines and approved protocols. The animal experiment was approved by the Animal Ethics Committee of Harbin Veterinary Research Institute of the Chinese Academy of Agricultural Sciences.

Systemic Lethal Infection

An overnight culture of *S. aureus* ATCC 33591 cells was washed and resuspended in PBS. Each mouse received an intraperitoneal (i.p.) injection (200 μL) containing the bacterial suspension (9×10^9 CFU). One hour after infection, the mice were divided into seven groups (10 mice per group). The mice were intravenously injected with either aspidinol or vancomycin (5, 15, or 25 mg/kg) or the vehicle alone (10% ethanol). The treatment was provided once daily for 3 days following infection. Mortality was monitored daily for 5 days, and the moribund mice were euthanized using CO_2 asphyxiation.

Systemic Non-lethal Infection

The infection protocol was carried out as described above (systemic lethal infection) with the following exceptions. Each mouse received an i.p. injection containing 2×10^7 CFU *S. aureus* ATCC 33591. The mice were divided into three groups (16 mice per group) and intravenously injected with either aspidinol, vancomycin (25 mg/kg), or vehicle (10% ethanol). The mice were treated once daily for 6 days. The mice were euthanized 24 h after the last administration, and the organs (including heart, lung, kidney, spleen, and liver) were excised, homogenized in MHA, and finally incubated at 37°C for 24 h for MRSA CFU counting. For evaluation of the extent of tissue damage and cellular response, histological analyses were also performed. Mice from the control group, vancomycin group, and aspidinol group that underwent the same infection protocol as the systemic non-lethal infection were submitted to histopathology examination after 6 days. The following organs were collected from each animal: heart, liver, spleen, lung, and kidneys. The tissues were fixed with 4% paraformaldehyde and then stained with hematoxylin–eosin.

RNA-Seq Transcriptomics

Staphylococcus aureus ATCC 33591 was grown to an OD_{600} of 0.4 from an initial absorbance of 0.01, and aspidinol was added to a final sub-MIC concentration (1 μg/mL). Samples were collected at 1-h post treatment and preserved with RNA protect (Qiagen, United States) following the manufacturer's instructions. Cells were pelleted by centrifugation at 5,000 *g* for 10 min at 4°C. The RNA was isolated using an RNeasy minikit (Qiagen, United States) in accordance with the manufacturer's instructions, with the following additions. The cell pellets were homogenized in 1 mL Tris-buffered saline (TBS) (20 mM Tris, pH 7.5) containing 0.4 mg of lysostaphin and incubated at 37°C for 15 min. Subsequently, 20 mg of lysozyme in TE buffer (20 mM Tris, pH 7.5, 2 mM EDTA, pH 7.8) was added, and the sample was incubated at 25°C for 10 min. Control samples were collected from an antibiotic-free culture, and each experiment was repeated three times.

Three independently prepared RNA samples from each strain were used for RNA-Seq. Illumina sequencing was performed by Shanghai Majorbio Bio-pharm Technology Co., Ltd. (Shanghai, China) using the Illumina Hiseq2000 Truseq SBS Kit v3-HS (200 cycles) and Miseq Reagent Kit V2 (500 cycle/600 cycle) (Illumina, Inc.). The data analyses were performed using edgeR software. Genes exhibiting twofold changes in expression, which were statistically significant as determined by Student's *t*-test ($p < 0.05$), were considered to be differentially expressed under the conditions indicated.

Real-Time PCR

To confirm the RNA-Seq data, we selected some genes that were downregulated and assessed their relative expression levels by real-time PCR. *S. aureus* ATCC 33591 cells were cultured in the same conditions as the RNA-Seq transcriptomics experiments. qRT-PCR was performed by a two-step process. These reactions were performed using the Applied qTOWER 2.2 (Analytik Jena, Jena, Germany) Real-Time PCR System by using the following cycle parameters: 95°C for 5 min, followed by 40 cycles of 95°C for 15 s, 55°C for 15 s, and 72°C for 15 s; and one dissociation step of 95°C for 1 min, 55°C for 30 s, and 95°C for 30 s. All measurements were independently conducted three times on two separate biological isolates. All of the primers and sequences are listed in **Supplementary Table S2.**

The melting curve analysis was performed immediately after amplification to verify the specificity of the PCR amplification products. Fluorescence was measured at the end of the annealing-extension phase of each cycle. A threshold value for the fluorescence of all samples was manually set. The reaction cycle at which the PCR product exceeds this fluorescence threshold was identified as the threshold cycle (CT). The relative quantitation was calculated by the $2^{-\Delta\Delta}$CT method.

Statistical Analysis

Statistical analyses were carried out using GraphPad Prism 5.0 (Graph Pad Software, LaJolla, CA). One-way model ANOVA was performed between the groups. In ANOVA, the observed variance is partitioned into components due to different explanatory variables. A level of $p < 0.05$ was considered to be statistically significant.

RESULTS

Antibacterial Activity of Aspidinol

The antimicrobial activity of aspidinol was tested against clinical isolates of *S. aureus*, including drug-resistant strains, the MICs and MBCs of which are given in **Table 1**. Aspidinol showed potent bactericidal activity against MSSA and MRSA, with MICs and MBCs ranging from 0.25 to 2 μg/mL and 0.5 to 4 μg/mL, respectively.

After confirming that aspidinol possessed excellent antimicrobial activity against *S. aureus*, we next assessed the killing kinetics of aspidinol. As depicted in **Figure 1A**, aspidinol also showed excellent bactericidal activity against *S. aureus*.

Cytotoxicity of Aspidinol

Cytotoxicity tests indicated that the toxicity of aspidinol toward macrophage cells (RAW264.7) was negligible. At 128 μg/mL, i.e., the highest dose tested, aspidinol showed no toxicity to RAW264.7 cells. The dose response curve of aspidinol in the cytotoxicity assay can be found in **Supplementary Figure S2**.

Aspidinol Efficiently Clears Intracellular Bacteria

Eliminating intercellular *S. aureus* has long been considered to be key to clinical success because *S. aureus* is capable of entering multiple mammalian cells, thereby evading the antibiotic therapy. The ability to internalize into mammalian cells might result in the long-term colonization of the host and explain clinical failures. Lehar et al. have confirmed this hypothesis, showing that three major antibiotics commonly used for clinical standard care (vancomycin, daptomycin, and linezolid) failed to kill the highly virulent community-acquired *S. aureus* ATCC 33591 strain (Lehar et al., 2015).

As aspidinol exhibited potent anti-MRSA activity, we explored the ability of aspidinol to permeate cellular membranes and kill MRSA located inside eukaryotic cells. To investigate the efficacy of aspidinol in eliminating intracellular MRSA, macrophage cells (RAW264.7) infected with *S. aureus* ATCC 33591 were employed. As depicted in **Figure 1B**, intracellular *S. aureus* ATCC 33591 exposed to aspidinol (20 μg/mL) were efficiently killed, and the intracellular bacteria decreased by 100-fold. In contrast, conventional antibiotics such as linezolid (20 μg/mL) and vancomycin (10 μg/mL) were shown to reduce the bacterial burden inside the infected macrophages by 5- to 10-fold. From the above data, aspidinol was confirmed to be capable of eradicating MRSA infection in macrophage cells.

Inhibitory Effect of Aspidinol on MRSA Biofilm Formation

The biofilms were stained with crystal violet after treatment with aspidinol, and the absorbance was measured at 570 nm for mass estimation. Compared to linezolid and vancomycin, aspidinol was not able to significantly reduce adherent biofilms of *S. aureus* ATCC 33591. At a concentration of 256 μg/mL, which corresponds to the 128-fold MIC, aspidinol reduced the biofilm mass by approximately by 30%. The control antibiotics, linezolid (256 μg/mL, i.e., 128-fold MIC) and vancomycin (128 μg/mL, i.e., 128-fold MIC), were able to reduce the biofilm mass by only 20% (**Figure 2A**).

The morphology of *S. aureus* ATCC 33591 biofilms on the surface of coverslips was observed using scanning electron microscope (SEM). Under a 2,000-fold magnification, the biofilm was shown to be composed of many multilayered MRSA colonies. The SEM analysis results were consistent with those of the crystal violet staining observations. At a concentration of 256 μg/mL of aspidinol, linezolid, and vancomycin, we observed a decrease in density of the MRSA biofilms (**Figure 2B**).

In Vivo Efficacy of Aspidinol

To determine the role of aspidinol against MRSA *in vivo*, both a lethal and a non-lethal systemic MRSA infection model were used. In the lethal systemic study, mice were infected intraperitoneally with MRSA ATCC 33591 (2.95×10^9 CFU per mouse). Both aspidinol and vancomycin provided significant protection from mortality (**Figure 3A**). The survival rate of infected mice varied in a concentration-dependent manner, with the survival rate improving dramatically when the dose of aspidinol increased. Approximately 80% of mice that received a higher dose of aspidinol (25 mg/kg) survived for 5 days. These results exhibited the *in vivo* activity of aspidinol in protecting mice from septicemic MRSA infection.

Next, the efficacy of aspidinol against MRSA ATCC 33591 in a non-lethal model was investigated. In brief, mice were first infected with a non-lethal dose of MRSA ATCC 33951 (4.20×10^7 CFU/mouse), and then each group of mice received two oral doses of aspidinol, vancomycin (25 mg/kg), or the vehicle alone. As depicted in **Figure 3B**, aspidinol and vancomycin produced a significant reduction in mean bacterial load in different organs. In particular, both treatments reduced the mean bacterial load by more than 1000-fold in the lung. The histopathological inspection 6 days after infection with the non-lethal dose of MRSA ATCC 33951 revealed no changes in the heart, spleen, and kidney. While the animals showed moderate histopathological alterations in lung and liver in the control

TABLE 1 | MIC and MBC of aspidinol against *Staphylococcus* strains.

Strains	Aspidinol	Oxacillin	Aspidinol	Oxacillin
	MIC (μg/mL)		MBC (μg/mL)	
MSSA standard strain ATCC 29213	0.5	0.25	1	0.5
MSSA clinical isolates (20 isolates)	0.25–2	0.25–1	0.25–4	0.5–2
MRSA standard strain ATCC 33591	2	128	4	>128
MRSA clinical isolates (19 isolates)	0.5–2	32 to >128	1–8	64 to >128

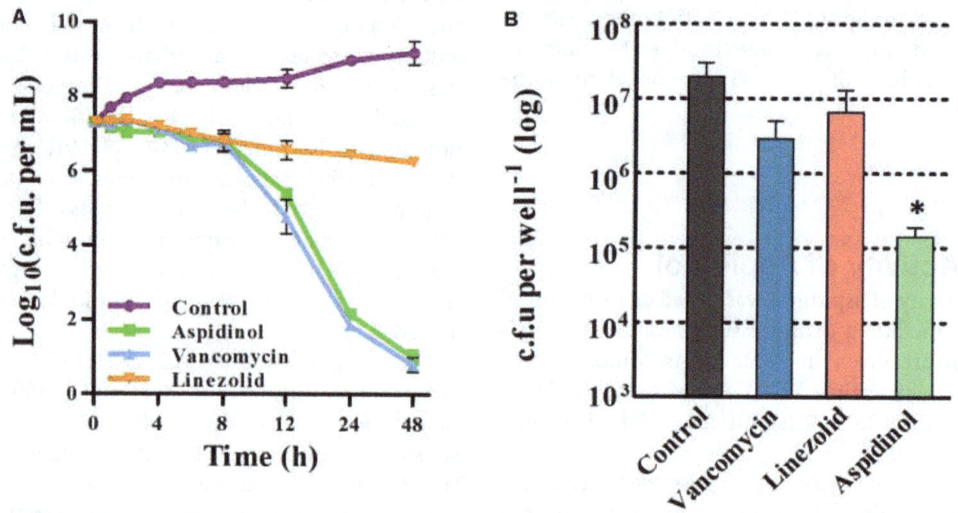

FIGURE 1 | Time-kill analysis and the intracellular bacterial killing activity of aspidinol. **(A)** Time-kill kinetics of aspidinol against *S. aureus* ATCC 33591. The error bars show the standard deviations of the results from three independent biological repeats. **(B)** *S. aureus* ATCC 33591-infected RAW264.7 cells were treated with aspidinol and control antibiotics (vancomycin or linezolid) for 24 h, and the percent bacterial reduction was calculated compared to that of the untreated control groups. The results are given as the mean ± SD (n = 3). Two-tailed Student's t-test was employed, and *p-values of ≤0.05 are considered to be significant.

group, after treatment with aspidinol or vancomycin, there were no obvious histopathological alterations (**Figure 3C**).

RNA-Seq

To better understand the mechanism of the anti-MRSA effect of aspidinol, the underlying differential expression of MRSA genes was analyzed after treatment with aspidinol.

A heatmap and volcano plot analyses revealed the differential gene expression for both untreated and treated MRSA (**Figures 4A,B**). A total of 2952 genes were identified; among these, 1147 genes were upregulated and 1183 were downregulated during aspidinol treatment. After quantile normalization of the FPKM values followed by Student's t-test at $p = 0.05$ and the selection of DEGs with at least a twofold change in their expression in response to aspidinol treatment, we identified 949 DEGs (456 upregulated and 493 downregulated) with highly significant expression patterns before and after the treatment. All the sequencing reads have been submitted to the NCBI short-read archive (SRA) with accession number SRP129492.

KEGG Pathway Analysis of the DEGs

KEGG pathway analysis was used to further clarify the biological function of aspidinol. Overall, DEGs were significantly enriched in 55 KEGG pathways, meeting the criteria of p-values <0.05 (**Figure 4C**, more clearer pictures can be found in **Supplementary Figure S1**). The KEGG pathways that showed the highest levels of significance were the lysine biosynthesis pathway (ko00300), the valine, leucine, and isoleucine biosynthesis pathways (ko00290), nitrogen metabolism (ko00910), galactose metabolism (ko00052), carbon metabolism (ko01200), and amino sugar and nucleotide sugar metabolism (ko00520), suggesting that these pathways may play important roles in the antibacterial processes of aspidinol.

Genes Involved in the Synthesis of Amino Acid

The analysis of genes downregulated by aspidinol in *S. aureus* ATCC 33591 showed a significant decrease in the expression of the genes involved in the synthesis of amino acids. The synthesis of amino acids is important for the survival of bacteria. Related genes that act in the synthesis of valine, leucine, isoleucine, and lysine were downregulated after treatment with aspidinol. Genes encoding important intermediates in amino acid synthesis, such as *ilvC* and *ilvD*, were also downregulated 3.47- and 4.73-fold, respectively. In addition, the leucine synthesis genes *leuABCD* were also downregulated 2.6-, 3.08-, 2.58-, and 2.49-fold, respectively. The gene *lysC*, which encodes an aspartate kinase, was downregulated 5.77-fold. In addition to amino acid biosynthesis, genes involved

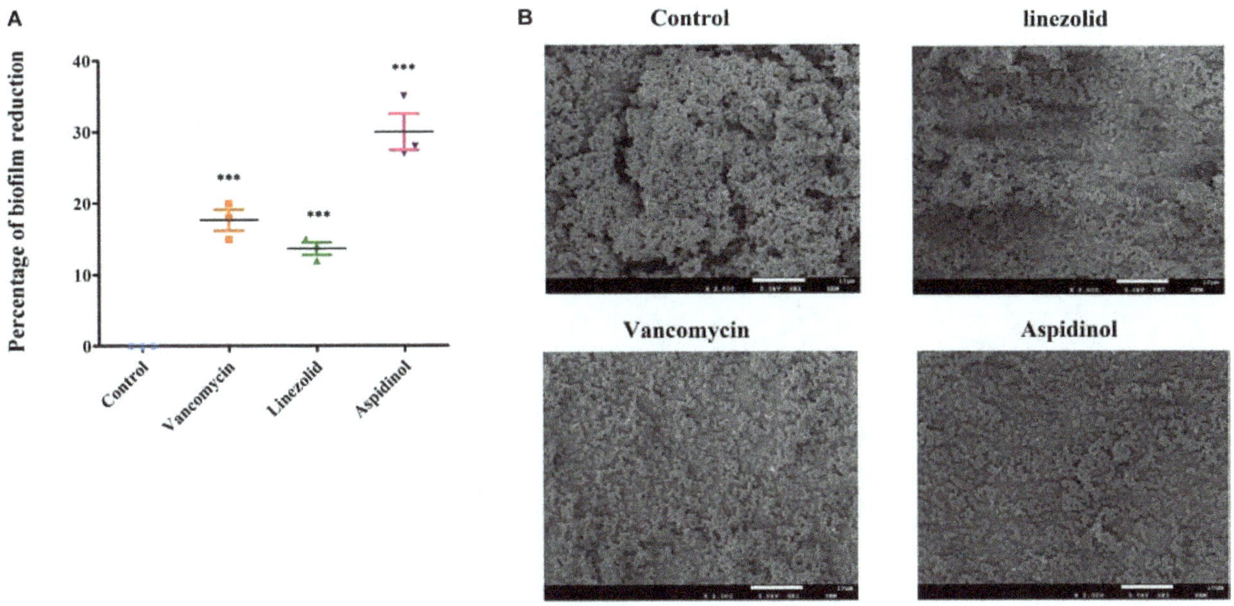

FIGURE 2 | Anti-biofilm activity of aspidinol. **(A)** The effects of aspidinol and antibiotics (linezolid and vancomycin) on established biofilms of *S. aureus* ATCC 33591 were evaluated. The pre-formed biofilms were treated with linezolid, vancomycin, or aspidinol and then stained with crystal violet. The optical density of the dissolved crystal violet was measured using a spectrophotometer. The values are the mean of the triplicate samples with standard deviation bars. The results are given as the mean ± SD (n = 3). Two-tailed Student's t-test was employed, and *** means p-values $\leq$ 0.005. **(B)** Scanning electron microscopy images showing the structure of MRSA biofilms treated with aspidinol and antibiotics at 24 h. Magnifications, ×2000.

in peptide import were also significantly downregulated. The genes *oppABCDF*, encoding a peptide transport system, were downregulated 1.15-, 7.37-, 3.68-, 2.30-, and 1.40-fold, respectively.

Genes Involved in Ribosome Synthesis

Four genes involved in structural components of ribosomes, 30S ribosomal protein S20 *rpsT* (−4.01-fold), 50S ribosomal protein L1 *rplA* (−4.34-fold), L20 *rplT* (−4.11-fold), and L32 (−2.33-fold), were downregulated after treatment with aspidinol. Nevertheless, three genes involved in structural components of ribosomes, 30S ribosomal protein S11 *rpsK* (2.3-fold), 50S ribosomal protein L17 *rplQ* (2.33-fold), and L7/L12 *SAV1268* (2.22-fold) were upregulated. In addition, some genes involved in ribosome synthesis were significantly changed. The gene expression of the ribosomal large subunit pseudouridine synthase D *rluD*, ribosomal-protein-serine N-acetyltransferase *rimL*, and ribosome-binding factor A *rbfA* decreased by 4.66-, 2.82−, and 2.9-fold, respectively. The ribosomal subunit interface protein *SAV0752* and ribosomal large subunit pseudouridine synthase B *SAV1493* were increased by 4.21- and 2.32-fold, respectively.

Repression of Genes Involved in Iron Transport and Key Virulence Factors

Aspidinol also significantly repressed genes involved in iron ABC transporter synthesis. The constituents of the ferrichrome ABC transporter system comprising *fhuABG* were downregulated by aspidinol 4.93-, 4.12-, and 3.87-fold, respectively. The genes encoding metal iron ABC transport *mtsABC* were downregulated 4.06-, 5.31-, and 8.59-fold, respectively. Heme transporter *IsdA* was downregulated 4.34-fold. After treatment with aspidinol, the repression of key virulence factors, exfoliative toxins *eta* and IgG-binding protein *sbi*, were downregulated 4.82- and 2.82-fold, respectively.

Genes Involved in the Metabolism of Energy

Aspidinol-treated *S. aureus* ATCC 700699 showed an increase in the expression of genes involved in basic metabolic processes, including metabolism of nitrogen, galactose, and carbon. The genes involved in nitrogen metabolism, including *nirBD*, *narGHJ*, and *arc*, were upregulated 5.36-, 4.68-, 4.68-, 3.81-, and 9.91-fold, respectively. The *lacABCDEFG* genes encoding a galactose-6-phosphate isomerase were upregulated 5.68-, 4.28-, 4.22-, 5.72-, 3.6-, 6.22-, and 5.54-fold, respectively. In addition, the carbon metabolism genes *sdaA*, *sdaB*, *lpd*, *prsA*, and *tdcB* were also upregulated 4.29-, 3.67-, 2.84-, 2.75-, and 5.1-fold, respectively.

Genes Involved in β-Lactam Resistance

Most genes related to the β-lactam resistance pathway were significantly downregulated after treatment with aspidinol, including beta-lactamase repressor *blaI*, beta-lactamase regulatory gene *blaR1*, and methicillin resistance regulatory genes *mecI* and *mecR1*, which are key genes attributed to drug resistance of β-lactam antibiotics. After treatment, *blaR1*, *blaI*, *mecR1*, *mecI* were downregulated 5.6-, 4.49-, 3.06-, and 4.35-fold, respectively, relative to their expression in the untreated control.

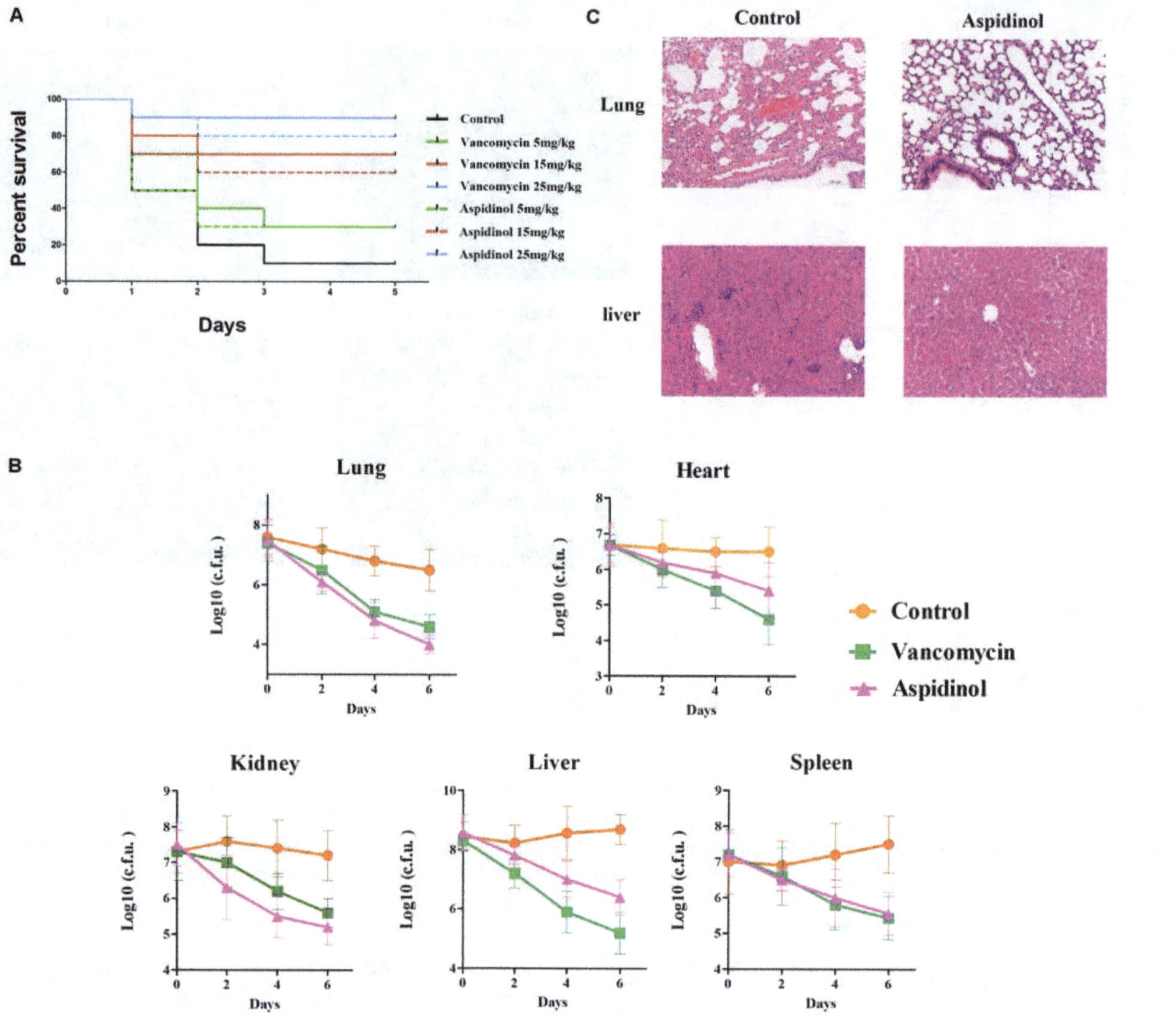

FIGURE 3 | Aspidinol is effective in a mouse model of MRSA septicemic infection. **(A)** Ten mice per group were infected (i.p.) with a lethal dose of *S. aureus* ATCC 33591 and intravenously injected with aspidinol, vancomycin (5, 15, or 25 mg/kg), or the vehicle alone for 5 days (one dose per day). Mice were monitored for 5 days and the percentage survival was calculated. The statistical significance was calculated in order to compare treated to control groups. **(B)** Six mice per group were infected (i.p.) with a non-lethal dose of *S. aureus* ATCC 33591 and intravenously injected with aspidinol, vancomycin (25 mg/kg) or the vehicle alone for 6 days (one dose per day). Twenty-four hours after the last treatment, the mice were euthanized, and their organs were excised and homogenized in TSB to count viable MRSA colonies. The number of CFUs from each mouse is plotted as individual points. Values are the mean of triplicate samples with standard deviation bars. **(C)** Histological evaluation of lung and liver of mice infected with *S. aureus* ATCC 33591 receiving no treatment or a treatment with aspidinol. Both lung and liver in the control group demonstrated acute inflammation; no apparent pathological changes were observed in the treatment group.

RNA-Seq Results Were Verified by qRT-PCR

A qRT-PCR assay was conducted to further validate transcriptional changes induced by aspidinol and observed in the RNA-seq experiments. After treatment with sub-MIC (1 μg/mL) of aspidinol, 30 different genes were chosen, including *oppABCDF*, *fhuABG*, and *ilvBCD* among others (**Figure 5**), to determine changes in their transcript accumulation. There was no obvious variation between qRT-PCR and transcriptomic data in the expression patterns except for *mtsA*. Although the exact fold change difference in expression for each gene by qRT-PCR was different from the RNA-seq data, similar trends were observed, which suggests that there is a relatively high consistency between the RNA-seq and qRT-PCR results.

DISCUSSION

Staphylococcus aureus, in particular MRSA, has acquired numerous antimicrobial resistance genes, rendering these isolates multi-resistant. This development of resistance and multi-resistance is likely to have the effect that the currently available antibiotics will not be as efficacious in the near future (Rodvold

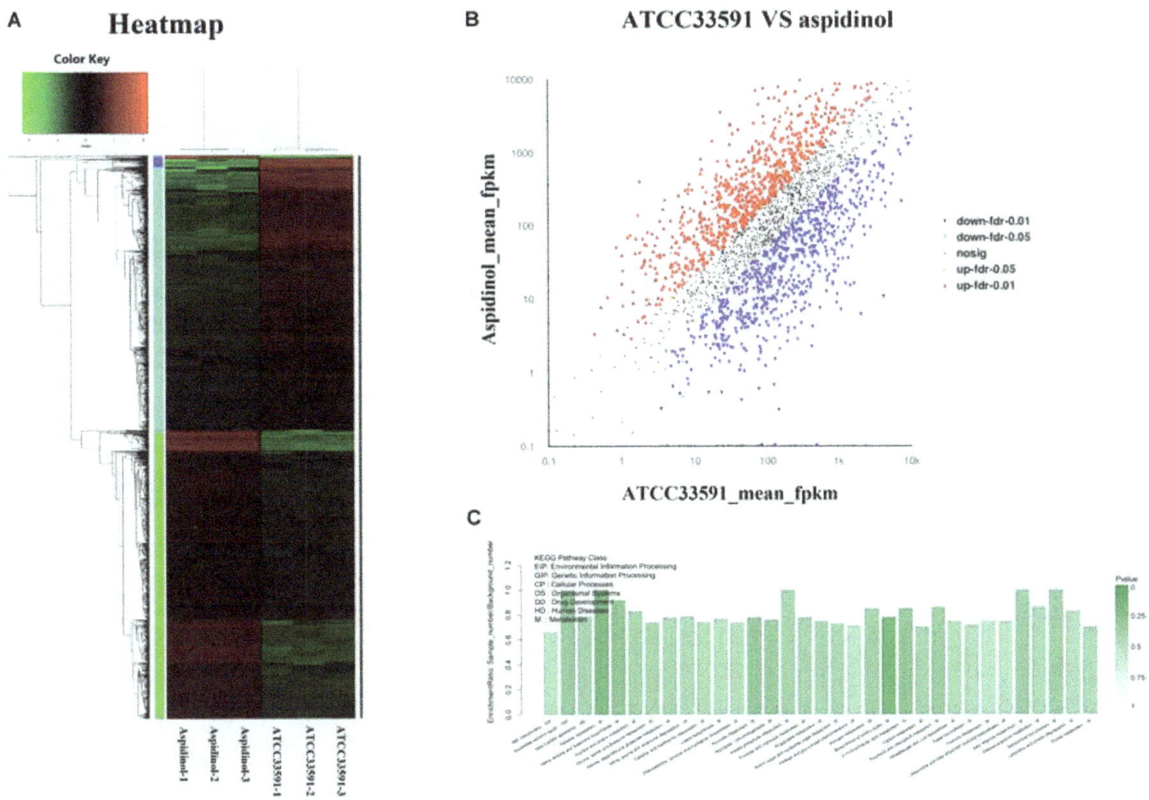

FIGURE 4 | RNA-Seq gene expression results for *S. aureus* ATCC 33591 cells treated and not treated with aspidinol. **(A)** A heatmap generated comparing aspidinol-treated cells to untreated control *S. aureus* ATCC 33591 cells is shown. Triplicate samples were used for each group. **(B)** Volcano plot analyses of unigenes in aspidinol and the ATCC 33591 group. **(C)** Differentially expressed genes enriched in the KEGG pathway.

and McConeghy, 2014; Shenoy et al., 2014; Stahlmann, 2014). Unfortunately, the development of novel antibiotics and their introduction into clinical use cannot keep pace with the emergence of resistant pathogens. Relatedly, pharmaceutical companies have increasingly withdrawn investment in the development of new antimicrobial agents. Despite this situation and the associated challenges to healthcare, new strategies, and alternative methods for anti-infective therapy need to be explored.

In preliminary experiments, aspidinol was chosen as a study object through antibacterial activity screening. Aspidinol exhibited an excellent anti-MRSA activity *in vitro* and no cytotoxicity. Time-kill assays revealed that the anti-MRSA effect of aspidinol was nearly identical to that seen with vancomycin and linezolid. In previous reports of Mu, two analogs of aspidinol, aspidinol C and D, were reported to have significant anti-MRSA activity. The MICs of aspidinol C and D against MRSA were 2 and 4 μg/mL, respectively (The structures of aspidinol, aspidinol C and D can be found in **Supplementary Figure S3**). However, there was no further in-depth study of aspidinol C and D except for determining their MIC value (Mu et al., 2012). Therefore, it could be speculated that aspidinol may also have excellent anti-MRSA activity due to it similar chemical structure. Indeed, compared with aspirinol C and D, aspirinol shows stronger anti-MRSA activity.

Once MRSA internalizes into eukaryotic cells, intracellular persistence will prolong the presence of the pathogen in the host and result in a weakening of the host defenses (Lemaire et al., 2008). Because of their inability to penetrate the cell membranes, most antibiotics, including vancomycin, cannot effectively combat intracellular MRSA (Garzoni and Kelley, 2009; Seleem et al., 2009; Tenover and Goering, 2009; Thangamani et al., 2015). Vancomycin has been reported to have a failure rate of greater than 40% in treating *S. aureus* pneumonia (Rubinstein et al., 2008). In this study, aspidinol exhibited excellent anti-MRSA activity inside macrophages; this activity was 100 times better than that of vancomycin. However, compared to vancomycin and linezolid, aspidinol did not significantly reduce adherent MRSA biofilms. This outcome suggests that aspidinol may be more suitable for systemic MRSA infectious diseases, such as septicemia, rather than skin infections.

The *in vivo* efficacy of aspidinol was assessed in two murine MRSA systemic infection models (non-lethal and lethal). Both the non-lethal and lethal mouse studies confirmed that aspidinol retains its antibacterial activity *in vivo*. The results were consistent with the results of the anti-MRSA activity *in vitro*, proving that aspidinol was able to effectively prevent and treat systemic infections caused by MRSA.

To better understand the pathway of the anti-MRSA effect of aspidinol, RNA-seq experiments were conducted. The analysis

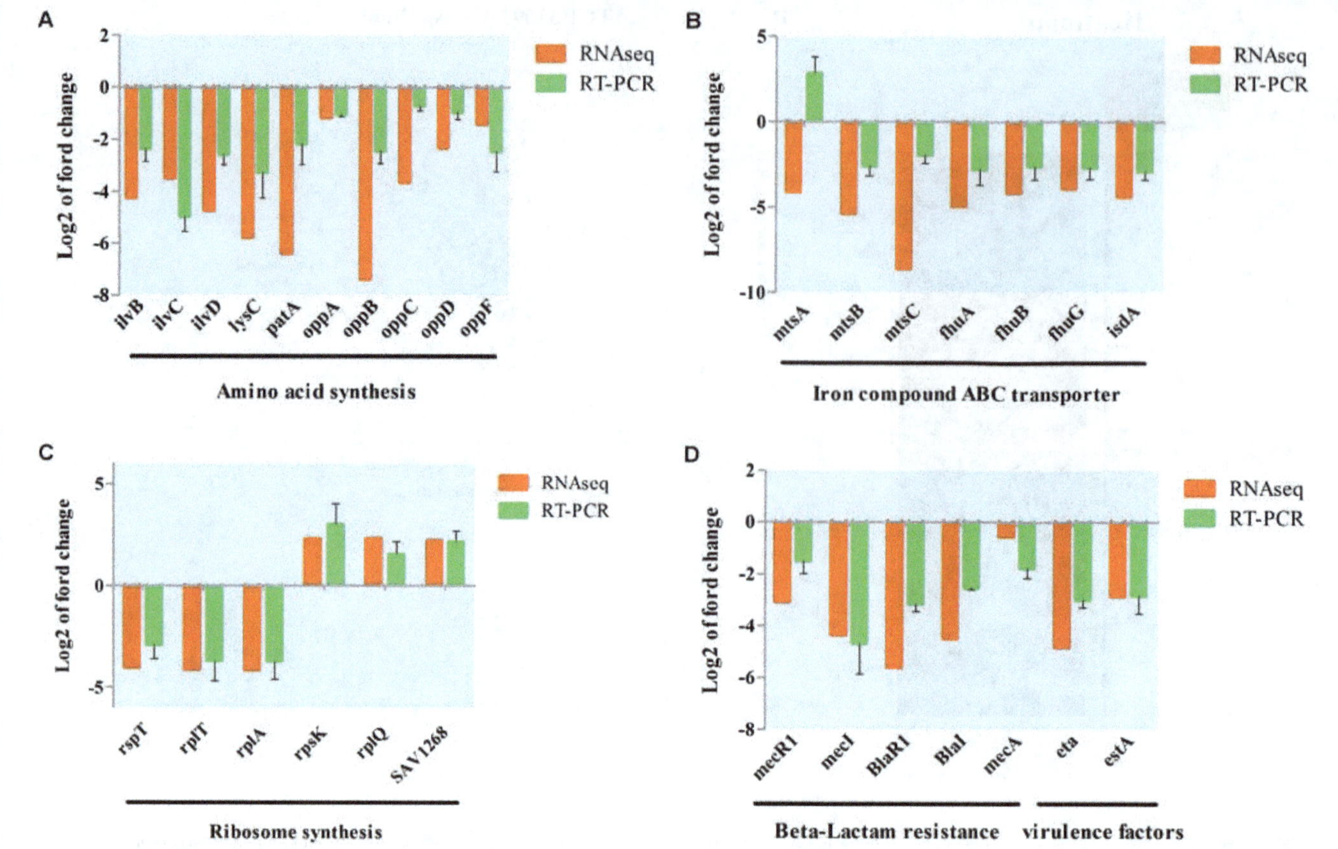

FIGURE 5 | Validation of RNA-seq data for selected genes by real-time PCR. **(A)** Differentially expressed genes involved in amino acid synthesis; **(B)** differentially expressed genes involved in iron ABC transporter synthesis; **(C)** differentially expressed genes involved in ribosome synthesis; **(D)** differentially expressed genes involved in beta-lactam resistance and virulence factor.

of transcriptomic changes caused by aspidinol treatment showed that the expression of a number of genes involved in ribosome synthesis was up- and downregulated upon treatment with aspidinol. The results indicated that ribosome synthesis was more likely to be inhibited after treatment with aspidinol and result in the inhibition of protein synthesis in bacteria. The increase in the expression of genes involved in ribosome synthesis may therefore be in response to stress. The inhibition of the formation of the ribosome, which is composed of the 30S and 50S subunits, is an important antibacterial mechanism, such as in linezolid (Colca et al., 2003; Ippolito et al., 2008; Wilson et al., 2008). Thus, the changes of genes involved in ribosome synthesis may contribute to the antimicrobial activity of aspidinol.

Iron transport was also found to be suppressed. With the possible exception of lactobacilli, all bacteria require iron for growth because it plays a vital role in the biological processes of bacteria (Sebulsky et al., 2000). MtsABC proteins were reported to be associated with metal binding and transmembrane transport. A metal solute-binding lipoprotein and an ATP-binding protein were encoded by *mtsA* and *mtsB*, respectively, while *mtsC* encodes a transmembrane permease protein (Sun et al., 2008, 2009; Zou et al., 2010). Thus, the *mtsABC* operon is also essential for the survival of bacteria (Janulczyk et al., 2003); *mtsA*, as a metal ion transporter, is responsible for iron release and transmembrane uptake and interacts with membrane components. The Fhu system is the best-characterized system in *S. aureus* for ferric hydroxamate uptake and is composed of up to five genes (Sebulsky et al., 2000). The genes *fhuC*, *fhuB*, and *fhuG* reside in an operon that encodes an ATP-binding cassette (ABC) transporter; *fhuC* encodes an ATPase at the inner side of the cytoplasmic membrane, and *fhuB* and *fhuG* are membrane-spanning proteins (Pramanik and Braun, 2006; Speziali et al., 2006). When treated with aspidinol, *mtsABC* and *fhuABCDF* are downregulated, resulting in decreased iron transport and further reducing the energy supply of ribosome synthesis, which also might contribute to MRSA killing.

Moreover, amino acid biosynthesis was downregulated after aspidinol treatment, including the leucine, isoleucine, and valine synthesis. Pathway analysis using the transcriptome data showed that the expression of the valine, leucine, and isoleucine biosynthesis system was decreased. The downregulated *ilv* and *leu* operons have been reported to encode leucine, isoleucine, and valine intermediates in the synthesis of these amino acids in *E. coli* (Miyanoiri et al., 2016). According to our results, we speculate that these operons may play the same role, although there are no reports regarding their function in *S. aureus*. Components of other amino acid pathways, such as *lysC*, were apparently downregulated by aspidinol; *lysC* is the primary gene for lysine biosynthesis and is involved in the biosynthesis of lysine from aspartic acid (Wiltshire and Foster, 2001; Nishi et al., 2004). In addition to amino acid biosynthesis, the *oppABCDF* genes were also downregulated in response to aspidinol. The Opp system is essential for the uptake of nutrients by bacteria (Gardan et al., 2009) and has been shown to supply bacteria with exogenous peptides that serve as an amino acid resource (Zhao et al., 2016). In this study, downregulation of amino acid biosynthesis pathways after treatment with aspidinol could be attributed to the killing of MRSA.

Aspidinol also significantly repressed genes involved in the virulence of MRSA. Following aspidinol treatment at sub-inhibitory concentrations, exfoliative toxin *eta* and IgG-binding protein *sbi* were measurably downregulated. Our data suggest that in addition to killing ATCC 33591, it is very likely that aspidinol reduced the virulence of the infecting bacterial cells as a secondary effect.

According to the data analysis, genes associated with β-lactam resistance were significantly reduced after treatment with aspidinol. Through the analysis of the transcription data, we found that the expression levels of genes associated with β-lactam resistance (*mecI*, *mecR1*, *blaZ*, and *blaR1*) were significantly reduced after treatment with aspidinol; *mecA* coding for PBP2a (a low affinity penicillin binding protein) is responsible for methicillin resistance in *S. aureus* and other staphylococci (Wilke et al., 2004; Staude et al., 2015). While transcription of *mecA* is regulated by *mecI* and *mecR1* (Wilke et al., 2004; Aedo and Tomasz, 2016), *blaR1* and *blaI* are involved in the regulation of *blaZ* (Thumanu et al., 2006). Based on our current understanding, blocking of *blaR1* and *mecR1* is helpful to restore the susceptibility of MRSA to β-lactam antibiotics. Hou et al. (2011) have designed specific anti-mecR1 and anti-blaR1 deoxyribozymes and confirmed their function in restoring the β-lactam susceptibility of MRSA.

According to the transcriptome data, the expression of *mecA* was decreased 0.52-fold, but there were no statistically significant differences. However, the RT-PCR results showed that *mecA* was downregulated 1.75-fold after treatment with aspidinol. Subsequently, a combination administration experiment was conducted to test whether a sub-MIC concentration of aspidinol was able to restore the susceptibility to β-lactams. In this experiment, oxacillin was co-administered with 1 μg/mL aspidinol, and the oxacillin MIC decreased from 256 to 0.5 μg/mL. This observation might provide a first hint toward the use of aspidinol as a combination drug to restore the β-lactam susceptibility. We theorize that aspidinol is able to inhibit the expression of *mecA*-related genes to restore susceptibility to β-lactam antibiotics.

Genes involved in some metabolic pathways, such as carbon metabolism and nitrogen metabolism, were upregulated after treatment with aspidinol, which could be attributed to metabolic disorders of bacteria in the process of dying.

Although the validation of the effects of aspidinol on metabolic pathways has been carried out by RT-PCR, further studies are still needed to more thoroughly understand the antibacterial mechanisms of aspidinol.

However, these data were not sufficient to fully elucidate the antibacterial mechanisms of aspidinol against MRSA. In future studies, we will focus on the identification of potential drug targets to clearly reveal the mechanism of action.

CONCLUSION

In this study, the anti-MRSA activity of aspidinol, both *in vitro* and *in vivo*, was reported for the first time. The mechanism of aspidinol's anti-MRSA effect was also investigated. In particular, RNA-seq was applied for the analysis of differentially expressed genes after treatment with aspidinol. When combined with verification experiments, the results suggest that the inhibition of the formation of ribosomes was the primary *S. aureus* cell-killing mechanism, and the inhibition of amino acid synthesis and the reduction of virulence factors were considered to be a secondary effect.

AUTHOR CONTRIBUTIONS

XH and SL responsible for experimental design. XH, QY, and ZD responsible for experimental operation. XH, WZ, and SY responsible for writing the manuscript. SS responsible for reviewing the manuscript.

FUNDING

The authors gratefully acknowledge the financial support from the Program for Natural Science Foundation of Heilongjiang Province of China (C2016063), China Postdoctoral Science Foundation (2016M591311), National Natural Science Foundation of China (31602100), and Central Public-interest Scientific Institution Basal Research Fund (1610302017007).

SUPPLEMENTARY MATERIAL

FIGURE S1 | Differentially expressed genes enriched in the KEGG pathway for *S. aureus* ATCC 33591 cells treated and not treated with aspidinol.

FIGURE S2 | Cell survival curve after treated with aspidinol.

FIGURE S3 | Chemical structure of aspidinol, aspidinol C and aspidinol D.

TABLE S1 | Strain list.

TABLE S2 | Primers used in this study.

REFERENCES

Aedo, S., and Tomasz, A. (2016). Role of the stringent stress response in the antibiotic resistance phenotype of methicillin-resistant *Staphylococcus aureus*. *Antimicrob. Agents Chemother.* 60, 2311–2317. doi: 10.1128/AAC.02697-15

Colca, J. R., Mcdonald, W. G., Waldon, D. J., Thomasco, L. M., Gadwood, R. C., Lund, E. T., et al. (2003). Cross-linking in the living cell locates the site of action of oxazolidinone antibiotics. *J. Biol. Chem.* 278, 21972–21979. doi: 10.1074/jbc.M302109200

Farah, S. I., Abdelrahman, A., North, E. J., and Chauhan, H. (2016). Opportunities and challenges for natural products as novel antituberculosis agents. *Assay Drug Dev. Technol.* 14, 29–38. doi: 10.1089/adt.2015.673

Gao, C., Guo, N., Li, N., Peng, X., Wang, P., Wang, W., et al. (2016). Investigation of antibacterial activity of aspidin BB against *Propionibacterium acnes*. *Arch. Dermatol. Res.* 308, 79–86. doi: 10.1007/s00403-015-1603-x

Gardan, R., Besset, C., Guillot, A., Gitton, C., and Monnet, V. (2009). The oligopeptide transport system is essential for the development of natural competence in *Streptococcus thermophilus* strain LMD-9. *J. Bacteriol.* 191, 4647–4655. doi: 10.1128/JB.00257-09

Garzoni, C., and Kelley, W. L. (2009). *Staphylococcus aureus*: new evidence for intracellular persistence. *Trends Microbiol.* 17, 59–65. doi: 10.1016/j.tim.2008.11.005

Guzman, J. D., Gupta, A., Evangelopoulos, D., Basavannacharya, C., Pabon, L. C., Plazas, E. A., et al. (2010). Anti-tubercular screening of natural products from Colombian plants: 3-methoxynordomesticine, an inhibitor of MurE ligase of *Mycobacterium tuberculosis*. *J. Antimicrob. Chemother.* 65, 2101–2107. doi: 10.1093/jac/dkq313

Hou, Z., Zhou, Y., Wang, H., Bai, H., Meng, J., Xue, X., et al. (2011). Co-blockade of mecR1/blaR1 signal pathway to restore antibiotic susceptibility in clinical isolates of methicillin-resistant *Staphylococcus aureus*. *Arch. Med. Sci.* 7, 414–422. doi: 10.5114/aoms.2011.23404

Huang, Y. H., Zeng, W. M., Li, G. Y., Liu, G. Q., Zhao, D. D., Wang, J., et al. (2014). Characterization of a new sesquiterpene and antifungal activities of chemical constituents from *Dryopteris fragrans* (L.) Schott. *Molecules* 19, 507–513. doi: 10.3390/molecules19010507

Ippolito, J. A., Kanyo, Z. F., Wang, D., Franceschi, F. J., Moore, P. B., Steitz, T. A., et al. (2008). Crystal structure of the oxazolidinone antibiotic linezolid bound to the 50S ribosomal subunit. *J. Med. Chem.* 51, 3353–3356. doi: 10.1021/jm800379d

Janulczyk, R., Ricci, S., and Bjorck, L. (2003). MtsABC is important for manganese and iron transport, oxidative stress resistance, and virulence of *Streptococcus pyogenes*. *Infect. Immun.* 71, 2656–2664. doi: 10.1128/IAI.71.5.2656-2664.2003

Lehar, S. M., Pillow, T., Xu, M., Staben, L., Kajihara, K. K., Vandlen, R., et al. (2015). Novel antibody-antibiotic conjugate eliminates intracellular *S. aureus*. *Nature* 527, 323–328. doi: 10.1038/nature16057

Lemaire, S., Olivier, A., Van Bambeke, F., Tulkens, P. M., Appelbaum, P. C., and Glupczynski, Y. (2008). Restoration of susceptibility of intracellular methicillin-resistant *Staphylococcus aureus* to beta-lactams: comparison of strains, cells, and antibiotics. *Antimicrob. Agents Chemother.* 52, 2797–2805. doi: 10.1128/AAC.00123-08

Mihu, M. R., Roman-Sosa, J., Varshney, A. K., Eugenin, E. A., Shah, B. P., Lee, H. H., et al. (2015). Methamphetamine alters the antimicrobial efficacy of phagocytic cells during methicillin-resistant *Staphylococcus aureus* skin infection. *MBio* 6:e1622-15. doi: 10.1128/mBio.01622-15

Miyanoiri, Y., Ishida, Y., Takeda, M., Terauchi, T., Inouye, M., and Kainosho, M. (2016). Highly efficient residue-selective labeling with isotope-labeled Ile, Leu, and Val using a new auxotrophic *E. coli* strain. *J. Biomol. NMR* 65, 109–119. doi: 10.1007/s10858-016-0042-0

Mu, Q., Zeng, C. H., Gibbons, S., and Osman, C. (2012). Aspidin Phenolic Compounds and Their Use in the Orparation of Anti-drug Resistant. CN Patent No. 102464578 A. Peking: State Intellectual Property Office of the People's Republic of China.

Nishi, H., Komatsuzawa, H., Fujiwara, T., Mccallum, N., and Sugai, M. (2004). Reduced content of lysyl-phosphatidylglycerol in the cytoplasmic membrane affects susceptibility to moenomycin, as well as vancomycin, gentamicin, and antimicrobial peptides, in *Staphylococcus aureus*. *Antimicrob. Agents Chemother.* 48, 4800–4807. doi: 10.1128/AAC.48.12.4800-4807.2004

Peng, B., Bai, R. F., Li, P., Han, X. Y., Wang, H., Zhu, C. C., et al. (2016). Two new glycosides from *Dryopteris fragrans* with anti-inflammatory activities. *J. Asian Nat. Prod. Res.* 18, 59–64. doi: 10.1080/10286020.2015.1121853

Pramanik, A., and Braun, V. (2006). Albomycin uptake via a ferric hydroxamate transport system of *Streptococcus pneumoniae* R6. *J. Bacteriol.* 188, 3878–3886. doi: 10.1128/JB.00205-06

Rennie, R. P. (2012). Current and future challenges in the development of antimicrobial agents. *Handb. Exp. Pharmacol.* 211, 45–65. doi: 10.1007/978-3-642-28951-4_4

Rodvold, K. A., and McConeghy, K. W. (2014). Methicillin-resistant *Staphylococcus aureus* therapy: past, present, and future. *Clin. Infect. Dis.* 58(Suppl. 1), S20–S27. doi: 10.1093/cid/cit614

Rubinstein, E., Kollef, M. H., and Nathwani, D. (2008). Pneumonia caused by methicillin-resistant *Staphylococcus aureus*. *Clin. Infect. Dis.* 46, S378–S385. doi: 10.1086/533594

Sebulsky, M. T., Hohnstein, D., Hunter, M. D., and Heinrichs, D. E. (2000). Identification and characterization of a membrane permease involved in iron-hydroxamate transport in *Staphylococcus aureus*. *J. Bacteriol.* 182, 4394–4400. doi: 10.1128/JB.182.16.4394-4400.2000

Seleem, M. N., Jain, N., Pothayee, N., Ranjan, A., Riffle, J. S., and Sriranganathan, N. (2009). Targeting *Brucella melitensis* with polymeric nanoparticles containing streptomycin and doxycycline. *FEMS Microbiol. Lett.* 294, 24–31. doi: 10.1111/j.1574-6968.2009.01530.x

Shenoy, E. S., Paras, M. L., Noubary, F., Walensky, R. P., and Hooper, D. C. (2014). Natural history of colonization with methicillin-resistant *Staphylococcus aureus* (MRSA) and vancomycin-resistant *Enterococcus* (VRE): a systematic review. *BMC Infect. Dis.* 14:177. doi: 10.1186/1471-2334-14-177

Speziali, C. D., Dale, S. E., Henderson, J. A., Vines, E. D., and Heinrichs, D. E. (2006). Requirement of *Staphylococcus aureus* ATP-binding cassette-ATPase FhuC for iron-restricted growth and evidence that it functions with more than one iron transporter. *J. Bacteriol.* 188, 2048–2055. doi: 10.1128/JB.188.6.2048-2055.2006

Stahlmann, R. (2014). Antibiotics for treatment of infections by methicillin-resistant *Staphylococcus aureus* (MRSA). *Pneumologie* 68, 676–684. doi: 10.1055/s-0034-1377747

Staude, M. W., Frederick, T. E., Natarajan, S. V., Wilson, B. D., Tanner, C. E., Ruggiero, S. T., et al. (2015). Investigation of signal transduction routes within the sensor/transducer protein BlaR1 of *Staphylococcus aureus*. *Biochemistry* 54, 1600–1610. doi: 10.1021/bi501463k

Sun, X., Baker, H. M., Ge, R., Sun, H., He, Q. Y., and Baker, E. N. (2009). Crystal structure and metal binding properties of the lipoprotein MtsA, responsible for iron transport in *Streptococcus pyogenes*. *Biochemistry* 48, 6184–6190. doi: 10.1021/bi900552c

Sun, X., Ge, R., Chiu, J. F., Sun, H., and He, Q. Y. (2008). Lipoprotein MtsA of MtsABC in *Streptococcus pyogenes* primarily binds ferrous ion with bicarbonate as a synergistic anion. *FEBS Lett.* 582, 1351–1354. doi: 10.1016/j.febslet.2008.03.020

Taylor, A. R. (2013). Methicillin-resistant *Staphylococcus aureus* infections. *Prim. Care* 40, 637–654. doi: 10.1016/j.pop.2013.06.002

Tenover, F. C., and Goering, R. V. (2009). Methicillin-resistant *Staphylococcus aureus* strain USA300: origin and epidemiology. *J. Antimicrob. Chemother.* 64, 441–446. doi: 10.1093/jac/dkp241

Thangamani, S., Younis, W., and Seleem, M. N. (2015). Repurposing clinical molecule ebselen to combat drug resistant pathogens. *PLoS One* 10:e0133877. doi: 10.1371/journal.pone.0133877

Thumanu, K., Cha, J., Fisher, J. F., Perrins, R., Mobashery, S., and Wharton, C. (2006). Discrete steps in sensing of beta-lactam antibiotics by the BlaR1 protein of the methicillin-resistant *Staphylococcus aureus* bacterium. *Proc. Natl. Acad. Sci. U.S.A.* 103, 10630–10635. doi: 10.1073/pnas.0601971103

Vandal, J., Abou-Zaid, M. M., Ferroni, G., and Leduc, L. G. (2015). Antimicrobial activity of natural products from the flora of Northern Ontario, Canada. *Pharm. Biol.* 53, 800–806. doi: 10.3109/13880209.2014.942867

VanEperen, A. S., and Segreti, J. (2016). Empirical therapy in methicillin-resistant *Staphylococcus aureus* infections: an up-to-date approach. *J. Infect. Chemother.* 22, 351–359. doi: 10.1016/j.jiac.2016.02.012

WHO (2017). *Global Priority List of Antibiotic-Resistant Bacteria to Guide Research, Discovery, and Development of New Antibiotics*. Available at:

http://www.who.int/medicines/publications/WHO-PPL-Short_Summary_25 Feb-ET_NM_WHO.pdf

Wilke, M. S., Hills, T. L., Zhang, H. Z., Chambers, H. F., and Strynadka, N. C. (2004). Crystal structures of the Apo and penicillin-acylated forms of the BlaR1 beta-lactam sensor of *Staphylococcus aureus*. *J. Biol. Chem.* 279, 47278–47287. doi: 10.1074/jbc.M407054200

Wilson, D. N., Schluenzen, F., Harms, J. M., Starosta, A. L., Connell, S. R., and Fucini, P. (2008). The oxazolidinone antibiotics perturb the ribosomal peptidyl-transferase center and effect tRNA positioning. *Proc. Natl. Acad. Sci. U.S.A.* 105, 13339–13344. doi: 10.1073/pnas.0804276105

Wiltshire, M. D., and Foster, S. J. (2001). Identification and analysis of *Staphylococcus aureus* components expressed by a model system of growth in serum. *Infect. Immun.* 69, 5198–5202. doi: 10.1128/IAI.69.8.5198-5202.2001

Woods, C., and Colice, G. (2014). Methicillin-resistant *Staphylococcus aureus* pneumonia in adults. *Expert Rev. Respir. Med.* 8, 641–651. doi: 10.1586/17476348.2014.940323

Zhang, Y., Luo, M., Zu, Y., Fu, Y., Gu, C., Wang, W., et al. (2012). Dryofragin, a phloroglucinol derivative, induces apoptosis in human breast cancer MCF-7 cells through ROS-mediated mitochondrial pathway. *Chem. Biol. Interact.* 199, 129–136. doi: 10.1016/j.cbi.2012.06.007

Zhao, D. D., Zhao, Q. S., Liu, L., Chen, Z. Q., Zeng, W. M., Lei, H., et al. (2014). Compounds from *Dryopteris fragrans* (L.) Schott with cytotoxic activity. *Molecules* 19, 3345–3355. doi: 10.3390/molecules19033345

Zhao, J., Cheah, S.-E., Roberts, K. D., Nation, R. L., Thompson, P. E., Velkov, T., et al. (2016). Transcriptomic analysis of the activity of a novel polymyxin against *Staphylococcus aureus*. *mSphere* 1:e00119-16. doi: 10.1128/mSphere.00119-16

Zhong, Z.-C., Zhao, D.-D., Liu, Z.-D., Jiang, S., and Zhang, Y.-L. (2017). A new human cancer cell proliferation inhibition sesquiterpene, dryofraterpene a, from medicinal plant *Dryopteris fragrans* (L.) Schott. *Molecules* 22:180. doi: 10.3390/molecules22010180

Zou, L., Wang, J., Huang, B., Xie, M., and Li, A. (2010). A solute-binding protein for iron transport in *Streptococcus iniae*. *BMC Microbiol.* 10:309. doi: 10.1186/1471-2180-10-309

12

Sirt1 Activation by Post-ischemic Treatment with Lumbrokinase Protects Against Myocardial Ischemia-Reperfusion Injury

Yi-Hsin Wang[1†], Shun-An Li[2†], Chao-Hsin Huang[3†], Hsing-Hui Su[4], Yi-Hung Chen[5,6], Jinghua T. Chang[1] and Shiang-Suo Huang[7,8]**

[1] Institute of Medicine, Chung Shan Medical University, Taichung, Taiwan, [2] Superintendent Office, Yuanli Lee's General Hospital, Lee's Medical Corporation, Miaoli, Taiwan, [3] Department of Internal Medicine, Dajia Lee's General Hospital, Lee's Medical Corporation, Taichung, Taiwan, [4] Department and Institute of Pharmacology, School of Medicine, National Yang-Ming University, Taipei, Taiwan, [5] Graduate Institute of Acupuncture Science and Research Center for Chinese Medicine and Acupuncture, China Medical University, Taichung, Taiwan, [6] Department of Photonics and Communication Engineering, Asia University, Taichung, Taiwan, [7] Department of Pharmacology and Institute of Medicine, Chung Shan Medical University, Taichung, Taiwan, [8] Department of Pharmacy, Chung Shan Medical University Hospital, Taichung, Taiwan

***Correspondence:**
Jinghua T. Chang
jinghuat@csmu.edu.tw
Shiang-Suo Huang
sshuang@csmu.edu.tw

† These authors have contributed equally to this work.

Lumbrokinase is used as an oral supplement to support and maintain healthy cardiovascular function, and to treat cardiovascular diseases in clinical for more than 10 years. Up until now, the mechanism of the cardioprotective effects of post-ischemic treatment with lumbrokinase has remained unclear. We therefore investigated the signaling pathways involved in the amelioration of myocardial ischemia-reperfusion (I-R) injury in rats treated with lumbrokinase 20 min after myocardial ischemia. Compared to vehicle-treated rats, post-ischemic treatment with lumbrokinase was associated with significant reductions in myocardial I-R-induced arrhythmias and myocardial damage, and an improvement in cardiac function. Moreover, lumbrokinase significantly upregulated levels of silent information regulator 1 (Sirt1). In addition, lumbrokinase significantly increased manganese-dependent superoxide dismutase expression, decreased Cleaved-Caspase-3 expression, and induced deacetylation of FoxO1. On the other hand, lumbrokinase also significantly downregulated levels of succinate dehydrogenase, cytochrome c oxidase, nuclear factor kappa B (NF-κB) and elevated levels of microtubule-associated protein light chain 3. Notably, the cardioprotective effects of lumbrokinase were abolished by administration of the specific Sirt1 inhibitor EX527. These findings demonstrate that post-ischemic treatment with lumbrokinase attenuates myocardial I-R injury through the activation of Sirt1 signaling, and thus enhances autophagic flux and reduces I-R-induced oxidative damage, inflammation and apoptosis.

Keywords: lumbrokinase, cardioprotection, ischemia, reperfusion, Sirt1

INTRODUCTION

Ischemic heart disease (IHD) is a leading cause of death and disability due to acute myocardial infarction, angina pectoris, or ischemic heart failure (Mendis et al., 2011). The main therapeutic intervention for IHD consists of thrombolytic therapy or primary percutaneous coronary intervention, which aims to reduce myocardial infarct size and improve clinical outcomes. However, the reperfusion of acutely ischemic myocardium can lead to further cardiomyocyte damage, known as myocardial ischemia-reperfusion (I-R) injury, involving clinical manifestations of arrhythmia, myocardial stunning, microvascular obstruction and myocardial necrosis (Hausenloy and Yellon, 2013).

Silent information regulator 1 (Sirt1) is a nicotinamide adenine dinucleotide (NAD)-dependent histone deacetylase that performs a wide variety of functions in different biologic systems. Sirt1 plays a protective role in the pathophysiology of vascular aging and age-related diseases including neurodegenerative diseases, cardiovascular disease, chronic kidney disease, osteoporosis and the metabolic syndrome (Guarente, 2011). Research has reported that activation of Sirt1 extends the lifespan and retards heart-related aging in mice fed a high-fat diet (Mitchell et al., 2014). Previous studies have demonstrated that activation of Sirt1 signaling mimics ischemic preconditioning and protects against myocardial I-R injury (Yamamoto and Sadoshima, 2011; Ding et al., 2015; Yamamoto et al., 2016; Yu et al., 2016). After myocardial I-R injury, the extent of myocardial infarction and the number of TUNEL-positive nuclei are significantly reduced in transgenic mice displaying a cardiac-specific overexpression of Sirt1 compared with non-transgenic mice (Hsu et al., 2010). In diabetic rats, upregulation of Sirt1 in the heart improved cardiac function and reduced infarct size to the same extent as that observed in non-diabetic animals following myocardial I-R injury, and this phenomenon was associated with reductions in serum creatine kinase-MB (CK-MB), lactate dehydrogenase (LDH) activities and cardiomyocyte apoptosis (Ding et al., 2015). Sirt1 also stimulates the expression of pro-survival molecules and negatively regulates the survival of pro-apoptotic molecules through the deacetylation of the forkhead box O (FoxO) family transcription factors, reducing oxidative damage and apoptosis in Sirt1 transgenic mice with myocardial I-R injury (Hsu et al., 2010; Yu et al., 2016). Thus, modulation of Sirt1 signaling is a potential therapeutic strategy in myocardial I-R injury.

Lumbrokinase, an extract of *Lumbricus rubellus*, was identified in the early 1990s (Mihara et al., 1991) as a group of bioactive proteolytic enzymes ranging in molecular weight from 25 to 32 kDa (Cho et al., 2004) that includes plasminogen activator and plasmin (Cooper and Balamurugan, 2010). The extrinsic plasminogen activator (e-PA) in lumbrokinase is similar to endogenous tissue plasminogen activator (t-PA) found in other species. Lumbrokinase can dissolve fibrin clots and convert plasminogen to plasmin by increasing endogenous t-PA activity. Moreover, lumbrokinase enzymes show thrombolytic activity only in the presence of fibrin. Thus, lumbrokinase is not associated with the excessive bleeding and heavy blood loss seen with streptokinase or urokinase, which may result in death (Delaney et al., 2007; Vernooij et al., 2009). In our previous study, pre-treatment with lumbrokinase 10 μg/kg significantly reduced ventricular arrhythmias and myocardial infarction in rats after myocardial I-R injury (Wang et al., 2016). We suggested that lumbrokinase has significant potential as a cardioprotective agent, regulating anti-inflammatory mechanisms that protect the heart against I-R injury (Wang et al., 2016). Oral lumbrokinase supplementation has been used in Japan, Korea, Canada and the United States to support and maintain healthy cardiovascular function. In addition, lumbrokinase is used clinically as a thrombolytic agent in China in the treatment of stroke and cardiovascular disease (Wang et al., 2013), the prevention of secondary ischemic stroke (Cao et al., 2013), and for the improvement of myocardial perfusion in stable angina (Kasim et al., 2009). Lumbrokinase has approved a phase III clinical trial that indicated the total effective rate was 88.21% and the significant response rate was 68.91% in treating ischemic cerebrovascular disease. However, the underlying molecular mechanism involved in the amelioration of myocardial I-R injury by post-ischemic treatment with lumbrokinase remains unclear. The aims of the present study were (1) to explore the effects of post-ischemic treatment with lumbrokinase in rats subjected to myocardial I-R injury, (2) investigate whether lumbrokinase treatment confers anti-inflammation, anti-oxidative and anti-apoptotic effects in myocardial I-R injury, and (3) examine whether Sirt1 signaling ameliorates myocardial I-R injury in rats.

MATERIALS AND METHODS

Animals

Six-week-old male Sprague-Dawley rats (LASCO Co., Charles River Technology, Taipei, Taiwan) weighing 250–300 g were housed in the Chung Shan Medical University Animal Center at an ambient temperature of 25 ± 1°C under a normal 12 h light-12 h dark cycle. The animals were fed with normal chow and given water *ad libitum*. All surgical procedures were reviewed and approved by the Chung Shan Medical University Institutional Animal Care and Use Committee. The study complied with the protocols outlined in the *Guide for the Care and Use of Laboratory Animals* issued in 2011 by the US National Research Council Committee. The animal study protocol was approved by the Institutional Animal Ethics Committee of Chung Shan Medical University, Taichung, Taiwan (IACUC 1431). All efforts were taken to minimize animal suffering and the numbers of sacrificed animals.

Myocardial Ischemia-Reperfusion Injury Model

Myocardial I-R injury was induced by temporary occlusion of the left anterior descending coronary artery, according to a previously described procedure (Wang et al., 2016). Slight modification of the procedure meant that the left anterior descending coronary artery was occluded by tightening of the ligature to induce ischemia for 30 min, followed by 3 h of reperfusion.

Experimental Groups

For this study, we referred to the effective dose of lumbrokinase used in our previous publication (Wang et al., 2016). Lumbrokinase (10 μg/kg; Canada RNA Biochemical Inc. Richmond, BC, Canada) or vehicle (sterile saline) was intravenously infused 20 min after occlusion of the left anterior decending coronary artery. The selective Sirt1 inhibitor EX527 (Sigma-Aldrich, St Louis, MO, United States) was intraperitoneally injected at a dose of 5 mg/kg 15 min after coronary artery occlusion (CAO). The dose of EX527 was based on previous study (Yu et al., 2017). The animals were randomly assigned to the following groups: (1) Sham-operated group (Sham); (2) Myocardial I-R+vehicle group (Vehicle); (3) Myocardial I-R+lumbrokinase group (LK); (4) Myocardial I-R+LK + EX527 group (LK+EX527).

Evaluation of Arrhythmias and Cardiac Function

Antiarrhythmic effects of lumbrokinase were evaluated during myocardial I-R injury, using the diagnostic criteria recommended by the Lambeth Convention (Curtis et al., 2013). The incidence and duration of ventricular tachycardia (VT) and ventricular fibrillation (VF) were determined in both surviving rats and those that died. In rats with irreversible VF, the duration of VF was recorded until mean BP was less than 15 mmHg. To evaluate the effect of lumbrokinase on cardiac function during myocardial I-R injury, a Millar catheter was inserted into the left ventricular cavity via the right common carotid artery and changes in the left ventricular systolic pressure (LVSP), left ventricular diastolic pressure (LVDP) and maximal slope of systolic pressure increment (max dP/dt) and diastolic decrement (min dP/dt) were continuously recorded using a Transonic Scisense Pressure Measurement system (SP200, Transonic Scisense Inc., Ontario, Canada).

Determination of Myocardial Infarct Size

Myocardial infarct size was determined by the double-staining technique using Evans blue and 2,3,5-triphenyltetrazolium chloride (TTC; Sigma-Aldrich, St Louis, MO, United States) (Bohl et al., 2009). At the end of the experiment, the coronary artery was re-occluded and 1% Evans blue solution was intravenously injected to stain non-ischemic myocardium and determine the area at risk. The heart was cut transversely into 2-mm-thick slices using a heart slicer matrix (Jacobowitz Systems, Zivic-Miller Laboratories Inc., Allison Park, PA, United States). Heart sections were stained with 2% TTC at 37°C for 30 min in darkness. The slices were placed in a solution with 10% formalin at room temperature for 1 day. Infarcted tissue slices were scanned and tissue weights were evaluated by distinguishing the normal myocardium (stained blue) from the area at risk and infarct area (unstained) in a TTC staining assay.

Determination of Myocardial Damage

Arterial blood collected from the carotid catheter in rats that survived after 30 min of ischemia and 3 h of reperfusion was centrifuged at 3,000 g for 10 min to isolate plasma and determine myocardial damage. Myocardial cellular damage was determined using automated clinical analyzers to measure plasma activities of LDH and CK-MB (ADVIA 1800, Siemens Healthcare Diagnostics Inc., NY, United States) and the levels of troponin I (Centaur, Siemens Healthcare Diagnostics Inc., NY, United States).

Protein Extraction and Western Blot Analysis

Myocardium samples from surviving rats at the end of experiment were homogenized with a tissue protein extraction reagent (Thermo Scientific, United States) containing a protease inhibitor cocktail (Sigma-Aldrich, St Louis, MO, United States). The homogenates were then centrifuged at 12,000 g for 10 min at 4°C. The supernatant was mixed with an equal volume of loading buffer and heated at 95°C for 10 min. The protein samples were subjected to SDS-PAGE and electrophoretically transferred onto PVDF protein sequencing membranes for 90 min. The membrane was blocked with 5% non-fat milk in PBS with 0.1% (v/v) Tween-20 (PBST) at room temperature for 1 h. The membrane was washed and blotted with the antibodies of Bax, Bcl-2, Beclin-1 (Abcam, United Kingdom), succinate dehydrogenase (SDH), cytochrome c oxidase (CcO), Caspase-3, Cleaved-Caspase-3, p-NF-κB, NF-κB, iNOS, FoxO1 (Cell Signaling, United States), Sirt1, Ac-FoxO1, manganese-dependent superoxide dismutase (MnSOD) (Santa Cruz, United States), COX-2 (Cayman Chemical, United States), LC3, p62, and β-actin (Novus, United States). The membrane was incubated with HRP-conjugated secondary antibody (Jackson ImmunoResearch Laboratories, United States) prior to chemiluminescence detection (Pierce, United States). Western blot analyses of protein expression were performed using two different samples from each treatment group and repeated at least three times (using the same samples), we thus obtained at least six values for each study group. And then, chose the lower value of sham group as standard, each of band intensity divide by the standard and multiplied by 100 to get % of sham.

Statistical Analysis

Data are expressed as the mean ± standard error of the mean (SEM). Differences between the groups in myocardial I-R-induced infarction, duration of arrthymias, cardiac function, and Western blot data were compared using one-way analysis of variance (ANOVA) and the variables were subsequently analyzed using Bonferroni's tests to determine any significant between-group differences. Between-group differences in VT and VF percentages were analyzed using the $\chi 2$ test and a significance level was set at 0.05 for each comparison.

RESULTS

Effects of Post-ischemic Treatment With Lumbrokinase on Cardiac Function

The effects of post-ischemic lumbrokinase treatment on myocardial I-R-induced cardiac dysfunction are shown in **Figure 1**. HR and MBP did not differ significantly amongst the groups. We measured LVSP, LVDP, max dP/dt and min dP/dt to detect cardiac systolic and diastolic function parameters. Baseline cardiac function parameters did not differ significantly amongst the sham-operated group, vehicle

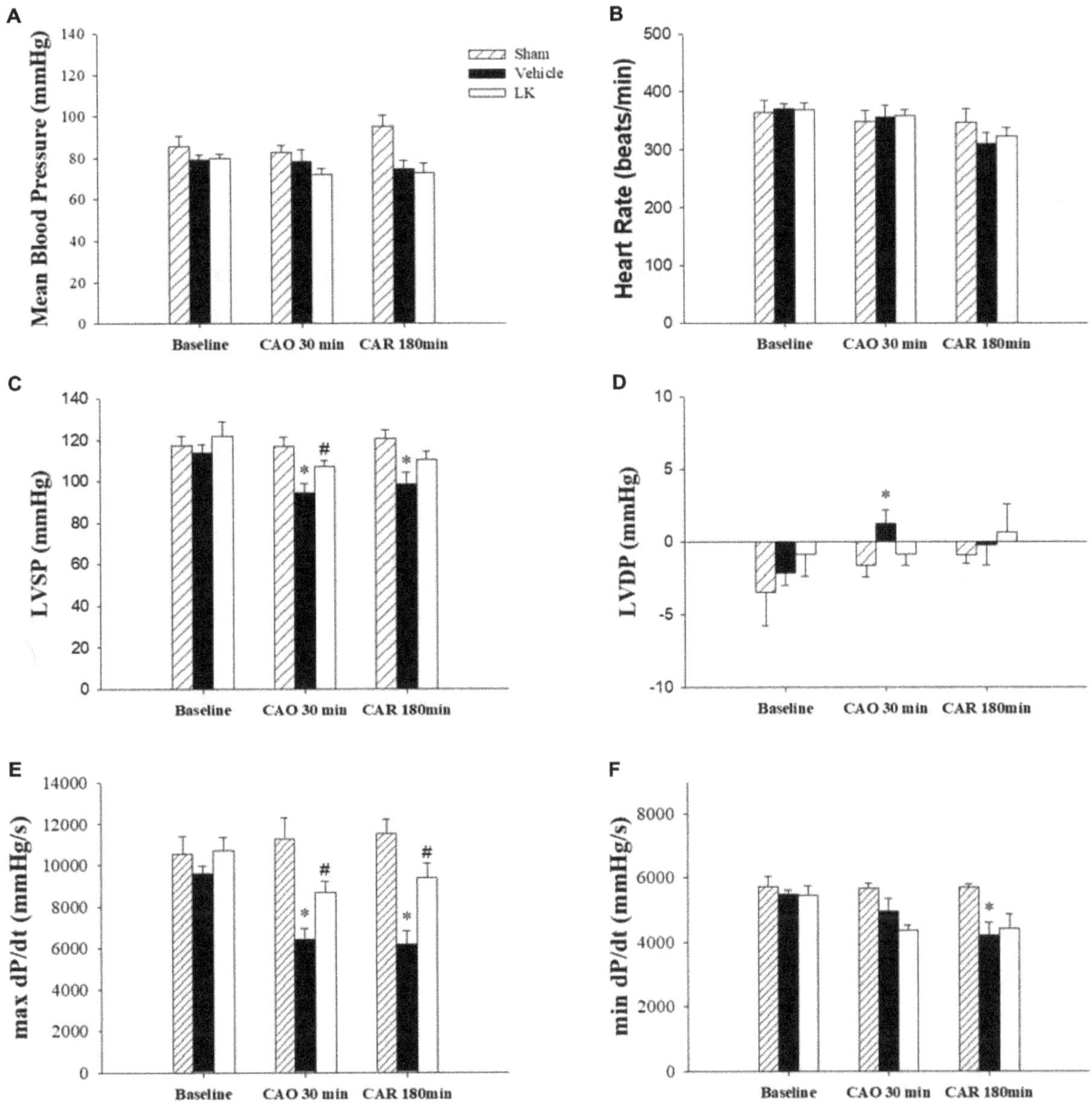

FIGURE 1 | Cardiac function parameters in I-R rats treated with vehicle or lumbrokinase. Post-ischemic treatment with vehicle or lumbrokinase (10 μg/kg) in rats subjected to myocardial I-R injury. **(A)** Mean blood pressure, **(B)** heart rate, **(C)** LVSP, **(D)** LVDP, **(E)** max dP/dt, and **(F)** min dP/dt were determined before CAO (baseline), 30 min after CAO (CAO 30 min), and 180 min after reperfusion (CAR 180 min). Each value is represented as the mean ± SEM (n = 4–8). $^{*}p < 0.05$ compared with the sham group; $^{\#}p < 0.05$ compared with the vehicle group.

group and LK group. As expected, LVSP, LVDP, max dP/dt, and min dP/dt in the vehicle group were significantly worse after 30 min of myocardial ischemia followed by 180 min of reperfusion, compared with measurements in the sham group. Post-ischemic lumbrokinase treatment significantly reversed cardiac function injury by significantly increasing the LVSP and max dP/dt after 30 min of myocardial ischemia and significantly increasing max dP/dt after myocardial I-R injury, compared with the vehicle group. We therefore suggest that post-ischemic treatment with lumbrokinase preserves cardiac function after myocardial I-R injury.

Effects of Post-ischemic Treatment With Lumbrokinase on Myocardial I-R-Induced Myocardial Damage and Rhythm Disturbances

The effects of post-ischemic treatment with lumbrokinase on infarct size after myocardial I-R injury were determined by Evans-blue/TTC staining. As shown in **Table 1**, there were no significant differences in the area at risk (AAR)/ventricle ratio amongst experimental groups, indicating that in each group, similar amounts of myocardium were at risk from left CAO. Compared to the sham group, 30 min of ischemia followed by 180 min of reperfusion resulted in severe myocardial injury. The infarct/AAR ratio was significantly reduced by post-ischemic treatment with lumbrokinase. We also measured LDH activity, a marker of tissue damage, CK-MB activity and troponin I levels, important indicators of the extent of myocardial cellular injury, to investigate the effects of post-ischemic lumbrokinase treatment on myocardial I-R-induced myocardial damage. LDH and CK-MB activities, as well as troponin I levels, were significantly higher in the vehicle group compared with the sham group. In comparison with vehicle-treated rats, LDH and CK-MB activities and troponin I levels in plasma were significantly decreased after post-ischemic lumbrokinase treatment. LDH and CK-MB activities and also troponin I levels were consistent with infarct size data.

The effects of post-ischemic lumbrokinase treatment on myocardial I-R-induced arrhythmias are shown in **Table 1**. In the vehicle group, the incidence of VT was 86% (26.4 ± 8.4 s) and incidence of VF was 36% (19.8 ± 8.6 s) during the period of myocardial I-R injury. Post-ischemic lumbrokinase administration significantly decreased the incidence of VT to 46% and VT duration to 3.8 ± 1.8 s, and the incidence of VF to 8% and duration to 0.9 ± 0.9 s compared with the vehicle group. These results indicate that post-ischemic treatment with lumbrokinase decreases myocardial I-R-induced rhythm disturbances.

Effects of Post-ischemic Treatment With Lumbrokinase on Sirt1 Protein Expression in Myocardial Tissue

As shown in **Figure 2**, Sirt1 protein expression was significantly decreased in the vehicle group compared with the sham group. Notably, post-ischemic treatment with lumbrokinase significantly increased Sirt1 protein expression in comparison with the vehicle group. As presented in **Figure 2C**, the Ac-FoxO1/FoxO1 ratio was significantly increased in the vehicle group compared with the sham group, while post-ischemic lumbrokinase treatment significantly decreased the Ac-FoxO/FoxO1 ratio compared with the vehicle group. These results suggest that post-ischemic treatment with lumbrokinase activates Sirt1 and induces deacetylation of FoxO1.

Effects of Post-ischemic Treatment With Lumbrokinase on Myocardial I-R-Induced Mitochondrial Oxidative Damage

Mitochondrial electron transport chain (ETC) deficiency induces reactive oxygen species (ROS) overproduction that may increase SDH and CcO activity in myocardial I-R injury (Muntean et al., 2016). We evaluated the role of mitochondrial oxidative damage in the cardioprotective effect of post-ischemic lumbrokinase treatment by evaluating the levels of SDH and CcO protein expression in rats subjected to myocardial I-R injury (**Figure 3**). We found that SDH and CcO levels were significantly increased after myocardial I-R injury compared with those in the sham group. Post-ischemic lumbrokinase treatment significantly attenuated SDH and CcO expression. We also assessed MnSOD protein expression to examine the effects of post-ischemic lumbrokinase treatment on oxidative stress (**Figure 3**). We found that MnSOD expression was significantly decreased after myocardial I-R injury compared with the sham-operated group. Post-ischemic lumbrokinase treatment significantly increased MnSOD expression compared with levels in the vehicle group. These results indicate that post-ischemic treatment with lumbrokinase attenuates myocardial I-R-induced mitochondrial oxidative damage.

TABLE 1 | Effects of post-ischemic lumbrokinase treatment in rats subjected to myocardial I-R injury.

		Sham (*n* = 6)	Vehicle (*n* = 13)	LK (*n* = 13)
Myocardial Infarction				
Ventricle (g)		0.78 ± 0.07	0.87 ± 0.05	0.86 ± 0.02
AAR (g)		–	0.55 ± 0.01	0.57 ± 0.01
AAR/Ventricle (%)		–	63.8 ± 2.89	65.8 ± 0.69
Infarct (g)		–	0.13 ± 0.004	0.11 ± 0.003#
Infarct/AAR (%)		–	23.6 ± 0.96	19.6 ± 0.59#
Cardiac Biomarkers				
LDH (U/L)		1083.0 ± 229.6	4290.0 ± 940.4*	3125.3 ± 577.4#
CK-MB (U/L)		4525.5 ± 1548.5	10053.6 ± 1285.9*	7209.8 ± 984.9#
Troponin-I (ng/mL)		1.07 ± 0.68	189.29 ± 52.68*	39.44 ± 19.00#
Arrthymias				
VT	Incidence (%)	–	86	46#
	Duration (sec)	–	26.4 ± 8.4	3.8 ± 1.8#
VF	Incidence (%)	–	36	8
	Duration (sec)	–	19.8 ± 8.6	0.9 ± 0.9#

*AAR, area at risk; LDH, lactate dehydrogenase; CK-MB, creatine kinase-MB; VT, ventricular tachycardia; VF, ventricular fibrillation. Values are shown as the mean ± SEM. *$p < 0.05$ compared with sham; #$p < 0.05$ compared with vehicle.*

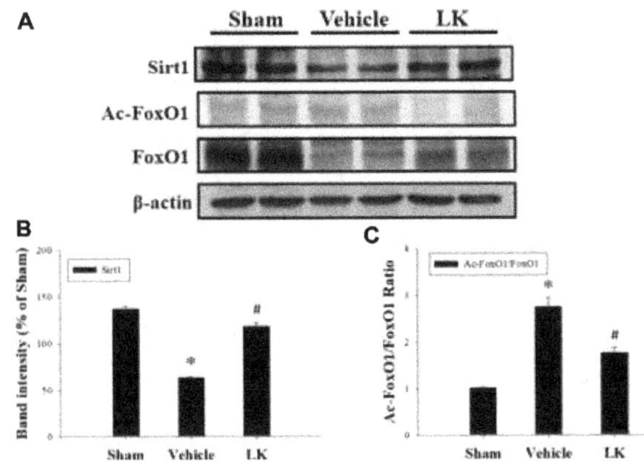

FIGURE 2 | Post-ischemic lumbrokinase treatment activated Sirt1 after myocardial I-R injury. Post-ischemic treatment with vehicle or lumbrokinase (10 μg/kg) in rats subjected to myocardial I-R injury. **(A)** Representative images of the Western blot results. Quantitative densitometric analysis of **(B)** Sirt1 protein expression and **(C)** the ratio of Ac-FoxO1 to FoxO1 in rat myocardium after myocardial I-R injury. Data are normalized with values from the sham group and presented as percentage rates. Each value is represented as the mean ± SEM (n = 3). $^*p < 0.05$ compared with the sham group; $^{\#}p < 0.05$ compared with the vehicle group.

Effects of Post-ischemic Treatment With Lumbrokinase on Myocardial I-R-Induced Cardiomyocyte Apoptosis

In order to investigate the anti-apoptotic effects of post-ischemic lumbrokinase treatment, we evaluated the expression of Bcl-2, Bax and Caspase-3 in rats subjected to myocardial I-R injury (**Figure 4**). Compared with the sham-operated group, the expression of Bax, the active form of caspase-3 and the Cleaved-Caspase-3/Pro-Caspase-3 ratio were significantly increased, while Bcl-2 expression and the Bcl-2/Bax ratio were significantly decreased in the vehicle group. The opposite trends were observed with post-ischemic lumbrokinase administration, with significant reductions in Bax, Cleaved-Caspase-3 expression and the Cleaved-Caspase-3/Pro-Caspase-3 ratio, and significant increases in Bcl-2 expression and the Bcl-2/Bax ratio in the myocardium. These results indicate that post-ischemic treatment with lumbrokinase attenuates myocardial I-R-induced cardiomyocyte apoptosis.

Effects of Post-ischemic Treatment With Lumbrokinase on Myocardial I-R-Induced Inflammation

We measured the protein expression levels of NF-κB, p-NF-κB, COX-2, and iNOS to assess the role played by inflammation on the effect of lumbrokinase post-ischemic treatment in rats subjected to myocardial I-R injury. As shown in **Figure 5**, we found significant increases in NF-κB, p-NF-κB, COX-2, and iNOS protein expression in the myocardium after myocardial I-R injury compared with the sham-operated animals. Levels of NF-κB, p-NF-κB, COX-2, and iNOS expression were significantly decreased by post-ischemic lumbrokinase treatment compared with levels in vehicle-treated animals. These results indicate that post-ischemic treatment with lumbrokinase attenuates myocardial I-R-induced inflammation.

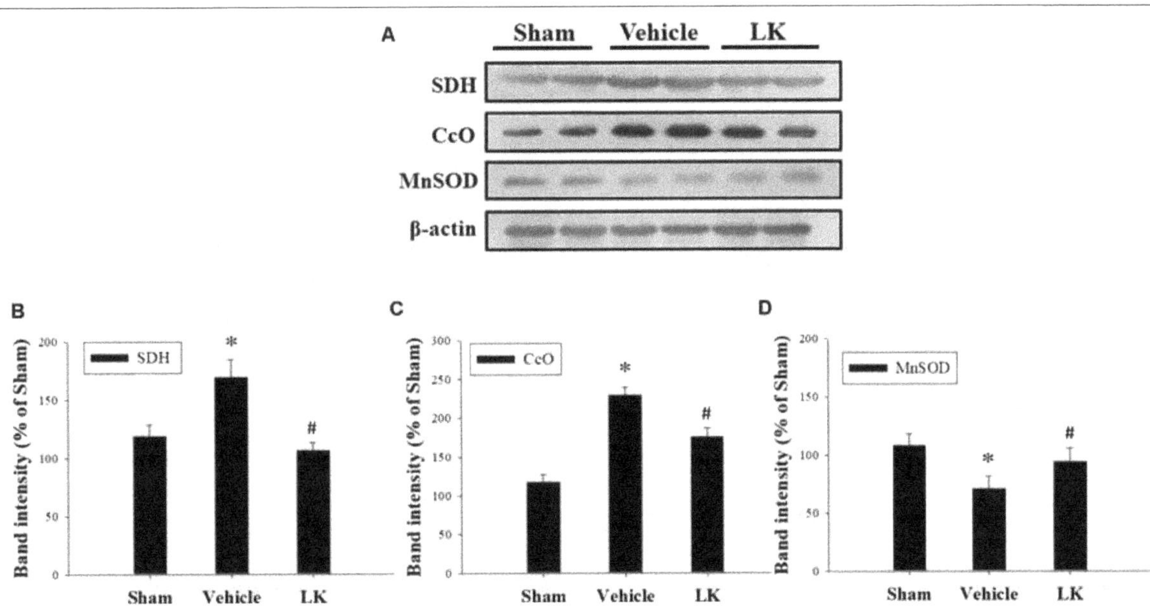

FIGURE 3 | Post-ischemic lumbrokinase treatment reduced mitochondrial oxidative stress induced by myocardial I-R injury. **(A)** Representative images of the Western blot results. Quantitative densitometric analysis of **(B)** SDH, **(C)** CcO, and **(D)** MnSOD protein expression in rat myocardium after myocardial I-R injury. Data are normalized with values from the sham group and presented as percentage rates. Each value is represented as the mean ± SEM (n = 3). $^*p < 0.05$ compared with the sham group; $^{\#}p < 0.05$ compared with the vehicle group.

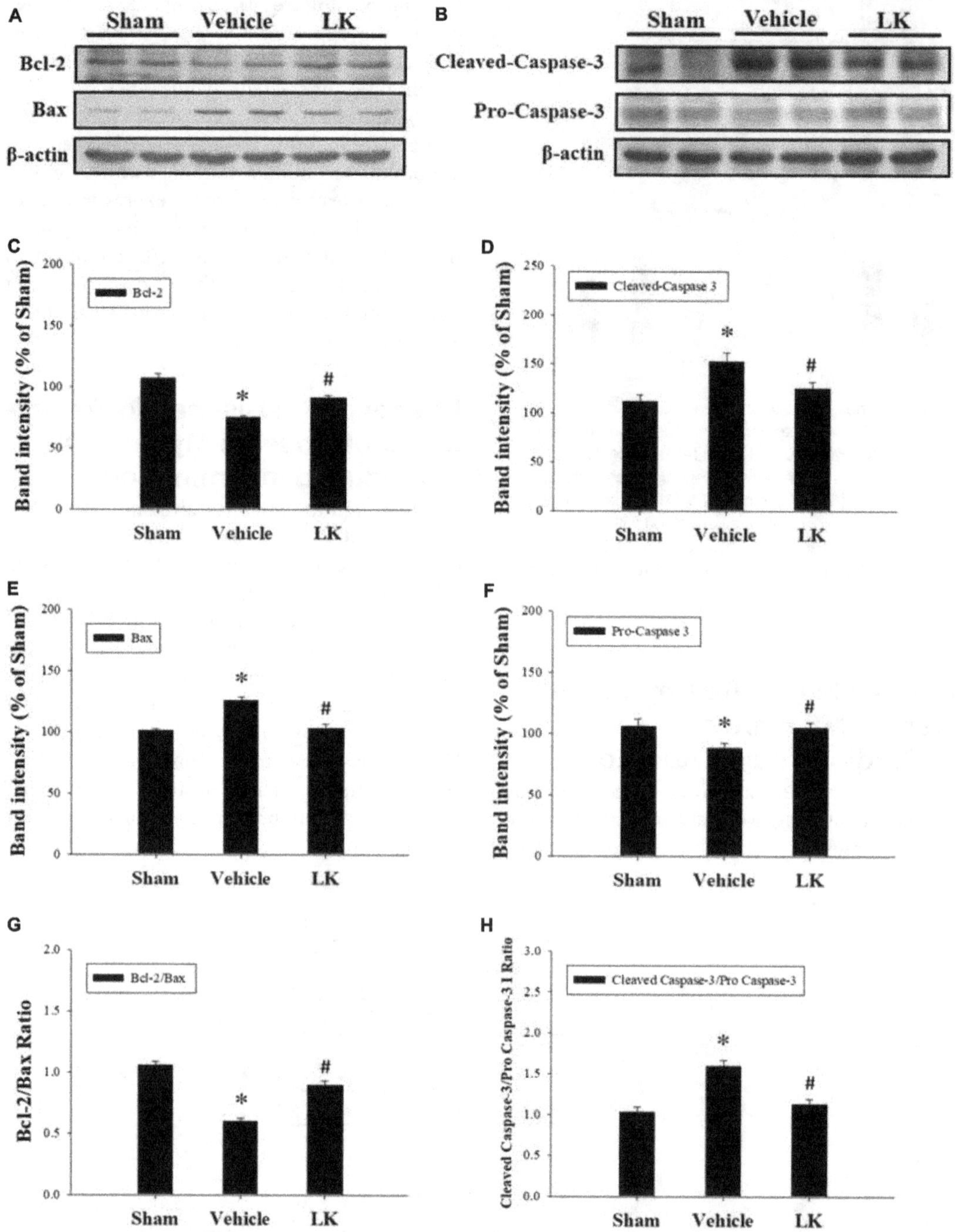

FIGURE 4 | Post-ischemic lumbrokinase treatment attenuated cardiomyocyte apoptosis in rats subjected to myocardial I-R injury. Representative immunoblot images of **(A)** Bcl-2 and Bax, and **(B)** Cleaved-Caspase-3 and Pro-Caspase-3. Quantitative densitometric analysis showing expression of **(C)** Bcl-2, **(D)** Bax, **(E)** the ratio of Bcl-2 to Bax, **(F)** Cleaved-Caspase 3 **(G)** Pro-Caspase-3 and **(H)** the ratio of Cleaved-Caspase 3 to Pro-Caspase-3 in rat myocardium after myocardial I-R injury. Data are normalized with values from the sham group and presented as percentage rates. Each value is represented as the mean ± SEM (n = 3). $^{*}p < 0.05$ compared with the sham group; $^{\#}p < 0.05$ compared with the vehicle group.

Effects of Post-ischemic Treatment With Lumbrokinase on Myocardial I-R-Induced Autophagy

We evaluated the levels of Beclin-1, p62, and LC3 expression to examine the role of autophagy in the effect of post-ischemic lumbrokinase treatment (**Figure 6**). We found that Beclin-1, p62, and LC3 expression were all significantly decreased after myocardial I-R injury compared with the sham-operated group, and that post-ischemic lumbrokinase treatment significantly increased the levels of these autophagy-related proteins after myocardial I-R injury compared with those in the vehicle group.

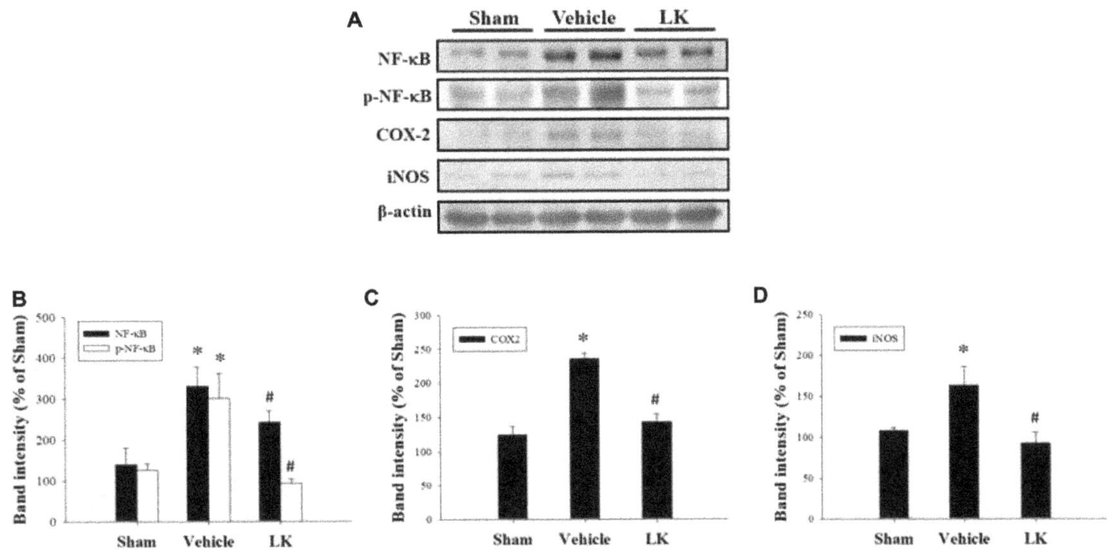

FIGURE 5 | Post-ischemic lumbrokinase treatment reduced levels of inflammation induced by myocardial I-R injury. **(A)** Representative images of the Western blot results. Quantitative densitometric analysis of **(B)** NF-κB and p-NF-κB, **(C)** COX-2, and **(D)** iNOS protein expression in rat myocardium after myocardial I-R injury. Data are normalized with values from the sham group and presented as percentage rates. Each value is represented as the mean ± SEM (n = 3). $^{*}p < 0.05$ compared with the sham group; $^{\#}p < 0.05$ compared with the vehicle group.

These results indicate that post-ischemic lumbrokinase treatment enhances autophagy.

Effects of Post-ischemic Treatment With Lumbrokinase and EX527 in Rats Subjected to Myocardial I-R Injury

Further to the above-mentioned results, we speculated that the post-ischemic cardioprotective effects of lumbrokinase are associated with Sirtl signaling. We therefore examined the effects of EX527, a selective Sirtl inhibitor, to investigate the mechanisms underlying lumbrokinase-induced effects. Firstly, the effects of post-ischemic treatment with lumbrokinase and EX527 on myocardial I-R-induced cardiac dysfunction are shown in **Figure 7**. Baseline cardiac function parameters did not differ significantly amongst these groups. In the LK, LVSP and max dP/dt values at CAO 30 min and the value of max dP/dt at 180 min after coronary artery reperfusion (CAR 180 min) were significantly increased compared with the vehicle group. In rats intraperitoneally injected with EX527 at 5 min before lumbrokinase administration, LVSP and max dP/dt values at CAO 30 min and max dP/dt at CAR 180 min were significantly decreased compared with those in the LK. Secondly, the influences of post-ischemic treatment with lumbrokinase and EX527 on myocardial I-R-induced myocardial damage are presented in **Figure 8**. In comparison with vehicle-treated rats, post-ischemic lumbrokinase treatment significantly reduced the infarct/AAR ratio, LDH, and CK-MB activities and troponin I levels in plasma collected at the end of the myocardial I-R procedure. In addition, we found that EX527 treatment abolished the protective effects of lumbrokinase by significantly increasing the infarct/AAR ratio, LDH, and CK-MB activities and the troponin levels in plasma determined after myocardial I-R, compared with the LK. Thirdly, the outcomes of lumbrokinase and EX527 on myocardial I-R-induced arrhythmias in rats are expressed in **Figure 8**. Post-ischemic administration with lumbrokinase significantly reduced the incidence of VT and the durations of VT and VF compared with the vehicle group. The anti-arrythmic effect of lumbrokinase was abolished by administration of EX527, which significantly increased the incidence of VT to 78% and the duration of VT to 16.8 ± 6.8 s compared with values in theLK. Based on the above results, we suggest that the cardioprotective effects of post-ischemic treatment with lumbrokinase may involve the Sirtl-related signaling pathway.

DISCUSSION AND CONCLUSION

The important findings of this study are as follows: first, we found that administration of lumbrokinase 20 min after ischemia significantly reduced the durations of VT and VF and the incidence of VT, improved cardiac function and decreased myocardial infarction, all of which are consistent with our findings that post-ischemic lumbrokinase treatment decreases plasma LDH, CK-MB activities and troponin I levels, which serve as indicators of myocardial damage. Second, we have demonstrated that post-ischemic lumbrokinase treatment decreased oxidative stress, inflammation and apoptosis after myocardial I-R injury. Lumbrokinase also increased autophagosome levels and activated Sirtl, which induced the deacetylation of FoxO1. Third, our results indicate that EX527, a specific Sirtl inhibitor, abolishes the cardioprotective effects of lumbrokinase. Importantly, this is the first study to suggest that

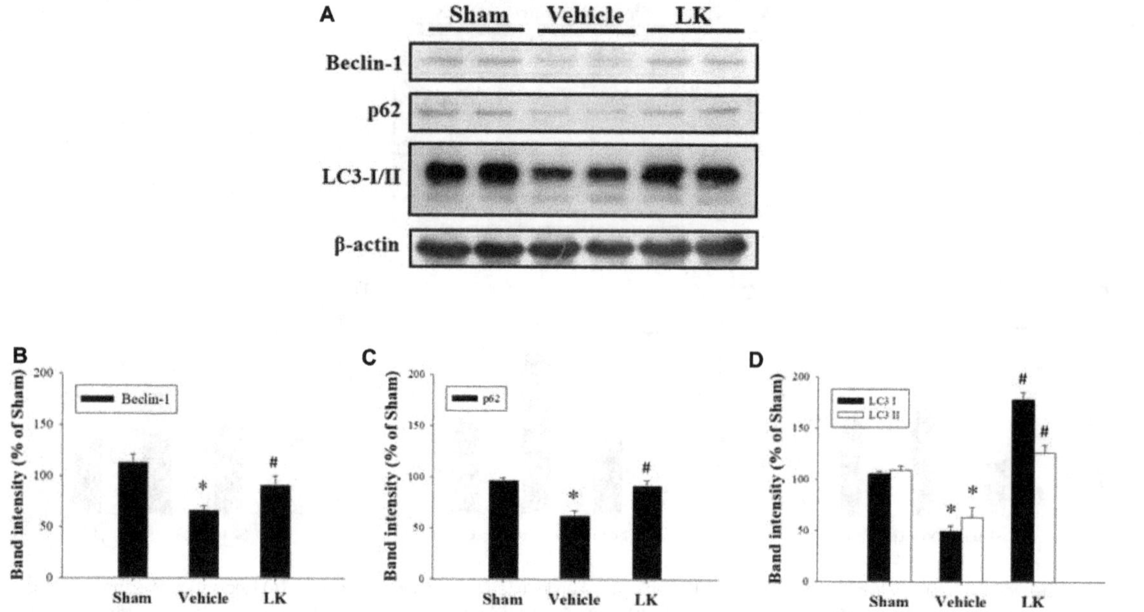

FIGURE 6 | Post-ischemic lumbrokinase treatment enhanced autophagic flux in rats subjected to myocardial I-R injury. **(A)** Representative images of the Western blot results. Quantitative densitometric analysis of **(B)** Beclin-1, **(C)** p62, and **(D)** LC3-I/II protein expression in rat myocardium after myocardial I-R injury. Data are normalized with values from the sham group and presented as percentage rates. Each value is represented as the mean ± SEM (n = 3). $^*p < 0.05$ compared with the sham group; $^\#p < 0.05$ compared with the vehicle group.

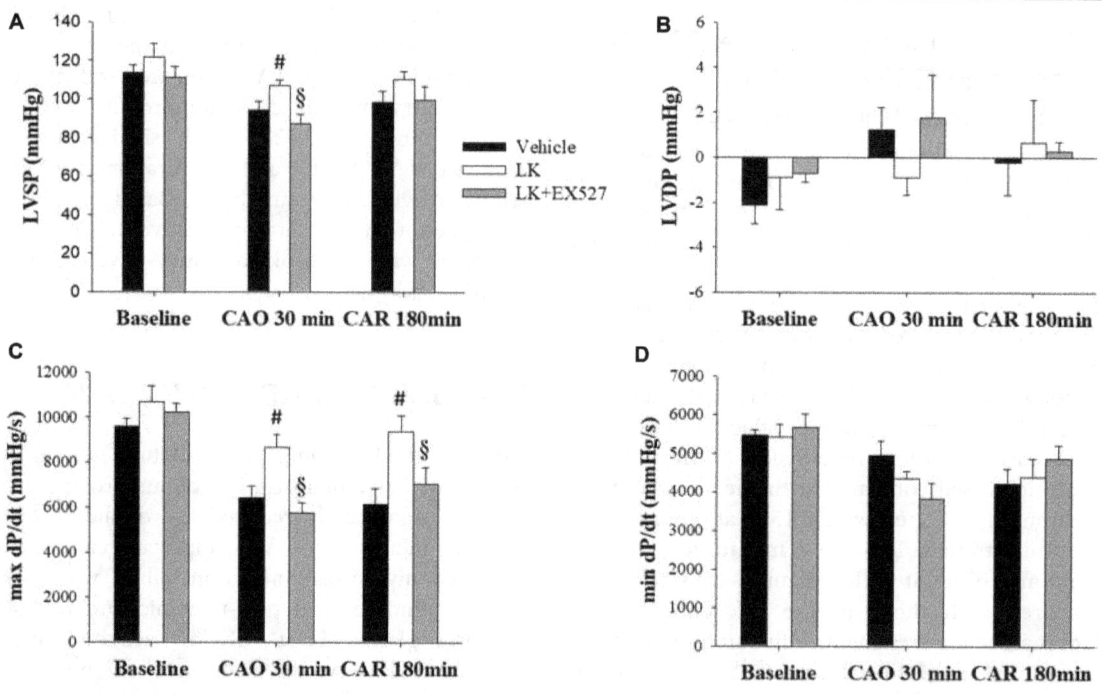

FIGURE 7 | Post-ischemic lumbrokinase treatment reserved myocardial ischemia-reperfusion injury induced cardiac dysfunction via Sirt1 activation. Post-ischemic treatment with vehicle or lumbrokinase (10 μg/kg) was given 20 min after coronal artery ligation; the Sirt1 specific inhibitor, EX527, was administered 15 min after coronal artery ligation. Cardiac function parameters were assessed by a pressure transducer catheter inserted into the LV via the carotid artery. **(A)** LVSP, **(B)** LVDP, **(C)** max dP/dt, and **(D)** min dP/dt were determined before CAO (baseline), 30 min after CAO (CAO 30 min), and 180 min after reperfusion (CAR 180 min). Each value is represented as the mean ± SEM (n = 4–10). $^\#p < 0.05$ compared with the vehicle group; $^\S p < 0.05$ compared with the LK group.

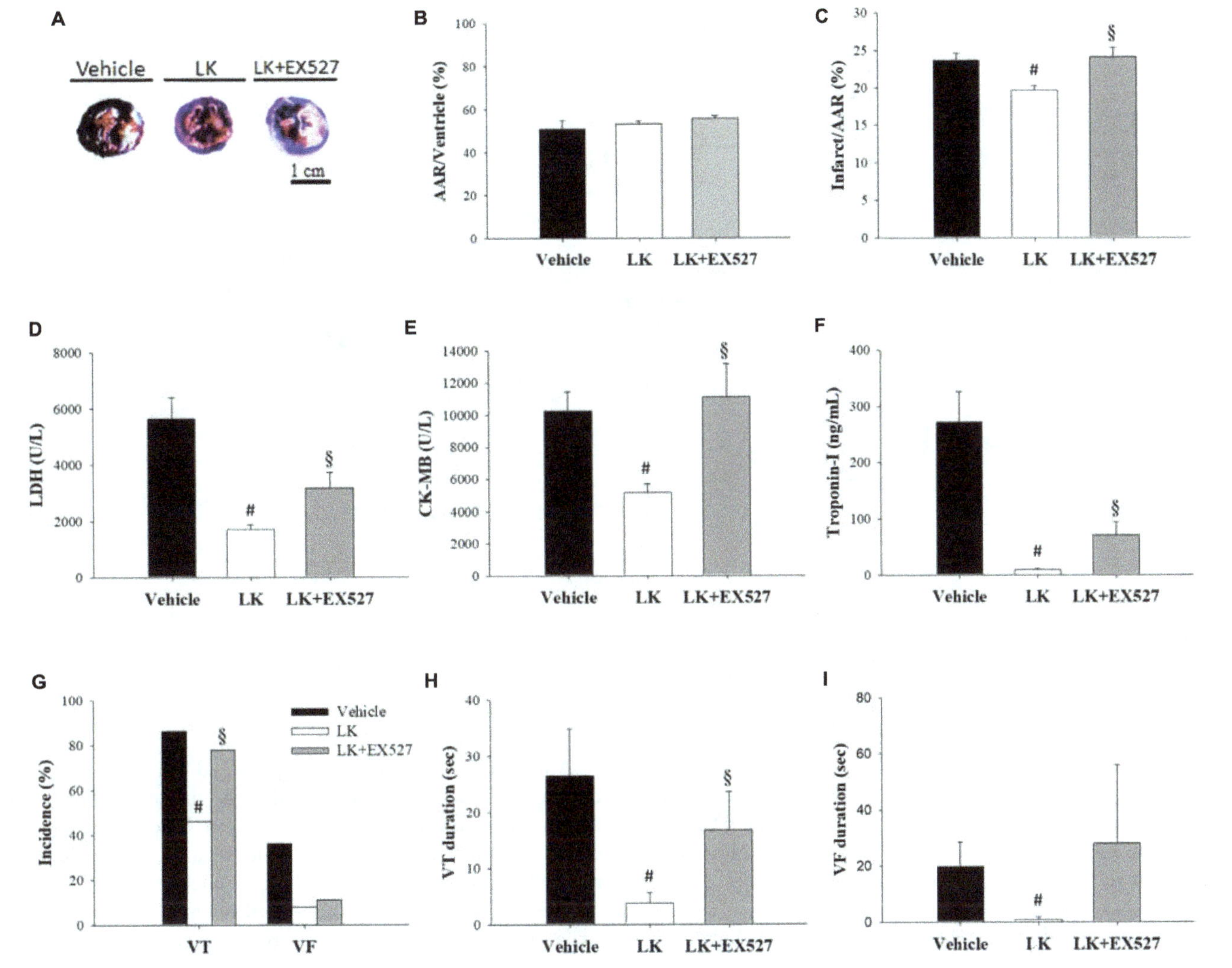

FIGURE 8 | Post-ischemic lumbrokinase treatment attenuated myocardial damage via the Sirt1 signaling pathway. Myocardial infarct size was evaluated by Evans blue/TTC staining. **(A)** Representative images of heart horizontal sections. The blue area depicts non-ischemic tissue, red plus white depicts at-risk tissue, white depicts infarcted tissue. **(B)** The area at risk (AAR) was measured relative to the ventricle and **(C)** the infarct was measured relative to the AAR. The activities of **(D)** LDH, **(E)** CK-MB, and the levels of **(F)** troponin-I were assessed by an automated clinical analyzer. **(G)** The incidence of VT and VF and the duration of **(H)** VT and **(I)** VF were monitored during 30 min of ischemia followed by 3 h of reperfusion. Each value is represented as the mean ± SEM (n = 4–13). $^{\#}p < 0.05$ compared with the vehicle group; $^{\S}p < 0.05$ compared with the LK group.

Sirt1 signaling plays a critical role in the cardioprotective effects of lumbrokinase when administered after myocardial ischemia. The data in **Figure 9** summarize the effect of post-ischemic treatment with lumbrokinase in rats subjected to myocardial I-R injury.

Previous studies have demonstrated that the reperfusion of ischemic myocardium induces the excessive generation of ROS, resulting in oxidative stress (Zhou et al., 2015). Mitochondrial ETC have been conventionally recognized as the major source of ROS, activating cytotoxic mechanisms responsible for cell death via apoptosis and necrosis during myocardial I-R injury (Brown and Griendling, 2015). ETC components are organized into five complexes (complex I, II, III, IV, and V), with each complex containing several different electron carriers. Although the main sources of ROS in the myocardial mitochondria are complexes I and III (Chen and Zweier, 2014), some studies have indicated that inhibition of SDH (complex II) or CcO (complex IV) may also reduce ROS generation (Drose et al., 2011; Chouchani et al., 2014; Yang et al., 2017). Our results show that levels of SDH and CcO expression are significantly increased in the myocardium after myocardial I-R injury. Post-ischemic lumbrokinase treatment significantly attenuated these increases. Interestingly, we also observed in this myocardial I-R injury model that MnSOD expression was significantly decreased in the myocardium after myocardial I-R injury and that post-ischemic lumbrokinase treatment significantly reversed this phenomenon. MnSOD is the main endogenous antioxidant enzyme that protects the heart from active oxygen species (Csanyi and Miller, 2014). This protection is necessary for preservation of ETC function and certain functions of the tricarboxylic acid (TCA) cycle. MnSOD is

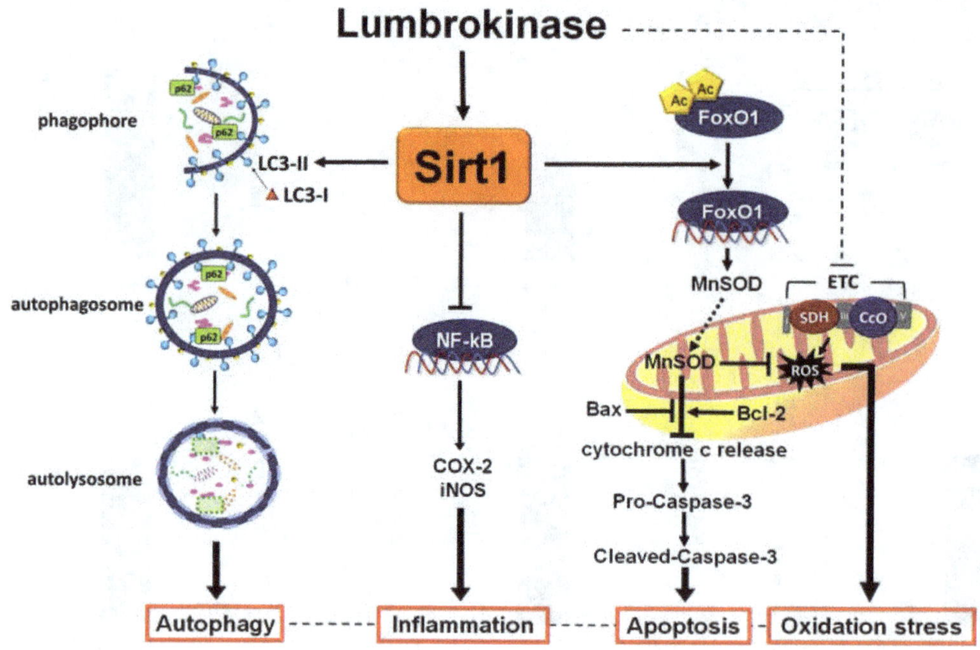

FIGURE 9 | Schematic diagram of the effects of post-ischemic lumbrokinase treatment in myocardial I-R injury. Post-ischemic lumbrokinase treatment attenuates myocardial I-R injury through the activation of Sirt1 signaling, inhibition of NF-κB expression and activation of FoxO1 and LC3, and thus reduces inflammation, oxidative stress and apoptosis, and enhances autophagy after myocardial I-R injury.

not only an essential cytoprotector against the deleterious effects of ROS but is also a mediator of mitochondrial ROS signaling through the generation of H_2O_2. Changes in MnSOD activity are associated with a variety of diseases, such as cardiovascular disease, cancer, the metabolic syndrome and the process of aging (Candas and Li, 2014).

It is well known that an imbalance between ROS production and elimination leads to inflammatory reaction in myocardial I-R injury (Xiong et al., 2010; Rodrigo et al., 2013). Subsequent ROS generation by polymorphonuclear neutrophils (PMNs) triggers inflammation, causing endothelial dysfunction and severe cardiac damage (Mittal et al., 2014; Valle Raleigh et al., 2017). The activation of the NF-κB signaling pathway plays a central role in the inflammatory processes that occur during myocardial I-R injury (Kitada et al., 2016). When exposed to I-R injury, various cytokines are released that trigger an inflammatory reaction and ROS overproduction leading to oxidative stress, which activates cytotoxic mechanisms responsible for cardiac dysfunction and cell death via apoptosis and necrosis (Yellon and Hausenloy, 2007; Steffens et al., 2009; Padfield et al., 2013; Yang et al., 2013; Brown and Griendling, 2015). In this study, we found that post-ischemic lumbrokinase treatment induces cardioprotective effects that are partly mediated by reducing the inflammatory response. The results of this present study show that post-ischemic lumbrokinase treatment in myocardial I-R injury significantly reduces levels of NF-κB, COX-2, and iNOS expression in the I-R myocardium. These findings suggest that post-ischemic treatment with lumbrokinase reduces inflammation after myocardial I-R injury.

Apoptosis is a process of programmed cell death that occurs in multicellular organisms, which is initiated shortly after the onset of myocardial infarction and becomes significantly enhanced during reperfusion (Gu et al., 2014). The Bcl-2 family of proteins acts as a critical checkpoint of apoptotic cell death. The anti-apoptotic members of this family, such as Bcl-2, interact with the pro-apoptotic members, such as Bax, which is required to regulate the process of cytochrome *c* release from the mitochondrion and modulate sensitivity to cell death signals (Letai, 2005). Caspases are a family of protease enzymes that are crucial mediators of programmed cell death. Initiator caspases activate executioner caspases that subsequently coordinate their activities to cleave the nuclear lamin and activate other enzymes (McIlwain et al., 2013). Caspase-3 is considered to be the most important of the executioner caspases. Once caspases are initially activated, there seems to be an irreversible commitment towards cell death (Elmore, 2007). In this study, we found that post-ischemic lumbrokinase treatment provided anti-apoptotic effects by increasing the Bcl-2/Bax ratio and decreasing the Cleaved-Caspase-3/Pro-Caspase-3 ratio after myocardial I-R injury. Notably, apoptosis and autophagy are important in cellular programmed death that occurs in myocardial I-R injury. Apoptosis can regulate autophagy; conversely, autophagy can regulate apoptosis (Gordy and He, 2012; Yonekawa and Thorburn, 2013). Autophagy is an important switch that protects cells from undergoing apoptosis (Green and Levine, 2014). LC3, p62, and Beclin-1 are the main autophagic indicators and are essential components for the formation of autophagosomes. At an early stage of autophagy, Beclin-1 is involved in the nucleation phase of phagopore formation, while the cytosolic

LC3-I form is converted into the lipidated LC3-II form associated with autophagosomal membranes, and p62 together with ubiquitinated proteins are transported to autophagosomes (Mizushima et al., 2010). Monitoring the conversion of LC3 is considered to be one of the most reliable ways to monitor autophagic flux, preferable to analysis of other components of the autophagic mechanism such as members of the initiation complex (i.e., Beclin-1) or autolysosome substrates (i.e., p62) (Ma et al., 2015). Deficiency of Beclin-1 and p62 lead to increase ROS levels and enhancement of cell death, while treatment with rapamycin or overexpression of Beclin-1 induce autophagy and have been shown to play a protective role in response to I-R (Gurusamy et al., 2009). In this study, we found that post-ischemic lumbrokinase treatment significantly increased autophagosome levels by increasing the levels of Beclin-1, p62, and LC3 expression after myocardial I-R injury. These results illustrate that post-ischemic lumbrokinase treatment enhances autophagy and thereby attenuates myocardial I-R-induced cardiomyocyte apoptosis.

Our results also show that post-ischemic administration with lumbrokinase increased Sirt1 expression and decreased the Ac-FoxO1/FoxO1 ratio. Sirt1 has the ability to deacetylate FoxO, leading to an upregulation in expression of genes involved in cell-protective processes. Researchers have reported that Sirt1 activation reduces oxidative stress and maintains mitochondrial function by deacetylating and activating some of the FoxO family proteins and synthesizing antioxidant enzymes, such as MnSOD and catalase (Brunet et al., 2004; El Assar et al., 2013). Furthermore, Sirt1 plays a beneficial role in myocardial I-R injury (Hsu et al., 2010; Yang et al., 2013). Not only does Sirt1 activation protect against myocardial I-R injury by upregulating antioxidants and anti-apoptotic molecules, but Sirt1 also downregulates pro-apoptotic molecules through the deacetylation of FoxO1 in Sirt1 transgenic mice (Hsu et al., 2010). In this study, treatment with lumbrokinase after ischemia significantly increased Sirt1 expression. Importantly, the upregulation of Sirt1 induced by post-ischemic lumbrokinase treatment reduced levels of the pro-apoptotic factor Bax and the apoptosis-related Cleaved-Caspase-3 protein, and increased anti-apoptotic Bcl-2 expression. Notably, inhibiting Sirt1 with EX527 abolished the cardioprotective effects of lumbrokinase. We therefore suggest that Sirt1 signaling is involved in the post-ischemic cardioprotective effects of lumbrokinase treatment.

Many mechanisms of lumbrokinase have been reported in the literatures. Lumbrokinase inhibits second-hand smoke-induced apoptotic signaling and cardiac fibrosis by blocking transforming growth factor beta (TGF-β) receptors and suppressing ERK1/2 activation, and thus modulates downstream molecular events (Liao et al., 2015). Lumbrokinase also reduces side-stream cigarette smoke-induced hippocampus apoptosis and autophagy by enhancing eNOS expression and inhibiting proinflammatory NF-κB/iNOS/COX-2 signaling activity (Huang et al., 2013). Previous studies have demonstrated protective effects of lumbrokinase against I-R injury. For instance, lumbrokinase has a neuroprotective effect via its anti-platelet activity, increasing c-AMP levels and reducing calcium release from calcium stores, and acts as an anti-thrombotic by inhibiting ICAM-1 expression, and displays anti-apoptotic activity via the activation of the JAK1/STAT1 pathway in the focal cerebral ischemia injury model (Ji et al., 2008). In our previous study, the cardioprotective effects of pretreatment with lumbrokinase appeared to correlate with its anti-inflammatory effects on I-R-induced expression of COX-2, iNOS, and MMP-9, which were mediated by TLR4 signaling through the JNK and NF-κB pathways (Wang et al., 2016). According to the results in this study, we consider that Sirt1 signaling plays a critical role in the cardioprotective effects of lumbrokinase when administered after myocardial ischemia. We observed that the post-ischemic lumbrokinase treatment attenuated myocardial I-R injury by activating Sirt1 signaling, and thus reduced I-R-induced levels of COX-2, iNOS, and NF-κB expression. Evidence suggests that Sirt1 regulates inflammatory responses through NF-κB deacetylation, and that TLR4 signaling pathways culminated in activation of the transcription factor NF-κB, which controls some factors involved in inflammation, such as proinflammatory cytokines (TNF-α and IL-1β), adhesion molecules, and enzymes such as iNOS and COX-2 (Yang et al., 2012; Fuentes-Antras et al., 2014). We speculate that NF-κB plays an important regulatory role in the crosstalk between anti-inflammatory action seen with lumbrokinase when given before or after myocardial I-R injury.

In conclusion, this study demonstrates that Sirt1 is a critical regulator in the post-ischemic cardioprotective effects of lumbrokinase in rats subjected to myocardial I-R injury. We provide evidence that post-ischemic lumbrokinase administration significantly attenuates infarct size, and improves ventricular arrhythmias and cardiac dysfunction resulting from myocardial I-R injury. Moreover, post-ischemic treatment with lumbrokinase activates Sirt1 and induces FoxO1 deacetylation, which enhances autophagic flux and reduces oxidative damage, inflammation and apoptosis after myocardial I-R-injury. In our previous study, we reported that pretreatment with lumbrokinase protects the heart through anti-inflammatory mechanisms against myocardial I-R injury (Wang et al., 2016). We believe that the use of lumbrokinase will provide a novel therapeutic strategy against myocardial I-R injury. It would be very interesting to explore the therapeutic effects of this dietary supplement in the amelioration of myocardial I-R injury in humans.

AUTHOR CONTRIBUTIONS

Y-HW and S-SH designed research. S-AL, C-HH, H-HS, and Y-HC conducted research and analyzed data. Y-HW, JC, and S-SH wrote the paper. All authors read and approved the final manuscript.

FUNDING

This work was supported financially by research grants from Chung Shan Medical University Hospital (CSH-2017-C-021) and Taiwan's Ministry of Science and Technology (MOST 103-2320-B-040-001-MY3 and MOST 106-2320-B-040-005) awarded to S-SH.

REFERENCES

Bohl, S., Medway, D. J., Schulz-Menger, J., Schneider, J. E., Neubauer, S., and Lygate, C. A. (2009). Refined approach for quantification of in vivo ischemia-reperfusion injury in the mouse heart. *Am. J. Physiol. Heart Circ. Physiol.* 297, H2054–H2058. doi: 10.1152/ajpheart.00836.2009

Brown, D. I., and Griendling, K. K. (2015). Regulation of signal transduction by reactive oxygen species in the cardiovascular system. *Circ. Res.* 116, 531–549. doi: 10.1161/CIRCRESAHA.116.303584

Brunet, A., Sweeney, L. B., Sturgill, J. F., Chua, K. F., Greer, P. L., Lin, Y., et al. (2004). Stress-dependent regulation of FOXO transcription factors by the SIRT1 deacetylase. *Science* 303, 2011–2015. doi: 10.1126/science.1094637

Candas, D., and Li, J. J. (2014). MnSOD in oxidative stress response-potential regulation via mitochondrial protein influx. *Antioxid. Redox Signal.* 20, 1599–1617. doi: 10.1089/ars.2013.5305

Cao, Y. J., Zhang, X., Wang, W. H., Zhai, W. Q., Qian, J. F., Wang, J. S., et al. (2013). Oral fibrinogen-depleting agent lumbrokinase for secondary ischemic stroke prevention: results from a multicenter, randomized, parallel-group and controlled clinical trial. *Chin. Med. J.* 126, 4060–4065.

Chen, Y. R., and Zweier, J. L. (2014). Cardiac mitochondria and reactive oxygen species generation. *Circ. Res.* 114, 524–537. doi: 10.1161/CIRCRESAHA.114.300559

Cho, I. H., Choi, E. S., Lim, H. G., and Lee, H. H. (2004). Purification and characterization of six fibrinolytic serine-proteases from earthworm *Lumbricus rubellus*. *J. Biochem. Mol. Biol.* 37, 199–205. doi: 10.5483/BMBRep.2004.37.2.199

Chouchani, E. T., Pell, V. R., Gaude, E., Aksentijevic, D., Sundier, S. Y., Robb, E. L., et al. (2014). Ischaemic accumulation of succinate controls reperfusion injury through mitochondrial ROS. *Nature* 515, 431–435. doi: 10.1038/nature13909

Cooper, E. L., and Balamurugan, M. (2010). Unearthing a source of medicinal molecules. *Drug Discov. Today* 15, 966–972. doi: 10.1016/j.drudis.2010.09.004

Csanyi, G., and Miller, F. J. Jr. (2014). Oxidative stress in cardiovascular disease. *Int. J. Mol. Sci.* 15, 6002–6008. doi: 10.3390/ijms15046002

Curtis, M. J., Hancox, J. C., Farkas, A., Wainwright, C. L., Stables, C. L., Saint, D. A., et al. (2013). The Lambeth Conventions (II): guidelines for the study of animal and human ventricular and supraventricular arrhythmias. *Pharmacol. Ther.* 139, 213–248. doi: 10.1016/j.pharmthera.2013.04.008

Delaney, J. A., Opatrny, L., Brophy, J. M., and Suissa, S. (2007). Drug drug interactions between antithrombotic medications and the risk of gastrointestinal bleeding. *CMAJ* 177, 347–351. doi: 10.1503/cmaj.070186

Ding, M., Lei, J., Han, H., Li, W., Qu, Y., Fu, E., et al. (2015). SIRT1 protects against myocardial ischemia-reperfusion injury via activating eNOS in diabetic rats. *Cardiovasc. Diabetol.* 14:143. doi: 10.1186/s12933-015-0299-8

Drose, S., Bleier, L., and Brandt, U. (2011). A common mechanism links differently acting complex II inhibitors to cardioprotection: modulation of mitochondrial reactive oxygen species production. *Mol. Pharmacol.* 79, 814–822. doi: 10.1124/mol.110.070342

El Assar, M., Angulo, J., and Rodriguez-Manas, L. (2013). Oxidative stress and vascular inflammation in aging. *Free Radic. Biol. Med.* 65, 380–401. doi: 10.1016/j.freeradbiomed.2013.07.003

Elmore, S. (2007). Apoptosis: a review of programmed cell death. *Toxicol. Pathol.* 35, 495–516. doi: 10.1080/01926230701320337

Fuentes-Antras, J., Ioan, A. M., Tunon, J., Egido, J., and Lorenzo, O. (2014). Activation of toll-like receptors and inflammasome complexes in the diabetic cardiomyopathy-associated inflammation. *Int. J. Endocrinol.* 2014:847827. doi: 10.1155/2014/847827

Gordy, C., and He, Y. W. (2012). The crosstalk between autophagy and apoptosis: where does this lead? *Protein Cell* 3, 17–27. doi: 10.1007/s13238-011-1127-x

Green, D. R., and Levine, B. (2014). To be or not to be? How selective autophagy and cell death govern cell fate. *Cell* 157, 65–75. doi: 10.1016/j.cell.2014.02.049

Gu, J., Fan, Y., Liu, X., Zhou, L., Cheng, J., Cai, R., et al. (2014). SENP1 protects against myocardial ischaemia/reperfusion injury via a HIF1alpha-dependent pathway. *Cardiovasc. Res.* 104, 83–92. doi: 10.1093/cvr/cvu177

Guarente, L. (2011). Franklin H. Epstein Lecture: Sirtuins, aging, and medicine. *N. Engl. J. Med.* 364, 2235–2244. doi: 10.1056/NEJMra1100831

Gurusamy, N., Lekli, I., Gorbunov, N. V., Gherghiceanu, M., Popescu, L. M., and Das, D. K. (2009). Cardioprotection by adaptation to ischaemia augments autophagy in association with BAG-1 protein. *J. Cell Mol. Med.* 13, 373–387. doi: 10.1111/j.1582-4934.2008.00495.x

Hausenloy, D. J., and Yellon, D. M. (2013). Myocardial ischemia-reperfusion injury: a neglected therapeutic target. *J. Clin. Invest.* 123, 92–100. doi: 10.1172/JCI62874

Hsu, C. P., Zhai, P., Yamamoto, T., Maejima, Y., Matsushima, S., Hariharan, N., et al. (2010). Silent information regulator 1 protects the heart from ischemia/reperfusion. *Circulation* 122, 2170–2182. doi: 10.1161/CIRCULATIONAHA.110.958033

Huang, C. Y., Kuo, W. W., Liao, H. E., Lin, Y. M., Kuo, C. H., Tsai, F. J., et al. (2013). Lumbrokinase attenuates side-stream-smoke-induced apoptosis and autophagy in young hamster hippocampus: correlated with eNOS induction and NFkappaB/iNOS/COX-2 signaling suppression. *Chem. Res. Toxicol.* 26, 654–661. doi: 10.1021/tx300429s

Ji, H., Wang, L., Bi, H., Sun, L., Cai, B., Wang, Y., et al. (2008). Mechanisms of lumbrokinase in protection of cerebral ischemia. *Eur. J. Pharmacol.* 590, 281–289. doi: 10.1016/j.ejphar.2008.05.037

Kasim, M., Kiat, A. A., Rohman, M. S., Hanifah, Y., and Kiat, H. (2009). Improved myocardial perfusion in stable angina pectoris by oral lumbrokinase: a pilot study. *J. Altern. Complement. Med.* 15, 539–544. doi: 10.1089/acm.2008.0506

Kitada, M., Ogura, Y., and Koya, D. (2016). The protective role of Sirt1 in vascular tissue: its relationship to vascular aging and atherosclerosis. *Aging* 8, 2290–2307. doi: 10.18632/aging.101068

Letai, A. (2005). Pharmacological manipulation of Bcl-2 family members to control cell death. *J. Clin. Invest.* 115, 2648–2655. doi: 10.1172/JCI26250

Liao, H. E., Lai, C. H., Ho, T. J., Yeh, Y. L., Jong, G. P., Kuo, W. H., et al. (2015). Cardio protective effects of lumbrokinase and dilong on second-hand smoke-induced apoptotic signaling in the heart of a rat model. *Chin. J. Physiol.* 58, 188–196. doi: 10.4077/CJP.2015.BAD277

Ma, S., Wang, Y., Chen, Y., and Cao, F. (2015). The role of the autophagy in myocardial ischemia/reperfusion injury. *Biochim. Biophys. Acta* 1852, 271–276. doi: 10.1016/j.bbadis.2014.05.010

McIlwain, D. R., Berger, T., and Mak, T. W. (2013). Caspase functions in cell death and disease. *Cold Spring Harb. Perspect. Biol.* 5:a008656. doi: 10.1101/cshperspect.a008656

Mendis, S., Pekka, P., Norrving, B., World Health Organization and World Heart Federation (2011). *Global Atlas on Cardiovascular Disease Prevention and Control.* Geneva: World Health Organization.

Mihara, H., Sumi, H., Yoneta, T., Mizumoto, H., Ikeda, R., Seiki, M., et al. (1991). A novel fibrinolytic enzyme extracted from the earthworm, *Lumbricus rubellus*. *Jpn. J. Physiol.* 41, 461–472. doi: 10.2170/jjphysiol.41.461

Mitchell, S. J., Martin-Montalvo, A., Mercken, E. M., Palacios, H. H., Ward, T. M., Abulwerdi, G., et al. (2014). The SIRT1 activator SRT1720 extends lifespan and improves health of mice fed a standard diet. *Cell Rep.* 6, 836–843. doi: 10.1016/j.celrep.2014.01.031

Mittal, M., Siddiqui, M. R., Tran, K., Reddy, S. P., and Malik, A. B. (2014). Reactive oxygen species in inflammation and tissue injury. *Antioxid. Redox Signal.* 20, 1126–1167. doi: 10.1089/ars.2012.5149

Mizushima, N., Yoshimori, T., and Levine, B. (2010). Methods in mammalian autophagy research. *Cell* 140, 313–326. doi: 10.1016/j.cell.2010.01.028

Muntean, D. M., Sturza, A., Danila, M. D., Borza, C., Duicu, O. M., and Mornos, C. (2016). The role of mitochondrial reactive oxygen species in cardiovascular injury and protective strategies. *Oxid. Med. Cell. Longev.* 2016:8254942. doi: 10.1155/2016/8254942

Padfield, G. J., Din, J. N., Koushiappi, E., Mills, N. L., Robinson, S. D., Cruden Nle, M., et al. (2013). Cardiovascular effects of tumour necrosis factor alpha antagonism in patients with acute myocardial infarction: a first in human study. *Heart* 99, 1330–1335. doi: 10.1136/heartjnl-2013-303648

Rodrigo, R., Libuy, M., Feliu, F., and Hasson, D. (2013). Oxidative stress-related biomarkers in essential hypertension and ischemia-reperfusion myocardial damage. *Dis. Markers* 35, 773–790. doi: 10.1155/2013/974358

Steffens, S., Montecucco, F., and Mach, F. (2009). The inflammatory response as a target to reduce myocardial ischaemia and reperfusion injury. *Thromb. Haemost.* 102, 240–247. doi: 10.1160/TH08-12-0837

Valle Raleigh, J., Mauro, A. G., Devarakonda, T., Marchetti, C., He, J., Kim, E., et al. (2017). Reperfusion therapy with recombinant human relaxin-2 (Serelaxin) attenuates myocardial infarct size and NLRP3 inflammasome following ischemia/reperfusion injury via eNOS-dependent mechanism. *Cardiovasc. Res.* 113, 609–619. doi: 10.1093/cvr/cvw246

Vernooij, M. W., Haag, M. D., Van Der Lugt, A., Hofman, A., Krestin, G. P., Stricker, B. H., et al. (2009). Use of antithrombotic drugs and the presence of cerebral microbleeds: the Rotterdam Scan Study. *Arch. Neurol.* 66, 714–720. doi: 10.1001/archneurol.2009.42

Wang, K. Y., Tull, L., Cooper, E., Wang, N., and Liu, D. (2013). Recombinant protein production of earthworm lumbrokinase for potential antithrombotic application. *Evid. Based Complement. Alternat. Med.* 2013:783971. doi: 10.1155/2013/783971

Wang, Y. H., Chen, K. M., Chiu, P. S., Lai, S. C., Su, H. H., Jan, M. S., et al. (2016). Lumbrokinase attenuates myocardial ischemia-reperfusion injury by inhibiting TLR4 signaling. *J. Mol. Cell Cardiol.* 99, 113–122. doi: 10.1016/j.yjmcc.2016.08.004

Xiong, J., Xue, F. S., Yuan, Y. J., Wang, Q., Liao, X., and Wang, W. L. (2010). Cholinergic anti-inflammatory pathway: a possible approach to protect against myocardial ischemia reperfusion injury. *Chin. Med. J.* 123, 2720–2726.

Yamamoto, T., and Sadoshima, J. (2011). Protection of the heart against ischemia/reperfusion by silent information regulator 1. *Trends Cardiovasc. Med.* 21, 27–32. doi: 10.1016/j.tcm.2012.01.005

Yamamoto, T., Tamaki, K., Shirakawa, K., Ito, K., Yan, X., Katsumata, Y., et al. (2016). Cardiac Sirt1 mediates the cardioprotective effect of caloric restriction by suppressing local complement system activation after ischemia-reperfusion. *Am. J. Physiol. Heart Circ. Physiol.* 310, H1003–H1014. doi: 10.1152/ajpheart.00676.2015

Yang, H., Zhang, W., Pan, H., Feldser, H. G., Lainez, E., Miller, C., et al. (2012). SIRT1 activators suppress inflammatory responses through promotion of p65 deacetylation and inhibition of NF-kappaB activity. *PLoS One* 7:e46364. doi: 10.1371/journal.pone.0046364

Yang, Y., Duan, W., Lin, Y., Yi, W., Liang, Z., Yan, J., et al. (2013). SIRT1 activation by curcumin pretreatment attenuates mitochondrial oxidative damage induced by myocardial ischemia reperfusion injury. *Free Radic. Biol. Med.* 65, 667–679. doi: 10.1016/j.freeradbiomed.2013.07.007

Yang, Z., Duan, Z., Yu, T., Xu, J., and Liu, L. (2017). Inhibiting cytochrome C oxidase leads to alleviated ischemia reperfusion injury. *Korean Circ. J.* 47, 193–200. doi: 10.4070/kcj.2016.0137

Yellon, D. M., and Hausenloy, D. J. (2007). Myocardial reperfusion injury. *N. Engl. J. Med.* 357, 1121–1135. doi: 10.1056/NEJMra071667

Yonekawa, T., and Thorburn, A. (2013). Autophagy and cell death. *Essays Biochem.* 55, 105–117. doi: 10.1042/bse0550105

Yu, L., Li, Q., Yu, B., Yang, Y., Jin, Z., Duan, W., et al. (2016). Berberine attenuates myocardial ischemia/reperfusion injury by reducing oxidative stress and inflammation response: role of silent information regulator 1. *Oxid. Med. Cell. Longev.* 2016:1689602. doi: 10.1155/2016/1689602

Yu, L., Li, S., Tang, X., Li, Z., Zhang, J., Xue, X., et al. (2017). Diallyl trisulfide ameliorates myocardial ischemia-reperfusion injury by reducing oxidative stress and endoplasmic reticulum stress-mediated apoptosis in type 1 diabetic rats: role of SIRT1 activation. *Apoptosis* 22, 942–954. doi: 10.1007/s10495-017-1378-y

Zhou, T., Chuang, C. C., and Zuo, L. (2015). Molecular characterization of reactive oxygen species in myocardial ischemia-reperfusion injury. *Biomed Res. Int.* 2015:864946. doi: 10.1155/2015/864946

13

Aqueous Extract of Black Maca Prevents Metabolism Disorder via Regulating the Glycolysis/Gluconeogenesis-TCA Cycle and PPARα Signaling Activation in Golden Hamsters Fed a High-Fat, High-Fructose Diet

Wenting Wan[1,2], Hongxiang Li[1,2], Jiamei Xiang[1,2], Fan Yi[3], Lijia Xu[1,2], Baoping Jiang[1,2]* and Peigen Xiao[1,2]*

[1] Institute of Medicinal Plant Development, Chinese Academy of Medical Sciences and Peking Union Medical College, Beijing, China, [2] Key Laboratory of Bioactive Substances and Resources Utilization of Chinese Herbal Medicine, Ministry of Education, Beijing, China, [3] School of Sciences/Key Laboratory of Cosmetic, China National Light Industry, Beijing Technology and Business University, Beijing, China

***Correspondence:**
Lijia Xu
xulijia@hotmail.com
Baoping Jiang
bpjiang@implad.ac.cn

Maca (*Lepidium meyenii* Walpers) has been used as a dietary supplement and ethnomedicine for centuries. Recently, maca has become a high profile functional food worldwide because of its multiple biological activities. This study is the first explorative research to investigate the prevention and amelioration capacity of the aqueous extract of black maca (AEM) on high-fat, high-fructose diet (HFD)-induced metabolism disorder in golden hamsters and to identify the potential mechanisms involved in these effects. For 20 weeks, 6-week-old male golden hamsters were fed the following respective diets: (1) a standard diet, (2) HFD, (3) HFD supplemented with metformin, or (4) HFD supplemented with three doses of AEM (300, 600, or 1,200 mg/kg). After 20 weeks, the golden hamsters that received daily AEM supplementation presented with the beneficial effects of improved hyperlipidemia, hyperinsulinemia, insulin resistance, and hepatic steatosis *in vivo*. Based on the hepatic metabolomic analysis results, alterations in metabolites associated with pathological changes were examined. A total of 194 identified metabolites were mapped to 46 relative metabolic pathways, including those of energy metabolism. In addition, via *in silico* profiling for secondary maca metabolites by a joint pharmacophore- and structure-based approach, a compound-target-disease network was established. The results revealed that 32 bioactive compounds in maca targeted 16 proteins involved in metabolism disorder. Considering the combined metabolomics and virtual screening results, we employed quantitative real-time PCR assays to verify the gene expression of key enzymes in the relevant pathways. AEM promoted glycolysis and inhibited gluconeogenesis via regulating the expression of key genes such as *Gck* and *Pfkm*. Moreover, AEM upregulated tricarboxylic acid (TCA) cycle flux by changing the concentrations of intermediates and increasing the mRNA levels of *Aco2*, *Fh,* and *Mdh2*. In addition, the lipid-lowering effects of AEM in both the serum and liver may be partly related to PPARα signaling activation, including enhanced fatty acid β-oxidation and lipogenesis pathway inhibition. Together, our data demonstrated that AEM intervention significantly improved lipid and glucose metabolism disorder by regulating the glycolysis/gluconeogenesis-TCA cycle and by modulating gene expression levels involved in the PPARα signaling pathway.

Keywords: maca (*Lepidium meyenii* Walpers), metabolism disorder, metabolomics, glycolysis/gluconeogenesis-TCA cycle, lipid metabolism

INTRODUCTION

Metabolism disorder are major symptoms in several pathological phenomena, like atherosclerotic cardiovascular disease and type 2 diabetes. Excess energy intake and concomitant obesity are the major drivers of this syndrome. By alleviating metabolism disorder, the onset of diabetes, atherosclerotic cardiovascular disease, and other associated comorbidities might be postponed. Currently, the recommended treatments for metabolic impairments are lifestyle changes, such as medicinal plant supplementation, caloric restriction, healthier foods, and increased physical activity (Grundy, 2016). Clinical trials have shown that medicinal plant supplements can reduce the likelihood of early-stage metabolism disorder progressing to type 2 diabetes (Jia et al., 2015). Nutraceutical interventions aimed at correcting metabolism disorder may be a promising option, but thus far, few natural products have been investigated. Traditional and folk edible herbal treatments are gaining attention for their health benefits and low toxicity and might be suitable for long-term supplementation in metabolism disorder.

Maca (*Lepidium meyenii* Walpers), known as "Peruvian ginseng," is an annual herbaceous plant of the Brassicaceae family, growing at elevations of over 4,000 m in the Andes region. This herb grows in a habitat with a harsh climate, such as intense cold, extremely intense sunlight, and strong winds (Gonzales et al., 2006). Maca is traditionally consumed fresh or dehydrated after being boiled in water or milk and can be made into juices, cocktails, alcoholic beverages, or maca coffee (Campos et al., 2013). Since the time of the Incas, maca has been used as an energizing and revitalizing food additive; has been recommended for malnutrition, convalescence, memory loss, fatigue, mental weakness, and insomnia; and has been used to regulate menstruation and lessen menopausal symptoms (Henry et al., 2016). Recently, maca attracted global attention when it was listed as safe to eat by the Food and Agriculture Organization. After several years of research and development, the safety and various pharmacological effects of maca have been increasingly recognized.

Metabolomic approaches have been widely applied to study metabolic changes in response to disease or interventions by the analysis of various biological samples, including blood, urine, and tissue. The power of metabolomic approaches has already been used to create profiles that create biomarkers for obesity-associated insulin resistance and to identify metabolites that correlate with diabetes under subclinical conditions, which is key for early detection and management (Sallese and Zhu, 2017). Recent advances in metabolomics suggest that it is possible to not only use this analytical technique to assess the holistic effects of nutritional intervention in metabolism disorder but also investigate the compound–target interactions and to analyze involved metabolic pathways (Puiggròs et al., 2015; Le et al., 2016; Li et al., 2016). Moreover, the natural product is delicate and complex, and its pharmacodynamics characteristics are regulated by different functional groups (Ma et al., 2017). As is known, the functional food discovery process based on natural products is risk-, time-, and cost-intensive. Several studies have confirmed the high success rates of computer-assisted tools, such as virtual screening, to increase the efficiency and efficacy of discovering lead structures in medicinal chemistry (Kitchen et al., 2004; Harvey, 2008). The combination of metabolomic approaches and virtual screening with multivariate data analysis can be used to evaluate pharmacodynamic effects and to understand the molecular mechanisms of the signaling pathways.

This research is the first to study the capacity of an aqueous extract of black maca (AEM) to prevent and improve high-fat, high-fructose diet (HFD)-induced metabolism disorder in golden hamsters. To assess the potential health benefits of AEM, a 20-week intervention study was conducted. We took advantage of recent developments in pharmacophore- and structure-based screening approaches to predict the potential active protein targets of AEM. In addition, mass spectrometry was used to obtain the metabolomic profile of the liver following AEM treatment, and several changes in the metabolic pathway were identified. Building on the success of the *in silico* target prediction and the capacity to quantitatively measure metabolome abundance, we used quantitative real-time PCR (qPCR) to verify the potential underlying molecular mechanisms. These results suggested that AEM may improve metabolism disorder via upregulating the glycolysis/gluconeogenesis-tricarboxylic acid (TCA) cycle pathway and enhancing the expression of genes involved in lipid metabolism.

MATERIALS AND METHODS

Plant Extract

Black maca powder was obtained from TTD International Pty Ltd. (QLD, Australia). An aqueous extract of maca powder was prepared according to traditional methods. The powder (500 g) was placed into a container with 2,000 ml of water, sonicated for 30 min, and then boiled for 2 h. Afterward, the aqueous extract was cooled to room temperature and filtered. Water (500 ml) was added to the filter residue, and the solution was boiled again for 2 h. The two filtrates were combined and concentrated to 416 ml. The concentrate, containing 1,200 mg/ml maca, was placed in small vials and stored in a refrigerator at 4°C until further use. Before the experiments, the concentrate was dissolved in aqueous solution to concentrations of 600 and 300 mg/ml. The nutritional composition of the AEM is shown in **Table 1**.

Animals and Diets

Forty-eight 6-week-old male golden hamsters (Vital River Laboratory Animal Technology Co., Ltd., Beijing, China) were housed in a temperature-controlled (22 ± 2°C) room in our animal center on a 12 h:12 h light–dark cycle with food and water available. The standard chow was composed of 28% protein, 12% lard, and 60% vegetable starch. The HFD contained 30% fructose, 0.5% cholesterol (CHO), 22% lard, 14.5% protein, and 33% vegetable starch. All the animal care procedures and interventions were performed in accordance with the Guidelines and Policies for Animal Surgery under the control of the Chinese Academy of Medical Sciences and Peking Union Medical College, Beijing, China (approval No: SLXD-2016052117) and were approved by the Institutional Animal Use and Care Committee (IACUC). All the animal experiments were conducted based on the recommendations for the care and use of laboratory animals proposed by the National Institutes of Health regulations.

Experimental Scheme

Golden hamsters were randomly divided into the following six treatment groups, with eight animals in each group:

(1) Control group (standard chow)
(2) HFD group (HFD)
(3) Metformin (Metf) group (daily instillation of 125 mg/kg metformin + HFD)
(4) Low dose of AEM (daily instillation of 300 mg/kg AEM + HFD)
(5) Middle dose of AEM (daily instillation of 600 mg/kg AEM + HFD)
(6) High dose of AEM (daily instillation of 1,200 mg/kg AEM + HFD)

The daily food intake of the golden hamsters in each group was recorded during the 20-week treatment period. The body weights of the golden hamsters in each group were noted weekly. At the end of the 20 weeks, after 12 h of fasting, the hamsters were euthanatized via pentobarbital. Blood samples were then taken from the abdominal aorta, and the serum was separated by centrifugation at 5,000 rpm for 10 min and stored at −20°C. Liver samples and epididymal white adipose tissue (WAT) were dissected at the time of death, sections from the same sample were prepared for histological examination, and liver subsections were frozen in liquid nitrogen for metabolomic analysis. All the serum and hepatic biochemical parameters were determined using appropriate kits (Biosino Bio-technology and Science Incorporation, Beijing, China) according to the manufacturer's instructions. The serum insulin levels were measured using a radio immunoassay kit (Beijing North Institute of Biological Technology, Beijing, China).

TABLE 1 | Nutritional composition in aqueous extract of black maca (AEM 1,200 mg/kg).

Item	Content
Energy (kJ/100 g)	56.144
Protein (g/100 g)	0.44
Fat (g/100 g)	0.4
Carbohydrate (g/100 g)	1.992
Potassium (mg/100 g)	283.36
Calcium (mg/100 g)	2.6
Ash (g/100 g)	0.368
Water (g/100 g)	396.8

Determination of Metabolic Parameters and Insulin Sensitivity

The homeostasis model of insulin resistance (HOMA-IR) was used with the following formulas: HOMA-IR = [Fasting insulin level (mU/ml)]*[Fasting serum glucose (mmol/l)]/22.5; and Insulin sensitivity index = 1/[Fasting insulin level (mU/ml)]*[Fasting serum glucose (mmol/l)].

Histological Examination

Livers and epididymal WAT were removed immediately and immersed in formalin solution for at least 24 h. Then, the samples were embedded in paraffin, and 5-μm-thick slices were sectioned and stained with hematoxylin and eosin (H&E). The images were observed with a light microscope (Olympus IX51, Tokyo, Japan).

Metabolite Profiling

Liver tissue extraction, pulse-acquire sequence, metabolite identification, and data processing were performed as described previously (Wan et al., 2017). The metabolomic analysis was performed on a Q Exactive Orbitrap (Thermo, United States) equipped with an amide column (Waters, CA, United States). The processed results were imported to MetaboAnalyst 3.0[1] for analysis.

In Silico Predictions

Through literature reviews, we collected the components and structures of maca (**Supplementary File S1**). All chemistries were used for target fishing with two databases: the PharmaDB database and a similarity ensemble approach (SEAware 1.7; SeaChange Pharmaceuticals, Inc., San Francisco, CA, United States). When PharmaDB was used, the chemical structures were prepared in SD format and converted from a 2D cdx file format to 3D models using Open Babel GUI version 2.3.2 (OpenBableGUI; Chris Morley, United States). Molecular energy was minimized using the Energy Minimization module of Discovery Studio version 4.5 (DS 4.5; Accelrys Inc.,

[1] http://www.metaboanalyst.ca

San Diego, CA, United States) under the Chemistry at Harvard Macromolecular Mechanics (CHARMM) force field (Yi et al., 2016). All pharmacophore models with the shape of the binding pocket were selected for virtual screening using the default settings of the Ligand Profiler module of DS 4.5. Ligand and pharmacophore fitness characteristics were assessed by the values and shape similarity of the molecules. When using SEAware, molecules were prepared in the SMILES format (Simplified Molecular Input Line Entry System[2]). The 2D structural similarity of each compound to each target's ligand set was quantified as an expectation value (Keiser et al., 2009). A compound-target-disease table was established via analyzing the hit targets, associated protein and diseases, and the interactions between these parameters.

RNA Isolation, cDNA Generation, and Quantitative Real-Time PCR (qPCR)

Total RNA was extracted from flash-frozen liver tissue using an RNAiso Plus kit (Takara BIO Inc., Dalian, China) and was reverse-transcribed with a PrimeScript RT reagent kit (Takara BIO Inc., Dalian, China) according to the manufacturer's instructions. qPCR was performed using SYBR Premix DimerEraser (Takara BIO Inc., Dalian, China) with a Fast Real-time PCR System 7500 (Applied Biosystems 7500 Fast Real-Time PCR System). Reaction conditions were as follows: heating to 95°C in 30 s, followed by 40 cycles at 95°C for 3 s, 55°C for 30 s and 72°C for 30 s. Each cDNA sample was tested with at least three independent replicates to check the data reproducibility. Data were analyzed using the $2^{-\Delta\Delta Ct}$ method. **Supplementary Table S1** contains the list of primers used for qPCR.

Statistical Analysis

Statistical analyses were performed in GraphPad Prism, Version 5.0 (GraphPad Software Inc., CA, United States) using Student's *t*-test. The data are expressed as the means ± standard errors of the mean (SEMs). In this paper, significant differences in multiple comparisons were identified at $P < 0.05$, $P < 0.01$, and $P < 0.001$.

[2]http://www.daylight.com/smiles

RESULTS

Effects of AEM on Body Weight, Food Intake, and Food Utilization

After 20 weeks, the golden hamsters in the control group consumed a total of 1,255.05 g of the normal diet; the HFD; Metf; and 300, 600, and 1,200 mg/kg AEM groups consumed 861.17; 922.67; and 969.37, 950.53, and 861.41 g of the HFD, respectively (**Supplementary Figure S1**). **Table 2** shows that food intake was substantially decreased in the HFD-fed golden hamsters compared with that in the hamsters fed a normal diet. The Metf and 300 and 600 mg/kg AEM groups presented with increased food intake, but the food intake of the 1,200 mg/kg AEM group was not affected. The food utilization rate was higher in the HFD group than that in the control group, while the Metf and AEM (300, 600, and 1,200 mg/kg) groups presented a clear, decreasing trend in this parameter (**Table 2**). Moreover, none of the initial body weights were different among the groups. After 20 weeks, compared with the normal diet, the HFD led to greater final body weight gain and a higher fat coefficient in the golden hamsters. The final body weight, total fat mass, and fat coefficient were significantly decreased in the Metf and AEM (1,200 mg/kg) groups compared with the HFD group.

Effects of AEM Intervention on Liver and Epididymal WAT

We evaluated the development of inflammation in epididymal WAT (**Figure 1A**). The histological analysis of the HFD-fed golden hamsters revealed a notable enlargement in adipocyte size (**Supplementary Figure S2**) and increased inflammation. However, AEM (300, 600, and 1,200 mg/kg) and metformin treatment attenuated this trend, resulting in adipocytes with a similar shape and size as those in the control group. In addition, H&E section staining revealed that compared with chow diet-fed golden hamsters, hamsters that received the long-term HFD presented with substantial liver lipid deposition. In contrast, AEM (300, 600, and 1,200 mg/kg) treatment and metformin ameliorated the lipid accumulation in the liver (**Figure 1B**). The liver coefficient is the ratio of the liver mass to the body mass and should be constant under normal conditions.

TABLE 2 | Effects of aqueous extract of black maca (AEM) and metformin on body weight, food intake, food utilization, and fat and liver coefficients in golden hamsters.

	Control	HFD	Metf	AEM 300	AEM 600	AEM 1200
Initial body weight (g)	102.35 ± 5.75	103.19 ± 5.02	102.77 ± 3.45	103.07 ± 4.99	103.39 ± 5.17	102.08 ± 5.54
Final body weight (g)	215.44 ± 19.55	216.88 ± 13.88	200.22 ± 14.67*	216.80 ± 14.22	215.40 ± 21.07	196.00 ± 19.98*
Body weight gain (g)	112.52 ± 21.11	114.79 ± 14.04	97.74 ± 14.08*	113.73 ± 10.35	112.01 ± 18.97	93.92 ± 20.19*
Food intake (g)	1255.05 ± 1.86	861.17 ± 1.58###	922.67 ± 1.75*	969.37 ± 1.44**	950.53 ± 1.17**	861.41 ± 1.33
Food utilization rate (%)	8.97 ± 1.68	13.33 ± 1.63###	10.59 ± 1.53**	11.73 ± 1.07*	11.78 ± 2.00	10.90 ± 2.34*
Total fat weight (g)	12.05 ± 2.06	13.10 ± 1.76	10.26 ± 1.38**	12.00 ± 1.69	13.02 ± 1.44	10.65 ± 1.40**
Fat coefficient (%)	5.65 ± 0.81	6.06 ± 0.95	5.15 ± 0.63*	5.50 ± 0.59	6.13 ± 0.77	5.59 ± 0.79
Liver weight (g)	6.10 ± 2.26	11.84 ± 1.68###	8.44 ± 0.98***	10.48 ± 0.80	11.38 ± 1.19	9.96 ± 1.35*
Liver coefficient (%)	2.78 ± 0.97	5.45 ± 0.61###	4.30 ± 0.44***	4.94 ± 0.26*	5.44 ± 0.57	5.10 ± 0.52

*Data are presented as the means ± SEMs. #P < 0.05, ##P < 0.01, ###P < 0.001 compared with the control group; *P < 0.05, **P < 0.01, ***P < 0.001 compared with the HFD model group, n = 6*

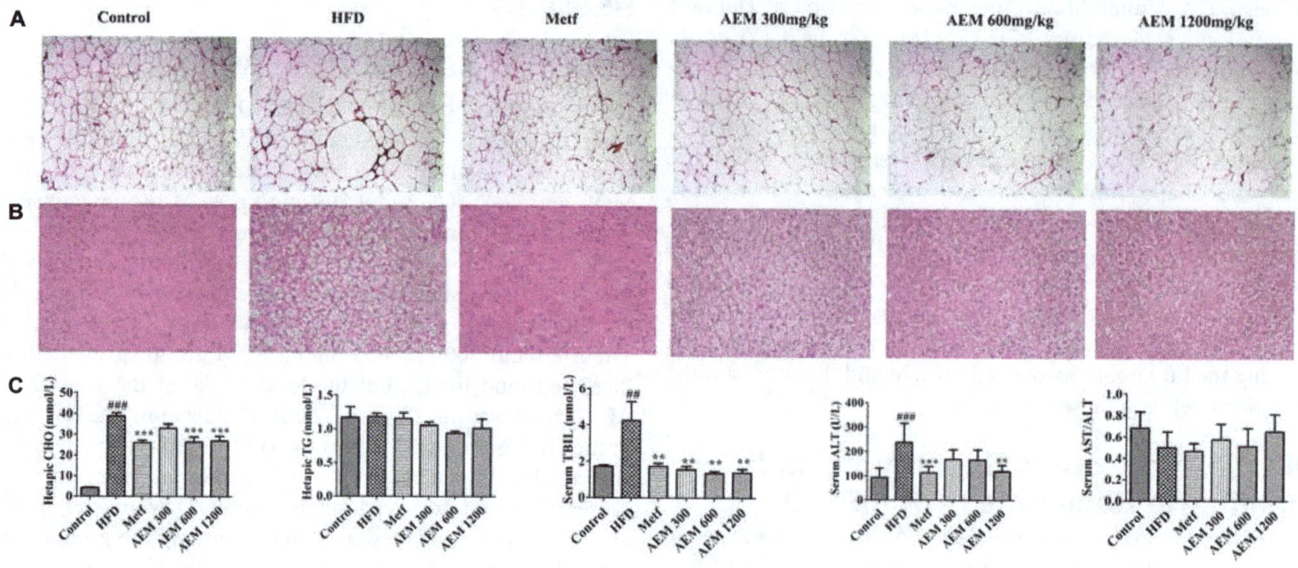

FIGURE 1 | Effects of aqueous extract of black maca (AEM) on the histology of epididymal white adipose tissue and liver and the hepatic lipid profiles in golden hamsters. **(A)** The epididymal white adipose tissue sections were stained with H&E. **(B)** The liver sections were stained with H&E. **(C)** The hepatic cholesterol (CHO), hepatic triglyceride (TG), serum total bilirubin (TIBL), serum aminotransferase (AST), and AST/alanine aminotransferase (ALT) levels were measured. Data are presented as the means ± SEMs. $^{\#}P < 0.05$, $^{\#\#}P < 0.01$, $^{\#\#\#}P < 0.001$ compared with the control group; $^{*}P < 0.05$, $^{**}P < 0.01$, $^{***}P < 0.0$ compared with the HFD model group, $n = 6$.

An increased liver coefficient indicates edema, inflammation, or hyperplasia in the liver tissue. **Table 2** shows that the liver weight and liver coefficient were significantly increased in the HFD group compared with the control group, while AEM (300 and 1,200 mg/kg) treatment changed this trend. We further measured the levels of hepatic triglycerides (TGs) and CHO and found that metformin and AEM (600 and 1,200 mg/kg) treatment markedly reduced the liver CHO content and that AEM (300, 600, and 1,200 mg/kg) caused a downward trend in TG levels (**Figure 1C**). In addition, the HFD led to higher serum total bilirubin (TBIL) levels, while the administration of different doses of AEM (300, 600, and 1,200 mg/kg) reversed this trend. Serum aminotransferase (AST) and alanine aminotransferase (ALT) levels reflect the degree of liver damage. The serum ALT levels in the HFD group were increased dramatically, but the values in the different AEM dose groups tended to be close to those of the control group. The AST/ALT ratio also showed that AEM did not damage the liver function of golden hamsters (**Figure 1C**).

Effects of AEM on Serum Biochemical Parameters

As shown in **Supplementary Figure S3**, compared with the normal diet, the HFD significantly increased the CHO, TG, high-density lipoprotein CHO (HDL-C), and low-density lipoprotein CHO (LDL-C) levels after 4 weeks. These results revealed that the golden hamsters developed significant hyperlipidemia after 4 weeks of the HFD feeding. During the 20 weeks of treatment, the serum TG, CHO, HDL-C, and LDL-C levels were low and stable in the control group but were comparatively much higher and continued to increase in the HFD group. After the AEM supplementation, both treated groups showed clear, dose-dependent decreases in serum lipid levels (**Figures 2A–D**). After 20 weeks, compared with the HFD group, both the AEM-treated groups presented with significant reductions in serum CHO and LDL-C levels (**Figures 2E,G**). Moreover, AEM supplementation (600 and 1,200 mg/kg) significantly reduced TG accumulation; this decreasing trend was also observed in the 300 mg/kg AEM group but was not significant (**Figure 2F**). Serum HDL-C levels were slightly but non-significantly decreased in all the AEM groups (**Figure 2H**).

Glucose and insulin levels were also measured over the course of this study (**Figures 2I–L**). Glucose levels remained unchanged among the HFD and AEM groups (**Figure 2I**). Serum insulin concentrations were significantly lower after 20 weeks of metformin and AEM treatment compared with these levels following the HFD treatment (**Figure 2J**). Compared with the HFD group, among the Metf and AEM (600 and 1,200 mg/kg) groups, the insulin sensitivity index was significantly increased (**Figure 2K**).

Protein–Ligand Docking

As shown in **Supplementary File S1**, 63 compounds from maca were collected by literature review: 56% of the compounds were alkaloids and macaenes (compounds A1–A35), 33% were glucosinolates (compounds J1–J21), and the others were sterols (compounds S1–S7). We chose six disease categories (obesity, insulin resistance, hyperinsulinemia, hyperglycemia, hyperlipidemia, and diabetes) closely related to glucose and lipid metabolism disorders to validate the medical actions and to identify maca compounds. **Supplementary Table S2** provides

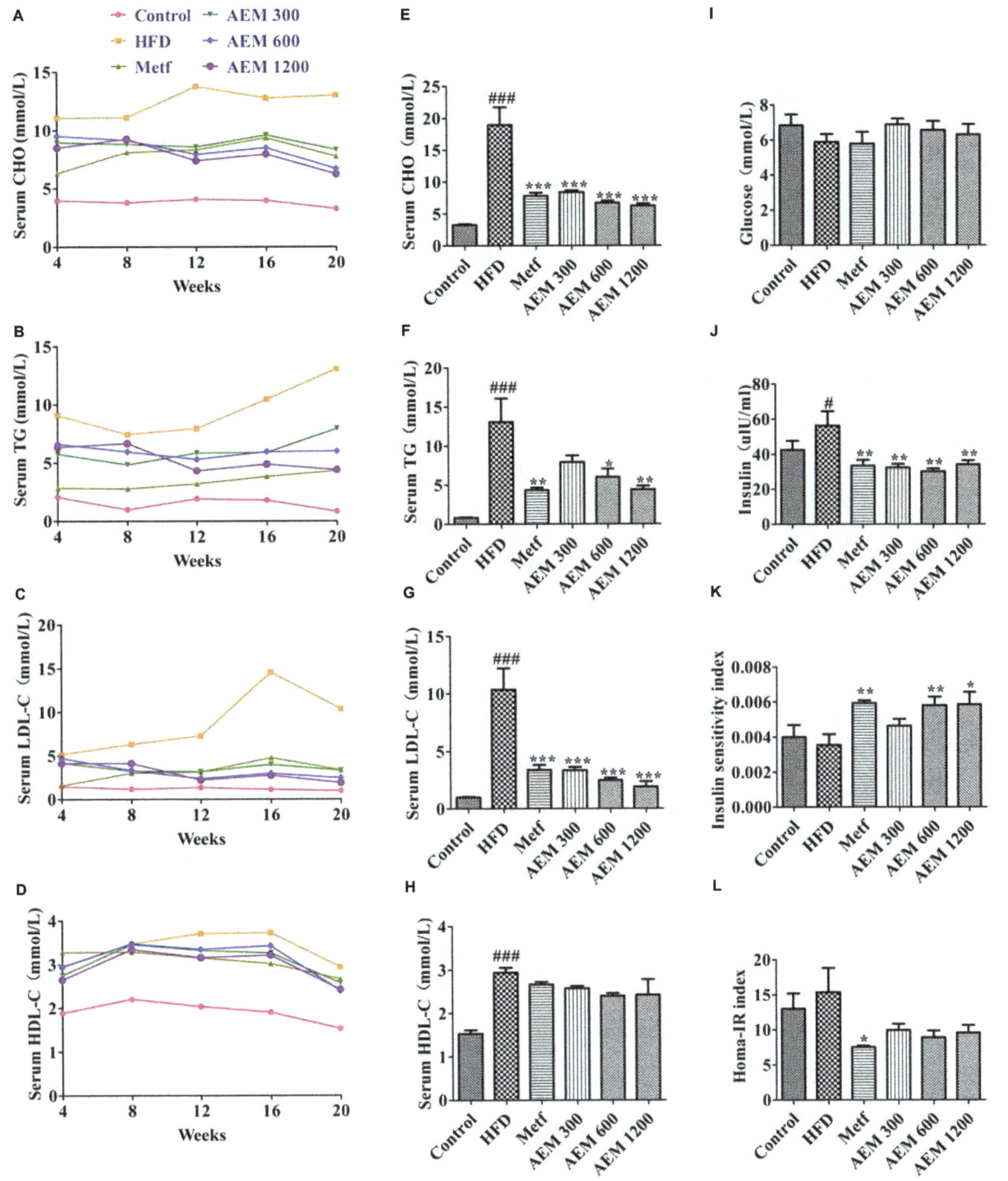

FIGURE 2 | Effects of aqueous extract of black maca (AEM) on the serum lipid, glucose, and insulin profiles in golden hamsters. Over 20 weeks, **(A)** serum cholesterol (CHO), **(B)** serum triglyceride (TG), **(C)** serum low-density lipoprotein CHO (LDL-C), and **(D)** high-density lipoprotein CHO (HDL-C) levels were tested. At the end of 20 weeks, **(E)** serum CHO, **(F)** serum TG, **(G)** serum LDL-C, **(H)** serum HDL-C, **(I)** serum glucose, and **(J)** serum insulin were measured. The calculated insulin sensitivity index **(K)** and HOMA-IR index **(L)** are displayed. Data are presented as the means ± SEMs. $^{\#}P < 0.05$, $^{\#\#}P < 0.01$, $^{\#\#\#}P < 0.001$ compared with the control group; $^{*}P < 0.05$, $^{**}P < 0.01$, $^{***}P < 0.001$ compared with the HFD model group, $n = 6$.

an overview of the compound-target-disease relationships. Fructose-1,6-bisphosphatase 1 (F16P1), which acts as a rate-limiting enzyme in gluconeogenesis, was determined by the alkaloids (A1, A12, A14, A16, A17, and A21) and the glucosinolate (J9). The alkaloids (A3, A7, A10, A12, A13, A23, A24, and A27) and the glucosinolates (J4 and J13) identified glycogen synthase kinase-3 beta (GSK3B). The glucosinolate (J10) and alkaloids (A6, A8, A14, A15, and A24) were connected to protein-tyrosine phosphatase 1B (PTN1). Peroxisome proliferator-activated receptor gamma (PPARγ), a key regulator of adipocyte differentiation and glucose homeostasis, was found by the alkaloids (A10, A11, A14, A15, A16, A24, and A25). We found that the glucosinolates (J10, J11, J12, and J14) and (J3, J4, J9, and J14) were associated with sodium/glucose cotransporter 1 (SC5A1) and sodium/glucose cotransporter 2 (SC5A2), respectively. The glucosinolate (J9) and sterols (S1, S2, S4, and S7) were related to acetyl-CoA acetyltransferase (THIL). Glucosinolates (J3, J4, J12, J13, J14, J15, and J16), (J15 and J16), (J4 and J9), and (J11) were separately found with aldose reductase (ALDR), dipeptidyl peptidase 4 (DPP4), corticosteroid 11-beta-dehydrogenase isozyme 1 (DHI1), and liver carboxylesterase 1 (EST1), respectively. The alkaloids (A13), (A7 and A25), and (A13 and A14) were separately involved with the bile acid receptor (FXR), lanosterol synthase (ERG7), and peroxisome proliferator-activated receptor alpha (PPARα), respectively. Oxysterols receptor LXR-beta (LXRβ) interacted with the alkaloid (A24) and sterol (S7); mitogen-activated protein kinase 14 (MK14) was identified by the sterol (S7) and glucosinolates (J4, J9, and J10).

Metabolomic Analysis and Pathway Impact Analysis

By MetaboAnalyst 3.0, a total of 194 identified metabolites were mapped to KEGG metabolic pathways for over-representation and pathway topology analyses. Ultimately, 46 relative metabolic pathways were identified (**Figure 3A**). The pathway impact factor was evaluated by the relative importance of the compounds. Arginine and proline metabolism, glyoxylate and dicarboxylate metabolism, the TCA cycle, and glycolysis/gluconeogenesis had the highest impact factors.

Metabolomics uses multivariate statistical tools on a data set acquired from an MS-coupled method to discriminate systematic variation using a subsequent supervised statistical analysis, such as orthogonal partial least-squares discriminatory analysis (OPLS-DA). This analysis clearly separates a data set into different groups, ultimately screening candidate metabolites for variation (And and Sturm, 2007). To gain an overview of the metabolic contents, OPLS-DA was performed among the different groups. As seen in the OPLS-DA score plot (**Figure 3B**), well-delineated clusters and separation trends among the control, HFD, and AEM-treated groups were observed. The results from the three different AEM dose groups mostly overlapped and significantly deviated from those of the HFD group, indicating that metabolic perturbation occurs and that AEM exerts an intervening effect on this disturbance. In addition, a well-fitted, two component OPLS-DA model was constructed to identify the differential metabolites that respond to the control vs. HFD group and the HFD vs. AEM (1,200 mg/kg) group. **Figure 3C** shows that the metabolic profile of the HFD-fed golden hamsters was fairly different from the profile of the control hamsters. A similar distinction was apparent between the HFD and AEM (1,200 mg/kg) groups (**Figure 3D**). The metabolomic pattern of the key metabolites, those with *P*-values < 0.05, are expressed as squares in the heatmap, which displays the normalized data values using carefully chosen color gradients (**Figures 3E,F**).

Effects of AEM on Hepatic mRNA Expression Related to Energy and Lipid Metabolism

To validate the aforementioned metabolic changes and *in silico* target prediction, the gene expression levels of key enzymes involved in glucose and lipid metabolism were assessed in liver tissues. PPARs, which serve as potential therapeutic targets for treating lipid metabolism disorder, and their downstream genes are involved in almost all aspects of lipid metabolism. As shown in **Figure 4**, the HFD feeding markedly reduced the hepatic mRNA levels of *Pparα* and its target genes. In contrast, AEM (1,200 mg/kg) supplementation upregulated the hepatic mRNA levels of *Pparα* (0.20-fold, $P < 0.01$), carnitine palmitoyltransferase 1 (*Cpt1*, 0.54-fold, $P < 0.01$), *Apoa1* (0.35-fold, $P < 0.001$), oxysterols receptor LXR-beta (*Lxrb*, 0.53-fold, $P < 0.001$), retinoic acid receptor alpha (*Rxra*, 1.92-fold, $P < 0.01$), and low-density lipoprotein receptor (*Ldlr*, 0.48-fold, $P < 0.05$), yet downregulated 3-hydroxy-3-methylglutaryl-coenzyme A reductase (*Hmgcr*, 0.73-fold, $P < 0.001$) and sterol regulatory element-binding protein 1 (*Srebp1*, 0.41-fold, $P < 0.01$). In addition, we checked the expression of selected genes involved in glycolysis/gluconeogenesis and the TCA cycle. AEM (1,200 mg/kg) upregulated the mRNA levels inhibited by the HFD, including ATP-dependent 6-phosphofructokinase (*Pfkl*, 1.23-fold, $P < 0.05$), phosphoglucomutases 2 and 3 (*Pgm2*, 0.84-fold, $P < 0.01$; *Pgm3*, 0.68-fold, $P < 0.01$), the succinate dehydrogenase complex, subunit A (*Sdha*, 0.73-fold, $P < 0.01$), phosphoenolpyruvate carboxykinase 1 (*Pepck*, 1.06-fold, $P < 0.01$), citrate synthase (*Cs*, 0.94-fold, $P < 0.001$), fetal hematoma (*Fh*, 0.67-fold, $P < 0.01$), glucokinase (*Gck*, 3.36-fold, $P < 0.001$), phosphofructokinase (*Pfkm*, 0.88-fold, $P < 0.001$), malate dehydrogenase (*Mdh2*, 1.89-fold, $P < 0.001$), fructose bisphosphatase 1 (*Fbp1*, 0.47-fold, $P < 0.001$), and aconitate hydratase, mitochondrial (*Aco2*, 1.24-fold, $P < 0.001$). Moreover, the expression of glycogen synthase kinase 3 beta (*Gsk3b*), a key regulatory enzyme in glucose metabolism, was significantly increased in the HFD group (1.69-fold, $P < 0.001$) but was decreased in the AEM (1,200 mg/kg) group (0.71-fold, $P < 0.001$).

Energy Metabolism

Metabolic disorder is closely associated with energy metabolism, including gluconeogenesis, glycogenolysis, and the TCA cycle. In the HFD group, the concentrations of the major TCA cycle intermediates increased. However, AEM (1,200 mg/kg)

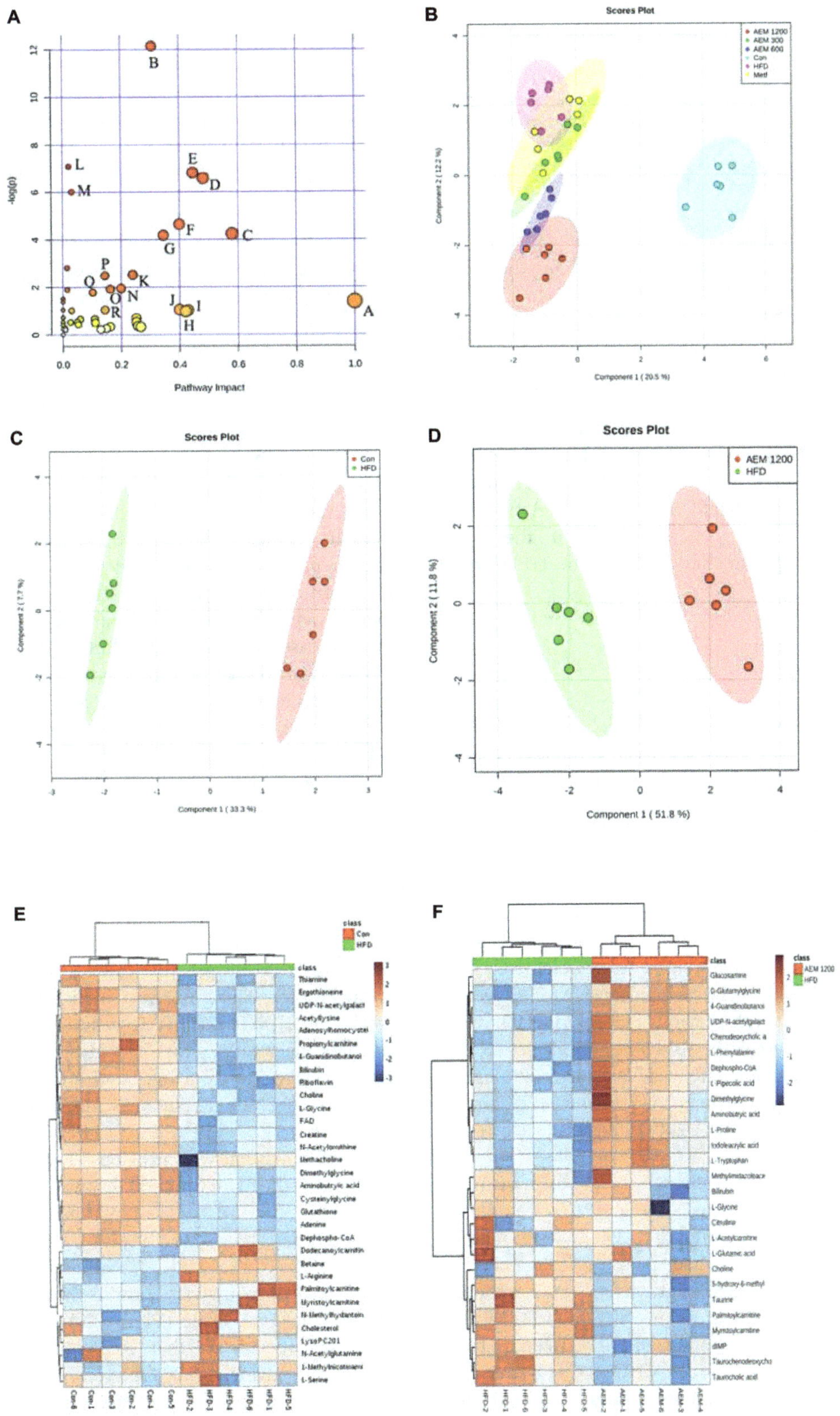

FIGURE 3 | Aqueous extract of black maca (AEM) regulated the disturbed metabolism. **(A)** Summary of pathway analysis with MetPA. A, D-Glutamine and D-glutamate metabolism; B, Arginine and proline metabolism; C, Glyoxylate and dicarboxylate metabolism; D, Glutathione metabolism; E, Nicotinate and

(Continued)

FIGURE 3 | Continued
nicotinamide metabolism; F, Thiamine metabolism; G, TCA cycle; H, Alanine, aspartate, and glutamate metabolism; I, Taurine and hypotaurine metabolism; J, Ascorbate and aldarate metabolism; K, Cysteine and methionine. **(B)** Orthogonal partial least-squares discriminant analysis (OPLS-DA) score plots for UPLC/MS data of all the groups. OPLS-DA score plots showed differences in the metabolic states in the control group (Con), the HFD model group (HFD), the metformin groups (Metf), the 300 mg/kg AEM group (AEM 300), the 600 mg/kg AEM group (AEM 600), and the 1,200 mg/kg AEM group (AEM 1200). **(C)** OPLS-DA score plot showing the difference in the metabolic state between the control group (Con) and the HFD model group (HFD). **(D)** OPLS-DA score plot showing the difference in the metabolic state between the HFD model group (HFD) and the 1,200 mg/kg AEM group (AEM 1200). **(E)** The heatmap of the correlation analysis of the key metabolites between the control group (Con) and the HFD model group (HFD). **(F)** The heatmap of the correlation analysis of the key metabolites between the HFD model group (HFD) and the 1,200 mg/kg AEM group (AEM 1200), $n = 6$.

supplementation reversed the disorder induced by the HFD. Decreased concentrations of citrate (0.38-fold, $P < 0.05$), *cis*-aconitate (0.82-fold, $P < 0.05$), and fumarate (0.66-fold, $P < 0.05$) were observed in the liver tissue. Furthermore, the HFD also interfered with the glycolysis/gluconeogenesis pathway, as evidenced by the increased fructose 6-phosphate (F6P, 1.75-fold, $P < 0.05$) level but decreased phosphoenolpyruvic acid (PEP, 0.32-fold, $P < 0.05$) and lactate (0.88-fold, $P < 0.05$) levels. The F6P (1.47-fold, $P < 0.05$), lactate (1.60-fold, $P < 0.001$), oxaloacetate (1.73-fold, $P < 0.05$), and succinate (1.93-fold, $P < 0.001$) levels were higher in the AEM (1,200 mg/kg) treatment group than those in the HFD group (**Figure 5A**).

DISCUSSION

After 20 weeks, the golden hamster model of metabolism disorder induced by HFD feeding was established, with substantially increased serum levels of biochemical indicators (including TG, CHO, LDL-C, and others). The model was very appropriate because golden hamsters respond consistently to dietary modulation and, compared with the profiles of other rodents, showed a close similarity to human lipoprotein profiles (Liao et al., 2015). In this paper, we found that supplemental AEM (1,200 mg/kg) did not alter food intake but significantly prevented the increased in body weight, liver weight, and fat weight that occurred in golden hamsters fed a HFD for 20 weeks. This finding was consistent with previous reports in which maca was demonstrated to decrease body mass index (Gonzales, 2010). In addition, the food utilization rate was markedly lower in the AEM (600 and 1,200 mg/kg) groups than in the HFD group. These results indicated that AEM (1,200 mg/kg) may accelerate metabolism in golden hamsters.

The occurrence of lipid and glucose metabolism disorder is often accompanied by increased TG and CHO contents and is most directly associated with the LDL-C level. Vecera et al. (2007) found that maca had positive influences on lipid, antioxidative, and glucose parameters in hereditary hypertriglyceridemic rats. In this study, we also found that after 20 weeks, AEM administration (300, 600, and 1,200 mg/kg) dose-dependently decreased the serum CHO, TG, LDL-C, and insulin levels to near-baseline control values. Although the insulin level was significantly increased in the HFD group and was decreased in all the AEM treatment groups, the concentration of glucose did not change substantially in any group. This result may suggest that in the HFD group, the glucose level was regulated by a high insulin content, which is consistent with the lower insulin sensitivity index. In contrast, compared with the HFD-fed golden hamsters, the AEM-supplemented (600 and 1,200 mg/kg) hamsters presented with not only a lower insulin level but also improved insulin sensitivity. These findings indicated that AEM reduces HFD-induced hyperlipidemia and hyperinsulinemia and improves insulin sensitivity.

Liver is the central organ for lipid, carbohydrate, and protein metabolic processes, which are closely associated with metabolic diseases. Serum AST and ALT levels sensitively reflect hepatocyte damage, and TBIL represents the secretion and excretion function of the liver. In the HFD group, the hepatic coefficient and the hepatic levels of CHO, ALT, and TBIL increased markedly; in addition, the pathological section analysis revealed the presence of non-alcoholic fatty liver disease. Our results revealed that AEM (300, 600, and 1,200 mg/kg) treatment significantly reversed these trends and alleviated the lipid accumulation in the liver. The comprehensive results revealed that AEM improved liver secretion and excretion, protected liver cells, and reduced the levels of hepatic CHO and TG accumulation caused by the HFD.

Virtual screening is a computational technique used in drug discovery and is becoming increasingly popular in pharmaceutical research. The screening process searches libraries of small molecules to identify structures that are most likely to bind a drug target, typically a protein receptor or an enzyme (Rester, 2008). In this context, among the 16 identified targets, FBP1, ALDR, PPARγ, and GSK3B were the most promising maca targets for preventing and improving lipid and glucose metabolism disorder. In addition, the active compounds identified more targets, such as macaene (A14), which fished the protein targets FBP1, PTN1, PPARγ, and PPARα. These results are consistent with previous reports that macamides and macaenes are the main functional constituents of maca (Gonzales et al., 2005). With the *in silico* target fishing screening results, we identified targets related to glycolysis/gluconeogenesis pathways, including FBP1 and GSK3β (**Supplementary Table S2**). In addition, pathway analysis showed that AEM supplementation impacted the TCA cycle (**Figure 3A**). Considering the above results, we speculated that AEM prevented and improved metabolic impairments via the glycolysis/gluconeogenesis-TCA cycle (**Figure 5B**). Moreover, the expression profiles of genes involved in the glycolysis/gluconeogenesis-TCA cycle were measured (**Figure 4**).

The liver is a major player in maintaining glucose homeostasis, controlling the balance between glucose levels in the bloodstream

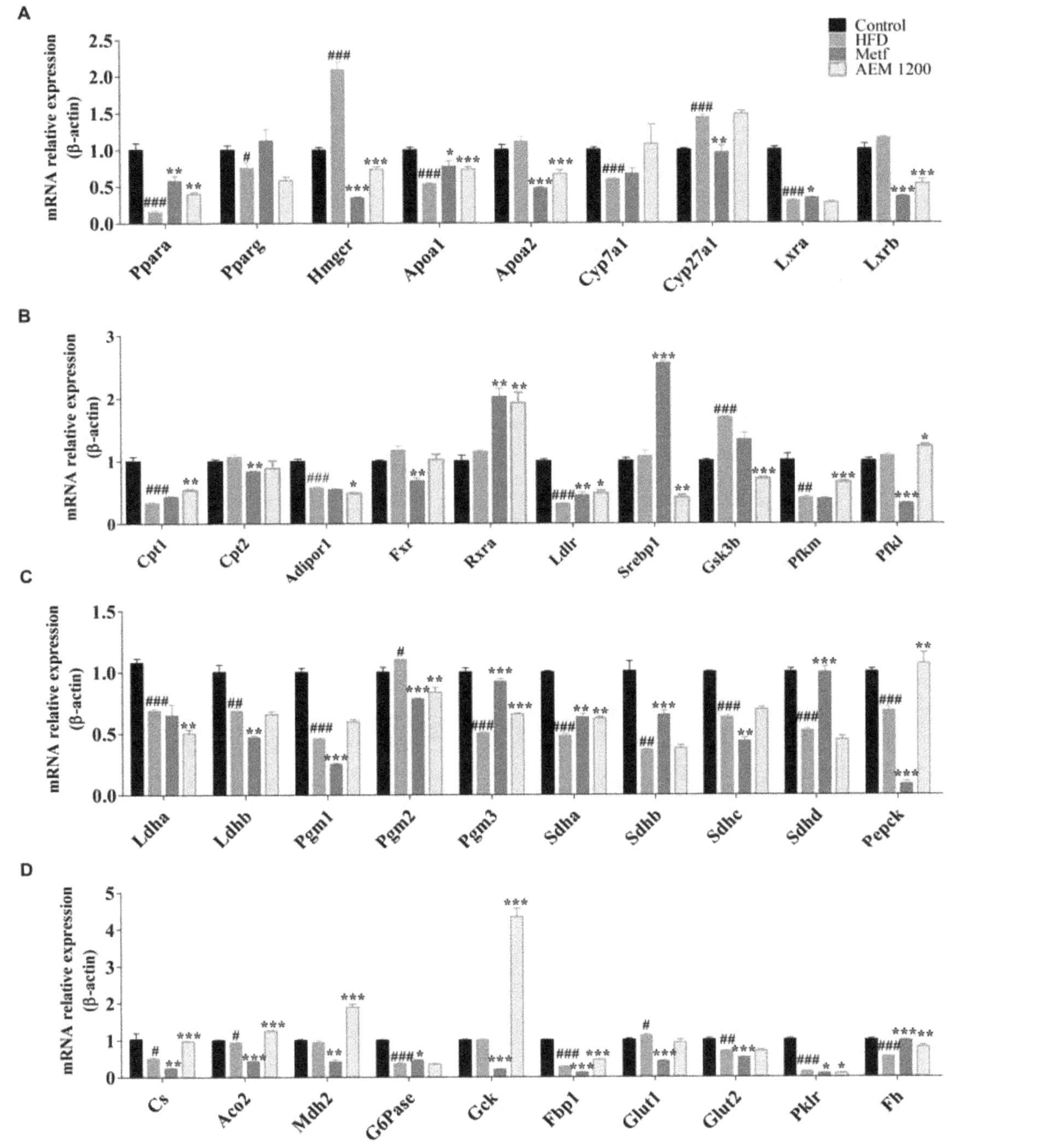

FIGURE 4 | (A–D) mRNA expression levels of hepatic genes involved in lipid metabolism and the glycolysis/gluconeogenesis-TCA cycle. The mRNA levels were determined using quantitative real-time PCR and were normalized to β-actin mRNA expression. Data are presented as the means ± SEMs. $^{\#}P < 0.05$, $^{\#\#}P < 0.01$, $^{\#\#\#}P < 0.001$ compared with the control group; $^{*}P < 0.05$, $^{**}P < 0.01$, $^{***}P < 0.001$ compared with the HFD model group, $n = 6$.

and in hepatocytes (Jiang and Zhang, 2003). A key method for controlling hepatic glucose production and consumption is the net TCA-glycolytic/gluconeogenic flux. By regulating the activity levels of key enzymes, the liver can switch from net hepatic glucose consumption to glucose output. Although glycolysis and gluconeogenesis share several enzymes that catalyze reversible reactions, the irreversible key steps are catalyzed by separate enzymes subjected to different regulations. Therefore, regulating these gluconeogenic enzymes and their glycolytic counterparts by allosteric effectors, gene expression levels, or covalent modifications is a mechanism for achieving a net flux toward gluconeogenesis or glycolysis in the liver (Sharabi et al., 2015). Glucose is phosphorylated by *Gck*, a liver-specific hexokinase, to generate glucose 6-phosphate

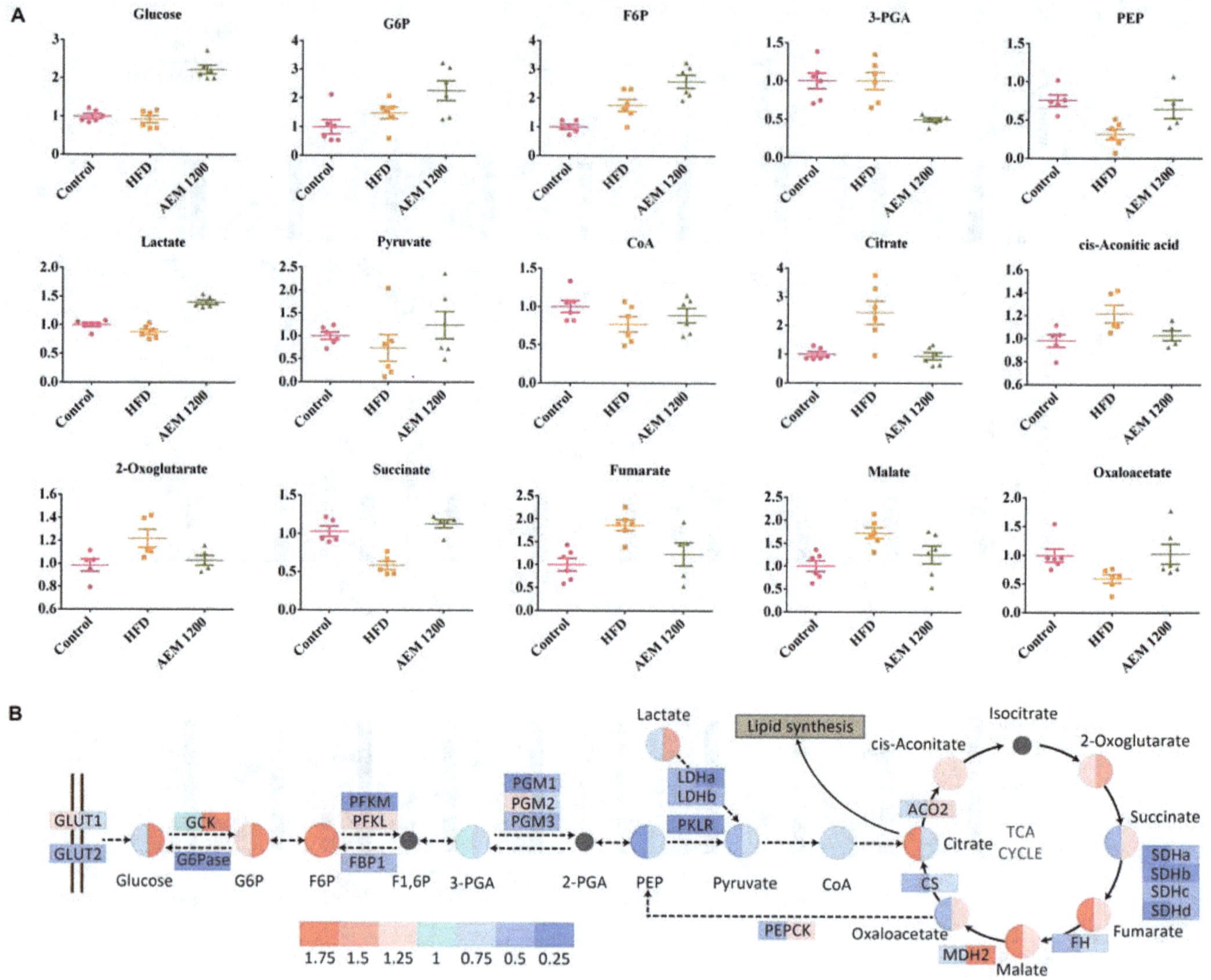

FIGURE 5 | Aqueous extract of black maca (AEM) influences the metabolism of the glycolysis/gluconeogenesis pathway and the TCA cycle. **(A)** The scatter plot of the relative quantities of the energy metabolites in liver samples from the treated and untreated groups. The *Y*-axis data were normalized according to the average value of the control. **(B)** Differential analysis of the glycolysis/gluconeogenesis pathway and the tricarboxylic acid (TCA) cycle among the control group (Con), the HFD model group (HFD), and the 1,200 mg/kg AEM group (AEM 1200). Log_2 fold changes of metabolites and the ratios of the average values of gene expression are color-coded, *n* = 5–6.

(G6P). *Gck* activity is regulated by its mRNA expression in hepatocytes (Peter et al., 2011). Compared with the HFD group, in the AEM (1,200 mg/kg) group, the mRNA expression level of *Gck* was increased more than twofold. The *Gck*-opposing gluconeogenic enzyme is *G6Pase*, and the HFD significantly decreased *G6Pase* expression. In addition, the highly significant accumulation of the G6P and F6P metabolic substrates in the AEM (1,200 mg/kg) group demonstrated that the dominant direction of the glucose/glucose-6-phosphate cycle was toward glycolytic flux. The F6P/F1, 6P substrate cycle is a major determinant of the net glycolytic or gluconeogenic flux. Thus, phosphofructokinase (*Pfkl* and *Pfkm*), the first committed step in glycolysis, together with its opposing gluconeogenic enzyme, *Fbp1*, controls the net glycolytic or gluconeogenic flux. Compared with the HFD group, the AEM (1,200 mg/kg) group presented with decreased *Fbp1* mRNA expression, while *Pfkm* gene expression was upregulated. The first step in glycogen breakdown is catalyzed by glycogen phosphorylase, and the final step in glycogen synthesis is catalyzed by glycogen synthase. GSK3 inhibits glycogen synthesis by suppressing glycogen synthase through inhibitory phosphorylation. Type 2 diabetes is strongly associated with decreases in insulin-stimulated glycogen synthase activity and glycogen synthesis and with increased GSK3 protein levels (Lee and Kim, 2007). Similarly, AEM (1,200 mg/kg) reversed the increased *Gsk3b* mRNA expression in the HFD group. In addition, lactate levels were increased, and the mRNA expression of *Ldha* was reduced in the AEM (1,200 mg/kg) group, which suggests an increased rate of glycolysis, consistent with a previous study (Chao et al., 2014; Le et al., 2016). Overall, these results indicated that AEM promotes glycolysis and inhibits gluconeogenesis.

The final products of fatty acid degradation and glycolysis are used in the TCA cycle (Friedrich, 2012). Due to the importance of this cycle in the central mitochondrial metabolic pathway, certain metabolic disturbances through this metabolic pathway have been reflected in obese and type 2 diabetic subjects (Satapati et al., 2012; Lu et al., 2013). Our metabolomic data revealed that the concentration change of six TCA cycle intermediates, citrate, 2-oxoglutarate, fumarate, malate, oxaloacetate, and succinate, were highly variable between the HFD and AEM (1,200 mg/kg) groups. Recently, Patterson et al. (2011) found that, compared with normal animals, type 2 diabetic rhesus macaques demonstrated a twofold higher level of citrate, which is consistent with our results. Furthermore, our qPCR results revealed that *Mdh2*, *Fh*, *Aco2*, *Sdha*, *Sdhb*, *Sdhd*, and *Cs* levels were downregulated in the HFD-fed golden hamsters, which likely contributed to the substantial malate, fumarate, and citrate accumulation. However, compared with the HFD group, the AEM (1,200 mg/kg)-treated group demonstrated lower levels of citrate, malate, and fumarate and high mRNA expression levels of *Sdha*, *Sdhd*, *Fh*, *Mdh2*, *Aco2*, and *Cs*. This result suggested that AEM increased TCA cycle flux by upregulating *Aco2*, *Fh*, *Cs*, *Sdha*, and *Mdh2* gene expression. Some studies have indicated that a reduced TCA cycle flux may be a metabolic adaptation that occurs during the metabolic progression of normal rats to diabetic phenotypes (Bakar et al., 2015; Zhou et al., 2015). In summary, via an array of mechanisms, our results indicated that AEM improves glucose metabolism disorder, specifically by upregulating the TCA cycle pathway.

From the biochemical data, we found that AEM affected hyperlipidemia, and the *in silico* target prediction identified genes related to lipid metabolism, especially PPARs. To elucidate the mechanism underlying the hypolipidemic effect of AEM, we assessed the expression profiles of hepatic genes involved in lipid metabolism. An increasing amount of evidence suggests that *Pparα* is a key regulator of lipid metabolism. Known *Pparα* target genes are involved in almost all aspects of lipid metabolism, including fatty acid uptake, binding, and oxidation; lipoprotein assembly; and lipid transport (Neve et al., 2000). Increases in the mRNA expression levels of *Pparα* and its target genes have also been identified as a mechanism for improving glucose and lipid metabolic disorders in high-fat diet-fed mice (Ding et al., 2013). In the AEM (1,200 mg/kg) group, the mRNA expression levels of *Pparα* and its downstream genes, including *Rxr* and *Cpt1*, were substantially upregulated, but *Hmgcr* and *Lxrb* were downregulated. Increased fatty acid β-oxidation leads to decreased serum TG concentrations in rodents (Reddy and Rao, 2005). In the AEM (1,200 mg/kg) consumption group, the increased *Pparα* mRNA expression upregulated the expression of *Cpt1* mRNA, which modulates fatty acid β-oxidation. This finding showed that AEM-reduced lipid synthesis may contribute to fatty acid β-oxidation. Positive correlations between *Lxrb* expression and the degrees of lipid accumulation, inflammation, and fibrosis in the livers of patients with non-alcoholic fatty liver have also been noted (Ahn et al., 2014). Thus, inhibiting the expression of *Lxrb* and its target genes reversed the high serum TG levels and improved steatosis in HFD-fed mice (Ding et al., 2012). *Srebp1c* plays a critical role in synthesizing lipids, suggesting that SREBP pathway inhibition might be a potential approach for treating obesity (Xiao and Song, 2013). In this paper, AEM reduced the expression levels of *Lxrb* and its target gene, *Srebp1*. In addition, the most important change at the mRNA level was found in the expression of *Hmgcr*, a rate-limiting enzyme in CHO synthesis. AEM (1,200 mg/kg) significantly reversed the increased *Hmgcr* transcript level in HFD-fed golden hamsters and, therefore, may reduce CHO synthesis. In summary, the above results are consistent with the lower serum and liver levels of CHO and TGs and demonstrate that the lipid-lowering effect of AEM may be partly related to the enhanced expression of genes involved in lipid metabolism through *Pparα* activation, fatty acid β-oxidation, and lipogenesis inhibition.

Limitations exist in this work. First, the studies on chemical compositions and the quantitative analysis were not sufficiently deep, restricting the comprehensiveness of the database used by virtual screening. In addition, further work is needed to determine the prevention effectiveness of AEM on metabolism disorder in clinical trials.

CONCLUSION

Our study first demonstrated that AEM supplementation positively affected lipid and glucose metabolism disorder prevention and amelioration in hamsters. A golden hamster model of metabolism disorder induced by feeding HFD was established, which shared many similarities with human lipid metabolism. Based on the serum biochemical and histopathological results, AEM appeared to significantly prevent the hyperlipidemia, hyperinsulinemia, insulin resistance, and non-alcoholic fatty liver caused by the HFD. For the first time, metabolomics, virtual screening, and qPCR were used together to reveal the complex pathogenesis underlying the protective effect of AEM on metabolic impairments. AEM promoted glycolysis and inhibited gluconeogenesis via regulating the expression levels of key genes such as *Gck*, *Fbp1*, and *Pfkm*. Moreover, AEM upregulated TCA cycle flux activity by changing the intermediate concentrations and increasing the mRNA levels of *Aco2*, *Fh*, *Cs*, *Sdha*, and *Mdh2*. In addition, the lipid-lowering effects of AEM in both the serum and liver may be partly related to PPARα signaling activation, including enhanced fatty acid β-oxidation and lipogenesis pathway inhibition. Together, our data demonstrated that the AEM intervention significantly improved metabolism disorder by regulating the glycolysis/gluconeogenesis-TCA cycle pathway and via modulating the expression levels of genes involved in the PPARα signaling pathway. Thus, AEM has the potential to be a dietary supplement for preventing or at least slowing lipid and glucose metabolism disorder progression. However, more studies and clinical trials are needed to support this hypothesis.

AUTHOR CONTRIBUTIONS

WW, LX, BJ, and PX: designed the experiments, supervised, and participated in the entire work. WW, HL, and JX: maintained and performed animal studies, biochemical analysis, metabonomics, and qPCR analysis. FY, JX, and HL: supported *in silico* analysis. WW, FY, and BJ: contributed to data analysis and writing and editing the manuscript. All the authors read and approved the final manuscript.

FUNDING

This work was supported by the National Natural Science Foundation of China (Nos. 81573576 and 81703223), the CAMS Innovation Fund for Medical Sciences (CIFMS 2016-I2M-1-012), the Beijing Natural Science Foundation (7182112), and the Beijing Technology and Business University Youth Scholars Fund (QNJJ2018-2).

ACKNOWLEDGMENTS

We thank the Metabolomics Facility at the Technology Center for Protein Sciences, Tsinghua University, for providing the facility support.

SUPPLEMENTARY MATERIAL

FIGURE S1 | Effects of aqueous extract of black maca (AEM) on the food intake and body weight of golden hamsters over 20 weeks. **(A)** Daily food intake of each golden hamster. **(B)** The body weight of each golden hamster over the 20 weeks. Data are presented as the means ± SEMs, $n = 6$.

FIGURE S2 | Number of epididymal white adipocytes per field of vision. The number of epididymal white adipocytes per field of vision was measured. Three fields of vision of each pathology sections were selected randomly. Each field of vision was observed at a magnification of 400×, $n = 4$.

FIGURE S3 | Effects of aqueous extract of black maca (AEM) on serum lipid profiles and glucose and insulin levels in golden hamsters over 20 weeks. **(A)** At the end of 4 weeks, serum CHO, TG, LDL, HDL, and glucose levels were tested. **(B)** At the end of 8 weeks, serum CHO, TG, LDL, HDL, and glucose levels were measured. **(C)** At the end of 12 weeks, serum CHO, TG, LDL, HDL, and glucose levels were tested. **(D)** At the end of 16 weeks, serum CHO, TG, LDL, HDL, and glucose levels were measured. Data are presented as the means ± SEMs. $^{\#}P < 0.05$, $^{\#\#}P < 0.01$, $^{\#\#\#}P < 0.001$ compared with the control group; $^{*}P < 0.05$, $^{**}P < 0.01$, $^{***}P < 0.001$ compared with the HFD model group, $n = 6$.

TABLE S1 | Hamster quantitative real-time PCR primer sequences.

TABLE S2 | Major compound-target-disease table for maca.

FILE S1 | The collection of chemical constituents of maca.

REFERENCES

Ahn, S. B., Jang, K., Jun, D. W., Lee, B. H., and Shin, K. J. (2014). Expression of liver X receptor correlates with intrahepatic inflammation and fibrosis in patients with nonalcoholic fatty liver disease. *Dig. Dis. Sci.* 59, 2975–2982. doi: 10.1007/s10620-014-3289-x

And, C. S., and Sturm, S. (2007). Analytical aspects of plant metabolite profiling platforms: current standings and future aims. *J. Proteome Res.* 6, 480–497. doi: 10.1021/pr0604716

Bakar, M. H. A., Sarmidi, M. R., Cheng, K. K., Khan, A. A., Suan, C. L., Huri, H. Z., et al. (2015). Metabolomics-the complementary field in systems biology: a review on obesity and type 2 diabetes. *Mol. Biosyst.* 11, 1742–1774. doi: 10.1039/C5MB00158G

Campos, D., Chirinos, R., Barreto, O., Noratto, G., and Pedreschi, R. (2013). Optimized methodology for the simultaneous extraction of glucosinolates, phenolic compounds and antioxidant capacity from maca (*Lepidium meyenii*). *Ind. Crops Prod.* 49, 747–754. doi: 10.1016/j.indcrop.2013.06.021

Chao, J., Huo, T., Cheng, H., Tsai, J., Liao, J., Lee, M., et al. (2014). Gallic acid ameliorated impaired glucose and lipid homeostasis in high fat diet-induced NAFLD mice. *PLoS One* 9:e96969. doi: 10.1371/journal.pone.0096969

Ding, X., Fan, S., Lu, Y., Zhang, Y., Gu, M., Zhang, L., et al. (2012). *Citrus ichangensis* peel extract exhibits anti-metabolic disorder effects by the inhibition of PPARγ and LXR signaling in high-fat diet-induced C57BL/6 mouse. *Evid. Based Complement. Alternat. Med.* 2012:678592. doi: 10.1155/2012/678592

Ding, X., Guo, L., Zhang, Y., Fan, S., Gu, M., Lu, Y., et al. (2013). Extracts of pomelo peels prevent high-fat diet-induced metabolic disorders in C57BL/6 Mice through activating the PPARα and GLUT4 pathway. *PLoS One* 8:e77915. doi: 10.1371/journal.pone.0077915

Friedrich, N. (2012). Metabolomics in diabetes research. *J. Endocrinol.* 215, 29–42. doi: 10.1530/JOE-12-0120

Gonzales, G. F. (2010). Maca: from the lost crop of the Incas to the miracle of the Andes. A food security study. Segurança Aliment. Nutricional, Camp. 17, 16–36.

Gonzales, G. F., Miranda, S., Nieto, J., Fernandez, G., Yucra, S., Rubio, J., et al. (2005). Red maca (*Lepidium meyenii*) reduced prostate size in rats. *Reprod. Biol. Endocrinol.* 3:5. doi: 10.1186/1477-7827-3-5

Gonzales, G., Singh, V., Govil, J., Ahmad, K., and Sharma, R. (2006). Biological effects of *Lepidium meyenii*, Maca, a plant from the highlands of Peru. *Nat. Prod.* 15, 209–234.

Grundy, S. M. (2016). Metabolic syndrome update. *Trends Cardiovasc. Med.* 26, 364–373. doi: 10.1016/j.tcm.2015.10.004

Harvey, A. L. (2008). Natural products in drug discovery. *Drug Discov. Today* 13, 894–901. doi: 10.1016/j.drudis.2008.07.004

Henry, O. M., Alina, M., Ewa, P., Marek, B., Sebastian, M., Bogdan, K., et al. (2016). Peruvian Maca (*Lepidium peruvianum*): (II) phytochemical profiles of four prime Maca phenotypes grown in two geographically-distant locations. *Int. J. Biomed. Sci.* 12, 9–24.

Jia, Y., Kim, S., Kim, J. Y., Kim, B., Wu, C., Lee, J. H., et al. (2015). Ursolic acid improves lipid and glucose metabolism in high-fat-fed C57BL/6J mice by activating peroxisome proliferator-activated receptor alpha and hepatic autophagy. *Mol. Nutr. Food Res.* 59, 344–354. doi: 10.1002/mnfr.201400399

Jiang, G., and Zhang, B. B. (2003). Glucagon and regulation of glucose metabolism. *Am. J. Physiol. Endocrinol. Metab.* 284, E671–E678. doi: 10.1152/ajpendo.00492.2002

Keiser, M. J., Setola, V., Irwin, J. J., Laggner, C., Abbas, A. I., Hufeisen, S. J., et al. (2009). Predicting new molecular targets for known drugs. *Nature* 462, 175–181. doi: 10.1038/nature08506

Kitchen, D. B., Decornez, H., Furr, J. R., and Bajorath, J. (2004). Docking and scoring in virtual screening for drug discovery: methods and applications. *Nat. Rev. Drug Discov.* 3, 935–949. doi: 10.1038/nrd1549

Le, L., Jiang, B., Wan, W., Zhai, W., Xu, L., Hu, K., et al. (2016). Metabolomics reveals the protective of Dihydromyricetin on glucose homeostasis by enhancing insulin sensitivity. *Sci. Rep.* 6:36184. doi: 10.1038/srep36184

Lee, J., and Kim, M. (2007). The role of GSK3 in glucose homeostasis and the development of insulin resistance. *Diabetes. Res. Clin. Pract.* 77(Suppl. 1), S49–S57. doi: 10.1016/j.diabres.2007.01.033

Li, M., Shu, X., Xu, H., Zhang, C., Yang, L., Zhang, L., et al. (2016). Integrative analysis of metabolome and gut microbiota in diet-induced hyperlipidemic rats treated with berberine compounds. *J. Transl. Med.* 14:237. doi: 10.1186/s12967-016-0987-5

Liao, C. C., Lin, Y. L., and Kuo, C. F. (2015). Effect of high-fat diet on hepatic proteomics of hamsters. *J. Agric. Food Chem.* 63, 1869–1881. doi: 10.1021/jf506118j

Lu, J., Xie, G., Jia, W., and Jia, W. (2013). Metabolomics in human type 2 diabetes research. *Front. Med.* 7, 4–13. doi: 10.1007/s11684-013-0248-4

Ma, Q., Li, P. L., Hua, Y. L., Ji, P., Yao, W. L., Zhang, X. S., et al. (2017). Effects of Tao-Hong-Si-Wu decoction on acute blood stasis in rats based on a LC-Q/TOF-MS metabolomics and network approach. *Biomed. Chromatogr.* 32:e4144. doi: 10.1002/bmc.4144

Neve, B. P., Fruchart, J., and Staels, B. (2000). Role of the peroxisome proliferator-activated receptors (PPAR) in atherosclerosis. *Biochem. Pharmacol.* 60, 1245–1250. doi: 10.1016/S0006-2952(00)00430-5

Patterson, A. D., Bonzo, J. A., Li, F., Krausz, K. W., Eichler, G. S., Aslam, S., et al. (2011). Metabolomics reveals attenuation of the SLC6A20 kidney transporter in nonhuman primate and mouse models of type 2 diabetes mellitus. *J. Biol. Chem.* 286, 19511–19522. doi: 10.1074/jbc.M111.221739

Peter, A., Stefan, N., Cegan, A., Walenta, M., Wagner, S., Konigsrainer, A., et al. (2011). Hepatic glucokinase expression is associated with lipogenesis and fatty liver in humans. *J. Clin. Endocrinol. Metab.* 96, E1126–E1130. doi: 10.1210/jc.2010-2017

Puiggròs, F., Canela, N., and Arola, L. (2015). Metabolome responses to physiological and nutritional challenges. *Curr. Opin. Food Sci.* 4, 111–115. doi: 10.1016/j.cofs.2015.06.001

Reddy, J. K., and Rao, M. S. (2005). Lipid metabolism and liver inflammation. II. Fatty liver disease and fatty acid oxidation. *Am. J. Physiol. Gastrointest. Liver Physiol.* 290, G852–G858. doi: 10.1152/ajpgi.00521.2005

Rester, U. (2008). From virtuality to reality - Virtual screening in lead discovery and lead optimization: a medicinal chemistry perspective. *Curr. Opini. Drug Discov. Devel.* 11, 559–568.

Sallese, A., and Zhu, J. (2017). Mass spectrometry based metabolomics: a novel analytical technique for detecting metabolic syndrome? *Bioanalysis* 9, 1623–1626. doi: 10.4155/bio-2017-0165

Satapati, S., Sunny, N. E., Kucejova, B., Fu, X., He, T., Mendezlucas, A., et al. (2012). Elevated TCA cycle function in the pathology of diet-induced hepatic insulin resistance and fatty liver. *J. Lipid Res.* 53, 1080–1092. doi: 10.1194/jlr.M023382

Sharabi, K., Tavares, C. D. J., Rines, A. K., and Puigserver, P. (2015). Molecular pathophysiology of hepatic glucose production. *Mol. Aspects Med.* 46, 21–33. doi: 10.1016/j.mam.2015.09.003

Vecera, R., Orolin, J., Skottova, N., Kazdova, L., Oliyarnik, O., Ulrichova, J., et al. (2007). The influence of maca (*Lepidium meyenii*) on antioxidant status, lipid and glucose metabolism in rat. *Plant Foods Hum. Nutr.* 62, 59–63. doi: 10.1007/s11130-007-0042-z

Wan, W., Jiang, B., Sun, L., Xu, L., and Xiao, P. (2017). Metabolomics reveals that vine tea (*Ampelopsis grossedentata*) prevents high-fat-diet-induced metabolism disorder by improving glucose homeostasis in rats. *PLoS One*12:e0182830. doi: 10.1371/journal.pone.0182830

Xiao, X., and Song, B. (2013). SREBP: a novel therapeutic target. *Acta Biochim. Biophys. Sin.* 45, 2–10. doi: 10.1093/abbs/gms112

Yi, F., Sun, L., Xu, L., Peng, Y., Liu, H., He, C., et al. (2016). *In silico* approach for anti-thrombosis drug discovery: P2Y1R structure-based TCMs screening. *Front. Pharmacol.* 7:531. doi: 10.3389/fphar.2016.00531

Zhou, C., Li, G., Li, Y., Gong, L., Huang, Y., Shi, Z., et al. (2015). A high-throughput metabolomic approach to explore the regulatory effect of mangiferin on metabolic network disturbances of hyperlipidemia rats. *Mol. biosyst.* 11, 418–433. doi: 10.1039/C4MB00421C

14

Mechanisms of Triptolide-Induced Hepatotoxicity and Protective Effect of Combined Use of Isoliquiritigenin: Possible Roles of Nrf2 and Hepatic Transporters

Zhenyan Hou[1,2], Lei Chen[1,2], Pingfei Fang[1,2], Hualin Cai[1,2], Huaibo Tang[3], Yongbo Peng[4], Yang Deng[5], Lingjuan Cao[1,2], Huande Li[1,2], Bikui Zhang[1,2] and Miao Yan[1,2]**

[1] Department of Pharmacy, The Second Xiangya Hospital, Central South University, Changsha, China, [2] Institute of Clinical Pharmacy, Central South University, Changsha, China, [3] Department of Pharmacy, Chemistry College, Xiangtan University, Xiangtan, China, [4] Molecular Science and Biomedicine Laboratory, College of Life Sciences, State Key Laboratory of Chemo, Bio-Sensing and Chemometrics, Hunan University, Changsha, China, [5] School of Pharmacy, Hunan University of Chinese Medicine, Changsha, China

***Correspondence:**
Bikui Zhang
505995@csu.edu.cn
Miao Yan
yanmiao@csu.edu.cn

Triptolide (TP), the main bioactive component of *Tripterygium wilfordii* Hook F, can cause severe hepatotoxicity. Isoliquiritigenin (ISL) has been reported to be able to protect against TP-induced liver injury, but the mechanisms are not fully elucidated. This study aims to explore the role of nuclear transcription factor E2-related factor 2 (Nrf2) and hepatic transporters in TP-induced hepatotoxicity and the reversal protective effect of ISL. TP treatment caused both cytotoxicity in L02 hepatocytes and acute liver injury in mice. Particularly, TP led to the disorder of bile acid (BA) profiles in mice livers. Combined treatment of TP with ISL effectively alleviated TP-induced hepatotoxicity. Furthermore, ISL pretreatment enhanced Nrf2 expressions and nuclear accumulations and its downstream NAD(P)H: quinine oxidoreductase 1 (NQO1) expression. Expressions of hepatic P-gp, MRP2, MRP4, bile salt export pump, and OATP2 were also induced. In addition, *in vitro* transport assays identified that neither was TP exported by MRP2, OATP1B1, or OATP1B3, nor did TP influence the transport activities of P-gp or MRP2. All these results indicate that ISL may reduce the hepatic oxidative stress and hepatic accumulations of both endogenous BAs and exogenous TP as well as its metabolites by enhancing the expressions of Nrf2, NQO1, and hepatic influx and efflux transporters. Effects of TP on hepatic transporters are mainly at the transcriptional levels, and changes of hepatic BA profiles are very important in the mechanisms of TP-induced hepatotoxicity.

Keywords: triptolide, hepatotoxicity, isoliquiritigenin, nuclear transcription factor E2-related factor 2, transporter, bile acid

INTRODUCTION

Triptolide, the main bioactive component of the traditional Chinese herb TwHF, possesses various pharmacological properties (Wang et al., 2004; Liu, 2011; Li X. et al., 2014). However, the clinical application of TP is limited due to its toxicities, especially its high incidence of hepatotoxicity and serious consequences.

With regard to the mechanisms of TP-induced hepatotoxicity, previous studies have indicated that oxidative stress damage induced by TP is important (Wang J. et al., 2013), which is shown by increased ROS levels and decreased content of GSH in the liver (Li J. et al., 2014; Li X. et al., 2014). Besides, since TP-induced hepatotoxicity is quantitatively correlated with the hepatic exposure to the parent drug, changes in pharmacokinetic profiles of TP may also influence its hepatotoxicity (Kong et al., 2015), and CYP3A-mediated metabolism of TP is a detoxification pathway (Xue et al., 2011). More recently, TP administration was found to increase the total bile acid (TBA) accumulation in rat livers (Jiang et al., 2016; Yang et al., 2017), and activation of the BA receptor (FXR) ameliorates the TP-induced liver injuries (Jin et al., 2015). Combined with the cholestatic symptoms of TP administration observed in clinics (Xue et al., 2009), we speculate that besides the hepatic accumulation of TP, mechanisms involved in the change of endogenous BA profiles may as well contribute to TP-induced hepatotoxicity.

Hepatic influx and efflux transporters localized to the canalicular or basolateral membrane of hepatocytes are responsible for the movement of endogenous and exogenous compounds (e.g., BAs, drugs, and metabolites) across the cellular membranes, thus playing a critical role in determining the drug toxicity and efficacy (Klaassen and Aleksunes, 2010; Corsini and Bortolini, 2013). Changes in either expressions or activities of transporters contribute to the variability in drug hepatic exposure as well as the hepatic endogenous chemical accumulation and BA-dependent or -independent bile flows (Hillgren et al., 2013; Pfeifer et al., 2014). Since TP is predominantly metabolized in the liver and mainly secreted in the bile (Liu et al., 2014), hepatic transporters play an important role in modulating TP-induced hepatotoxicity and may serve as the treatment target. It has been proved that TP is the substrate of P-gp (ABCB1, MDR1) rather than a BCRP (ABCG2) (Zhuang et al., 2013). Inhibition of the expression and function of P-gp augments the TP-induced liver injuries (Kong et al., 2015). However, apart from P-gp, whether other hepatic transporters participate in TP transport and further hepatotoxicity has not been investigated, such as the efflux transporters MRPs (ABCCs) and the influx transporters OATPs, both of which have wide substrate specificity and are identified to be very important in clinical practice (Hillgren et al., 2013). On the other hand, whether TP causes disorders of hepatic BA profiles by modulating the BA transporter expressions or activities has not been made clear.

Nuclear receptors are transcription factors involved in the maintenance of BA homeostasis and drug disposition by regulating phase I and phase II metabolism as well as phase 0 and phase III transports (Zollner et al., 2010). Among them, Nrf2 is the primary player in the cell defense system and may activate the expressions of antioxidant enzymes, detoxification enzymes, and transporters such as MRPs and BSEP (ABCB11) (Klaassen and Reisman, 2010), promoting the antioxidation, detoxification, and elimination of harmful xenobiotics and BA homeostasis, thus protecting against the DILI (Weerachayaphorn et al., 2012; Kamisako et al., 2014; Zhang et al., 2017). Activation of Nrf2 can protect against TP-induced hepatotoxicity by combating the oxidative stress (Li J. et al., 2014), indicating that activation of Nrf2 and its downstream protective genes may be effective in preventing TP-induced liver injuries.

Licorice (*Glycyrrhiza uralensis*) is usually used as a unique "guide drug" in China to improve the efficacy and reduce the toxicity of other ingredients (Wang X. et al., 2013). Its main bioactive compounds have been used in combination with TwHF/TP to reduce the hepatotoxicity in clinical practice (Li X. et al., 2014). Our previous studies have demonstrated that ISL is the most potent Nrf2 inducer among the four compounds derived from licorice and can activate Nrf2 downstream cytoprotective enzymes and transporters (Gong et al., 2015). We also show that ISL may protect against TP-induced oxidative stress in HepG2 cells and mouse livers via Nrf2 activation (Cao et al., 2016a,b). Based on our previous studies, the present study aims to further explore the role of Nrf2 and hepatic transporters in TP-induced hepatotoxicity and the protective effects of ISL by interfering with the endogenous system (BA transport) or directly altering the transport of xenobiotic toxins from the liver.

Abbreviations: ALP, alkaline phosphatase; ALT, alanine aminotransferase; ANOVA, analysis of variance; ARE, antioxidant responsive element; AST, aspartate aminotransferase; BA, bile acid; BCRP, breast cancer resistance protein; BMR, benzbromarone; BSEP, bile salt export pump; CA, cholic acid; CAD, collision gas; CAR, constitutive androstane receptor; CDCA, chenodeoxycholic acid; CPA, cyproterone acetate; CUR, curtain gas; CYP3A, cytochrome P450 3A; DCA, deoxycholic acid; DILI, drug-induced liver injury; DMEM, Dulbecco Modified Eagle Medium; DMSO, dimethyl sulfoxide; $E_217\beta G$, estradiol-17-β-D-glucuronide; ECL, electrochemiluminescence; ESI, electrospray ionization; FBS, fetal bovine serum; FXR, farnesoid X receptor; GA, glycyrrhetinic acid; GCA, glycocholic acid; GCDCA, glycochenodeoxycholic acid; GDCA, glycodeoxycholic acid; GLCA, glycolithocholic acid; GSH, reduced glutathione; GUDCA, glycoursodeoxycholic acid; H&E, hematoxylin & eosin; HDCA, hyodeoxycholic acid; HEK293, human embryonic kidney 293; IC50, half maximal inhibitory concentration; IS, internal standard; ISL, isoliquiritigenin; KCZ, ketoconazole; LC-MS/MS, liquid chromatography-tandem mass spectrometry; LCA, lithocholic acid; LDH, lactate dehydrogenase; MRM, multiple reaction monitoring; MRP, multidrug resistance protein; MTT, 3-(4, 5-dimethylthiazol-2-yl)-2, 5-diphenyltetrazolium bromide; NA, not applicable; NMQ, N-methyl quinidine; NQO1, NAD(P)H: quinine oxidoreductase 1; Nrf2, nuclear transcription factor E2-related factor 2; OATP, organic anion transporting polypeptide; P-gp, P-glycoprotein; *SD*, standard deviation; tBHQ, *tert*-butylhydroquinone; TBM, tolbutamide; TCA, taurocholic acid; TCDCA, taurochemodeoxycholic acid; TDCA, taurodeoxycholic acid; THDCA, taurohyodeoxycholic acid; TLCA, taurolithocholic acid; TP, triptolide; TUDCA, tauroursodeoxycholic acid; TwHF, *Tripterygium wilfordii* Hook F; UDCA, ursodeoxycholic acid; UR, uptake ratio; VT, vesicular transport.

MATERIALS AND METHODS

Chemicals and Reagents

Isoliquiritigenin (purity > 99%) and TP (purity ≥ 98%) were purchased from On-Road Biotechnology Co., Ltd. (Changsha,

China); tBHQ, DMSO, MTT, E217βG, GA, KCZ, BMR, and TBM were purchased from Sigma-Aldrich (St. Louis, MO, United States). TP, ISL, and tBHQ were dissolved in DMSO and stored at −20°C before use. The concentration of DMSO in the experiments never exceeded 0.1% (v/v). tBHQ, an Nrf2 inducer, was used as the positive control. CPA was obtained from the National Institute for Food and Drug Control (Beijing, China). NMQ was obtained from GemoMembrane (Yokohama, Japan). Nrf2-siRNA, negative control siRNA, and transfection reagents were obtained from Santa Cruz Biotechnology (Santa Cruz, CA, United States). Human MDR1 and human MRP2 vesicle products and VT assay reagent kits were from GemoMembrane (Yokohama, Japan). BAs were as follows: CA, DCA, CDCA, UDCA, HDCA, TCDCA, and TUDCA were from On-Road Biotechnology Co., Ltd. (Changsha, China); LCA, TCA, TDCA, TLCA, THDCA, GCA, GDCA, GLCA, GCDCA, and GUDCA were from Sigma-Aldrich (St. Louis, MO, United States). The antibodies included anti-Nrf2 (sc-722, Santa Cruz), anti-NQO1 (ab28947, Abcam), anti-P-gp (ab170904, Abcam), anti-MRP2 (ab203397, Abcam), anti-MRP4 (#12705, Cell Signaling Technology), anti-GAPDH (#MAB374, Merck Millipore), and anti-Lamin B2 (#12255, Cell Signaling Technology). All other reagents were of analytical reagent grade.

Cell Culture

Human normal L02 hepatocytes obtained from the Cell Bank of the Chinese Academy of Sciences (Shanghai, China) were cultured in DMEM (Gibco, Grand Island, NY, United States) supplemented with 10% (v/v) FBS (BI, Israel) in a humidified incubator at 37°C with 5% CO_2. The cells were treated with 50 nM TP for 24 h with or without 12 h ISL pretreatment. In all experiments, the cells were plated at an appropriate density according to the experimental design and grown for 24 h before the treatment.

For the cellular uptake assays, HEK293 cells stably expressing OATP1B1 (HEK293-OATP1B1), OATP1B3 (HEK293-OATP1B3), or respective vector control cells (HEK293-MOCK) were obtained from GemoMembrane (Yokohama, Japan) and cultured in DMEM (Gibco, Grand Island, NY, United States) supplemented with 10% (v/v) FBS (Gibco, Grand Island, NY, United States) and 1% antibiotics (100 μg/mL streptomycin/100 U/mL penicillin mix) (Gibco, Grand Island, NY, United States) in a humidified incubator at 37°C with 5% CO_2.

Cell Viability Assay

The cell viability was determined by MTT assay according to our previous studies (Cao et al., 2016a). L02 cells (2.5×10^4 cells/well) were seeded in 24-well plates and treated with TP, ISL, or ISL + TP. Percent viability was defined as the relative absorbance of the treated cells versus the control cells. Morphological changes were detected with a light microscope (Nikon TS100, 10× magnification).

Nrf2-siRNA Transient Transfection

L02 cells were transiently transfected with a mixture of transfection reagents and Nrf2-siRNA or negative control siRNA according to the manufacturer instructions. The cells were further treated as designed for cell viability assay 48 h after the transfection.

Animal Treatments and Hepatotoxicity Assessments

All animal experiments were conducted according to the Regulations of Experimental Animal Administration issued by the State Committee of Science and Technology of China, with the approval of the Ethics Committee in the Experimental Animal Center of Hunan SJA Laboratory Animal Co. Ltd. (Changsha, China). All procedures were performed under urethane anesthesia, and all efforts were made to minimize the suffering.

Healthy male ICR mice, weighing 18–22 g, were provided by Hunan SJA Laboratory Animal Co. Ltd. (Changsha, China). The mice were kept at 22–25°C and humidity 50 ± 10% with a 12 h light-dark cycle and had free access to food and water. Thirty mice were randomly assigned to five groups (six in each group) and were respectively given the following treatments: (1) vehicle control, (2) TP (1.0 mg/kg), (3) ISL (25 mg/kg) + TP (1.0 mg/kg), (4) ISL (50 mg/kg) + TP (1.0 mg/kg), and (5) ISL (50 mg/kg). TP was injected intraperitoneally (i.p.), while ISL via oral gavage. The dosage of TP and ISL was decided based on our previous studies (Gong et al., 2015; Cao et al., 2016b). The mice received either 0.5% (w/v) CMC-Na or ISL once daily for 7 days consecutively. One hour after the final treatment, the mice were treated with TP ($1.0\ mg{\cdot}kg^{-1}$, i.p.) or corresponding vehicles. Six hours after the TP administration, the mice were given either 0.5% (w/v) CMC-Na or ISL again. In all treatment groups, the mice were anesthetized 24 h after the TP injection. Blood samples were collected, and the liver of each mouse was collected and weighed. The degree of liver injury was assessed by H&E staining and serum biochemical parameters, including ALT, AST, ALP, and LDH and analyzed on an automatic clinical analyzer (7600, HITACHI Ltd., Tokyo, Japan).

Quantitative Real-Time PCR

Total RNA was extracted with trizol reagent (Invitrogen Life Technologies, Carlsbad, CA, United States) according to the manufacturer's instruction before being converted to cDNA with the PrimeScript^{TM} RT reagent Kit with gDNA Eraser (Takara, Japan). The cDNAs were analyzed with ABI Prism 7900HT (Applied Biosystems, United States) using an SYBR Premix Ex Taq (Takara, Japan). Each sample was run in duplicate and the results were normalized to the level of GAPDH mRNA. The primers were as follows: human MRP2 forward 5′-TGAGCAAGTTTGAAACGCACAT-3′ and reverse 5′-AGCTCTTCTCCTGCCGTCTCT-3′, mouse Bsep forward 5′-ACTCAGTGATTCTTCGCAGTGT-3′ and reverse 5′-CAAAGAAGCCAACTCGAGCG-3′, mouse Oatp2 forward 5′-TGATCGGACCAATCCTTGGC-3′ and reverse 5′-TCACAATGAAGCCGAGCCAC-3′, and the human and mouse GAPDH primers (Millipore, United States).

Western Blot

The samples were lyzed with RIPA buffer (CW biotech, Beijing, China). Nuclear and cytoplasmic proteins were prepared with NE-PER nuclear and cytoplasmic extraction reagents (Pierce Biotechnology, Rockford, IL, United States) according to the manufacturer's instruction. The same amounts of protein were loaded and separated by 10% SDS-PAGE electrophoresis and transferred to PVDF membranes. After being blocked in 5% nonfat milk in 0.05% Tween-20/tris-buffered saline for 1 h at room temperature, the membranes were incubated overnight at 4°C with relevant primary antibodies. The immunoblots were then incubated with species-specific secondary antibodies at room temperature. The membranes were developed with an ECL kit (Advansta, United States) according to manufacturer's protocol.

Vesicular Transport (VT) Assay

The VT assay was conducted as described in the VT Kit protocol (GenoMembrane, Yokohama, Japan). To determine whether TP inhibited the transport activities of P-gp and MRP2, human P-gp vesicles or human MRP2 vesicles were incubated with the test solution containing TP (0.01, 0.1, 1, 10, and 100 μM), the relative positive control, and the relative substrate with ATP or AMP at 37°C for 10 min. KCZ and BMR were used as positive inhibitors of P-gp and MRP2, respectively. NMQ, the substrate of P-gp, was analyzed by fluorescence measurement at λ_{ex} 355 nm and λ_{em} 460 nm (Molecular Devices i3-R, CA, United States). $E_2 17\beta G$, the substrate of MRP2, was analyzed with LC-MS/MS. To determine whether TP was a substrate of MRP2, human MRP2 vesicles were incubated with the test solution containing TP (0.01, 0.1, 1, 10, and 100 μM) or $E_2 17\beta G$ serving as the positive control, with ATP or AMP at 37°C for 10 min. The vesicular accumulation of TP or $E_2 17\beta G$ was measured by LC-MS/MS.

Cellular Uptake Assay

To determine whether TP was a substrate of OATP1B1 or OATP1B3, HEK293-OATP1B1, HEK293-OATP1B3, and HEK293-MOCK cells were incubated with the test solution containing TP (0, 1, 10, and 100 μM) or $E_2 17\beta G$ in the uptake buffer at 37°C for 10 min. Then the cells were washed three times with ice-cold uptake buffer and lyzed with the TBM solution to be used as the IS in the following analysis. The intracellular accumulation of TP or $E_2 17\beta G$ was measured by LC-MS/MS, and the protein concentration of each sample was determined by bicinchoninic acid assay (Pierce BCA protein assay kit, Thermo Scientific, Rockford, IL, United States).

LC-MS/MS for BAs, TP, and $E_2 17\beta G$

Sample Preparation

To analyze 16 BAs in the mouse liver, 0.1 g liver tissue was weighed and added to 800 μL 75% acetonitrile. After the homogenation, 100 μL homogenate was added into 300 μL IS solution. The mixture was vortexed for 3 min before centrifugation at 15000 rpm at 4°C for 10 min. Then the supernatant was collected and injected to the LC-MS/MS system.

To analyze TP or $E_2 17\beta G$ in the vesicles, 50 μL 80% methanol was added to each well to dissolve the vesicles after washing and filtering. The obtained solution was centrifuged at 2000 rpm at 4°C for 2 min. These operations were repeated once. Then precooled methanol containing the relative IS was added to the supernatant. After centrifugation at 12000 rpm at 4°C for 5 min, the supernatant was collected and injected to the LC-MS/MS system.

To analyze TP in the HEK293 cells, precooled methanol containing the relative IS was added to the digested cells. After centrifugation at 12000 rpm at 4°C for 5 min, the supernatant was collected and injected to the LC-MS/MS system.

Instrumentation

An LC-20A HPLC system (SHIMADZU, Kyoto, Japan) coupled with a 4000 triple-quadrupole mass spectrometer (AB SCIEX, Framingham, MA, United States) was used to quantify BAs, TP, and $E_2 17\beta G$, respectively (Deng et al., 2015). For 16 BAs' analysis, the separation was performed on an Xtimate^{TM} C_{18} column (2.1 mm × 150 mm, 3 μm, Welch, United States) analytical column connected with a top C_{18} column (Guard cartridge System, United States). The column temperature was 40°C. CPA (20 μg/mL) and GA (250 ng/mL) mixture solution was used as the IS. The gradient system consisted of solvent A (0.005% formic acid containing 7 mmol/L ammonium acetate) and solvent B (methanol) at a flow rate of 0.25 mL/min, and the gradient program was as follows: 60% B (0–2.0 min), 95% B (13.0–17.3 min), and 60% B (17.4–27.3 min). The mass spectrometer was used in MRM function in the ESI-negative mode. Other MS parameters were as follows: CUR 30.0 psi; medium CAD; ionspray voltage 5500.0 V; and ion source temperature 550.0°C.

For TP analysis, a Phenomenex Synergi Hydro RP column (2.0 mm × 30 mm, 4 μm, Phenomenex, United States) at 40°C was used for chromatographic separation. TBM was used as the IS. The gradient system consisted of solvent A (0.1% formic acid) and solvent B (methanol containing 0.1% formic acid) at 0.5 mL/min, and the gradient program was as follows: 30% B (0 min), 85% B (0.5–1.0 min), and 30% B (1.01–2.0 min). The mass spectrometer was used in MRM function in the ESI-positive mode. Other MS parameters were as follows: CUR 20.0 psi; CAD 6 psi; ionspray voltage 5000.0 V; and ion source temperature 500.0°C.

For $E_2 17\beta G$ analysis, a Diamonsil C_{18} (2) column (4.6 mm × 50 mm, 5 μm, Diamonsil, United States) at 40°C was used for the chromatographic separation. TBM was used as the IS. The gradient system consisted of solvent A (0.05% ammonia) and solvent B (acetonitrile) at 0.85 mL/min, and the gradient program was as follows: 5% B (0 min), 70% B (2.0–2.5 min), and 5% B (2.51–3.3 min). The mass spectrometer was used in MRM function in the ESI-negative mode. Other MS parameters were as follows: CUR 20.0 psi; CAD 6 psi; ionspray voltage -4500.0 V; and ion source temperature 500.0°C.

Statistical Analysis

The transport activity was expressed as pmol/min/mg protein. The ATP-dependent uptake of probe compound was calculated by subtracting the measured value of uptake in the absence of

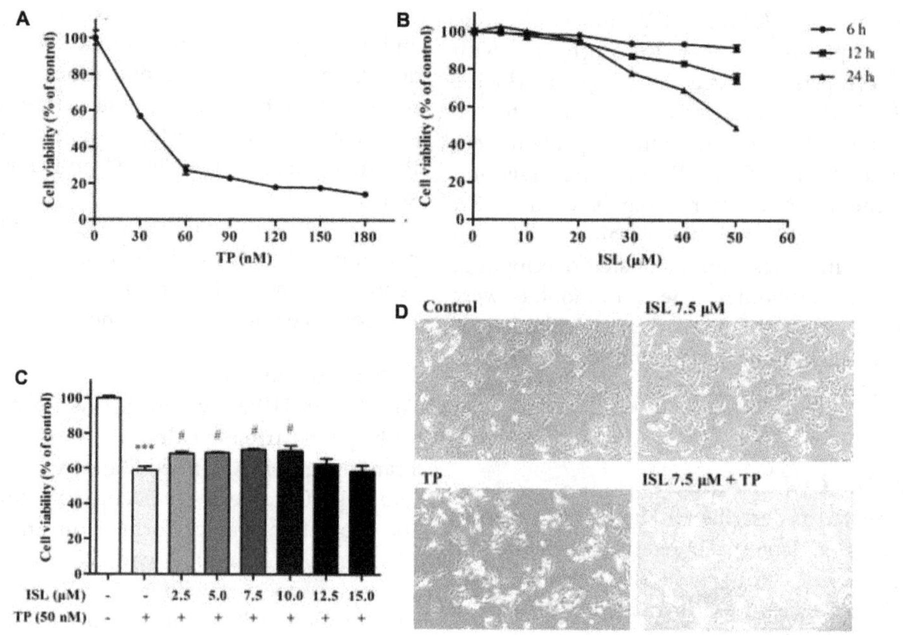

FIGURE 1 | Effects of triptolide (TP), isoliquiritigenin (ISL), or ISL + TP on the viability and morphological changes of L02 cells. **(A)** L02 cells were treated with TP at various concentrations for 24 h. **(B)** L02 cells were treated with ISL at various concentrations for 6, 12, and 24 h. **(C)** L02 cells were pretreated with indicated ISL concentrations for 12 h followed by TP (50 nM, 24 h) treatment. **(D)** L02 cells were pretreated with 7.5 μM ISL for 12 h followed by TP (50 nM, 24 h) treatment. Cell morphological changes were detected by a light microscope (10 × magnification). The cell viability was determined by MTT assay. Data were presented as means ± standard error (*SE*) (*n* = 3); ****P* < 0.001 vs. the control group, #*P* < 0.05 vs. the TP group, and ###*P* < 0.001 vs. the TP group.

ATP from the value of uptake in the presence of ATP. The ATP-dependent transport of probe compound was set as 100%. To determine the effect of the test compounds, we calculated the ratio of the ATP-dependent uptake of probe compound in the absence and presence of the test compound resulting in normalized ATP-dependent transport (%). The UR in the VT assay was calculated by the transport activity in the presence of ATP dividing that in the presence of AMP, and that in the cellular uptake assay was calculated by the transport activity in OATP-expressing cells dividing that in the control cells. If the UR ≥ 2, the test drug is considered as a substrate of the transporter.

All experiments were conducted in duplicate. The data were presented as the means ± standard error (SE) or the means ± standard derivation (SD). Statistical analyses were performed with SPSS 20.0 for Windows (SPSS Inc., Chicago, IL, United States) or GraphPad Prism 5.0 software (GraphPad Software Inc., United States). One-way ANOVA followed by Dunnett's *t*-test assessed the statistical significance of the difference between the mean values. A $P \leq 0.05$ was considered significantly different.

RESULTS

ISL Protected L02 Hepatocytes Against TP-Induced Cell Death

Triptolide treatment alone for 24 h impaired the cell viability in a dose-dependent manner (**Figure 1A**). TP 50 nM was used in subsequent experiments, which was close to the IC50. ISL treatment alone showed no obvious cytotoxicity at 0–15 μM, but a time- and dose-dependent decrease of cell viability at 15–50 μM (**Figure 1B**). ISL pretreatment significantly attenuated the TP-induced reduction in cell viability at 2.5–10 μM. The protective effect was dose-dependent between 2.5 and 7.5 μM, and reached the maximum at 7.5 μM of ISL treatment (**Figure 1C**). Besides, TP treatment alone caused the cell detachment and distortion, while ISL pretreatment partially prevented cells from such changes (**Figure 1D**).

Role of Nrf2 in ISL Protection Against TP-Induced Hepatotoxicity in L02 Cells

After confirming the effect of TP and ISL as well as the concentration and time of drug use, we further explored the mechanisms behind it. As shown in **Figures 2A–D**, protein levels of the total Nrf2, cytoplasmic Nrf2, and NQO1 decreased after the TP treatment, while the nuclear Nrf2 expression was induced. Compared with the TP-injured group, the total and nuclear Nrf2 and NQO1 protein levels were significantly increased after ISL (7.5 μM) or tBHQ (15 μM) pretreatment.

To further determine whether the ISL protection against TP-induced L02 injuries was Nrf2-dependent, Nrf2-siRNA was transfected into L02 cells. Nrf2-siRNA transfection led to a significant knockdown of Nrf2 at both mRNA and protein levels, while negative control siRNA had no effect on Nrf2 expressions (**Figures 2E,F**). Nrf2 knockdown significantly reduced the cell

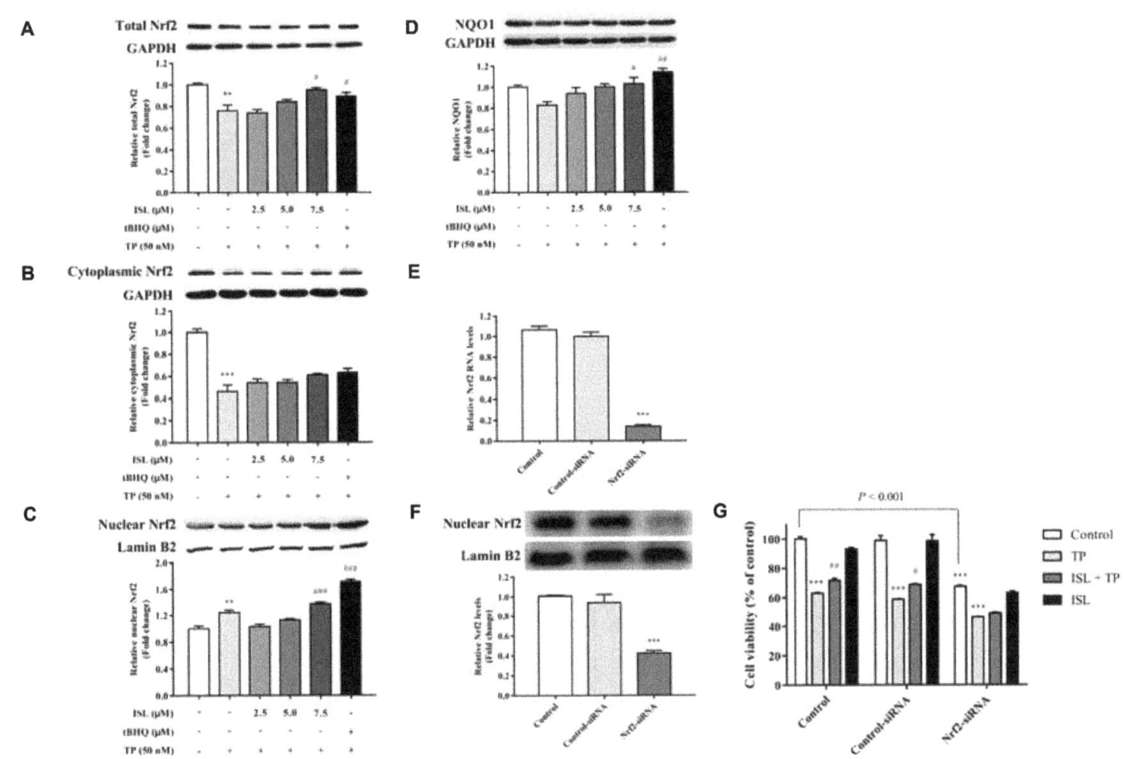

FIGURE 2 | Role of nuclear transcription factor E2-related factor 2 (Nrf2) in TP-induced cell death and ISL-induced protective effects. Effects of TP, ISL, or ISL + TP on the protein levels of **(A)** total, **(B)** cytoplasmic, and **(C)** nuclear Nrf2 and **(D)** NAD(P)H: quinine oxidoreductase 1 (NQO1) in L02 cells. Cells were treated with 50 nM TP with or without 2.5, 5, and 7.5 μM ISL pretreatment. The tBHQ (15 μM) was used as an Nrf2 inducer. Cell lysates were analyzed by Western blot. Role of Nrf2 in the protection against TP-induced cytotoxicity in L02 cells. Cells were transiently transfected with Nrf2-siRNA or Control-siRNA before TP, ISL, or ISL + TP treatment. **(E)** RT-PCR analysis of Nrf2 mRNA levels 48 h after the transfection. **(F)** Western blot analysis of nuclear Nrf2 protein levels 72 h after the transfection. **(G)** Cell viability determined by MTT assay. Data were presented as means ± *SE* ($n = 3$); $^{**}P < 0.01$ vs. the control group, $^{***}P < 0.001$ vs. the control group, $^{\#}P < 0.05$ vs. the TP group, $^{\#\#}P < 0.01$ vs. the TP group, and $^{\#\#\#}P < 0.001$ vs. the TP group.

viabilities, and ISL treatment did not significantly protect Nrf2-siRNA transfected cells from TP-induced injuries (**Figure 2G**).

Effect of TP and ISL Treatment on Expressions of MRP2, MRP4, and P-gp in L02 Cells

We detected the changes in the expression levels of Nrf2-regulated and -nonregulated transporters after the TP and ISL treatment. MRP2 mRNA levels of TP-injured groups significantly decreased, and decrease in MRP4 protein levels was insignificant, while ISL pretreatment increased MRP2 mRNA levels in a concentration-dependent manner (**Figures 3A,B**). ISL pretreatment significantly increased MRP4 protein levels at 7.5 μM, but tBHQ had no induction effect on MRP4. TP treatment induced P-gp expressions in L02 cells, and ISL pretreatment intensified this induction (**Figure 3C**).

Protective Effect of ISL on TP-Induced Liver Injury in Mice

The results of *in vitro* studies were validated *in vivo*. The liver indexes, histopathology, and serum biochemical indices were analyzed to determine the degree of liver injury. The liver index significantly increased in the TP-injured group, while ISL combined treatment decreased the liver index though the result was not statistically significant (**Table 1**).

In the TP-injured group, the serum activities of ALT, AST, and LDH significantly increased, and combined ISL treatment significantly reduced the serum ALT and AST activities (**Table 2**).

Histopathological analysis showed that the liver sections of the TP group showed a derangement of the hepatic cord and large areas of hydropic degeneration, compared with those of the control group. Nucleolysis and further hepatic parenchymal necrosis and some inflammatory cells infiltration were also seen in the TP group, but not in the positive control group. The severity of histopathological lesion was significantly decreased in the ISL + TP treatment group, showing less hepatocyte degeneration, and the hydropic degeneration was mostly near the central vein (**Figure 4**).

Role of Nrf2 in ISL Protection Against TP-Induced Hepatotoxicity in Mice

The total, cytoplasmic, and nuclear Nrf2 expressions were also detected in the mouse livers. As shown in **Figure 5**, TP administration reduced the total and nuclear levels of Nrf2,

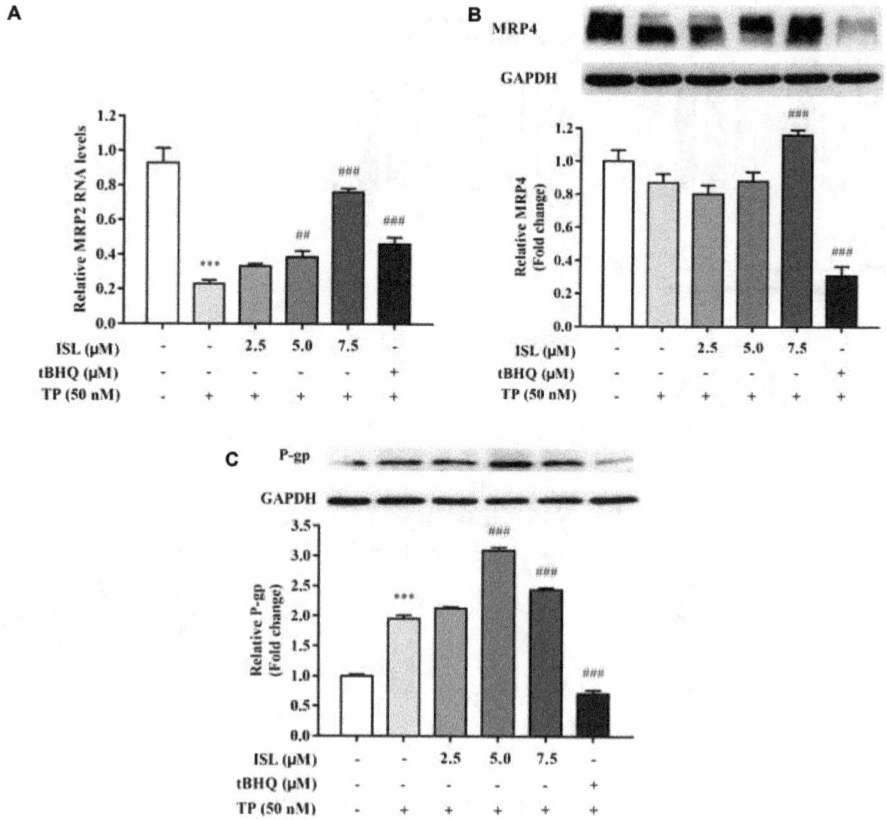

FIGURE 3 | ISL pretreatment induced expressions of **(A)** MRP2, **(B)** MRP4, and **(C)** P-gp to protect against TP-induced cytotoxicity. L02 cells were treated with 50 nM TP with or without 2.5, 5, and 7.5 μM ISL pretreatment. The *tert*-butylhydroquinone (15 μM) was used as an Nrf2 inducer. RT-PCR was used to analyze mRNAs and proteins by Western blot. Data were presented as means ± *SE* ($n = 3$);$^{***}P < 0.001$ vs. the control group, $^{\#\#}P < 0.01$ vs. the TP group, and $^{\#\#\#}P < 0.001$ vs. the TP group.

while combined ISL treatment induced the expressions of total, cytoplasmic, and nuclear Nrf2 as well as its downstream Nqo1.

Effect of TP and ISL Administration on the Expression of Hepatic Transporters in Mice

Protein levels of Mrp2 decreased in the TP-injured group, and combined ISL treatment caused a dramatic increase in the Mrp2 expression (**Figure 6A**). Combined ISL treatment also dose-dependently increased the protein levels of Mrp4 and P-gp (**Figures 6B,C**).

TABLE 1 | Effects of triptolide (TP), isoliquiritigenin (ISL), or ISL + TP on the liver indexes [means ± standard deviation (*SD*), $n = 5$–6].

Group	Liver weight (g)	Weight (g)	Liver index (%)
Control	1.28 ± 0.15	26.32 ± 1.53	4.87 ± 0.31
TP	1.69 ± 0.12	27.16 ± 1.04	6.23 ± 0.26***
25 mg/kg ISL + TP	1.53 ± 0.06	26.25 ± 1.94	5.85 ± 0.41
50 mg/kg ISL + TP	1.62 ± 0.12	27.58 ± 1.30	5.87 ± 0.22
50 mg/kg ISL	1.27 ± 0.12	26.87 ± 1.70	4.73 ± 0.30

$^{***}P < 0.0001$ vs. the control group.

Significant decrease in the mRNA levels of Bsep and Oatp2 was found in the TP-injured group, and combined ISL treatment resulted in an increase in the expressions of Bsep and Oatp2 (**Figures 6D,E**).

Changes of Hepatic Bile Acid Profiles in Mouse Livers

To further validate the role of transporters, the hepatic concentrations of 16 BAs were analyzed. Concentrations of LCA, GDCA, GCDCA, and GUDCA were under the lower limit of detections. TP administration dramatically increased the hepatic concentrations of CA, HDCA, TCA, and THDCA, compared with the control group, while the hepatic CA and THDCA, accumulation significantly reduced in ISL combined treatment (**Figure 7**). Besides, ISL combined treatment increased the concentrations of CDCA and UDCA in the mouse livers compared with those of the TP-treatment group.

TP Did Not Inhibit the Transport Activities of P-gp and MRP2

After determining changes in the transporter expressions, we further investigated whether TP inhibited the activity of human

TABLE 2 | Blood chemistry of male ICR mice administered TP, ISL, or both (mean ± SD, n = 5–6).

Group	ALT (U/L)	AST (U/L)	ALP (U/L)	LDH (U/L)
Control	30.23 ± 1.83	95.28 ± 13.15	128.00 ± 11.01	1091.96 ± 122.93
TP	59.73 ± 31.65*	214.30 ± 81.68***	113.23 ± 14.43	1567.90 ± 330.94**
25 mg/kg ISL + TP	32.87 ± 3.45#	166.33 ± 17.57	110.07 ± 26.02	1658.67.07 ± 203.40
50 mg/kg ISL + TP	28.97 ± 1.30#	144.10 ± 8.24#	103.66 ± 12.77	1393.36 ± 143.62
50 mg/kg ISL	30.17 ± 4.48	121.70 ± 26.35	147.63 ± 11.58	1255.03 ± 120.71

*ALT, alanine aminotransferase; AST, aspartate aminotransferase; ALP, alkaline phosphatase; LDH, lactate dehydrogenase. *P < 0.05 vs. the control group, **P < 0.001 vs. the control group, ***P < 0.0001 vs. the control group, and #P < 0.05 vs. the TP group.*

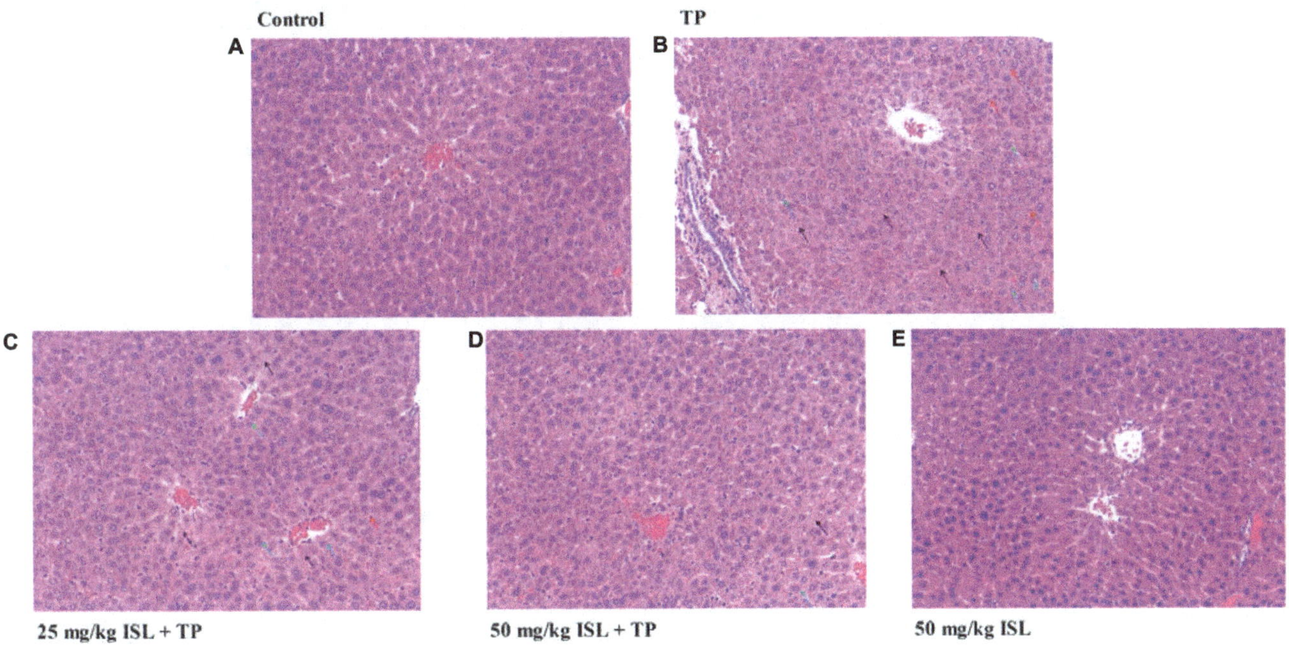

FIGURE 4 | Photomicrographs (× 200) of hematoxylin & eosin-stained liver sections obtained from the **(A)** control, **(B)** TP (1.0 mg/kg), **(C)** ISL (25 mg/kg) + TP (1.0 mg/kg), **(D)** ISL (50 mg/kg) + TP (1.0 mg/kg), and **(E)** ISL (50 mg/kg) groups. Green arrows indicate hepatocellular hydropic degeneration, black arrows indicate necrosis, and red arrows indicate inflammatory cell infiltration.

P-gp or MRP2. The UR of the substrate in the VT systems was 3.31 and 59.53 for P-gp and MRP2 vesicles, both greater than 2, indicating that the VT systems were running well. The relative transport of NMQ in the positive control group was 11.05% ± 2.53% for P-gp and 12.80% ± 0.81% for MRP2 vesicles. The relative transport of the substrates was not influenced by TP co-incubation, indicating that TP had no effect on the P-gp or MRP2 mediate transport in the vesicles (**Figures 8A,B**).

TP Was Not Transported by MRP2, OATP1B1, or OATP1B3

The UR of $E_2 17\beta G$, a substrate of MRP2, OATP1B1, and OATP1B3 which served as the positive control, was more than 2. TP concentrations in the vesicles or cells were under the lower limit of quantification when the incubation TP concentration was 0.1, 1, and 10 μM, respectively. The UR of 100 μM TP was less than 2 in the MRP2, OATP1B1, and OATP1B3 transport systems, indicating that TP was not a substrate of MRP2, OATP1B1, or OATP1B3 (**Figures 8C–E**).

DISCUSSION

Since TP-induced liver injury is always acute clinically (Xu et al., 2013), in this study, we established acute hepatotoxicity models by single-dose TP treatment in both L02 cells and ICR mice. Our data showed that TP treatment induced hepatic damage both *in vitro* and *in vivo*, indicating successful modeling and relieving effect of ISL combined treatment, which is consistent with our previous studies (Cao et al., 2016a,b). The present study for the first time used human normal L02 hepatocytes rather than hepatoma cells or rodent hepatocytes, which is as close to clinical practice as possible, since there are differences in physiological conditions as well as distributions and expression levels of transporters between human normal hepatocytes and hepatoma cells or rodent hepatocytes (Nicolaou et al., 2012; Le Vee et al., 2013).

As is known to all, antioxidants may react with MTT reagents and interfere with the results. However, in the present study, the ISL solution was removed and the cells were washed with

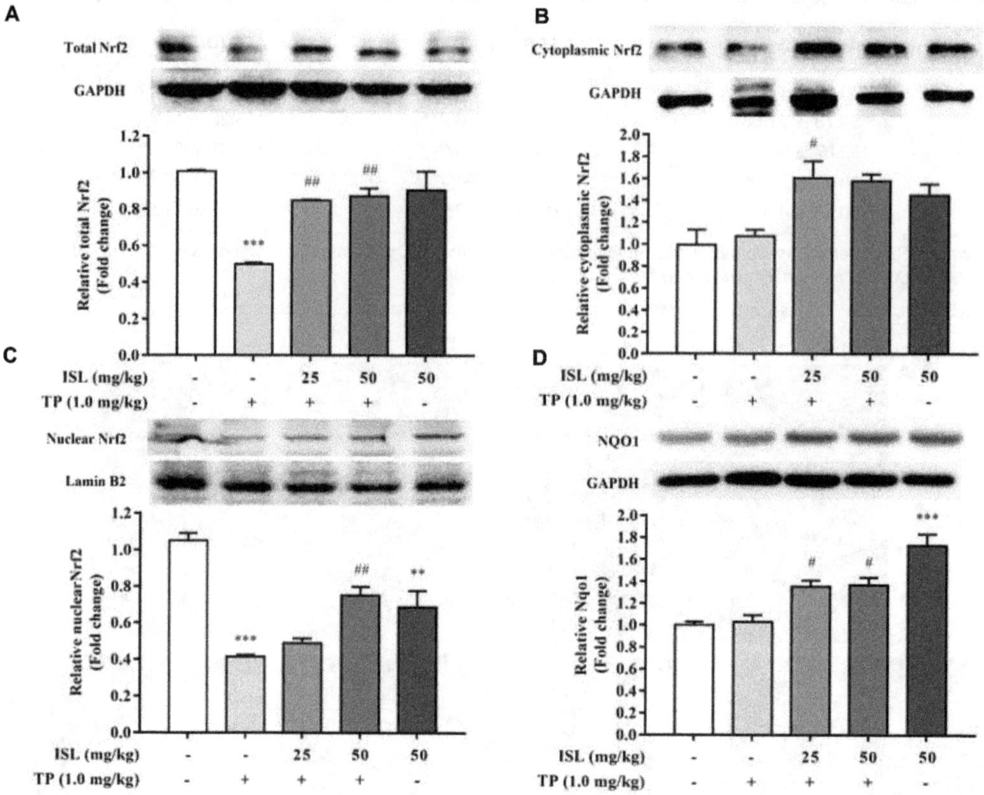

FIGURE 5 | Effects of TP, ISL, or ISL + TP on protein levels of **(A)** total, **(B)** cytoplasmic, and **(C)** nuclear Nrf2 and **(D)** Nqo1 in mouse livers. Cell lysates were analyzed by Western blot. Data were presented as means ± *SE* (*n* = 5); $^{**}P < 0.01$ vs. the control group, $^{***}P < 0.001$ vs. the control group, $^{\#}P < 0.05$ vs. the TP group, and $^{\#\#}P < 0.01$ vs. the TP group.

PBS twice before adding MTT to each well. To determine the protective effect of ISL on TP-induced cell death, the cells were preincubated with ISL, then ISL was removed and TP was added. Hence, ISL had no direct contact with MTT during the whole study, so it did not influence the results of the MTT assay.

Alanine aminotransferase is mainly distributed in the liver, whose increase is a sensitive marker of acute liver injury. AST is mainly distributed in the heart and followed by the liver. Obviously bigger increase in the AST than in the ALT is observed in the following conditions:

(1) When cardiomyocyte injuries appear, such as TP-induced cardiotoxicity (Yang et al., 2016).
(2) When prejaundill occurs. Clinical symptoms of TP-induced liver injuries include jaundice (Xue et al., 2009), and Zhang et al. (2018) found that *tripterygium wilfordii* significantly increased the total bilirubin in rat serum, which may be related to the changes in transporter expressions.
(3) When the mitochondria are injured, a large amount of AST may leak into the serum, so the big increase in the AST may be a sign of serious liver injury.

In addition, the serum level of LDH is a sign of cell necrosis or apoptosis, during which LDH may leak out from the cells since the membrane is broken (Zhou and Ho, 2014). The serum activities of LDH were not reduced after the combined ISL treatment compared with those of the TP-injured group, and it was not obviously increased, suggesting the cytotoxic effect of ISL. However, LDH is widely distributed in all organs, so increase in the serum LDH levels does not necessarily mean ISL induced liver injuries; it is possible that ISL may have side effect on other organs. Unfortunately, there are very few toxicological evaluations reported on ISL. Mahalingam et al. (2016) proved that ISL inhibited the growth of antral follicle and sex steroid synthesis in adult mouse ovaries. Several studies investigated the anticancer effect of ISL and showed that ISL could kill cancer cells by inducing the apoptotic pathways or disturbance of redox status (Sun et al., 2013; Zhou and Ho, 2014). It was reported that the decreased ROS caused by ISL might lead to redox imbalance and reductive stress. To adapt to this state, Nrf2 could be significantly decreased. Thus, ISL may induce the oxidative stress by disturbing the redox status (Sun et al., 2013). That may be the reason why low-dose ISL did not induce nuclear Nrf2 in L02 cells and why the serum levels of LDH was not reduced compared with those of the TP-injured group with ISL combined treatment. Further studies are needed to verify the target-organ toxicity or side effects (Peng et al., 2015). Anyway, the hepatoprotective effect of ISL is definite and outstanding (Kuang et al., 2017), and the levels of ALT and AST, the two sensitive markers of acute liver injuries, are significantly reversed

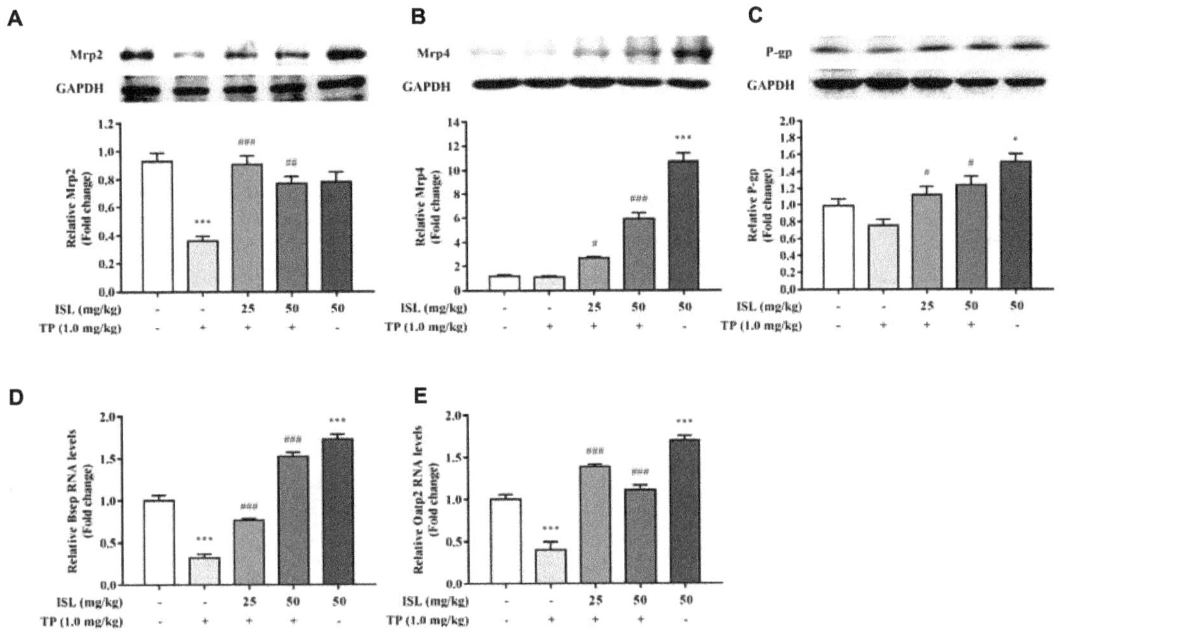

FIGURE 6 | Effects of TP, ISL, or ISL + TP on the protein levels of **(A)** MRP2, **(B)** MRP4, and **(C)** P-gp and the mRNA levels of **(D)** Bsep and **(E)** Oatp2 in mouse livers. Cell lysates were analyzed by Western blot and mRNAs by RT-PCR. Data were presented as means ± *SE* ($n = 5$); $^{*}P < 0.05$ vs. the control group,$^{***}P < 0.001$ vs. the control group, $^{\#}P < 0.05$ vs. the TP group, and $^{\#\#\#}P < 0.001$ vs. the TP group.

by ISL combined treatment, implying the hepatoprotective effect of ISL.

We try to explain the mechanisms behind it. Our previous studies have explored the total Nrf2 expression levels in HepG2 cells and mouse livers after TP and ISL treatment (Cao et al., 2016a,b), while as a nuclear transcription factor, Nrf2 was translocated into the nucleus to activate the target protective gene transcription (Suzuki et al., 2013). The present study determined the total, cytoplasmic, and nuclear Nrf2 protein levels as well as its downstream antioxidant NQO1, which is regarded as a prototypical Nrf2-target gene whose induction implies the activation of a host of other Nrf2-regulated cytoprotective genes (Yates et al., 2007). Our results showed that compared with the TP-injured group, ISL pretreatment significantly enhanced the total and nuclear Nrf2 as well as NQO1 expressions *in vitro* and *in vivo*, indicating that Nrf2 is more stabilized with ISL combined treatment, accumulated into the nucleus, and has activated its target protective genes. The increased expression of cytoplasmic Nrf2 is not statistically significant. Since Nrf2 is translocated into the nucleus and plays a protective role, the increased nuclear translocation of Nrf2 may lead to a relative decrease in the cytoplasmic Nrf2 expression level. When Nrf2 was knocked down by siRNA, TP-induced cytotoxicity in the L02 cells was enhanced, and the protective effect of ISL was diminished, further proving the role of Nrf2 in TP-induced hepatotoxicity and the protective effect of ISL. However, the Nrf2 influence was relatively low. **Figure 2G** shows that in the control group, ISL pretreatment improved the cell viability by 8.8% compared with that of the TP-injured group, while the cell viability in the Nrf2-siRNA group improved by 2.8%. Although ISL pretreatment still had some recovering effect on the cell viabilities after Nrf2-siRNA transfections, this protection diminished a lot. The remaining protective effect may be due to other nuclear factors and non-Nrf2-regulated transporters. Our present study also investigated the role of P-gp and OATPs in the protective effect of ISL on TP-induced hepatotoxicity. P-gp exports TP from the hepatocytes, and OATPs import BAs into the hepatocytes. Alterations of these two transporter expressions by ISL lead to low concentrations of TP and BAs in the liver, which is also an efficient way to alleviate TP-induced hepatotoxicity. Besides, increased nuclear Nrf2 level in the TP-injured group *in vitro* is an adaptive activation to alleviate or delay the TP-induced injury, since it was unable to completely eliminate the toxicity which was related to the time or dosage of TP treatment (Li J. et al., 2014; Xi et al., 2017; Zhou et al., 2017).

Considering that Nrf2 is the primary player in the inducible cell defense system, much interest is shown in identifying and developing Nrf2 activators for therapeutic use (Suzuki et al., 2013). Some of the most promising Nrf2 inducers include SFN, oltipraz, BHA, natural triterpenoid oleanolic acid, and synthetic triterpenoids (CDDO, CDDO-Me, and CDDO-Im), all of which have been shown to be able to protect the liver in different models of oxidative and electrophilic stress by activating the Nrf2 expressions (Klaassen and Reisman, 2010). As a flavonoid contains multiple phenolic hydroxyl groups, ISL also shows great antioxidant effect (Chin et al., 2007). Our previous studies show that ISL is the most potent ARE-luciferase inducer among the four main components of licorice, and it may increase the Nrf2 protein level and nuclear accumulation. Park et al. (2016) have also proved that ISL can function as a hepatic protectant

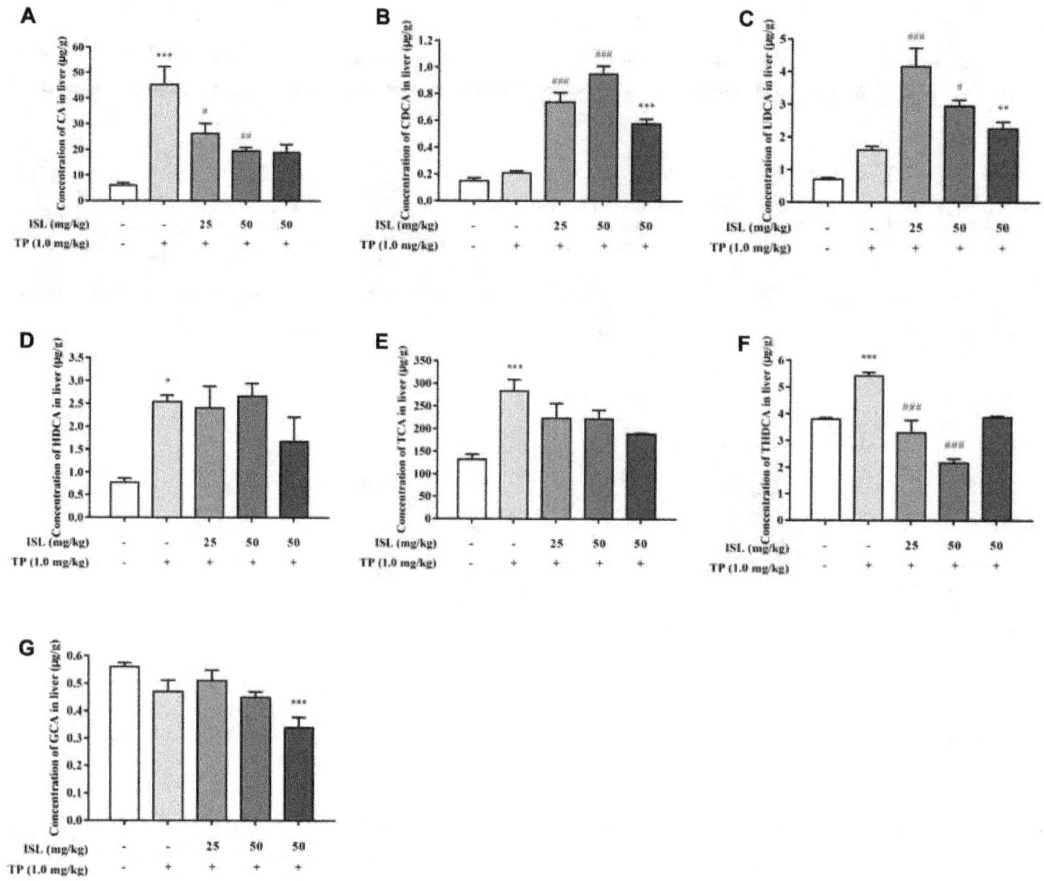

FIGURE 7 | Effects of TP, ISL, or ISL + TP on the hepatic bile acid (BA) profiles. Significant changes of hepatic concentration after TP or ISL administration were found in **(A)** CA, **(B)** CDCA, **(C)** UDCA, **(D)** HDCA, **(E)** TCA, **(F)** THDCA and **(G)** GCA. Concentrations of 16 BAs in mouse livers were quantified by liquid chromatography-tandem mass spectrometry. Data were presented as means ± SE (n = 4–6); $^{*}P < 0.05$ vs. the control group, $^{**}P < 0.01$ vs. the control group, $^{***}P < 0.001$ vs. the control group, $^{\#}P < 0.05$ vs. the TP group, $^{\#\#}P < 0.01$ vs. the TP group, and $^{\#\#\#}P < 0.001$ vs. the TP group.

by inducing the antioxidant genes through extracellular signal-regulated kinase-mediated Nrf2 pathway both *in vitro* and *in vivo*. Therefore, ISL may be a novel Nrf2-activating drug with hepatoprotective effect, but the molecular mechanisms through which ISL counteracts with Nrf2 need further clarification. In the present study, induction of nuclear Nrf2 by ISL does not imply oxidative stress; in contrast, it implies antioxidant effects on TP-induced hepatotoxicity. Moreover, the reduction of ROS and induction of GSH in our preliminary study also proved its protective effect (Cao et al., 2016a). Clearly, duration of exposure and dose selection are critical parameters to assess safe levels of TP and ISL. Further studies are needed to conduct an ISL risk assessment by evaluating three main data sets: animal toxicology data, human intervention studies, and published case reports and publicly available adverse event reports, to get the optimal exposure time and dose and to prevent the adverse effect of ISL (Yates et al., 2017). As a key regulator of detoxification and BA metabolism, Nrf2 induces a series of hepatic efflux transporters that aid in the elimination of potentially harmful endo- and xenobiotics (Klaassen and Reisman, 2010; Zhang et al., 2017). Since TP-induced hepatotxicity is correlated with its hepatic exposure and BA accumulation which may lead to cholestatic symptoms (Kong et al., 2015; Jiang et al., 2016; Yang et al., 2017), and licorice and its main constitutes have been proved to induce the expressions of an array of Nrf2 downstream transporters and inhibit chelostasis (Wang X. et al., 2013; Gong et al., 2015), we measured changes in the expression of hepatic transporters after TP and ISL treatment. TP treatment reduced the expressions of MRP2 *in vitro* and *in vivo*, while ISL combined treatment reversed this effect. MRP2 is an Nrf2 downstream transporter that locates in the canalicular membrane and exports many substrates including multiple drugs and its phase II conjugates as well as BAs (Csanaky et al., 2009; Klaassen and Reisman, 2010). It plays a major role in the formation of BA-independent bile flow, which is important for excretion of endobiotic and xenobiotic toxins (Klaassen and Aleksunes, 2010; Nicolaou et al., 2012). Hence, alterations in the expression of MRP2 may get involved in TP-induced hepatotoxicity and ISL-induced protective effect, resulting in changes in the hepatic accumulation of potential toxins. Compared with the TP-injured group, ISL combined treatment also increased the protein level of MRP4, a transporter that exports BAs and drugs/metabolites

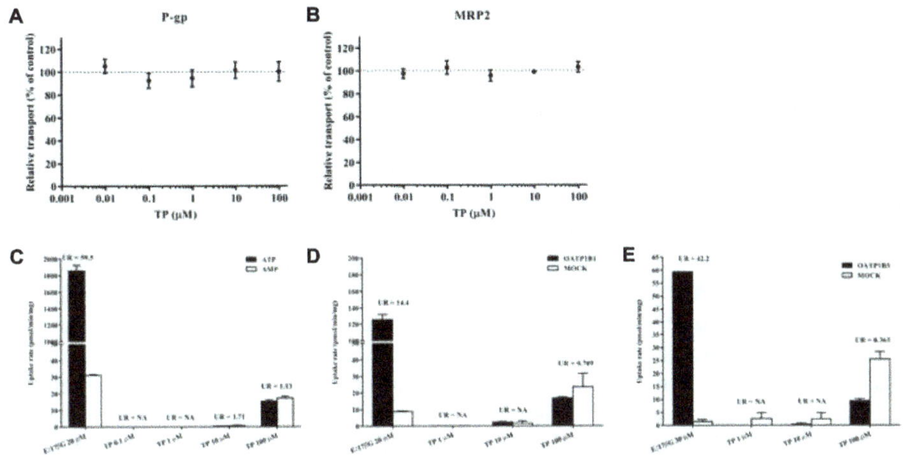

FIGURE 8 | *In vitro* transport assay to determine the interaction between TP and hepatic transporters. **(A,B)** Effects of TP on P-gp and MRP2-mediated transports in the vesicular transport (VT) assay. TP was incubated with relative membrane vesicles and substrates at 37°C for 10 min. N-methyl quinidine was used as the positive control. The ATP-dependent transport in the absence of TP was set as 100%. **(C–E)** Uptake of TP by MRP2 in the VT assay as well as OATP1B1 and OATP1B3 in human embryonic kidney 293 cells. Membrane vesicles or cells were incubated with TP at 37°C for 10 min. $E_2 17\beta G$ was used as the positive control. Uptake ratio (UR) in the MRP2 vesicles was calculated by the transport activity in the presence of ATP dividing that in the presence of AMP. UR in the OATP-expressing cells was calculated by the transport activity in OATP-expressing cells dividing that in the control cells. Data were presented as means ± *SE* (*n* = 3).

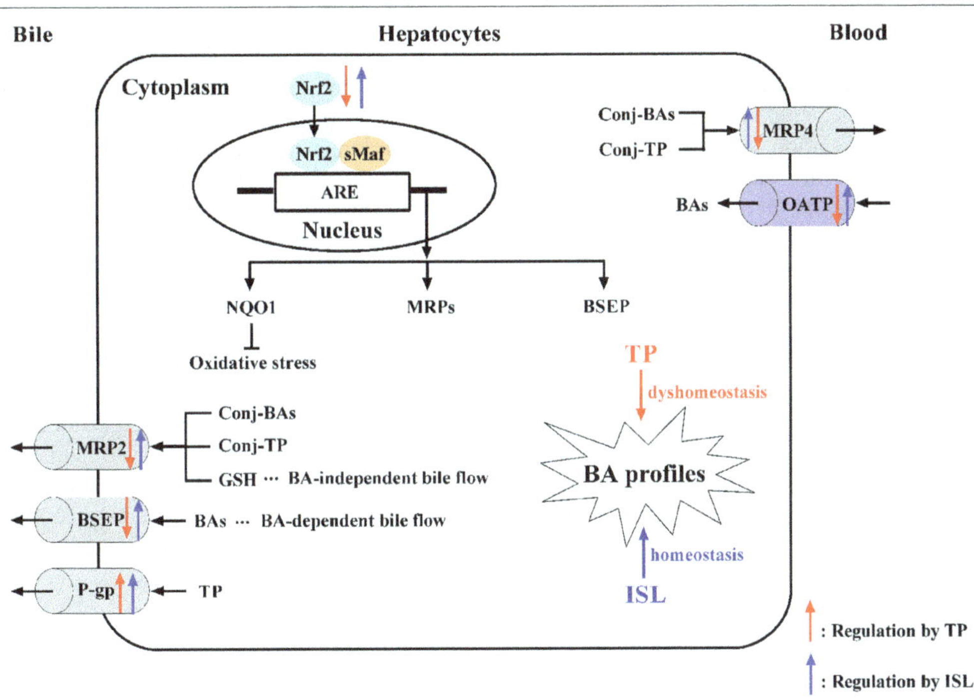

FIGURE 9 | The proposed mechanism of TP-induced hepatotoxicity and ISL combined treatment protecting against TP-induced liver injury. ARE, antioxidant responsive element; BA, bile acid; BSEP, bile salt export pump; conj, conjugated; GSH, reduced glutathione; ISL, isoliquiritigenin; MRP, multidrug resistance protein; NQO1, NAD(P)H: quinine oxidoreductase 1; Nrf2, nuclear transcription factor E2-related factor 2; OATP, organic anion transporting polypeptide; P-gp, P-glycoprotein; sMaf, small Maf proteins; TP, triptolide.

across the hepatic basolateral membranes, resulting in a further elimination of toxins from the liver (Hillgren et al., 2013). In addition, decrease in MRP4 expression level in L02 cells in the TP-injured group was not statistically significant, which might be the result of a compensatory role of MRP4 when MRP2 was impaired (Hillgren et al., 2013). Notably, pretreatment with tBHQ, an Nrf2 inducer, did not increase the MRP4 protein level *in vitro*, which may be attributed to the fact that besides Nrf2, many other nuclear factors are also involved in the regulation of MRP4 expressions, especially the CAR as a key regulator (Zollner et al., 2010). Considering that the Nrf2-regulated Bsep mediates the rate-limiting step of BA transport across hepatocytes (Nicolaou et al., 2012; Hillgren et al., 2013), we also measured the expression of Bsep *in vivo*. TP administration reduced the Bsep mRNA levels, implying a disruption of BA homeostasis, while combined ISL treatment improved the Bsep mRNA levels and led to a protective effect. In addition, since TP is a substrate of P-gp (Zhuang et al., 2013), the protein level of P-gp has also been measured, showing that ISL combined treatment induced P-gp expressions, which may help eliminate TP from the liver into the bile. Apart from the hepatic efflux transporters, we also detected the mRNA level of mouse Oatp2, a hepatic influx transporter with a broad substrate specificity, involved in the enterohepatic recycling of BAs (Obaidat et al., 2012). We found that TP administration reduced Oatp2 expression while ISL combined treatment induced it, suggesting a role of Oatp2 in TP-induced hepatotoxicity and the protective effect of ISL.

Given the alterations in the expressions of hepatic transporters and the reported results that TP administration increased TBA accumulation in rat livers (Jiang et al., 2016; Yang et al., 2017), we further validated whether changes in the expressions of transporters have any effect on hepatic BA accumulation by analyzing the profile of individual BAs in mouse livers with our previously established LC-MS/MS method. The results showed that TP induced 4 out of the 16 BAs, which may result in a cholestatic phenotype, while ISL combined treatment decreased the hepatic accumulation of CA and THDCA, which relieved TP-induced BA disorder. What is more, ISL combined treatment increased the hepatic concentration of CDCA and UDCA. Increase in UDCA might be cytoprotective by lowering the intracellular TCDCA, which is thought to be cytotoxic due to its hydrophilic nature (Guo et al., 2016). It has been reported that CDCA and UDCA can alleviate 17α-ethinylestradiol-induced cholestasis in rats, and UDCA can stimulate biliary secretion, upregulate the expression of Bsep and Mrp2, and stabilize Bsep protein in the apical membrane (Li et al., 2016). Hence, the increase in CDCA and UDCA levels induced by ISL may also have a protective effect on the TP-induced liver injury. The proposed mechanism is shown in **Figure 9**.

Above we have validated that TP and ISL treatment changed the expression of hepatic transporters. Since changes in transporter activities may also contribute to various drug and BA exposure and response, we tried to determine whether TP inhibited the activities of human P-gp and MRP2, or whether TP interacted with them. The reason for choosing these two transporters is that P-gp exports TP, and MRP2 has a wide range of substrates and its expression is inhibited by TP, so inhibition of P-gp and MRP2 transport may lead to the accumulation of TP or other substrates and finally result in hepatotoxicity. The VT assay utilizing inverted membrane vesicles enables direct interaction of a transporter with the compounds added to the reaction buffer. Therefore, it is a high-throughput *in vitro* method to identify the substrates, inhibitors, or modulators of transporters (Kidron et al., 2012), and can also avoid the compensatory effects between transporters. Our results showed that TP was not an inhibitor of P-gp or MRP2, suggesting that the effect of TP on transporters is at transcription levels, which is usually more powerful than that at functional levels (Kong et al., 2015).

Furthermore, we explored whether TP could be transported by several hepatic transporters and contribute to the hepatic TP accumulation. We found that TP was not a substrate of MRP2, OATP1B1, or OATP1B3, suggesting that these transporters mainly contributed to the hepatic accumulation of BAs but not TP. Besides, phase II metabolites of TP rather than the parent drug may be transported by MRP2, which may also contribute to the TP-induced hepatotoxicity.

CONCLUSION

Nrf2 and hepatic influx and efflux transporters play important roles in TP-induced hepatotoxicity and ISL-induced protective effect by modulating the hepatic BA profiles as well as the accumulation of TP and its metabolites. We also confirm that TP is not the substrate of MRP2, OATP1B1, or OATP1B3, nor does it inhibit the transport activity of MRP2 or P-gp, thus shedding new lights on TP-related drug–drug interactions as well as the mechanisms of TP-induced hepatotoxicity.

AUTHOR CONTRIBUTIONS

ZH, BZ, and MY designed the experiments. ZH, LeC, PF, HC, HT, and YP conducted the experiments. ZH, LeC, YD, and LiC analyzed the data. ZH, BZ, and MY wrote the paper. HL proposed the research idea. All authors contributed to the editing of the paper and to scientific discussions.

FUNDING

This work was supported by the National Natural Science Foundation of China (Grant Nos. 81573686 and 81473411).

REFERENCES

Cao, L., Li, H., Yan, M., Li, Z., Gong, H., Jiang, P., et al. (2016a). The protective effects of isoliquiritigenin and glycyrrhetinic acid against triptolide-induced oxidative stress in HepG2 cells involve Nrf2 activation. *Evid. Based Complement. Alternat. Med.* 2016:8912184. doi: 10.1155/2016/8912184

Cao, L., Yan, M., Ma, Y., Zhang, B., Fang, P., Xiang, D., et al. (2016b). Isoliquiritigenin protects against triptolide-induced hepatotoxicity in mice through Nrf2 activation. *Pharmazie* 71, 394–397. doi: 10.1691/ph.2016.6535

Chin, Y. W., Jung, H. A., Liu, Y., Su, B. N., Castoro, J. A., Keller, W. J., et al. (2007). Anti-oxidant constituents of the roots and stolons of licorice (*Glycyrrhiza glabra*). *J. Agric. Food Chem.* 55, 4691–4697. doi: 10.1021/jf0703553

Corsini, A., and Bortolini, M. (2013). Drug-induced liver injury: the role of drug metabolism and transport. *J. Clin. Pharmacol.* 53, 463–474. doi: 10.1002/jcph.23

Csanaky, I. L., Aleksunes, L. M., Tanaka, Y., and Klaassen, C. D. (2009). Role of hepatic transporters in prevention of bile acid toxicity after partial hepatectomy in mice. *Am. J. Physiol. Gastrointest. Liver Physiol.* 297, G419–G433. doi: 10.1152/ajpgi.90728.2008

Deng, Y., Zhang, B., Yan, M., Gong, H., Liu, S., Fang, P., et al. (2015). Determination of 16 bile acids in Nrf2 wild-type and knockout mice liver by using LC-MS/MS method. *Chin. Hosp. Pharm. J.* 35, 283–288.

Gong, H., Zhang, B., Yan, M., Fang, P., Li, H., Hu, C., et al. (2015). A protective mechanism of licorice (*Glycyrrhiza uralensis*): isoliquiritigenin stimulates detoxification system via Nrf2 activation. *J. Ethnopharmacol.* 162, 134–139. doi: 10.1016/j.jep.2014.12.043

Guo, Y., Zhang, Y., Huang, W., Selwyn, F. P., and Klaassen, C. D. (2016). Dose-response effect of berberine on bile acid profile and gut microbiota in mice. *BMC Complement. Altern. Med.* 16:394. doi: 10.1186/s12906-016-1367-7

Hillgren, K. M., Keppler, D., Zur, A. A., Giacomini, K. M., Stieger, B., Cass, C. E., et al. (2013). Emerging transporters of clinical importance: an update from the international transporter consortium. *Clin. Pharmacol. Ther.* 94, 52–63. doi: 10.1038/clpt.2013.74

Jiang, Z., Huang, X., Huang, S., Guo, H., Wang, L., Li, X., et al. (2016). Sex-related differences of lipid metabolism induced by triptolide: the possible role of the LXRα/SREBP-1 signaling pathway. *Front. Pharmacol.* 7:87. doi: 10.3389/fphar.2016.00087

Jin, J., Sun, X., Zhao, Z., Wang, W., Qiu, Y., Fu, X., et al. (2015). Activation of the farnesoid X receptor attenuates triptolide-induced liver toxicity. *Phytomedicine* 22, 894–901. doi: 10.1016/j.phymed.2015.06.007

Kamisako, T., Tanaka, Y., Kishino, Y., Ikeda, T., Yamamoto, K., Masuda, S., et al. (2014). Role of Nrf2 in the alteration of cholesterol and bile acid metabolism-related gene expression by dietary cholesterol in high fat-fed mice. *J. Clin. Biochem. Nutr.* 54, 90–94. doi: 10.3164/jcbn.13-92

Kidron, H., Wissel, G., Manevski, N., Häkli, M., Ketola, R. A., Finel, M., et al. (2012). Impact of probe compound in MRP2 vesicular transport assays. *Eur. J. Pharm. Sci.* 46, 100–105. doi: 10.1016/j.ejps.2012.02.016

Klaassen, C. D., and Aleksunes, L. M. (2010). Xenobiotic, bile acid, and cholesterol transporters: function and regulation. *J. Pharmacol. Exp. Ther.* 62, 1–96. doi: 10.1124/pr.109.002014

Klaassen, C. D., and Reisman, S. A. (2010). Nrf2 the rescue: effects of the antioxidative/electrophilic response on the liver. *Toxicol. Appl. Pharmacol.* 244, 57–65. doi: 10.1016/j.taap.2010.01.013

Kong, L., Zhuang, X., Yang, H., Yuan, M., Xu, L., and Li, H. (2015). Inhibition of P-glycoprotein gene expression and function enhances triptolide-induced hepatotoxicity in mice. *Sci. Rep.* 5:11747. doi: 10.1038/srep11747

Kuang, Y., Lin, Y., Li, K., Song, W., Ji, S., Qiao, X., et al. (2017). Screening of hepatoprotective compounds from licorice against carbon tetrachloride and acetaminophen induced HepG2 cells injury. *Phytomedicine* 34, 59–66. doi: 10.1016/j.phymed.2017.08.005

Le Vee, M., Jouan, E., Stieger, B., and Fardel, O. (2013). Differential regulation of drug transporter expression by all-trans retinoic acid in hepatoma HepaRG cells and human hepatocytes. *Eur. J. Pharm. Sci.* 48, 767–774. doi: 10.1016/j.ejps.2013.01.005

Li, J., Shen, F., Guan, C., Wang, W., and Sun, X. (2014). Activation of Nrf2 protects against triptolide-induced hepatotoxicity. *PLoS One* 9:e100685. doi: 10.1371/journal.pone.0100685

Li, X., Jiang, Z., and Zhang, L. (2014). Triptolide: progress on research in pharmacodynamics and toxicology. *J. Ethnopharmacol.* 155, 67–79. doi: 10.1016/j.jep.2014.06.006

Li, X., Yuan, Z., Liu, R., Hassan, H. M., Yang, H., Sun, R., et al. (2016). UDCA and CDCA alleviate 17α-ethinylestradiol-induced cholestasis through PKA-AMPK pathways in rats. *Toxicol. Appl. Pharmacol.* 311, 12–25. doi: 10.1016/j.taap.2016.10.011

Liu, J., Zhou, X., Chen, X. Y., and Zhong, D. F. (2014). Excretion of [3H]triptolide and its metabolites in rats after oral administration. *Acta Pharmacol. Sin.* 35, 549–554. doi: 10.1038/aps.2013.192

Liu, Q. (2011). Triptolide and its expanding multiple pharmacological functions. *Int. Immunopharmacol.* 11, 377–383. doi: 10.1016/j.intimp.2011.01.012

Mahalingam, S., Gao, L. Y., Eisner, J., Helferich, W., and Flaws, J. A. (2016). Effects of isoliquiritigenin on ovarian antral follicle growth and steroidogenesis. *Reprod. Toxicol.* 66, 107–114. doi: 10.1016/j.reprotox.2016.10.004

Nicolaou, M., Andress, E. J., Zolnerciks, J. K., Dixon, P. H., Williamson, C., and Linton, K. J. (2012). Canalicular ABC transporters and liver disease. *J. Pathol.* 226, 300–315. doi: 10.1002/path.3019

Obaidat, A., Roth, M., and Hagenbuch, B. (2012). The expression and function of organic anion transporting polypeptides in normal tissues and in cancer. *Annu. Rev. Pharmacol. Toxicol.* 52, 135–151. doi: 10.1146/annurev-pharmtox-010510-100556

Park, S. M., Lee, J. R., Ku, S. K., Cho, I. J., Byun, S. H., Kim, S. C., et al. (2016). Isoliquiritigenin in licorice functions as a hepatic protectant by induction of antioxidant genes through extracellular signal-regulated kinase-mediated NF-E2-related factor-2 signaling pathway. *Eur. J. Nutr.* 55, 2431–2444. doi: 10.1007/s00394-015-1051-6

Peng, F., Du, Q. H., Peng, C., Wang, N., Tang, H. L., Xie, X. M., et al. (2015). A review: the pharmacology of isoliquiritigenin. *Phytother. Res.* 29, 969–977. doi: 10.1002/ptr.5348

Pfeifer, N. D., Hardwick, R. N., and Brouwer, K. L. R. (2014). Role of hepatic efflux transporters in regulating systemic and hepatocyte exposure to xenobiotics. *Annu. Rev. Pharmacol. Toxicol.* 54, 509–535. doi: 10.1146/annurev-pharmtox-011613-140021

Sun, C., Zhang, H., Ma, X. F., Zhou, X., Gan, L., Liu, Y. Y., et al. (2013). Isoliquiritigenin enhances radiosensitivity of HepG2 cells via disturbance of redox status. *Cell Biochem. Biophys.* 65, 433–444. doi: 10.1007/s12013-012-9447-x

Suzuki, T., Motohashi, H., and Yamamoto, M. (2013). Toward clinical application of the Keap1–Nrf2 pathway. *Trends Pharmacol. Sci.* 34, 340–346. doi: 10.1016/j.tips.2013.04.005

Wang, B., Ma, L., Tao, X., and Lipsky, P. E. (2004). Triptolide, an active component of the Chinese herbal remedy *Tripterygium wilfordii* Hook F, inhibits production of nitric oxide by decreasing inducible nitric oxide synthase gene transcription. *Arthritis Rheum.* 50, 2995–3003. doi: 10.1002/art.20459

Wang, J., Jiang, Z., Ji, J., Wang, X., Wang, T., Zhang, Y., et al. (2013). Gene expression profiling and pathway analysis of hepatotoxicity induced by triptolide in Wistar rats. *Food Chem. Toxicol.* 58, 495–505. doi: 10.1016/j.fct.2013.04.039

Wang, X., Zhang, H., Chen, L., Shan, L., Fan, G., and Gao, X. (2013). Liquorice, a unique "guide drug" of traditional Chinese medicine: a review of its role in drug interactions. *J. Ethnopharmacol.* 150, 781–790. doi: 10.1016/j.jep.2013.09.055

Weerachayaphorn, J., Mennone, A., Soroka, C. J., Harry, K., Hagey, L. R., Kensler, T. W., et al. (2012). Nuclear factor-E2-related factor 2 is a major determinant of bile acid homeostasis in the liver and intestine. *Am. J. Physiol. Gastrointest. Liver Physiol.* 302, G925–G936. doi: 10.1152/ajpgi.00263.2011

Xi, C., Peng, S., Wu, Z., Zhou, Q., and Zhou, J. (2017). Toxicity of triptolide and the molecular mechanisms involved. *Biomed. Pharmacother.* 90, 531–541. doi: 10.1016/j.biopha.2017.04.003

Xu, L., Qiu, Y., Xu, H., Ao, W., Lam, W., and Yang, X. (2013). Acute and subacute toxicity studies on triptolide and triptolide-loaded polymeric micelles following intravenous administration in rodents. *Food Chem. Toxicol.* 57, 371–379. doi: 10.1016/j.fct.2013.03.044

Xue, J., Jia, X. B., Tan, X. B., and Hao, K. (2009). Study on hepatotoxicity induced by *Tripterygium wilfordii* and its thoughts of assessment based on ADME/Tox. *Chin. Tradit. Herb. Drugs* 40, 655–658.

Xue, X., Gong, L., Qi, X., Wu, Y., Xing, G., Yao, J., et al. (2011). Knockout of hepatic P450 reductase aggravates triptolide-induced toxicity. *Toxicol. Lett.* 205, 47–54. doi: 10.1016/j.toxlet.2011.05.003

Yang, J., Sun, L., Wang, L., Hassan, H. M., Wang, X., Hylemon, P. B., et al. (2017). Activation of Sirt1/FXR signaling pathway attenuates triptolide-induced hepatotoxicity in rats. *Front. Pharmacol.* 8:260. doi: 10.3389/fphar.2017.00260

Yang, Y. Q., Wang, W. W., Xiong, Z. W., Kong, J. M., Qiu, Y. W., Shen, F. H., et al. (2016). Activation of SIRT3 attenuates triptolide-induced toxicity through closing mitochondrial permeability transition pore in cardiomyocytes. *Toxicol. In Vitro* 34, 128–137. doi: 10.1016/j.tiv.2016.03.020

Yates, A. A., Erdman, J. W., Shao, A., Dolan, L. C., and Griffiths, J. C. (2017). Bioactive nutrients - Time for tolerable upper intake levels to address safety. *Regul. Toxicol. Pharmacol.* 84, 94–101. doi: 10.1016/j.yrtph.2017.01.002

Yates, M. S., Tauchi, M., Katsuoka, F., Flanders, K. C., Liby, K. T., Honda, T., et al. (2007). Pharmacodynamic characterization of chemopreventive triterpenoids as exceptionally potent inducers of Nrf2-regulated genes. *Mol. Cancer Ther.* 6, 154–162. doi: 10.1158/1535-7163.MCT-06-0516

Zhang, Q. C., Li, Y. Q., Liu, M. Z., Duan, J., Zhou, X. P., and Zhu, H. X. (2018). Compatibility with *Panax notoginseng* and *Rehmannia glutinosa* alleviates the hepatotoxicity and nephrotoxicity of *Tripterygium wilfordii* via modulating the pharmacokinetics of triptolide. *Int. J. Mol. Sci.* 19:E305. doi: 10.3390/ijms19010305

Zhang, W., Chen, L., Feng, H., Wang, W., Cai, Y., Qi, F., et al. (2017). Rifampicin-induced injury in HepG2 cells is alleviated by TUDCA via increasing bile acid transporters expression and enhancing the Nrf2-mediated adaptive response. *Free Radic. Biol. Med.* 112, 24–35. doi: 10.1016/j.freeradbiomed.2017.07.003

Zhou, L., Zhou, C., Liang, X., Feng, Z., Liu, Z., Wang, H., et al. (2017). Self-protection against triptolide-induced toxicity in human hepatic cells via Nrf2-ARE-NQO1 pathway. *Chin. J. Integr. Med.* 23, 929–936. doi: 10.1007/s11655-017-2546-6

Zhou, Y. L., and Ho, W. S. (2014). Combination of liquiritin, isoliquiritin and isoliquirigenin induce apoptotic cell death through upregulating p53 and p21 in the A549 non-small cell lung cancer cells. *Oncol. Rep.* 31, 298–304. doi: 10.3892/or.2013.2849

Zhuang, X. M., Shen, G. L., Xiao, W. B., Tan, Y., Lu, C., and Li, H. (2013). Assessment of the roles of P-glycoprotein and cytochrome P450 in triptolide-induced liver toxicity in sandwich-cultured rat hepatocyte model. *Drug Metab. Dispos.* 41, 2158–2165. doi: 10.1124/dmd.113.054056

Zollner, G., Wagner, M., and Trauner, M. (2010). Nuclear receptors as drug targets in cholestasis and drug-induced hepatotoxicity. *Pharmacol. Ther.* 126, 228–243. doi: 10.1016/j.pharmthera.2010.03.005

15

Phospholipase Cγ2 Signaling Cascade Contribute to the Antiplatelet Effect of Notoginsenoside Fc

*Yingqiu Liu[1], Tianyi Liu[2], Kevin Ding[3], Zengyuan Liu[1], Yuanyuan Li[1], Taotao He[1], Weimin Zhang[1], Yunpeng Fan[1], Wuren Ma[1], Li Cui[4] and Xiaoping Song[1]**

[1] Laboratory of Traditional Chinese Veterinary Medicine, College of Veterinary Medicine, Northwest A&F University, Yangling, China, [2] Department of Neurosurgery, The First Hospital of Jilin University, Changchun, China, [3] University of Illinois at Urbana–Champaign, Urbana, IL, United States, [4] Department of Neurosciences, University of California, San Diego School of Medicine, La Jolla, CA, United States

***Correspondence:**
Xiaoping Song
sxpxbnl@163.com

Scope: Bleeding, the main drawback of clinically used chemical anti-thrombotic drug is resulted from the unidirectional suppression of platelet activity. Therefore, dual-directional regulatory effect on platelet is the main preponderance of *Panax notoginseng* over these drugs. The dual-directional regulatory effect should be ascribed to the resourceful *Panax notoginseng* saponins (PNS). Clarifying the mechanism of main PNS in both inhibiting and promoting platelet aggregation will give a full outlook for the dual-directional regulatory effect. The present study is aimed at explaining the mechanism of Notoginsenoside Fc (Fc), a main PNS, in inhibiting platelet aggregation.

Methods: In the *in vitro* study, after incubating platelets with Fc and m-3M3FBS, platelet aggregation was triggered by thrombin, collagen or ADP. Platelet aggregation was measured by aggregometer. Phospholipase Cγ2 (PLCγ2) and protein kinase C (PKC) activities were studied by western blotting. Diacylglycerol (DAG), thromboxane B_2 (TXB_2) and 1,4,5-inositol trisphosphate (IP_3) concentrations were measured by corresponding ELISA kits. Calcium concentrations ($[Ca^{2+}]$) were estimated through the fluorescence intensity emitted from Fluo-4. In the *in vivo* study, thrombus model was induced by $FeCl_3$. The effect of Fc on thrombosis was evaluated by measurement of protein content and observation of injured blood vessel.

Results: thrombin, collagen and ADP induced platelet aggregation were all suppressed by incubating platelets with Fc. Platelet PLCγ2 and subsequent DAG-PKC-TXA_2 and IP_3 were down-regulated by Fc as well. However, the basal $[Ca^{2+}]$ in platelet was not altered by Fc. Nevertheless, thrombin triggered activation of PLCγ2 and subsequent DAG-PKC-TXA_2 and IP_3-$[Ca^{2+}]$ were all abolished by Fc. Fc also attenuated platelet aggregation and PLCγ2 signaling activation induced by PLC activator, m-3M3FBS. In the *in vivo* study, $FeCl_3$ induced thrombosis in rat femoral artery was significantly alleviated by administration of Fc.

Conclusion: The results above suggested the antiplatelet and antithrombotic effects of Fc are carried out through oppression of PLCγ2 and subsequent DAG-PKC-TXA_2 and IP_3-[Ca^{2+}]. The present study provided theoretical support for new anti-thrombotic drug exploitation by *Panax notoginseng*.

Keywords: *Panax notoginseng*, Notoginsenoside Fc, platelet aggregation, antiplatelet effect, thrombosis, phospholipase Cγ2

INTRODUCTION

Platelets are cells in mammal blood, formed from the cytoplasm of bone marrow megakaryocytes (Hartwig and Italiano, 2003). They play important role in a serious of physiological and pathological processes, such as hemostasis, inflammation responses and thrombosis. In normal condition, the main function of platelet is hemostasis. But in the pathological conditions, platelet aggregation was excessively triggered by a series of stimulators in the vascular microenvironment, which may result in thrombosis (Ruggeri and Mendolicchio, 2007). Thrombosis, the foremost precipitating factor for cardiovascular disease, threatened a great many people's lives during the past decades. Platelet is the primary target for treatment of thrombotic diseases (Mackman, 2008).

Many antiplatelet drugs have been used in clinic for treatment of thrombotic diseases. The dominating defect for the clinically used chemical antiplatelet drugs is the drawback of bleeding, which result from the unidirectional inhibition of platelet aggregation. During antiplatelet therapy, bleeding threatens people's lives more serious than thrombus itself (Meadows and Bhatt, 2007; Généreux et al., 2015). Although, attempts have been done for discovering new targets and new compounds for antiplatelet drug development, by simply down-regulate platelet aggregation, the defect of bleeding is still ineluctable (Mackman, 2008; Zhang et al., 2015).

Panax notoginseng, a plant mainly produced from Yunnan province of China, has been used as a Traditional Chinese Medicine for 100s of years because of its amazing stasis dispersing and hemostatic effects. Traditionally, the medicinal part of the plant is dried root and rhizome (under-ground part), which called "Sanqi." According to the Traditional Chinese Medicinal theory, thrombosis implies the syndrome of blood stasis. As a result, stasis dispersing and hemostatic drugs are the most appropriate for treatment of thrombosis (Liao, 2000). Sanqi, the best-known stasis dispersing and hemostatic drug, has amazing dual-directional regulatory effect on platelets. Therefore, the distinctive advantage of Sanqi over chemical antiplatelet drugs is removing stasis without bleeding. In addition, Sanqi have a powerful capacity in inhibiting platelet aggregation, which is superior to aspirin (Wang et al., 2016). As a result, Sanqi have good potential to be explored for anti-thrombotic therapy.

However, the price of Sanqi is so high that any drug developed from it would be hardly afforded for most patients. Meanwhile, more than 90% of the over-ground parts of *Panax notoginseng* were abolished, despite the leaves and flowers of *Panax notoginseng* also showed fantastic stasis dispersing and hemostatic effects (Ke et al., 2010). In Yunnan, the over-ground parts of *Panax notoginseng* are more popular for indigenes. The leaves and flowers were made into tea, food and wine. Recent years, since the leaves and flowers of *Panax notoginseng* attracted attentions of researchers, they have been made into nourishment, toothpaste and so on.

Preventive treatment is quite advocated by Traditional Chinese Medicine. It implies preventing disease from occurring and preventing disease from exacerbating (Liang and Yin, 2010). Compared with take drugs, prevent disease by daily food and tea is the easiest way for preventive treatment. Because the price of Sanqi is quite high, utilization of the over-ground part of *Panax notoginseng* instead is a good way for reducing the cost. Pharmacodynamics studies have demonstrated similar functions of *Panax notoginseng* leaves and flowers with Sanqi, including anti-thrombosis, wound healing, anti-hyperlipidemia, anti-depression, anti-inflammation and so on. By drinking *Panax notoginseng* tea made from leaves and flowers, thrombus formation was prevented and the symptoms of thrombotic diseases were relieved a lot. Therefore, food, tea and nourishment made from the leaves and flowers of *Panax notoginseng* will be good resource for thrombotic diseases preventive treatment.

The dual-directional regulatory effect of *Panax notoginseng* on platelets should be ascribed to the resourceful PNS (Wang et al., 2004; Yuan et al., 2011; Gao et al., 2014). Until now, over 70 saponins have been isolated from *Panax notoginseng*. Among them, Fc, Ginsenoside Rg1, Rg2, Rg3, Rh2, Re, and Rd were proved capable in inhibiting platelet aggregation. On the other hand, Ft1, Notoginsenoside Fe and protopanaxadiol are effective in promoting platelet aggregation (Gao et al., 2014). Compared with Sanqi, the leaves and flowers are richer in PNS. Furthermore, the content of most effective antiplatelet compound Fc (**Figure 1**) is the richest in leaves and flowers of *Panax notoginseng*, compared with in roots (Zhou et al., 2017).

Despite the stasis dispersing and hemostatic effect of *Panax notoginseng* is well-known, the mechanism on how the dual-directional regulatory effect been balanced remains to be clarified. Uncovering the molecular mechanisms of main PNS will be quite helpful for clarifying that. Since Fc is the saponin exerts strongest antiplatelet effect among the PNS, the present study

---

Abbreviations: [Ca^{2+}], calcium concentration; DAG, diacylglycerol; Fc, Notoginsenoside Fc; Ft1, notoginsenoside Ft1; IP_3, 1,4,5-inositol trisphosphate; PAR, protease activator receptor; PIP_2, phosphatidylinositol 4,5-bisphosphate; PKC, protein kinase C; PLCγ2, phospholipase Cγ2; PNS, *Panax notoginseng* saponins; TXA_2, thromboxane A_2; TXB_2, thromboxane B_2; WP, washed platelets.

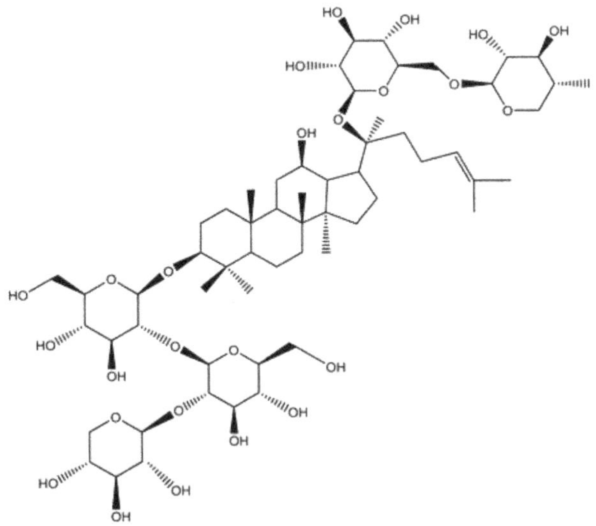

Notoginsenoside Fc

FIGURE 1 | Chemical structure of Notoginsenoside Fc.

aimed at uncovering the mechanism of Fc in inhibiting platelet aggregation.

MATERIALS AND METHODS

Materials

Fc standard was acquired from Shanghai Shifeng Biological Technology CO., LTD. (Shanghai, China). Collagen was purchased from Chrono-log (Havertown, PA, United States). Thrombin, ADP, clopidogrel and m-3M3FBS were obtained from Sigma–Aldrich (St. Louis, MO, United States). Fluo-4 AM indicator was obtained from Invitrogen (Carlsbad, CA, United States). Protease inhibitor and phosphatase inhibitor cocktail tablets were from Roche Diagnostics (Indianapolis, IN, United States). Phospho antibody for PLCγ2, Phospho antibody for PKC substrate and β-actin were purchased from Cell Signaling Technology (Beverly, MA). Immobilon western detection reagents, HRP-conjugated anti-rabbit and anti-mouse IgG were from Genshare Biological (Xi'an, Shaanxi, China). DAG, TXB_2 and IP_3 kits were purchased from R&D Systems (Minneapolis, MN, United States). Pierce™ BCA Protein Assay Kit was from Pierce Biotechnology (Rockford, IL, United States). All the chemicals used were purchased from standard suppliers.

Animals

All animal experiments were approved by the Ethics Committee of Northwest A&F University. Male SD rats (5–6 weeks of age) were purchased from Dossy Experimental Animals CO., LTD. (Xi'an, Shaanxi, China) and acclimated for 1 week before the experiments. The laboratory animal facility was maintained at a constant temperature and humidity with a 12 h light/dark cycle. Food and water were provided *ad libitum*.

Washed Platelets Preparation

The method for WP preparation was the same as before (Liu et al., 2013). Briefly, blood was withdrawn from the abdominal aorta of rats anesthetized with ether. Acid-citrate-dextrose (66.6 mM citric acid, 85 mM trisodium citrate, 111 mM glucose) was used as anticoagulant (Acid-citrate-dextrose: blood = 1: 6). Then, the blood was centrifuged at 150 × *g* for 10 min. After that, the upper layer platelet rich plasma was centrifuged (150 × *g*) for another 10 min and washed once with washing buffer (138 mM NaCl, 2.8 mM KCl, 0.8 mM $MgCl_2$, 0.8 mM Na_2HPO_4, 10 mM HEPES, 0.55 mM glucose, 22 mM trisodium citrate, 0.35% BSA, pH 6.5). Finally, the platelet pellets were suspended in suspension buffer (138 mM NaCl, 2.8 mM KCl, 0.8 mM $MgCl_2$, 0.8 mM Na_2HPO_4, 10 mM HEPES, 5.6 mM glucose, 1 mM $CaCl_2$, 0.3% BSA, pH 7.4) to a final concentration of 2×10^8 platelets/ml.

Platelet Aggregation Study

Platelet aggregation experiments were performed in a LBY-NJ4 platelet aggregometer (Techlink Biomedical). After treated with testing materials, WP aggregation was induced by different stimulators (thrombin, collagen, ADP, or m-3M3FBS). The stimulators were used in the minimal concentrations inducing submaximal aggregation.

Platelet PLCγ2 and PKC Activity Study

The activity of PLCγ2 and PKC were examined by conventional western blot analysis by suitable antibodies. After treatment with testing materials, platelets were precipitated by centrifugation (12,000 × *g*, 2 min). Then platelets were lysed by lysis buffer (50 μM HEPES, 50 μM NaCl, 50 μM sucrose, 1% Triton X-100, protease inhibitor cocktail, and phosphatase inhibitor cocktail). Protein contents were measured by a Pierce™ BCA Protein Assay Kit from Pierce Biotechnology. The lysates were used as western blotting samples. Western blotting experiment procedures were same as everyone known. The activity of PLCγ2 and PKC were assessed by the phosphorylation of PLCγ2 and a 47 kDa protein of PKC substrate, respectively. Because there is no antibody available for measuring the total protein of PLCγ2 and PKC substrate of rats, β-actin was used as internal reference for protein loaded. Result images were obtained and analyzed with ChemiDoc XRS+ system and Image Lab software (Bio-Rad Laboratories, Hercules, CA, United States).

Platelet Calcium Concentration ([Ca^{2+}]) Study

Intracellular [Ca^{2+}] was studied by Fluo-4 AM with a Live Cell Imaging System equipped with TIRF microscope, EMCCD Andor ultra888 and sCMOS Andor zyla4.2Plus (Andor, Belfast, NIR, ENG). Platelets were incubated in washing buffer containing 1 μM Fluo-4 AM and 1% BSA for 30 min. After washing by centrifugation, platelets were suspended in suspension buffer and treated with testing materials. Pictures were taken by the Live Cell Imaging System in a time dependent order. The intracellular [Ca^{2+}] were evaluated by analyzing the fluorescence intensity of the pictures.

Platelet IP_3, DAG and Thromboxane A_2 (TXA_2) Evaluation

The amount of IP_3, DAG and TXA_2 were evaluated by IP_3, DAG and TXB_2 ELISA assay kits from R&D Systems (Minneapolis, MN, United States), respectively. After incubating WP with indicated materials, reaction was stopped in ice bath. IP_3, DAG and TXA_2 content were measured according to the instruction of the test kits.

In vivo Thrombus Study

The method for *in vivo* thrombus study was in accordance with Chinatsu Sakata's study (Sakata et al., 2017). Rats were grouped randomly and i.p. injected with saline, Fc (50 mg/kg) or clopidogrel (5 mg/kg). The *in vivo* anti-thrombotic effect of Fc was evaluated with a $FeCl_3$ arterial thrombosis rat model. Briefly, the rats were anesthetized by i.p. injection of sodium pentobarbital (30 mg/kg). After detach the femoral artery from the surrounding tissues, a filter paper (1 mm × 1 mm) saturated with 20% $FeCl_3$ was applied to the artery for 20 min. The injured artery was isolated, observed and photographed under a LECIA M165FC Stereo Microscope (LECIA, Solms, Hesse, GER). Then, the thrombus was isolated gently and dissolved in NaOH (0.5 M). The size of a thrombus was evaluated by the protein content, which was measured by a BCA protein assay kit (Pierce Biotechnology, Rockford, IL, United States).

Statistical Analyses

Mean and SEM were calculated for all experimental groups. Data were analyzed by One-way Analysis of Variance followed by Dunn's test, to determine the statistically significant differences. Statistical analyses were performed by SigmaStat Software Ver. 3.5 (Systat Software, San Jose, CA, United States). $P < 0.05$ were considered as statistically significant.

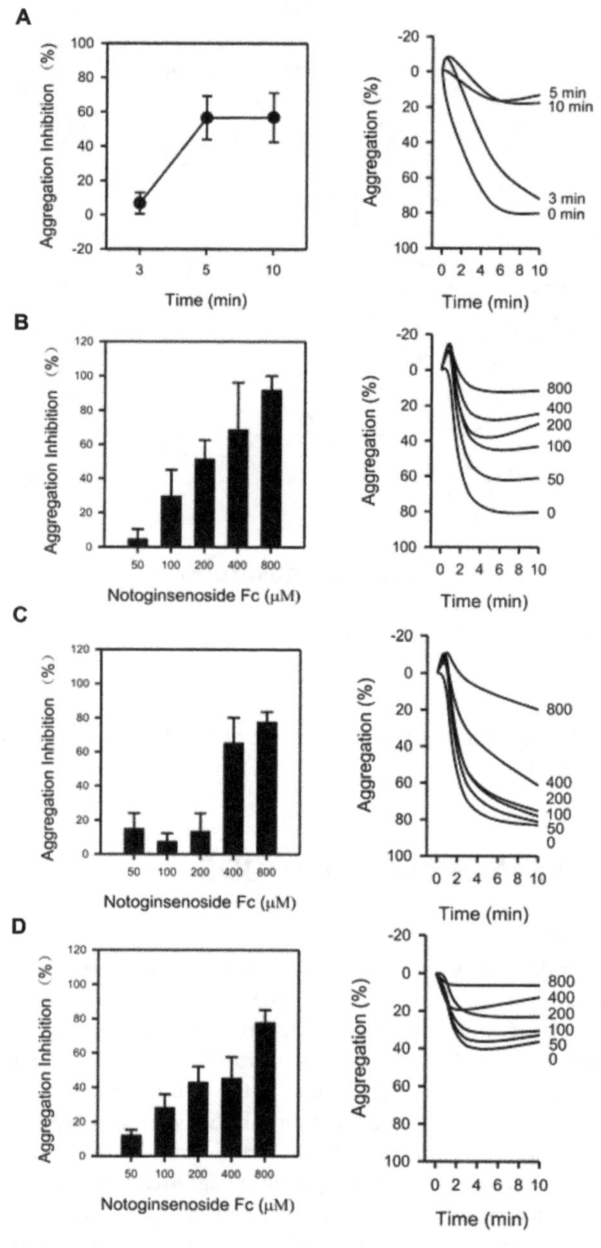

FIGURE 2 | Antiplatelet effect of Fc. **(A)** After incubating WP with Fc (400 μM) for indicated times (3, 5, 10 min), platelet aggregation was induced by thrombin. To determine the dose-dependent antiaggregatory effect of Fc, WP were incubated with indicated concentrations (50, 100, 200, 400, 800 μM) of Fc for 5 min. Platelet aggregation was induced by either thrombin **(B)**, collagen **(C)**, or ADP **(D)**. Tracing graphs represent the percentage of platelet aggregation variation after treated with stimulators. Values are mean ± SEM (n = 3 for **A**; n = 3~4 for **B** and **C**; n = 3~5 for **D**).

RESULTS

Fc Inhibited Platelet Aggregation Induced by Various Stimulators

The impact of Fc on platelet aggregation was examined. To determine the appropriate incubating time for the study, several time points (3, 5, and 10 min) were tested against thrombin. The anti-platelet effect of Fc (400 μM) was peaked at 5 min (**Figure 2A**). As a result, 5 min was used in the following study. After that, the concentration dependent antiplatelet effect for Fc was investigated. Treatment of WP with Fc resulted in proportional suppression of thrombin induced platelet aggregation, with an IC_{50} of 204.38 μM (**Figure 2B**). Consistent with these results, by pretreatment of WP with increasing concentrations (50, 100, 200, 400, and 800 μM) of Fc, platelet aggregation induced by collagen (**Figure 2C**) and ADP (**Figure 2D**) were all inhibited dose-dependently, with IC_{50} of 379.93 and 295.89 μM, respectively. According to these results, Fc can inhibit various stimulators induced platelet aggregation, and most effective to thrombin.

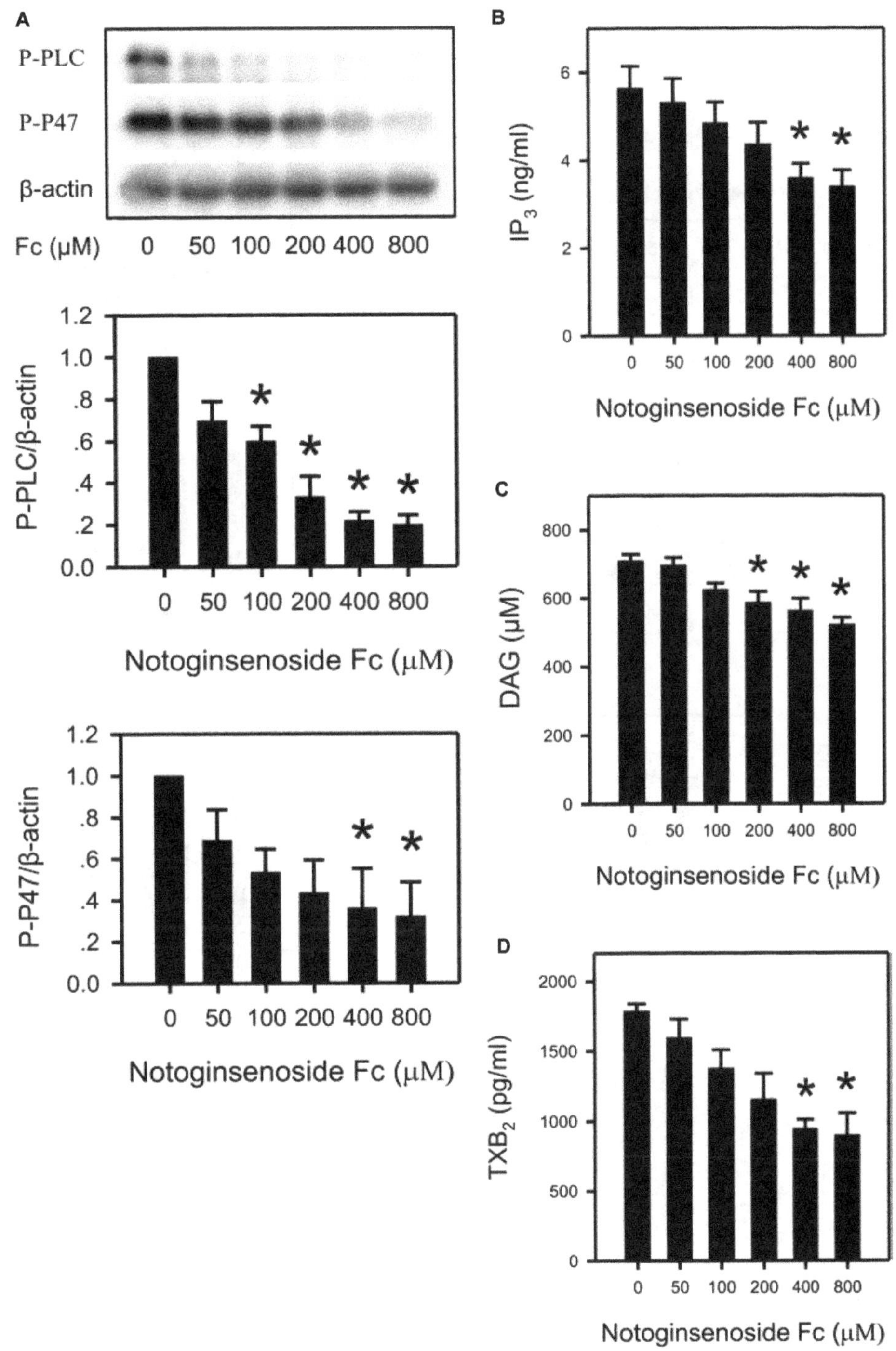

FIGURE 3 | Suppression of platelet PLCγ2 cascade by Fc. **(A)** After incubating WP with different concentrations of Fc, platelet PLCγ2 and PKC activity were evaluated according to the phosphorylation of PLCγ2 and P47. β-actin was used as a loading control. Platelet content of IP_3, DAG and TXB_2 were measured by ELISA kits. WP was incubated with the indicated concentrations of Fc, and platelet IP_3 **(B)**, DAG **(C)**, and TXB_2 **(D)** concentrations were assessed. Values are mean ± SEM ($n = 3$ for **A**; $n = 5$ for **B**; $n = 4$ for **C,D**). $^*P < 0.05$ versus control.

Fc Down Regulated the PLCγ2 Cascade in Platelet

To confirm the involvement of the PLCγ2 cascade in the antiplatelet effect of Fc, the following indexes were measured: P-PLCγ2, DAG, IP_3, P-P47 (a protein reflect PKC activity), TXB_2 (a metabolite of TXA_2) and $[Ca^{2+}]$. By incubating platelets with increasing concentrations of Fc, phosphorylation of PLCγ2 and P47 were reduced dose-dependently (**Figure 3A**). In addition,

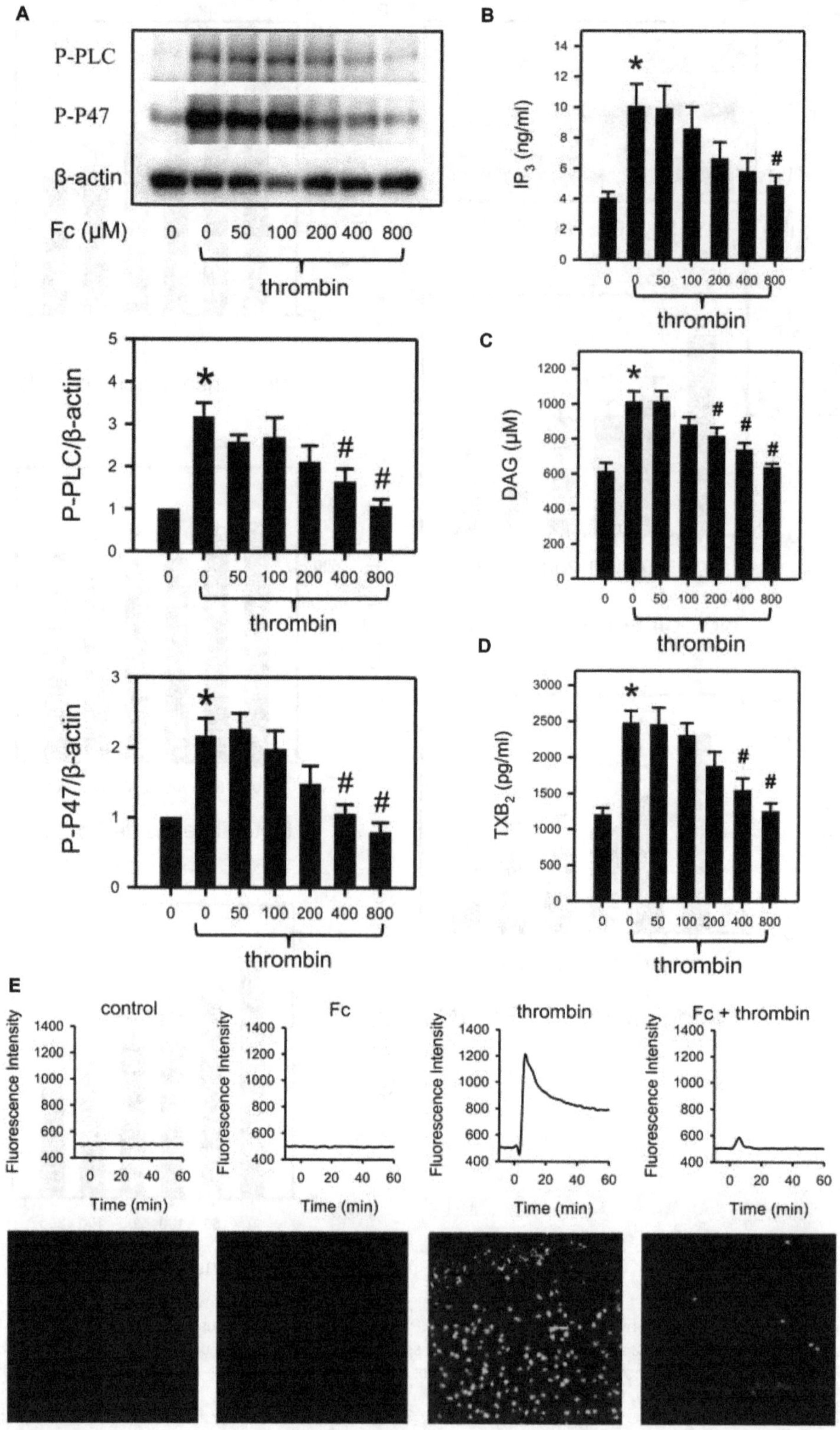

FIGURE 4 | Prevention of thrombin induced activation of PLCγ2 cascade by Fc. After incubating with different concentrations of Fc, WP was treated with thrombin for 3 min. **(A)** The phosphorylation of PLCγ2 and P47 in platelet were measured with western blotting. β-actin was used as a loading control. Platelet IP_3 **(B)**, DAG **(C)** and TXB_2 **(D)** concentrations were assessed by corresponding ELISA kits. **(E)** Variation in $[Ca^{2+}]$ was assessed by detecting the fluorescence intensity emitted from intracellular Fluo-4. The images are from the peak point of each experiment. Tracings were from representative results in three independent experiments. Values are mean ± SEM (n = 6 for **A**; n = 4 for **B,C**; n = 3 for **D**). $^{*}P < 0.05$ versus control; $^{\#}P < 0.05$ versus thrombin only.

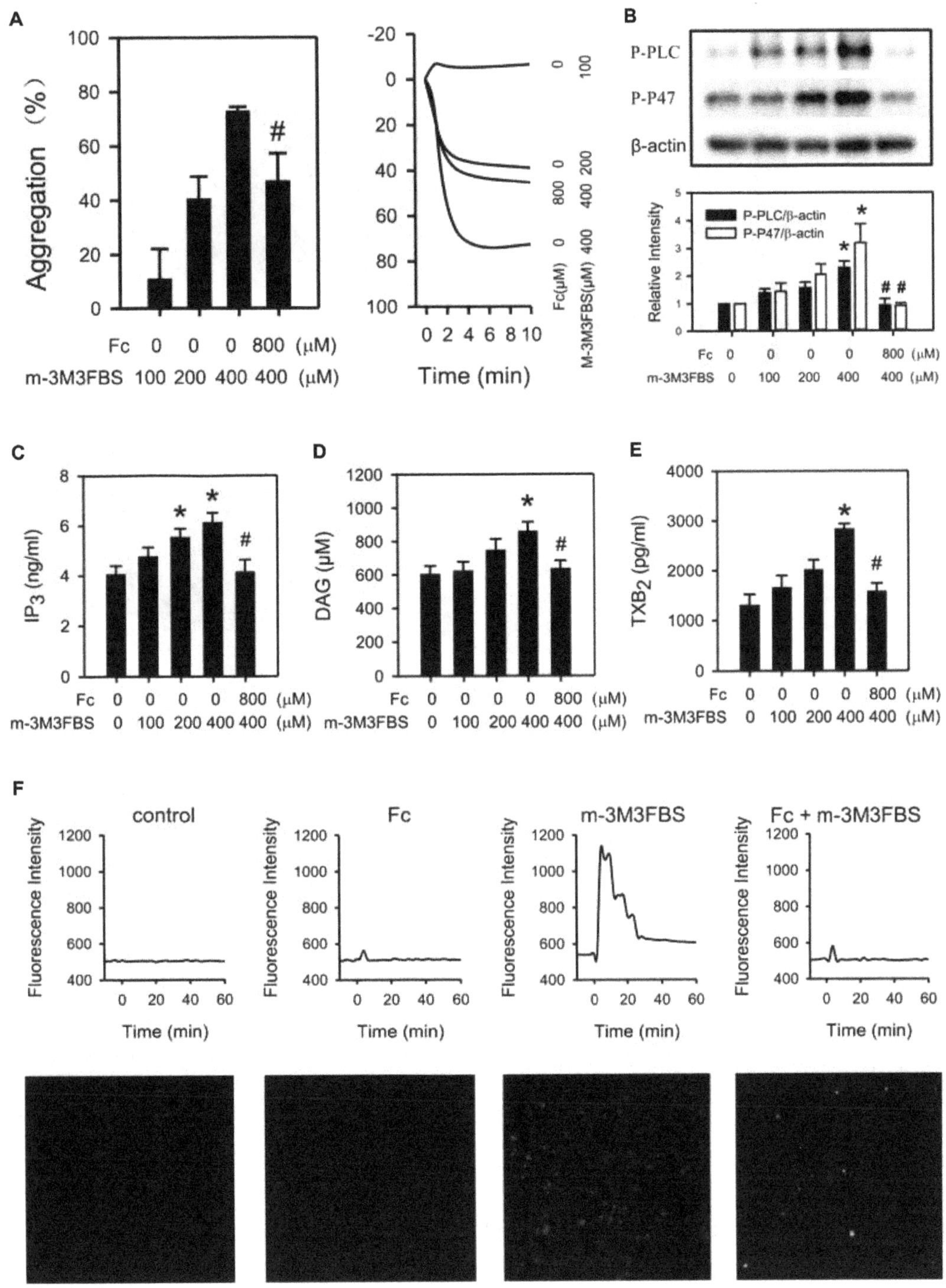

FIGURE 5 | Involvement of PLCγ2 cascade in the antiplatelet effect of Fc. WP were treated with either increasing concentrations of m-3M3FBS (100, 200, 400 μM) or m-3M3FBS (400 μM) followed Fc (800 μM). **(A)** Platelet aggregation was assessed by a 4-channed aggregometer. **(B)** The phosphorylation of PLCγ2 and P47 of platelet were measured with western blotting. β-actin was used as a loading control. Platelet IP_3 **(C)**, DAG **(D)**, and TXB_2 **(E)** concentrations were assessed by ELISA kits. **(F)** $[Ca^{2+}]$ was assessed by the fluorescence intensity from intracellular Fluo-4. The images are from the peak point of each experiment. Tracings were from representative results in three independent experiments. Values are mean ± SEM (n = 6~11 for **A**; n = 3~4 for **B–E**). $^{*}P < 0.05$ versus control; $^{\#}P < 0.05$ versus 400 μM m-3M3FBS only.

platelet IP_3, DAG and TXB_2 content were also decreased by Fc in a dose-dependent manner (**Figures 3B–D**). However, the alteration in intra-platelet $[Ca^{2+}]$ was not observed (**Figure 4E**). This may due to the sensitivity of the fluorescence dye (Fluo-4 AM). Because the basal $[Ca^{2+}]$ in resting platelets was too low to discern a further decrease.

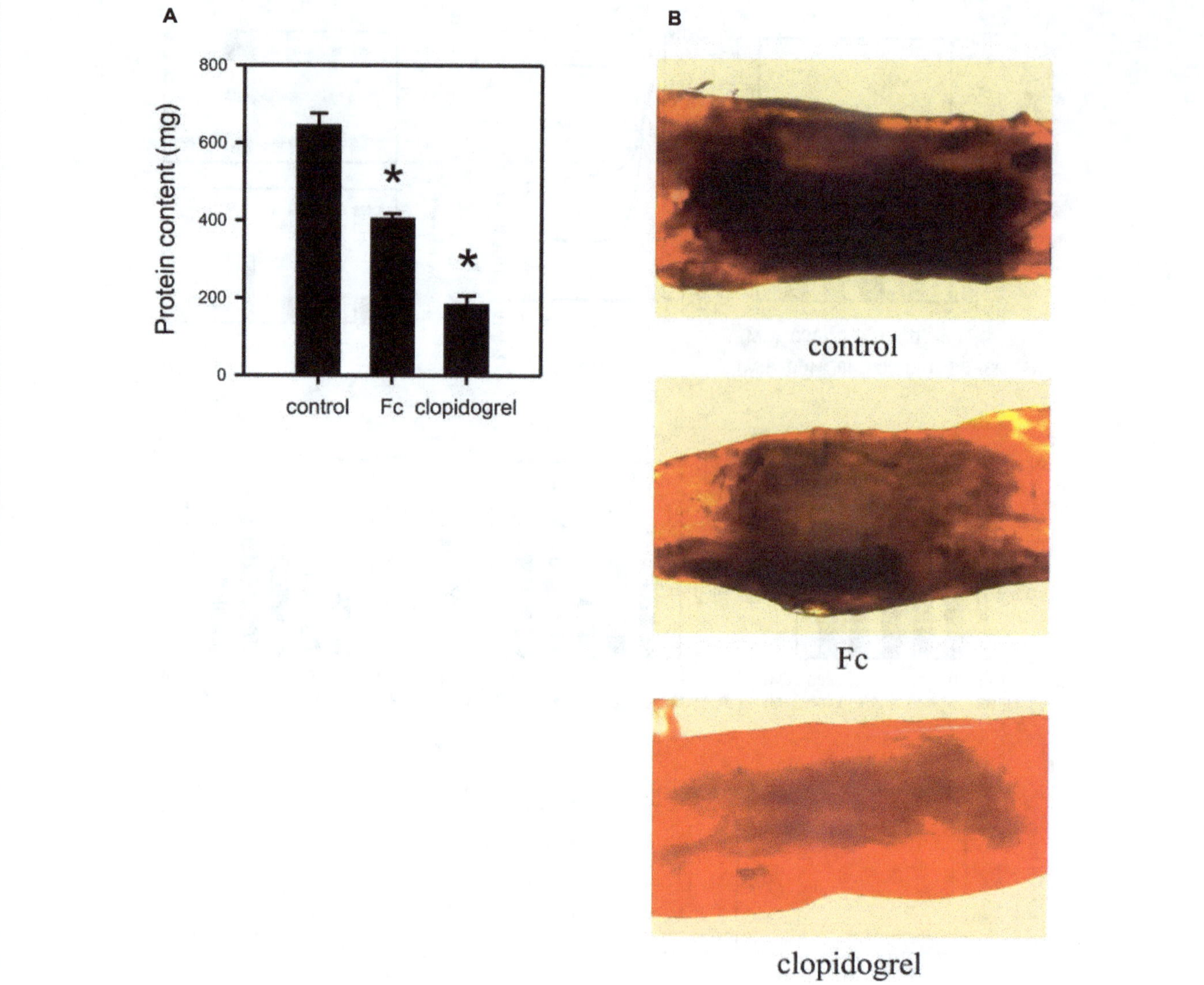

FIGURE 6 | *In vivo* anti-thrombotic effect of Fc. Rats were i.p. injected with saline, Fc or clopidogrel. 2 h later, a filter paper saturated with 20% $FeCl_3$ was applied to the isolated femoral artery for 20 min. Then the injured arteries were isolated for observation under microscope and measurement of thrombus protein content. **(A)** The bar graph indicates the protein contents in $FeCl_3$ induced thrombus of each group. **(B)** The representative graphs showed the artery condition after injured by $FeCl_3$. Values are mean ± SEM (n = 6 for control and Fc group; n = 3 for clopidogrel group). $^*P < 0.05$ versus control.

Fc Abolished Thrombin Induced PLCγ2 Cascade Activation

Thrombin induced platelet aggregation was most sensitive to Fc. As a result, we demonstrated the involvement of the PLCγ2 cascade in the anti-platelet effect of Fc against thrombin. In accordance with the previous study, thrombin can activate platelet PLCγ2, P47 (**Figure 4A**); upregulate IP_3 (**Figure 4B**), DAG (**Figure 4C**), TXB_2 (**Figure 4D**), and $[Ca^{2+}]$ (**Figure 4E**). By pre-incubation with increasing concentrations of Fc, thrombin induced platelet aggregation (**Figure 2B**) and activation of PLCγ2 cascade, including increase in $[Ca^{2+}]$, were downregulated dose-dependently (**Figure 4**). This proved our conjecture that Fc can decrease platelet $[Ca^{2+}]$ when it high enough to be detected.

Fc Attenuated m-3M3FBS Induced Platelet Aggregation and PLCγ2 Cascade Activation

M-3M3FBS (100, 200, 400 μM), direct PLC activator, activated PLCγ2 (**Figure 5B**) and induced platelet aggregation (**Figure 5A**) in a dose-dependent manner. Meanwhile, m-3M3FBS induced PLCγ2 activation was abolished by Fc (**Figure 5B**). And platelet aggregation was partially restored by pretreatment of Fc (**Figure 5A**). This demonstrated Fc can inhibit platelet aggregation through preventing m-3M3FBS induced PLCγ2 activation. In addition, m-3M3FBS increased P-P47, IP_3, DAG, TXB_2 and [Ca^{2+}] were prevented by Fc as well (**Figures 5B–F**). The above results proved that Fc inhibit platelet aggregation through oppression the activation of PLCγ2 and subsequent DAG-PKC-TXA_2 and IP_3-Ca^{2+}.

Fc Alleviated *in vivo* Thrombus Formation

To evaluate the *in vivo* anti-thrombotic effect of Fc, a $FeCl_3$ thrombosis model was employed. By i.p. injection of Fc, thrombus protein content was decreased from 647.10 ± 72.30 mg to 406.38 ± 28.77 mg, although not as strong as clopidogrel (**Figure 6A**). $FeCl_3$ injured blood vessels were also observed under a microscope. The dark part influencing blood vessel's transparency was thrombus. Fc administration significantly decreased the thickness of thrombus (**Figure 6B**). This indicated Fc not only can inhibit *in vitro* platelet aggregation, but also can alleviate *in vivo* thrombus formation.

DISCUSSION

Although antiplatelet drugs have been frequently used in the clinic, the problems of bleeding kept push people to develop new drugs for controlling thrombus growth. In this process, a series of targets for antiplatelet drugs have been suggested, most of which are platelet receptors. Collagen, a stimulator released from damaged blood vessel, induces platelet aggregation through activation of glycoprotein VI and integrin $\alpha_2\beta_1$ receptors. ADP is a platelet activator can be secreted both externally and internally. It activates platelet through $P2Y_{12}$ and $P2Y_1$ receptors. Thrombin, the most potent platelet activator, predominately activate platelets by protease activator receptor 1 (PAR_1) and PAR_4 (Coughlin, 2005; Leger et al., 2006). The receptors for thrombin, collagen and ADP are different, but there is a well-known pathway involved in all the three stimulators induced platelet aggregation: PLCγ2 activation improves hydrolyzation of PIP_2 into IP_3 and DAG, which in turn contribute to Ca^{2+} release, PKC activation and TXA_2 increase (Si-Tahar et al., 1996; Liu et al., 2005; Ragab et al., 2007; Stegner and Nieswandt, 2011). Thrombin, collagen and ADP trigger PLCγ2 cascade activation through PAR, glycoprotein VI and $P2Y_1$ receptors, respectively (**Figure 7**).

In the present study, Fc inhibited platelet aggregation induced by thrombin, collagen and ADP (**Figure 2**). Therefore, it is quite possible that PLCγ2 and its downstream signaling are related with antiplatelet effect. Indeed, by measurement of PLCγ2 and PKC activities, IP_3, DAG, PKC and TXA_2 concentrations were down-regulated by Fc dose dependently (**Figure 3**). However, a decrease in [Ca^{2+}] was not observed by Fc treatment. This is because the basal level of [Ca^{2+}] in platelets was not high enough to see a further decrease. This was proved by testing the influence of Fc on thrombin stimulated platelets. According to the result, PLCγ2 and PKC activities, IP_3, DAG, PKC, TXA_2 and Ca^{2+} concentrations raised by thrombin were all abolished by pretreatment of Fc (**Figure 4**).

Although Fc can restore thrombin induced platelet aggregation and activation of PLCγ2 cascade, the relationship between the anti-platelet effect and PLCγ2 cascade is still not clear yet. Since thrombin induced platelet aggregation is quite complicated, PLCγ2 cascade is only part of it. To exclude the interfuse of other pathway, a direct PLC activator, m-3M3FBS, was employed (Bae et al., 2003). As we expected, PLCγ2 activity in platelets were enhanced by m-3M3FBS dose-dependently. And the increase in light transmission detected by aggregometer usually happens in platelet aggregation were triggered by m-3M3FBS as well. However, m-3M3FBS induced platelet aggregation was only partially restored by Fc (**Figure 5**). This may because of the non-specific effect of m-3M3FBS. Indeed, platelet aggregation induced by m-3M3FBS through activation of PLC is related with the increase in light transmittance of platelets. But it may also occur during platelet apoptosis (Shcherbina and Remold-O'Donnell, 1999; Stivala et al., 2017). It is reported that m-3M3FBS can affect a serious of apoptosis related proteins: up-regulate pro-apoptotic Bax, down-regulate anti-apoptotic

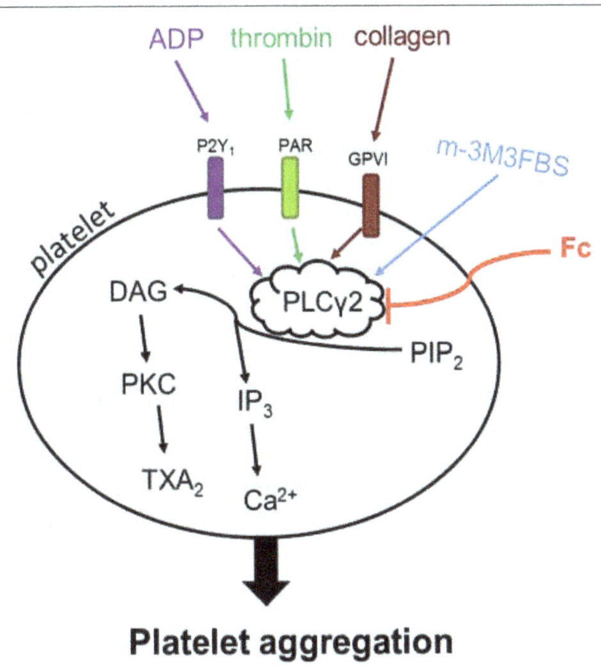

FIGURE 7 | Mechanism of Fc inhibits platelet aggregation. Thrombin, collagen and ADP activate PLCγ2 signaling cascade through PAR, GPVI and $P2Y_1$ receptors, respectively. PLCγ2 promotes the hydrolyzation of PIP_2 to DAG and IP_3 in platelets. The increase in platelet DAG and IP_3 subsequently up-regulate PKC activity, TXA_2 content and [Ca^{2+}]. m-3M3FBS triggers activation of PLCγ2 and downstream signaling directly. Fc can abolish platelet aggregation induced by thrombin, collagen, ADP, as well as m-3M3FBS, through preventing the activation of PLCγ2 signaling. Arrows indicate the activation of target molecules or stimulation of production. Blunt line means target inhibition. The difference in color demonstrates different stimulators triggered effects.

Bcl-2, activate caspase and promote release of cytochrome C (Lee et al., 2005). In addition, PLC was classified into 6 families, including PLCβ, PLCγ, PLCδ, PLCε, PLCζ, and PLCη (Nakamura and Fukami, 2017). Except PLCγ2, PLCβ3 also relates with platelet aggregation (Lee et al., 2014; Pradhan et al., 2017). Therefore, PLCβ3 may also contribute to m-3M3FBS induced platelet aggregation. However, specific activator for PLCγ2 is still not available. After all, m-3M3FBS induced activation of PLCγ2 and subsequent DAG-PKC-TXA_2 and IP_3-$[Ca^{2+}]$ were almost completely abolished by Fc (**Figure 5**). Therefore, PLCγ2 cascade indeed responsible to the antiplatelet effect of Fc.

By a single administration of Fc, $FeCl_3$ induced thrombosis in rat femoral artery was significantly alleviated (**Figure 6**). Although the anti-thrombotic potency of Fc is not as strong as clopidogrel, chronic administration may be a safer way for preventive treatment of thrombotic diseases. After all, the key point for new antiplatelet drug development is no longer high potency anymore. As we know, the strong unidirectional antiplatelet effect will result in serious bleeding. Safety is the predominant advantage of *Panax notoginseng* over clinical antiplatelet drugs (Rao et al., 2005; Bittl et al., 2016; Moon et al., 2018). By treatment of *Panax notoginseng*, when Fc exerts its effect on platelets, other saponins may provide complementary or eliminatory assistance. For instance, Ft1, another saponin from over-ground part of *Panax notoginseng*, was proved to have effect in promoting platelet aggregation by activating $P2Y_{12}$ receptors (Gao et al., 2014). Therefore, a hypothesis was put forward: as main saponins in over-ground part of *Panax notoginseng*, Ft1 and Fc may be the predominant compositions for the dual-directional regulatory effect on platelet. To clarify the way to balance the dual-directional regulatory effect and comprehensive impact of them on platelet and thrombus, further research is required.

The effect of PNS on inhibiting platelet aggregation has been mentioned in many studies. PNS can inhibit platelet aggregation through PPAR-γ/PI3K/Akt/eNOS pathway (Shen et al., 2017), $[Ca^{2+}]$, ERK_2/p38 (Qi et al., 2016), COX (Wang et al., 2016), FAK, NF-κB (Yuan et al., 2011). Whereas, most of them didn't mention any single saponin, but only investigated the complex PNS. Which single saponin stimulated the above signals is still unknown. The hemostatic effect of *Panax notoginseng* is well known, but no systematic study about it yet. Gao et al. (2014) screened several saponins and conclude only Notoginsenoside Ft1, Notoginsenoside Fe and protopanaxadiol are effective in increase ADP induced platelet aggregation. Among them, only Ft1 was demonstrated to activate platelet through $P2Y_{12}$ receptors. The effect of Notoginsenoside Fe and protopanaxadiol were not further studied (Gao et al., 2014). Based on these studies, it is hard to elaborate the mechanism of the dual-directional regulatory effect of *Panax notoginseng*. Therefore, our group is trying to investigate the effect and mechanism of more single saponins on platelet. After that, the dual-directional effect of *Panax notoginseng* can be clarified.

The present study demonstrated the mechanism of the antiplatelet effect of Fc, a main functional saponin in leaves and flowers of *Panax notoginseng*. This can provide theoretical basis for utilization of over-ground part of the plant. Attentions should be paid to the dual-directional regulatory effect of *Panax notoginseng* on platelets, which may be a new perspective for thrombotic disease treatment.

AUTHOR CONTRIBUTIONS

YqL, LC, and XS designed the research. YqL, TL, ZL, YyL, and TH performed the experiments. YqL, KD, WZ, YF, and WM analyzed the data. YqL, LC, and KD wrote the manuscript.

FUNDING

This work was supported by "National Natural Science Foundation of China" (Grant No. 31802230); "China Postdoctoral Science Foundation" (Grant No. 2016M602882); "Agro-Scientific Research in the Public Interest" (Grant No. 201303040), and "the Fundamental Research Funds for the Central Universities" (Grant No. 2452017297).

ACKNOWLEDGMENTS

The research was also technically supported by "Life Science Research Core Services (LSRCS) of Northwest A&F University."

REFERENCES

Bae, Y. S., Lee, T. G., Park, J. C., Hur, J. H., Kim, Y., Heo, K., et al. (2003). Identification of a compound that directly stimulates phospholipase C activity. *Mol. Pharmacol.* 63, 1043–1050. doi: 10.1124/mol.63.5.1043

Bittl, J. A., Baber, U., Bradley, S. M., and Wijeysundera, D. N. (2016). Duration of dual antiplatelet therapy: a systematic review for the 2016 ACC/AHA guideline focused update on duration of dual antiplatelet therapy in patients with coronary artery disease: a report of the american college of cardiology/american heart association task force on clinical practice guidelines. *J. Am. Coll. Cardiol.* 68, 1116–1139. doi: 10.1016/j.jacc.2016.03.512

Coughlin, S. R. (2005). Protease-activated receptors in hemostasis, thrombosis and vascular biology. *J. Thromb. Haemost.* 3, 1800–1814. doi: 10.1111/j.1538-7836.2005.01377.x

Gao, B., Huang, L., Liu, H., Wu, H., Zhang, E., Yang, L., et al. (2014). Platelet P2Y(1)(2) receptors are involved in the haemostatic effect of notoginsenoside Ft1, a saponin isolated from *Panax notoginseng*. *Br. J. Pharmacol.* 171, 214–223. doi: 10.1111/bph.12435

Généreux, P., Giustino, G., Witzenbichler, B., Weisz, G., Stuckey, T. D., Rinaldi, M. J., et al. (2015). Incidence, predictors, and impact of post-discharge bleeding after percutaneous coronary intervention. *J. Am. Coll. Cardiol.* 66, 1036–1045. doi: 10.1016/j.jacc.2015.06.1323

Hartwig, J., and Italiano, J. Jr. (2003). The birth of the platelet. *J. Thromb. Haemost.* 1, 1580–1586. doi: 10.1046/j.1538-7836.2003.00331.x

Ke, Y., Jiang, J. Y., Wang, X. Z., Zeng, X. Y., and Zhu, C. Y. (2010). Effect of total saponins from rhizomes and flowers of *Panax notoginseng* on tumor cell induced platelet aggregation. *Zhong Yao Cai* 33, 96–99.

Lee, J. J., Cho, W. K., Kwon, H., Gu, M., and Ma, J. Y. (2014). Galla rhois exerts its antiplatelet effect by suppressing ERK1/2 and PLC beta phosphorylation. *Food Chem. Toxicol.* 69, 94–101. doi: 10.1016/j.fct.2014.03.032

Lee, Y. N., Lee, H. Y., Kim, J. S., Park, C., Choi, Y. H., Lee, T. G., et al. (2005). The novel phospholipase C activator, m-3M3FBS, induces monocytic leukemia cell apoptosis. *Cancer Lett.* 222, 227–235. doi: 10.1016/j.canlet.2004.09.017

Leger, A. J., Covic, L., and Kuliopulos, A. (2006). Protease-activated receptors in cardiovascular diseases. *Circulation* 114, 1070–1077. doi: 10.1161/CIRCULATIONAHA.105.574830

Liang, Z. H., and Yin, D. Z. (2010). Preventive treatment of traditional chinese medicine as antistress and antiaging strategy. *Rejuv Res.* 13, 248–252. doi: 10.1089/rej.2009.0867

Liao, F. (2000). Herbs of activating blood circulation to remove blood stasis. *Clin. Hemorheol. Microcirc* 23, 127–131.

Liu, J., Pestina, T. I., Berndt, M. C., Jackson, C. W., and Gartner, T. K. (2005). Botrocetin/VWF-induced signaling through GPIb-IX-V produces TxA2 in an alpha IIb beta 3- and aggregation-independent manner. *Blood* 106, 2750–2756. doi: 10.1182/blood-2005-04-1667

Liu, Y., Oh, S. J., Chang, K. H., Kim, Y. G., and Lee, M. Y. (2013). Antiplatelet effect of AMP-activated protein kinase activator and its potentiation by the phosphodiesterase inhibitor dipyridamole. *Biochem. Pharmacol.* 86, 914–925. doi: 10.1016/j.bcp.2013.07.009

Mackman, N. (2008). Triggers, targets and treatments for thrombosis. *Nature* 451, 914–918. doi: 10.1038/nature06797

Meadows, T. A., and Bhatt, D. L. (2007). Clinical aspects of platelet inhibitors and thrombus formation. *Circ. Res.* 100, 1261–1275. doi: 10.1161/01.RES.0000264509.36234.51

Moon, J. Y., Franchi, F., Rollini, F., and Angiolillo, D. J. (2018). The quest for safer antithrombotic treatment regimens in patients with coronary artery disease: new strategies and paradigm shifts. *Expert Rev. Hematol.* 11, 5–12. doi: 10.1080/17474086.2018.1400378

Nakamura, Y., and Fukami, K. (2017). Regulation and physiological functions of mammalian phospholipase C. *J. Biochem.* 161, 315–321. doi: 10.1093/jb/mvw094

Pradhan, S., Khatlani, T., Nairn, A. C., and Vijayan, K. V. (2017). The heterotrimeric G protein G beta(1) interacts with the catalytic subunit of protein phosphatase 1 and modulates G protein-coupled receptor signaling in platelets. *J. Biol. Chem.* 292, 13133–13142. doi: 10.1074/jbc.M117.796656

Qi, H., Huang, Y., Yang, Y., Dou, G., Wan, F., Zhang, W., et al. (2016). Anti-platelet activity of panaxatriol saponins is mediated by suppression of intracellular calcium mobilization and ERK2/p38 activation. *BMC Complem. Altern. Med.* 16:978034. doi: 10.1186/s12906-016-1160-7

Ragab, A., Séverin, S., Gratacap, M. P., Aguado, E., Malissen, M., Jandrot-Perrus, M., et al. (2007). Roles of the C-terminal tyrosine residues of LAT in GPVI-induced platelet activation: insights into the mechanism of PLC gamma 2 activation. *Blood* 110, 2466–2474. doi: 10.1182/blood-2007-02-075432

Rao, S. V., O'Grady, K., Pieper, K. S., Granger, C. B., Newby, L. K., Van de Werf, F., et al. (2005). Impact of bleeding severity on clinical outcomes among patients with acute coronary syndromes. *Am. J. Cardiol.* 96, 1200–1206. doi: 10.1016/j.amjcard.2005.06.056

Ruggeri, Z. M., and Mendolicchio, G. L. (2007). Adhesion mechanisms in platelet function. *Circ. Res.* 100, 1673–1685. doi: 10.1161/01.RES.0000267878.97021.ab

Sakata, C., Suzuki, K. I., Morita, Y., and Kawasaki, T. (2017). Additive antithrombotic effect of ASP6537, a selective cyclooxygenase (COX)-1 inhibitor, in combination with clopidogrel in guinea pigs. *Eur. J. Pharmacol.* 798, 72–76. doi: 10.1016/j.ejphar.2017.01.015

Shcherbina, A., and Remold-O'Donnell, E. (1999). Role of caspase in a subset of human platelet activation responses. *Blood* 93, 4222–4231.

Shen, Q., Li, J., Zhang, C., Wang, P., Mohammed, A., Ni, S., et al. (2017). *Panax notoginseng* saponins reduce high-risk factors for thrombosis through peroxisome proliferator activated receptor-gamma pathway. *Biomed. Pharmacother.* 96, 1163–1169. doi: 10.1016/j.biopha.2017.11.106

Si-Tahar, M., Renesto, P., Falet, H., Rendu, F., and Chignard, M. (1996). The phospholipase C protein kinase C pathway is involved in cathepsin G-induced human platelet activation: comparison with thrombin. *Biochem. J.* 313, 401–408. doi: 10.1042/bj3130401

Stegner, D., and Nieswandt, B. (2011). Platelet receptor signaling in thrombus formation. *J. Mol. Med.* 89, 109–121. doi: 10.1007/s00109-010-0691-5

Stivala, S., Gobbato, S., Infanti, L., Reiner, M. F., Bonetti, N., Meyer, S. C., et al. (2017). Amotosalen/ultraviolet A pathogen inactivation technology reduces platelet activatability, induces apoptosis and accelerates clearance. *Haematologica* 102, 1650–1660. doi: 10.3324/haematol.2017.164137

Wang, J., Xu, J., and Zhong, J. B. (2004). Effect of radix notoginseng saponins on platelet activating molecule expression and aggregation in patients with blood hyperviscosity syndrome. *Zhongguo Zhong Xi Yi Jie He Za Zhi* 24, 312–316.

Wang, M. M., Xue, M., Xu, Y. G., Miao, Y., Kou, N., Yang, L., et al. (2016). Panax notoginseng saponin is superior to aspirin in inhibiting platelet adhesion to injured endothelial cells through COX pathway in vitro. *Thromb. Res.* 141, 146–152. doi: 10.1016/j.thromres.2016.03.022

Yuan, Z., Liao, Y., Tian, G., Li, H., Jia, Y., Zhang, H., et al. (2011). *Panax notoginseng* saponins inhibit Zymosan A induced atherosclerosis by suppressing integrin expression, FAK activation and NF-kappaB translocation. *J. Ethnopharmacol.* 138, 150–155. doi: 10.1016/j.jep.2011.08.066

Zhang, D., Gao, Z. G., Zhang, K., Kiselev, E., Crane, S., Wang, J., et al. (2015). Two disparate ligand-binding sites in the human P2Y1 receptor. *Nature* 520, 317–321. doi: 10.1038/nature14287

Zhou, X., Chen, L. L., Xie, R. F., Lam, W., Zhang, Z. J., Jiang, Z. L., et al. (2017). Chemosynthesis pathway and bioactivities comparison of saponins in radix and flower of *Panax notoginseng* (Burk.) F.H. *Chen. J. Ethnopharmacol.* 201, 56–72. doi: 10.1016/j.jep.2016.11.008

16

Ninjin'yoeito Improves Behavioral Abnormalities and Hippocampal Neurogenesis in the Corticosterone Model of Depression

*Kenta Murata[1], Nina Fujita[1], Ryuji Takahashi[1] and Akio Inui[2]**

[1] *Kampo Research Laboratories, Kracie Pharma, Ltd., Tokyo, Japan,* [2] *Pharmacological Department of Herbal Medicine, Kagoshima University Graduate School of Medical and Dental Sciences, Kagoshima, Japan*

Correspondence:
Akio Inui
inui@m.kufm.kagoshima-u.ac.jp

Ninjinyoeito (NYT), a traditional Chinese medicine consisting of 12 herbs, is designed to improve fatigue, cold limbs, anorexia, night sweats, and anemia. Recently, NYT was reported to improve cognitive outcome and depression in patients with Alzheimer's disease. However, little is known about how NYT alleviates depression and cognitive dysfunction. In this study, we investigated the effects and mechanisms of NYT in a corticosterone (CORT)-induced model of depression. Chronic NYT treatment ameliorated the depressive-like behaviors induced by CORT treatment in three types of behavioral tests. In addition, chronic NYT treatment also improved memory disruptions induced by CORT in both the Y-maze and novel object recognition tests, without affecting locomotor activity. Furthermore, we also showed that NYT treatment attenuated the CORT-induced reduction in cell proliferation and immature neuronal cell numbers in mouse hippocampal dentate gyrus. These results suggest that NYT has therapeutic effects on CORT-induced behavioral abnormalities and inhibition of hippocampal neurogenesis.

Keywords: ninjinyoeito, depression, neurogenesis, corticosterone, neuronal progenitor cell

INTRODUCTION

Depression is one of the most common mood disorders in modern society. It is estimated that about 1% of the population will be affected by major depression at least once during their lifetime (Rao et al., 2004). Although extensive studies have led to various hypotheses regarding the molecular mechanisms underlying depression, the pathogenesis of depression remains to be fully clarified. One hypothesis concerns the hypothalamic-pituitary-adrenal (HPA)-axis, which is well known to play a critical role in the pathogenesis of mood disorders (de Kloet et al., 2005, 2006). Under normal conditions, glucocorticoid levels in blood are sensitively regulated by the HPA-axis via negative feedback. However, in stressful situations, persistently high concentrations of glucocorticoids in the blood causes dysregulation of the HPA-axis, induces atrophy in the central nervous system, and even aggravates depression (Murphy, 1997; Sapolsky, 2000). Based on these findings, the chronic corticosterone (CORT) exposure model is widely used to induce depressive-like behavioral and neurochemical changes in rodents (Gourley et al., 2008). Recent work suggests that elevated glucocorticoid levels induces behavioral disorder and decreases cell proliferation in the hippocampal dentate gyrus, and that these changes are reversed by chronic antidepressant treatment. In addition, the efficacy of some antidepressants, such as fluoxetine, is abrogated by X-irradiation, which inhibits hippocampal neurogenesis (David et al., 2009). Thus, improving hippocampal neurogenesis is considered to be one of the most important strategies for the development of antidepressant medicines.

Ninjinyoeito (NYT), a traditional Chinese medicine described in Ho-chi-chü-fang, is designed to improve fatigue, cold limbs, anorexia, night sweats, and anemia. For that reason, NYT has been administered to elderly people in Traditional Oriental medicine. NYT is composed of 12 herbs: ginseng, astragalus root, angelica root, rehmannia root, atractylodes root, poria sclerotium, peony root, cinnamon bark, citrus unshiu peel, polygala root, schisandra fruit, and glycyrrhiza. In basic research, NYT was reported to improve memory impairments and the reduction of serotonin and 5-hydroxyindole-3-acetic in the olfactory bulb lesion mouse model (Song et al., 2001). NYT was also reported to improve demyelination and increase the number of oligodendrocytes in aged or cuprizone-treated rodents (Kobayashi et al., 2003; Seiwa et al., 2007). Another report suggested that NYT increased nerve growth factor in astrocytes (Yabe et al., 2003). In addition to basic research, a recent clinical trial revealed that NYT treatment improved cognitive outcome and Alzheimer's disease-related depression in patients with Alzheimer's disease (Kudoh et al., 2016). Although the action of NYT in the central nervous system is being clarified by some animal model studies, little is known about how NYT alleviates depression and cognitive disorder.

Here, we investigated how NYT may improve depression and cognitive disorder using the chronic CORT-induced model of depression.

MATERIALS AND METHODS

Animals

Five-week-old male C57BL/6 mice (SLC, Shizuoka, Japan) were used in these experiments. Animals were housed at 24 ± 2°C under a 12-h light–dark cycle (lights on from 8:00 to 20:00) with *ad libitum* access to food and water. Behavioral experiments were performed between 9:00 and 18:00. All efforts were made to minimize both the suffering of and the number of animals used. The experimental protocol was reviewed and approved by the Experimental Animal Care Committee of Kracie Pharma, Ltd. (Toyama, Japan).

Plant Materials and Preparation of the Extract

Ninjinyoeito is composed of twelve dried medical herbs, including rehmannia root, Japanese angelica root, atractylodes rhizome, poria sclerotium, ginseng, cinnamon bark, polygala root, peony root, citrus unshiu peel, astragalus root, glycyrrhiza, and schisandra fruit (**Table 1**), and is supplied by Kracie Pharma, Ltd. as a dried extract powder. Each plant material was identified by external morphology and authenticated by marker compounds of plant specimens according to the method of Japanese Pharmacopeia and our company's standard. The extract powder (lot no. 15112017) was suspended in distilled water immediately before use and was administered orally at a dose of 500 or 1000 mg/kg body-weight/day.

TABLE 1 | Medical herb composition of NYT.

Common name	Botanical name	weight (g)
Rehmannia Root	Rehmannia glutinosa (Gaertn.) Libosch. ex Fisch. & C.A. Mey.	4
Japanese Angelica root	Angelica acutiloba (Siebold & Zucc.) Kitag.	4
Atractylodes Rhizome	Atractylodes japonica Koidz. ex Kitam.	4
Poria Sclerotium	Wolfiporia cocos Ryvarden et Gilbertson	4
Ginseng	Panax ginseng C.A.Mey.	3
Cinnamon Bark	Cinnamomum cassia (L.) J.Presl	2.5
Polygala Root	Polygala tenuifolia Willd.	2
Peony Root	Paeonia lactiflora Pall.	2
Citrus Unshiu Peel	Citrus unshiu Markowicz	2
Astragalus Root	Astragalus membranaceus (Fisch.) Bunge	1.5
Glycyrrhiza	Glycyrrhiza uralensis Fisch.	1
Schisandra Fruit	Schisandra chinensis (Turcz.) Baill.	1

High-Performance Liquid Chromatography Analysis of NYT

Ninjinyoeito extract was mixed and shaken with 50% MeOH and the supernatant was subjected to high-performance liquid chromatography (HPLC) analysis. The three-dimensional HPLC profile of NYT was obtained using a Shimazu LC-30AD liquid chromatography equipped with an SPD-M30A detector with scanning for a range of 230–400 nm and a reversed-phase column (Shim-pack XR-ODSIII, 2.0 mm i.d. × 50 mm, 1.6 mm, Column temperature: 40°). The column was equipped with solvent A (0.1% formic acid in acetonitrile) and solvent B (0.1% formic solution), and the ratio of solvent A was increased by 5% over 16 min, 70% over 1 min, and 5% over 1 min, with a flow rate at 0.5 mL/min.

Drug Treatment

Five-week-old male C57BL6 mice were used for chronic oral CORT exposure. Mice were divided into 5 groups: control group (n = 10), CORT-treated group (n = 10), CORT + NYT (500 or 1000 mg/kg)-treated group (n = 10), CORT + imipramine-treated group (n = 10). Mice were administered CORT (100 μg/mL; Sigma-Aldrich, St. Louis, MO, United States) in place of drinking water for 14 days. Animal were weaned with 50 μg/mL CORT for 3 days and then with 25 μg/mL CORT for 3 days to allow for gradual recovery of endogenous corticosterone secretion. NYT (500 or 1000 mg/kg/day) was orally administered once daily from day 21 to day 49. As a positive control, imipramine (10 mg/kg/day, intraperitoneally (i.p.); Wako Pure Chemical, Osaka, Japan) was administered once daily. Subsequent behavioral tests were performed on days 50–64 and brain samples were collected on day 65. On the days behavioral tests were performed, the drugs were administered 30 min before the tests. A 5-bromo-2-deoxyuridine (BrdU) solution (50 mg/kg/day, i.p.; Sigma-Aldrich) was administered from day 15 to day 19.

Open Field Test

Each mouse was placed in the periphery of the open field apparatus (width 30 cm × length 30 cm × height 30 cm). The total distance traveled in the arena and the time spent in the center zone (width 15 cm × length 15 cm) was recorded for 10 min using a video tracking system, ANY-maze (Muromachi Kikai Co., Ltd., Japan).

Tail Suspension Test

We performed the tail suspension test as described in a previous report (Can et al., 2012). Briefly, the tails of mice were suspended with a piece of adhesive tape 50 cm above the floor with climbstoppers (clear plastic cylinder, 3 cm length, 1 cm outside diameter, 0.5 cm inside diameter), and animal behavior was recorded for 6 min. As a test parameter, the latency to immobility and the total immobility time in the last 4 min were measured manually in a blinded manner. Small movements that were confined to the front legs, but without the involvement of the hind legs, were counted as immobility. Additionally, oscillations and pendulum-like swings that were due to the momentum gained during the earlier mobility bouts were also counted as immobility. The latency to immobility was determined as the time required for the mouse to first cease all movement for > 5 s.

Forced Swim Test

Mice were placed in a glass cylinder (height, 30 cm; diameter, 15 cm) filled with water (23 ± 2°C) to a 15-cm depth for 6 min. Mice were judged to be immobile when they floated passively in the water, making only small movements to maintain their body balance or to keep their heads above the water. As a test parameter, the latency to immobility and the total immobility and mobility time during the last 4 min were measured manually in a blinded manner. The latency to immobility was determined as the time required for the mouse to first cease all movement for > 2 s.

Sucrose Preference Test

Animals were habituated to drinking water from two bottles for 2 days. Mice were deprived of water for 14 h before the test, and the test was carried out on the following morning at 10:00. In the sucrose preference test, two pre-weighed bottles [one containing tap water and the other containing a 1% (w/v) sucrose solution] were presented to each animal for 4 h. The position of the water and sucrose bottles (left or right) was switched every 2 h. The bottles were weighed again, and the weight difference represented the animal's intake from each bottle. The sum of the volume of water plus sucrose intake was defined as the total volume intake, and sucrose preference was expressed as the percentage of sucrose intake relative to the total intake.

Y-Maze Test

The Y-maze apparatus has three arms at 120° angles (width 8 cm × length 30 cm × height 15 cm) extending from a central space (8 × 8 cm). Each mouse was placed in one arm and allowed to explore freely for 8 min to assess the rate of spontaneous alternation, defined as consecutive entries into three different arms without repetition. The spontaneous alternation percentage was calculated by the equation [successive entries/(total arm entries −1) × 100].

Novel Object Recognition Test

Each mouse was placed in the open-field apparatus after being habituated to the apparatus (without objects) for 15 min prior to the training session. At the end of each trial, the mouse was removed from the arena, and the arena was cleaned with 70% ethanol solution and dried with paper towels. Object recognition was scored by the amount of time spent with each object (defined as time spent with the nose directed to the object and/or with forelimbs touching the object). In the training session (T1: 10 min), two similar objects (left and right: cubes) were placed in a symmetrical position 5 cm away from the wall. In the retention session (T2: 10 min), two dissimilar objects were presented [one a cube (familiar), as before, and the other a new object, a cylinder (novel)]. The time spent exploring each object was recorded during T1 and T2. All mice were tested with a 2-h interval between T1 and T2.

Cell Culture

Adult mouse hippocampal progenitor/stem cells (NPCs) were isolated from the dentate gyrus of 5-week-old C57BL/6 mice as previously described (Babu et al., 2011). Briefly, mice were euthanized with isoflurane and decapitated with surgical scissors. The area of the dentate gyrus was isolated under the microscope, and the tissue was incubated with an enzyme mixture (2.5 U/mL papain, 1 U/mL dispase, 250 U/mL DNase) for 20 min at 37°C and triturated to obtain a single-cell suspension. NPCs were isolated from the cell mixture by using 22% vol/vol Percoll solution (GE Healthcare Japan, Tokyo, Japan) and centrifugation. Isolated NPCs were re-suspended in Neurobasal A (Thermo Fisher Scientific, Waltham, MA, United States) supplemented with 2% B27 (Sigma-Aldrich), 2 mM glutamine, 20 ng/ml epidermal growth factor (EGF), and 20 ng/mL fibroblast growth factor (FGF)-2 (Miltenyi Biotec, Bergisch Gladbach, Germany). Cells were dispersed and passaged weekly and cells passaged 2–4 times were used for experiments.

Cell Proliferation Assay

Isolated NPCs were seeded at 1.5×10^3 cells/well in 96-well plates coated with poly-D-lysine (PDL)/laminin and then incubated for 24 h. NPCs were cultured for 72 h in the presence of 20 μM CORT and/or NYT in proliferation solution. The synthetic nucleotide BrdU (10 μM; Sigma-Aldrich) was added to the medium 4 h before treatment cessation. NPCs were fixed with 4% paraformaldehyde for 30 min at room temperature.

Immunohistochemistry

Mice were anesthetized with isoflurane and perfused with saline until the outflow was clear, then immediately perfused with 4% paraformaldehyde for 10 min. Brains were removed and post-fixed in the same fixative for 24 h at 4°C. Paraffin-embedded tissue (thickness, 10 μm) was used for immunohistochemical identification of Ki67-, BrdU-, doublecortin (DCX)-, and glial fibrillary acidic protein (GFAP)-positive cells. Formalin-fixed, paraffin-embedded tissue sections were deparaffinized and hydrated. For BrdU immunostaining, the sections were incubated with 2N hydrochloric acid (HCl) for 30 min. Endogenous peroxidase was inhibited by incubation with freshly prepared 3% hydrogen peroxide (H_2O_2) with methanol. The sections were treated with citrate buffer at 121°C for 10 min. Non-specific staining was blocked with 5% goat serum for 60 min at room temperature. The sections were then incubated with rabbit polyclonal anti-DCX antibody (1:400; Abcam, Cambridge, MA, United States), rabbit polyclonal anti-GFAP antibody (1:200; Cell Signaling Technology, Danvers, MA, United States), rabbit polyclonal anti-Ki67 antibody (1:400; Abcam), or mouse monoclonal anti-BrdU (1:400, Cell Signaling Technology) at 4°C. Staining was developed with diaminobenzidine (Sigma-Aldrich) substrate and the cell density was calculated by dividing the number of cells counted by the volume of the counted area and averaged per animal. For the *in vitro* study, NPCs incorporating BrdU were incubated with 2 N HCl for 30 min at 37°C. NPCs were washed in phosphate buffered saline (PBS) and blocked with 10% normal goat serum for 60 min at room temperature. Subsequently, the NPCs were incubated overnight at 4°C with mouse monoclonal anti-BrdU antibody (1:1000; Cell Signaling Technology, Danvers, MA, United States). After being washed in PBS, the cells were reacted with Alexa Fluor 594 goat anti-mouse IgG (1:1000; Invitrogen, Carlsbad, CA, United States) for 1 h at room temperature. Nuclei were stained with Hoechst 33342 (1:2000; Invitrogen) for 20 min in the dark. The proliferation rate was calculated by dividing the number of BrdU-positive cells by the total cell number.

Statistical Analysis

All data are expressed as mean ± standard error of the mean (SEM). Statistical comparisons were performed using a one-way analysis of variance (ANOVA) followed by a Student's *t*-test or Dunnett's test. The Student's *t*-test was used to analyze the differences between the two groups in **Figures 1–5**. Dunnett's *post hoc* test was used for the results shown in **Figure 6**. Differences with $p < 0.05$ were considered statistically significant.

RESULTS

HPLC Analysis of NYT

Figure 1 shows a 3D-HPLC profile of NYT along with a chemical analysis. Chemical makers, such as paeoniflorin, hesperidin, and glycyrrhizic acid, were used for quality control.

Effect of Treatment With NYT on CORT-Induced Behavioral Abnormalities

To investigate the effect and mechanism of action of NYT on depressive-like behaviors, we used the chronic CORT-induced model of depression, which is widely used for depression

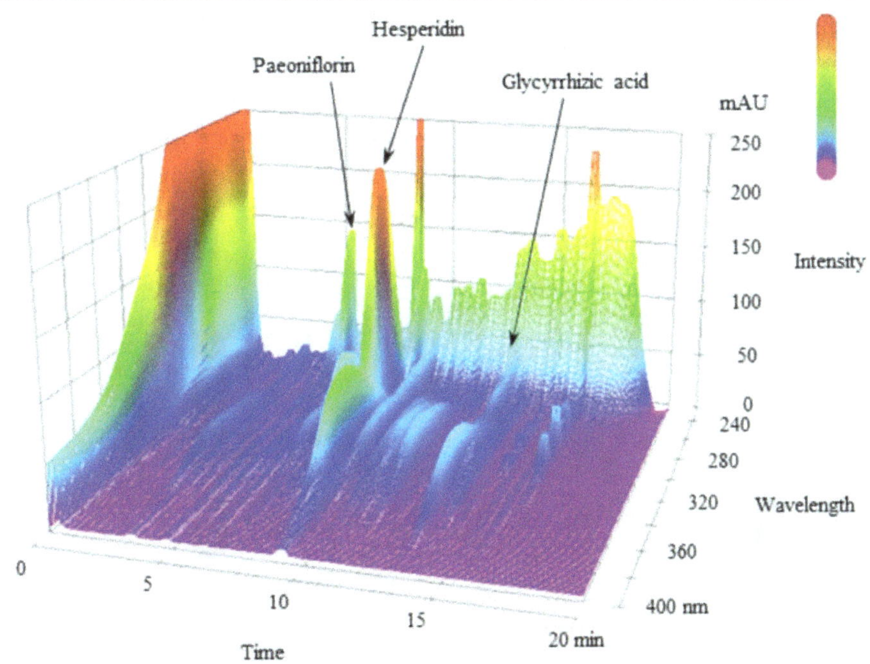

FIGURE 1 | 3D-HPLC profile of NYT. Each chemical marker (paeoniflorin, hesperidin, and glycyrrhizic acid) in the HPLC profile was identified by comparison with retention times and UV spectra (230–400 nm) of their reference standards.

research. To induce the depressive-like symptoms, C57BL/6 mice were treated with CORT in their drinking water for 3 weeks. After CORT treatment finished, mice were treated with NYT or imipramine for 4 weeks, and we examined whether NYT improved CORT-induced behavioral abnormalities by performing behavioral tests.

We first evaluated the effect of a 4-week treatment with NYT on spontaneous locomotor activity and anxiety-related behavior in mice. For this purpose, we performed the open field test for 10 min. In the open field test, chronic exogenous CORT treatment tended to decrease the total distance traveled, but this effect was not significant. Long-term CORT treatment had no effect on the time spent in the center zone. In addition, NYT treatment had no effect on either the total distance traveled or the time spent in the center zone compared with the vehicle-treated group. Treatment with imipramine also did not have any effect on either the total distance traveled or the time spent in the center zone (**Figures 2A,B**).

We next evaluated the effect of a 4-week treatment with NYT on CORT-induced depressive-like behavior. For this purpose, we used three behavioral tests: the tail suspension test, the forced swim test, and the sucrose preference test. In the tail suspension test, chronic exogenous CORT treatment significantly increased the immobility time compared with the control group; this increase continued for 4 weeks after completion of the CORT treatment. In addition, a 4-week treatment with NYT and imipramine significantly decreased immobility time compared with the vehicle-treated group (**Figure 3A**). The latency to immobility was also increased in the NYT and imipramine-treated groups, but there was no difference between the control and CORT-treated groups (**Figure 3C**). In the forced swim test, chronic exogenous CORT treatment significantly increased immobility time compared with the control group; this increase continued for 4 weeks after completion of the CORT treatment. However, chronic exogenous CORT treatment had no effect on the latency to immobility compared with the control group. NYT (500 mg/kg) increased the latency to immobility, but NYT did not improve total immobility time (**Figures 3D,E**). In the sucrose preference test, chronic exogenous CORT treatment significantly decreased the sucrose consumption rate compared with the control group. In addition, treatment with NYT and imipramine significantly improved the sucrose consumption rate (**Figure 3F**).

We further evaluated the effect of NYT on memory disruption in the CORT-induced depression model. For this purpose, we used two behavioral tests: the Y-maze test and the novel object recognition test. In the Y-maze test, chronic exogenous CORT treatment significantly decreased spontaneous alternations, but the number of total arm entries was unchanged compared with the control group. On the other hand, a 4-week treatment with NYT significantly improved spontaneous alternations compared with the vehicle-treated group (**Figures 4A,B**). In the novel object recognition test, mice treated with CORT could not distinguish between familiar and novel objects but the control and NYT-treated groups spent more time with the novel object. The total exploration time was significantly decreased by CORT treatment, but NYT treatment did not improve this when compared with the vehicle-treated group (**Figures 4C,D**).

These results indicate that NYT improves the depressive-like behaviors and memory disruption induced by CORT treatment without affecting locomotor activity.

Effect of NYT on CORT-Induced Inhibition of Hippocampal Neurogenesis in the CORT-Induced Depression Model

To investigate the mechanisms underlying the effects of NYT in this depression model, we focused on adult hippocampal neurogenesis, which contributes to the action of antidepressants. To evaluate the effect of NYT on hippocampal neurogenesis, we measured the BrdU-, Ki67-, DCX-, and GFAP-positive cell numbers in the mouse hippocampal dentate gyrus 4 weeks after NYT treatment started. To evaluate the effect on cell survival, we first measured the BrdU-positive cell number in the dentate gyrus. The mice were treated with 50 mg/kg BrdU for 5 days

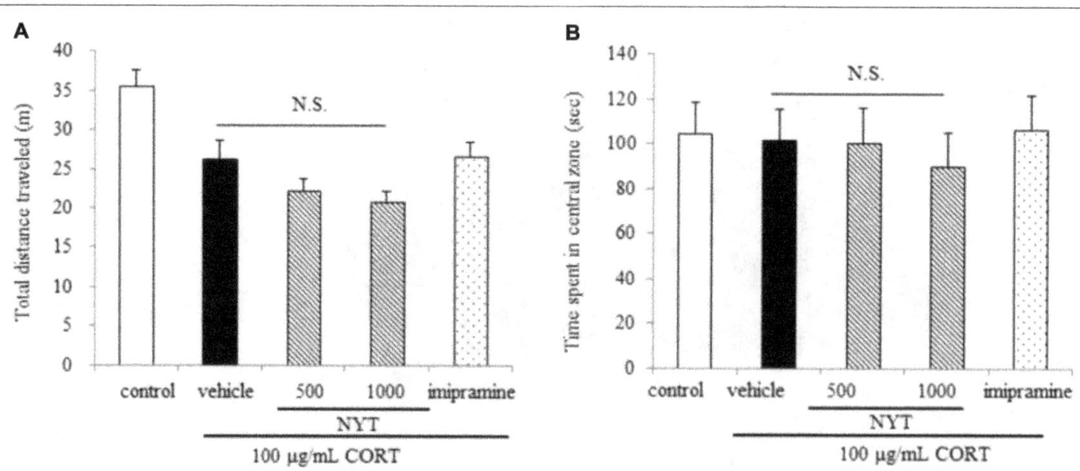

FIGURE 2 | Effect of NYT on locomotor activity and anxiety-like behavior in CORT-treated mice. Effect of repeated treatment with NYT on the total distance traveled **(A)** and the time spent in the center zone **(B)** in the open field test. Data are expressed as mean ± SEM (n = 9–10).

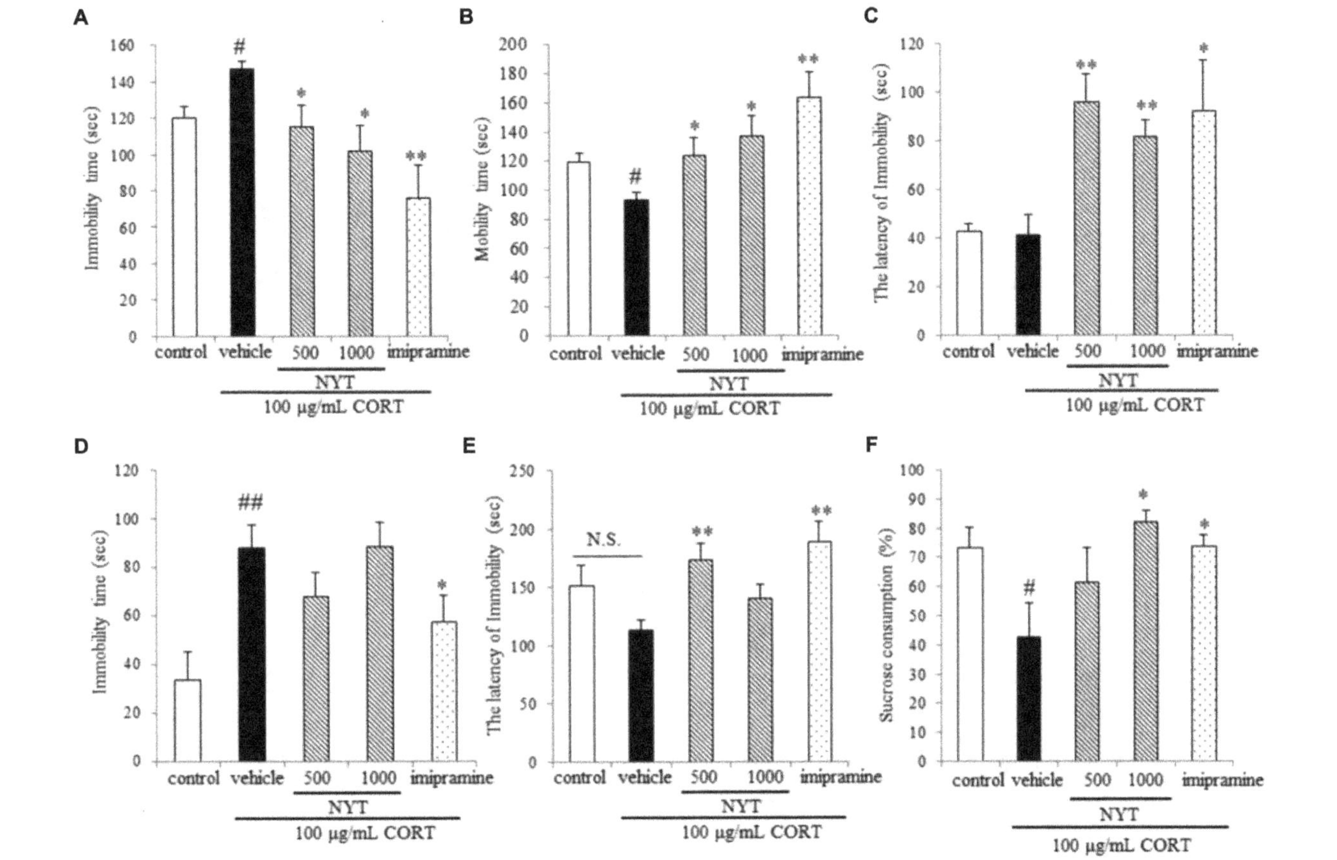

FIGURE 3 | Effect of NYT on depressive-like behaviors in CORT-treated mice. Effect of repeated treatment with NYT on the immobility time **(A)**, mobility time **(B)**, and latency to immobility **(C)** in the tail suspension test. Effect of repeated treatment with NYT on the duration **(D)** and the latency to immobility **(E)** in the forced swim test. **(F)** Effect of repeated treatment with NYT on the sucrose consumption rate in the sucrose preference test. Data are expressed as the mean ± SEM (n = 9–10). $^{\#}p < 0.05$, $^{\#\#}p < 0.01$ vs. the control group; $^{*}p < 0.05$, $^{**}p < 0.01$ vs. the vehicle-treated group, Student's t-test.

before NYT treatment started. Chronic CORT treatment did not change the number of BrdU-positive cells in the dentate gyrus compared with the control group. In addition, 1000 mg/kg NYT treatment tended to increase the number of BrdU-positive cells in the dentate gyrus compared with the vehicle-treated group, but this increase was not statistically significant (**Figure 5A**). This result indicates that NYT treatment did not affect the cell survival rate in the mouse hippocampal dentate gyrus.

To evaluate the effect on cell proliferation, we next measured the number of endogenous mitotic marker Ki67-positive cells in the dentate gyrus. As a result, chronic CORT treatment continued to decrease the number of Ki67-positive cells for 6 weeks after completion of the CORT treatment. The decrease in the Ki67-positive cell number was improved by 4 weeks of NYT treatment (**Figure 5B**). This result indicates that NYT treatment improved cell proliferation in the mouse hippocampus.

We also measured DCX- and GFAP-positive cell numbers in the dentate gyrus. DCX is broadly expressed in neuroblasts and immature neurons in neurogenic regions of the adult brain (Gleeson et al., 1999; Brown et al., 2003). GFAP is an intermediate filament expressed in astrocytes. GFAP is also expressed in the neural stem cells with radial glia-like morphology in the subgranular zone of dentate gyrus, so we counted the GFAP positive cell number in dentate gyrus except subgranular zone. In agreement with other reports (Hill et al., 2015), chronic CORT treatment reduced the number of DCX-positive cells in the dentate gyrus of the adult mouse hippocampus. The decrease in the DCX-positive cell number was improved by 4 weeks of NYT treatment (**Figures 6A,B**). On the other hand, chronic CORT and NYT treatment did not change the number of GFAP-positive cells in the dentate gyrus (**Figures 6C,D**). These results suggest that NYT treatment attenuated the CORT-induced inhibition of hippocampal neurogenesis.

Effect of NYT on CORT-Induced Inhibition of NPC Proliferation as Assessed Using an *in vitro* Assay

To examine whether NYT directly affects NPC proliferation, we isolated NPCs from the adult mouse hippocampus as described in the Materials and Methods. We found that CORT treatment reduced the ratio of BrdU-positive cells to total cells, and this reduction was inhibited by treatment with NYT in a dose-dependent manner (**Figures 7A,B**). These results indicate that

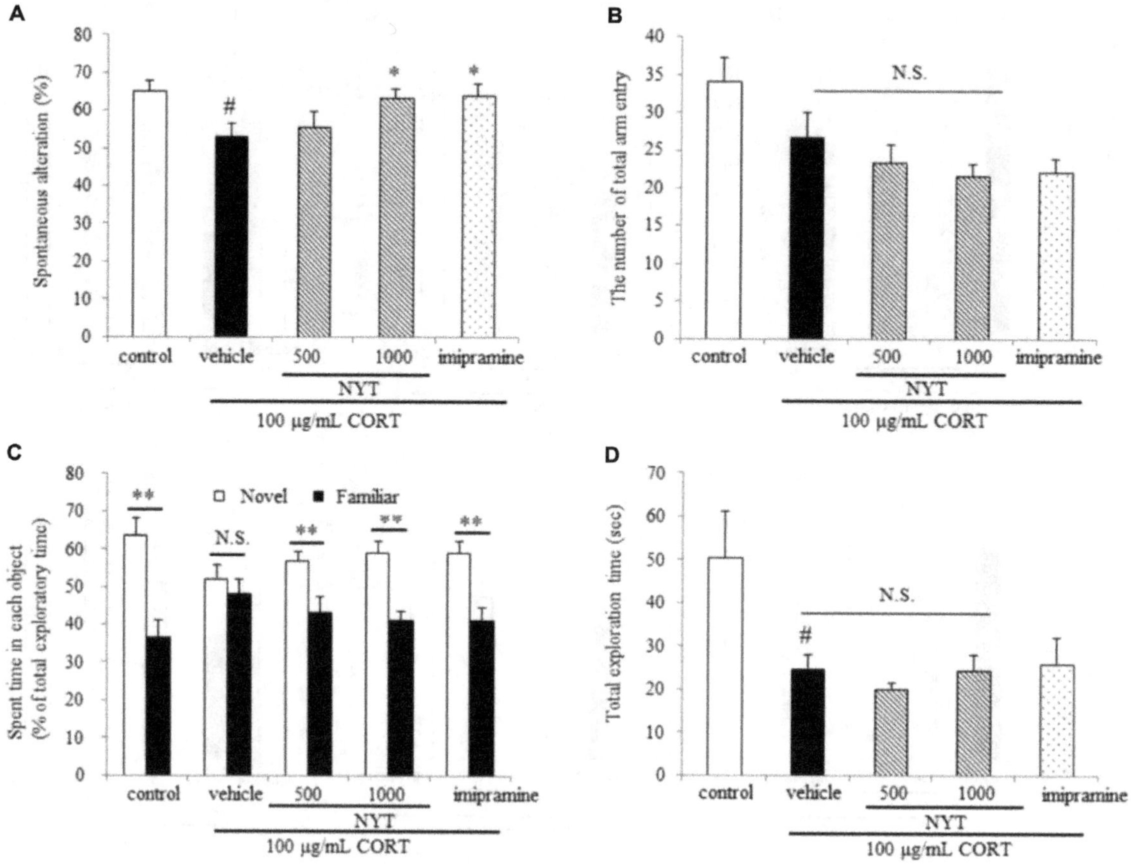

FIGURE 4 | Effect of NYT on memory impairment in CORT-treated mice. Effect of repeated treatment with NYT on spontaneous alternations **(A)** and the number of total arm entries **(B)** in the Y-maze test. #p < 0.05 vs. the control group; *p < 0.05 vs. the vehicle-treated group, Student's t-test. Effect of repeated treatment with NYT on the time spent with each object in the novel recognition test and total exploration time **(C)** is the time spent with each object and **(D)** is the total exploration time in novel object recognition test. Data are expressed as the mean ± SEM (n = 9–10). **p < 0.01 vs. the time spent with a familiar object, Student's t-test.

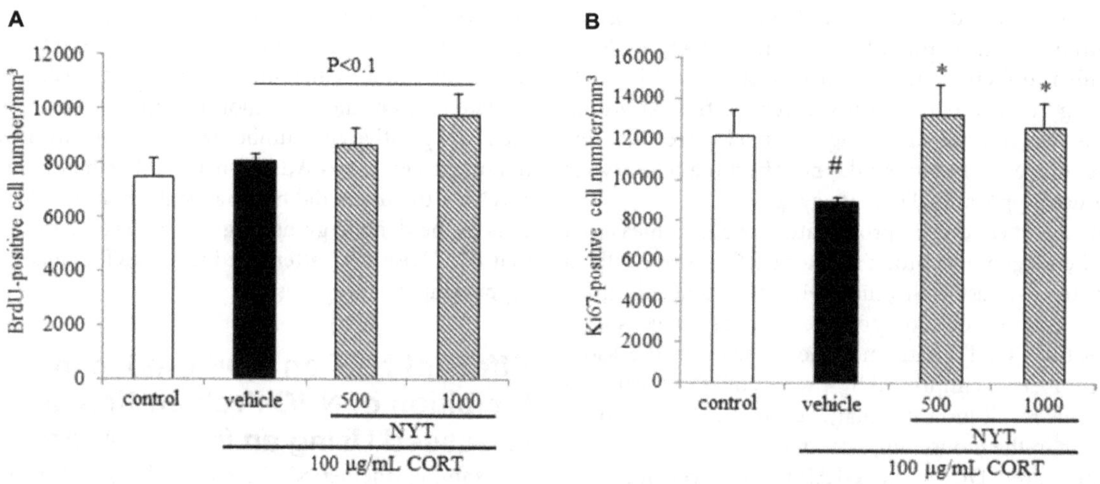

FIGURE 5 | Effect of NYT on cell survival and proliferation in the mouse hippocampus. Effect of repeated treatment with NYT on cell survival and cell proliferation in the dentate gyrus of the mouse hippocampus. Quantitative analyses of the density of BrdU-positive cells **(A)** and Ki67-positive cells **(B)** in the hippocampus. Data are expressed as the mean ± SEM (n = 5). $^{\#}p$ < 0.05 vs. the control group; *p < 0.05 vs. the vehicle-treated group, Student's t-test.

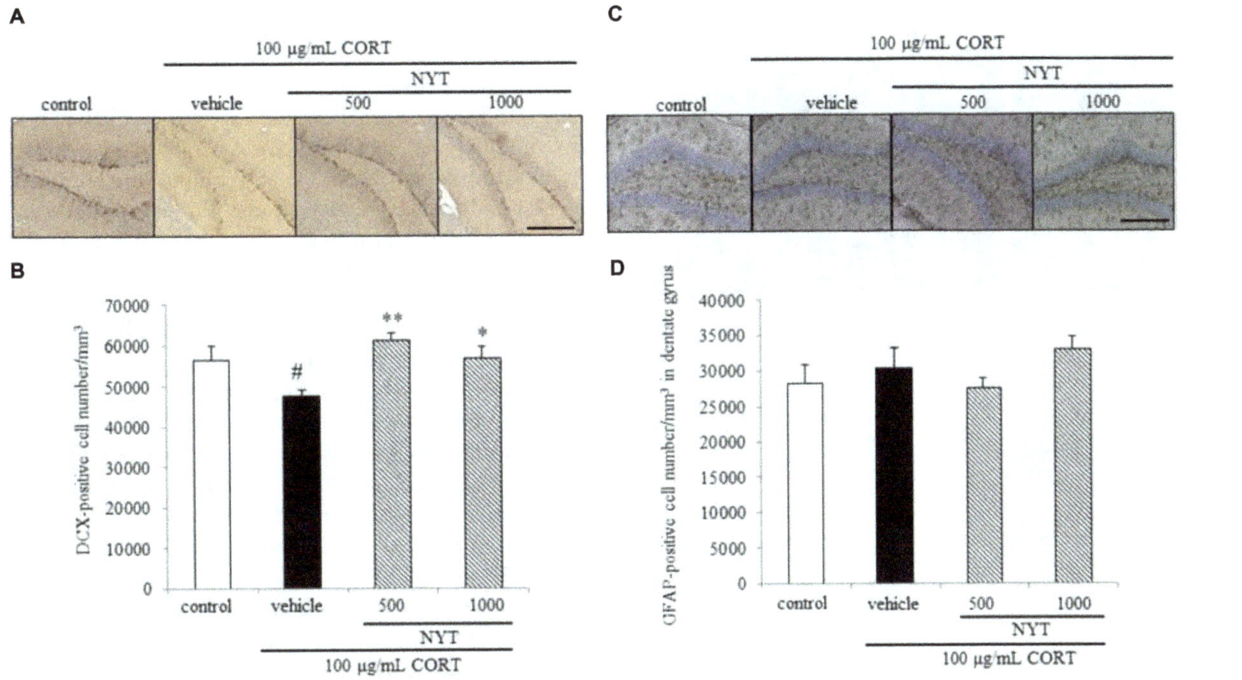

FIGURE 6 | Effect of NYT on the number of immature neurons and astrocytes in the mouse hippocampus. Effect of repeated treatment with NYT on the density of DCX- and GFAP-positive cells (cells/mm^3) in the dentate gyrus of the mouse hippocampus. **(A)** Representative image of DCX staining in the hippocampus. Scale bar = 200 μm. **(B)** Quantitative analyses of the total number of DCX-positive cells in the hippocampus. **(C)** Representative image of GFAP staining in the hippocampus. Scale bar = 200 μm. **(D)** Quantitative analyses of the total number of GFAP-positive cells in the hippocampus. Data are expressed as the mean ± SEM (n = 3–4). $^{\#}p < 0.05$ vs. the control group; $^{*}p < 0.05$, $^{**}p < 0.01$ vs. the vehicle-treated group, Student's t-test.

NYT directly attenuates the reduction in NPC proliferation induced by CORT treatment.

DISCUSSION

Here we showed NYT treatment improved CORT-induced behavioral abnormalities and inhibition of hippocampal neurogenesis.

Depressive disorder is characterized by low mood and/or anhedonia, combined with several cognitive and vegetative symptoms. Chronic stress and HPA-axis dysfunction are generally considered risk factors for the development of psychiatric disorders, including major depression. In addition, stress and stress hormone also impair hippocampal-dependent forms of memory in humans and mice (de Kloet et al., 1999). For example, the administration of stress levels of cortisol to normal human subjects selectively impairs verbal declarative memory without affecting non-verbal memory (Newcomer et al., 1994). Furthermore, a previous study showed that the depressive-like behaviors induced by chronic CORT treatment lasted for at least 3 weeks after treatment finished (Shibata et al., 2015). For these reasons, chronic CORT treatment appears to model a depressive-like state and the memory disruption observed in patients with depression, and the CORT-induced depression model in rodents is considered to be suitable for evaluating the therapeutic effect of drugs for depression. In accordance with a previous study, long-term CORT treatment continued to affect the behavior of mice for 4 weeks after completion of the treatment in the present study. We also showed that NYT treatment increased the latency to immobility in both the tail suspension test and forced swim test, and ameliorated the CORT-induced increase in immobility time in the tail suspension test, but not the forced swim test. We also showed that NYT treatment improved the sucrose consumption rate in the sucrose preference test (**Figure 3**). The latency to immobility has been used to detect the efficacy of fluoxetine, antagonists of glutamate receptors, and cytidine in rats (Contreras et al., 2001; Carlezon et al., 2002; Padovan and Guimarães, 2004), and psychostimulants, such as amphetamine, were reported to have no effects on the duration or latency to immobility in the forced swim test (Castagné et al., 2009). These results suggest that NYT has therapeutic effects on depressive-like symptoms in the CORT-induced depression model. The previous report also showed that fluoxetine treatment affected only the latency but not the duration of immobility in C57BL/6 mice in the forced swim test (Castagné et al., 2009). In another report, fluoxetine was reported to ameliorate the CORT-induced increase in immobility time duration in the tail suspension test but not in the forced swim test (Sawamoto et al., 2016). NYT treatment was previously reported to increase serotonin content in the cerebral cortex and substantia nigra in olfactory bulb lesion mice (Song et al., 2001). Therefore, the mechanism of action of NYT in the CORT-induced depression model might be similar to that of fluoxetine,

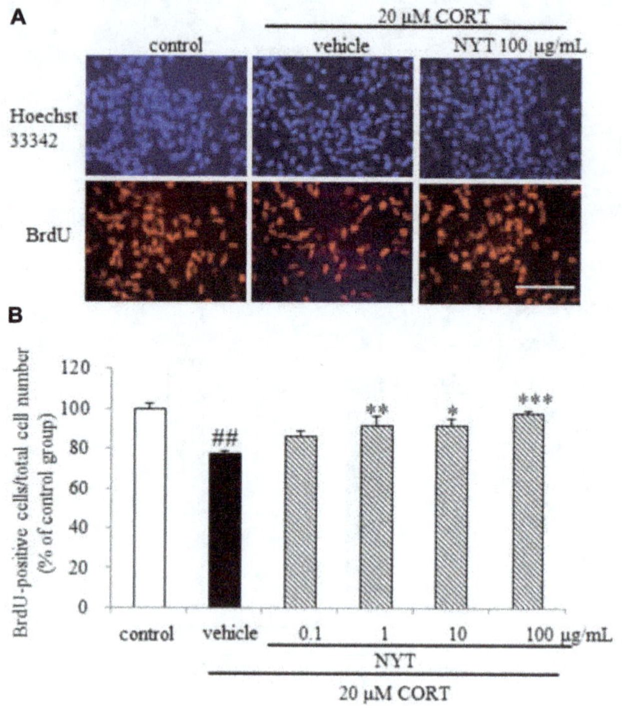

FIGURE 7 | Effect of NYT on CORT-induced inhibition of hippocampal neurogenesis in an *in vitro* model. The dose response of NYT on CORT-induced inhibition of proliferation assessed using BrdU incorporation in the presence of bFGF. **(A)** Representative fluorescence microscopic images of Hoechst 33342 (blue) and BrdU (red) staining after 72-h treatment of NPCs. Scale bar = 100 μm. **(B)** Quantitative analyses of the number of Hoechst 33342- and BrdU-positive cells after 72-h treatment of cells. Data are expressed as the mean ± SEM (n = 4). $^{\#\#}p < 0.01$ vs. the control group, Student's t-test. $^{*}p < 0.05$, $^{**}p < 0.01$, $^{***}p < 0.001$ vs. the vehicle-treated group, Dunnett's test.

in part. Furthermore, we showed that NYT treatment improved CORT-induced memory disruptions in the Y-maze and novel object recognition tests, without affecting locomotor activity (**Figures 2, 4**).

The selective serotonin reuptake inhibitors (SSRIs) and serotonin-norepinephrine reuptake inhibitors are widely used for first-line treatment of depressive disorders. The efficacy of these drugs led to the monoamine hypothesis of depression, which postulates a pathophysiological role of decreased monoamine levels in depression. However, SSRIs do not show beneficial effects until 2 weeks and the effects do not peak until 6–9 weeks after the start of treatment (Artigas et al., 1996; Gardier et al., 1996). In this regard, the requirement for hippocampal neurogenesis for the effects of antidepressants has been investigated using X-irradiation to disrupt hippocampal neurogenesis in the rodent brain (Santarelli et al., 2003). According to previous reports, the dependence of the behavioral effects of antidepressants on neurogenesis is affected by many factors, such as the genetic background of the animals, nature of the antidepressant, and type of behavioral paradigm. In C57BL/6 mice, the behavioral effect of fluoxetine is dependent on hippocampal neurogenesis in the novelty-suppressed feeding test, but not in the forced swim test (David et al., 2009). Since CORT crosses the blood-brain barrier, and the hippocampus is enriched with corticosteroid receptors, certain hippocampal functions are susceptible to disruption by stress (Lucassen et al., 2015). Glucocorticoids and antidepressants have been reported to modulate adult neurogenesis in opposing directions, and hippocampal neurogenesis is required for treatment in the CORT-induced depression model. Previous reports showed that chronic CORT exposure affected the proliferation of progenitor cells in the dentate gyrus of the hippocampus, but not the survival and maturation of newborn cells in C57BL/6 mice (David et al., 2009). Here, we showed that chronic CORT treatment reduced the number of Ki67- and DCX-positive cells, but not BrdU- and GFAP-positive cells in the dentate gyrus. In addition, 4 weeks of treatment with NYT improved the reduction of Ki67- and DCX-positive cell numbers, but had no effect on BrdU- and GFAP-positive cell numbers in the dentate gyrus (**Figures 5, 6**). In addition, we also showed that NYT treatment ameliorated the CORT-induced inhibition of proliferation in an *in vitro* assay (**Figure 7**). In previous reports, chronic CORT treatment decreased the proliferating cell number at 21 days after CORT treatment started (David et al., 2009). However, CORT treatment might have no effect on the proliferating cell number before NYT treatment started because CORT treatment did not change the BrdU-positive cell number in comparison to the control group in the present study. This difference might be derived from the difference in mouse species or protocol used. Immunostaining for DCX reflects the sum of neuronal differentiation and survival of migratory young neurons born 4–14 days before staining. On the other hand, GFAP is expressed in astrocytes, and the number of newborn cells becoming GFAP-positive is only a fraction of the total pool of GFAP-positive cells. In the present study, CORT treatment affected only the DCX-positive cell number, not the GFAP-positive cell number, which might be a result of the different expression times of each marker. Therefore, the effect of NYT on the differentiation of newborn cells into neurons remains unclear in the present study. However, these results indicate that one of the effects of NYT on depressive-like behaviors might in part be related to the improvement of neurogenesis inhibition.

Adult hippocampal neurogenesis under stress is regulated by several signaling pathways activated by glucocorticoids, including the nitric oxide (NO) signaling pathway. A previous study showed that treatment with a synthetic NO synthase (NOS) inhibitor, such as N(G)-nitro-L-arginine methyl ester (L-NAME), improved depressive-like behaviors and hippocampal neurogenesis in mice, and chronic inhibition of NOS increased cell proliferation and had no effect on cell death in the dentate gyrus of the rat hippocampus (Park et al., 2003; Moreno-López et al., 2004). These results suggests that NO may inhibit cell proliferation in the dentate gyrus. There are three different forms of NOS that account for NO production; neuronal NOS (nNOS), inducible NOS (iNOS), endothelial NOS. A previous study showed that CORT treatment increased iNOS but not nNOS expression in the hippocampal dentate gyrus, and an iNOS specific inhibitor improved CORT-induced inhibition of hippocampal neurogenesis (Pinnock et al., 2007). On the other hand, NYT was reported to inhibit activation of nuclear factor kappa-light-chain-enhancer of activated B cells (NF-κB) signaling and iNOS induction induced by interleukin-1beta (IL-1 β) in hepatocytes (Tanaka et al., 2014). In addition, Panax ginseng extract, a component of NYT, was reported to exert antidepressant effects via inhibition of NF-κB activation and iNOS induction (Choi et al., 2018). Although we did not investigate the signaling pathway involved in neurogenesis, NYT might improve hippocampal neurogenesis via inhibition of iNOS induction. However, further experiments are needed to clarify the mechanisms mediating the actions of NYT.

CONCLUSION

This study shows that NYT treatment improves depressive-like behaviors and memory impairments in the chronic CORT exposure model. In addition, NYT also blocks the inhibition of proliferation of hippocampal NPCs induced by CORT in *in vivo* and *in vitro* models. Our findings suggest that these behavioral improvements may be associated with increased hippocampal neurogenesis. Moreover, these results suggest that NYT may be a promising therapeutic agent for depression.

AUTHOR CONTRIBUTIONS

KM, NF, RT, and AI contributed to the conception and design of the study. KM conducted all experiments, analyzed the data, and wrote the manuscript. NF, RT, and AI revised the manuscript. All authors gave final approval for the version of the manuscript that has been submitted for publication.

REFERENCES

Artigas, F., Romero, L., de Montigny, C., and Blier, P. (1996). Acceleration of the effect of selected antidepressant drugs in major depression by 5-HT1A antagonists. *Trends Neurosci.* 19, 378–383. doi: 10.1016/S0166-2236(96)10037-10030

Babu, H., Claasen, J.-H., Kannan, S., Rünker, A. E., Palmer, T., and Kempermann, G. (2011). A protocol for isolation and enriched monolayer cultivation of neural precursor cells from mouse dentate gyrus. *Front. Neurosci.* 5:89. doi: 10.3389/fnins.2011.00089

Brown, J. P., Couillard-Després, S., Cooper-Kuhn, C. M., Winkler, J., Aigner, L., and Kuhn, H. G. (2003). Transient expression of doublecortin during adult neurogenesis. *J. Comp. Neurol.* 467, 1–10. doi: 10.1002/cne.10874

Can, A., Dao, D. T., Terrillion, C. E., Piantadosi, S. C., Bhat, S., and Gould, T. D. (2012). The tail suspension test. *J. Vis. Exp.* 59:e3769. doi: 10.3791/3769

Carlezon, W. A., Pliakas, A. M., Parow, A. M., Detke, M. J., Cohen, B. M., and Renshaw, P. F. (2002). Antidepressant-like effects of cytidine in the forced swim test in rats. *Biol. Psychiatry* 51, 882–889. doi: 10.1016/S0006-3223(01)01344-0

Castagné, V., Porsolt, R. D., and Moser, P. (2009). Use of latency to immobility improves detection of antidepressant-like activity in the behavioral despair test in the mouse. *Eur. J. Pharmacol.* 616, 128–133. doi: 10.1016/j.ejphar.2009.06.018

Choi, J. H., Lee, M. J., Jang, M., Kim, H.-J., Lee, S., Lee, S. W., et al. (2018). Panax ginseng exerts antidepressant-like effects by suppressing neuroinflammatory response and upregulating nuclear factor erythroid 2 related factor 2 signaling in the amygdala. *J. Ginseng Res.* 42, 107–115. doi: 10.1016/j.jgr.2017.04.012

Contreras, C. M., Rodriguez-Landa, J. F., Gutiérrez-García, A. G., and Bernal-Morales, B. (2001). The lowest effective dose of fluoxetine in the forced swim test significantly affects the firing rate of lateral septal nucleus neurones in the rat. *J. Psychopharmacol. Oxf. Engl.* 15, 231–236. doi: 10.1177/026988110101500401

David, D. J., Samuels, B. A., Rainer, Q., Wang, J.-W., Marsteller, D., Mendez, I., et al. (2009). Neurogenesis-dependent and -independent effects of fluoxetine in an animal model of anxiety/depression. *Neuron* 62, 479–493. doi: 10.1016/j.neuron.2009.04.017

de Kloet, C. S., Vermetten, E., Geuze, E., Kavelaars, A., Heijnen, C. J., and Westenberg, H. G. M. (2006). Assessment of HPA-axis function in posttraumatic stress disorder: pharmacological and non-pharmacological challenge tests, a review. *J. Psychiatr. Res.* 40, 550–567. doi: 10.1016/j.jpsychires.2005.08.002

de Kloet, E. R., Joëls, M., and Holsboer, F. (2005). Stress and the brain: from adaptation to disease. *Nat. Rev. Neurosci.* 6, 463–475. doi: 10.1038/nrn1683

de Kloet, E. R., Oitzl, M. S., and Joëls, M. (1999). Stress and cognition: are corticosteroids good or bad guys? *Trends Neurosci.* 22, 422–426.

Gardier, A. M., Malagié, I., Trillat, A. C., Jacquot, C., and Artigas, F. (1996). Role of 5-HT1A autoreceptors in the mechanism of action of serotoninergic antidepressant drugs: recent findings from in vivo microdialysis studies. *Fundam. Clin. Pharmacol.* 10, 16–27. doi: 10.1111/j.1472-8206.1996.tb00145.x

Gleeson, J. G., Lin, P. T., Flanagan, L. A., and Walsh, C. A. (1999). Doublecortin is a microtubule-associated protein and is expressed widely by migrating neurons. *Neuron* 23, 257–271. doi: 10.1016/S0896-6273(00)80778-3

Gourley, S. L., Kiraly, D. D., Howell, J. L., Olausson, P., and Taylor, J. R. (2008). Acute hippocampal brain-derived neurotrophic factor restores motivational and forced swim performance after corticosterone. *Biol. Psychiatry* 64, 884–890. doi: 10.1016/j.biopsych.2008.06.016

Hill, A. S., Sahay, A., and Hen, R. (2015). Increasing adult hippocampal neurogenesis is sufficient to reduce anxiety and depression-like behaviors. *Neuropsychopharmacology* 40, 2368–2378. doi: 10.1038/npp.2015.85

Kobayashi, J., Seiwa, C., Sakai, T., Gotoh, M., Komatsu, Y., Yamamoto, M., et al. (2003). Effect of a traditional Chinese herbal medicine, Ren-Shen-Yang-Rong-Tang (Japanese name: ninjin-Youei-To), on oligodendrocyte precursor cells from aged-rat brain. *Int. Immunopharmacol.* 3, 1027–1039. doi: 10.1016/S1567-5769(03)00101-102

Kudoh, C., Arita, R., Honda, M., Kishi, T., Komatsu, Y., Asou, H., et al. (2016). Effect of ninjin'yoeito, a Kampo (traditional Japanese) medicine, on cognitive impairment and depression in patients with Alzheimer's disease: 2 years of observation. *Psychogeriatrics* 16, 85–92. doi: 10.1111/psyg.12125

Lucassen, P. J., Oomen, C. A., Naninck, E. F. G., Fitzsimons, C. P., van Dam, A.-M., Czeh, B., et al. (2015). Regulation of adult neurogenesis and plasticity by (early) stress, glucocorticoids, and inflammation. *Cold Spring Harb. Perspect. Biol.* 7:a021303. doi: 10.1101/cshperspect.a021303

Moreno-López, B., Romero-Grimaldi, C., Noval, J. A., Murillo-Carretero, M., Matarredona, E. R., and Estrada, C. (2004). Nitric oxide is a physiological inhibitor of neurogenesis in the adult mouse subventricular zone and olfactory bulb. *J. Neurosci.* 24, 85–95. doi: 10.1523/JNEUROSCI.1574-03.2004

Murphy, B. E. (1997). Antiglucocorticoid therapies in major depression: a review. *Psychoneuroendocrinology* 22(Suppl. 1), S125–S132.

Newcomer, J. W., Craft, S., Hershey, T., Askins, K., and Bardgett, M. E. (1994). Glucocorticoid-induced impairment in declarative memory performance in adult humans. *J. Neurosci.* 14, 2047–2053. doi: 10.1523/JNEUROSCI.14-04-02047.1994

Padovan, C. M., and Guimarães, F. S. (2004). Antidepressant-like effects of NMDA-receptor antagonist injected into the dorsal hippocampus of rats. *Pharmacol. Biochem. Behav.* 77, 15–19. doi: 10.1016/j.pbb.2003.09.015

Park, C., Sohn, Y., Shin, K. S., Kim, J., Ahn, H., and Huh, Y. (2003). The chronic inhibition of nitric oxide synthase enhances cell proliferation in the adult rat hippocampus. *Neurosci. Lett.* 339, 9–12. doi: 10.1016/S0304-3940(02)01422-2

Pinnock, S. B., Balendra, R., Chan, M., Hunt, L. T., Hunt, L. T., Turner-Stokes, T., et al. (2007). Interactions between nitric oxide and corticosterone in the regulation of progenitor cell proliferation in the dentate gyrus of the adult rat. *Neuropsychopharmacology* 32, 493–504. doi: 10.1038/sj.npp.1301245

Rao, R. V., Ellerby, H. M., and Bredesen, D. E. (2004). Coupling endoplasmic reticulum stress to the cell death program. *Cell Death Differ.* 11, 372–380. doi: 10.1038/sj.cdd.4401378

Santarelli, L., Saxe, M., Gross, C., Surget, A., Battaglia, F., Dulawa, S., et al. (2003). Requirement of hippocampal neurogenesis for the behavioral effects of antidepressants. *Science* 301, 805–809. doi: 10.1126/science.1083328

Sapolsky, R. M. (2000). Glucocorticoids and hippocampal atrophy in neuropsychiatric disorders. *Arch. Gen. Psychiatry* 57, 925–935. doi: 10.1001/archpsyc.57.10.925

Sawamoto, A., Okuyama, S., Yamamoto, K., Amakura, Y., Yoshimura, M., Nakajima, M., et al. (2016). 3,5,6,7,8,3,4-heptamethoxyflavone, a citrus flavonoid, ameliorates corticosterone-induced depression-like behavior and restores brain-derived neurotrophic factor expression, neurogenesis, and neuroplasticity in the Hippocampus. *Molecules* 21:541. doi: 10.3390/molecules21040541

Seiwa, C., Yamamoto, M., Tanaka, K., Fukutake, M., Ueki, T., Takeda, S., et al. (2007). Restoration of FcRgamma/Fyn signaling repairs central nervous system demyelination. *J. Neurosci. Res.* 85, 954–966. doi: 10.1002/jnr.21196

Shibata, S., Iinuma, M., Soumiya, H., Fukumitsu, H., Furukawa, Y., and Furukawa, S. (2015). A novel 2-decenoic acid thioester ameliorates corticosterone-induced depression- and anxiety-like behaviors and normalizes reduced hippocampal signal transduction in treated mice. *Pharmacol. Res. Perspect.* 3:e00132. doi: 10.1002/prp2.132

Song, Q.-H., Toriizuka, K., Iijima, K., Watanabe, K., and Cyong, J.-C. (2001). Effect of Ninjin-yoei-to (Rensheng-Yangrong-Tang), a Kampo medicine, on brain monoamine and nerve growth factor contents in mice with olfactory bulb lesions. *Journa Tradit. Med.* 18, 64–70.

Tanaka, Y., Kaibori, M., Miki, H., Oishi, M., Nakatake, R., Tokuhara, K., et al. (2014). Japanese kampo medicine, ninjinyoeito, inhibits the induction of iNOS gene expression in proinflammatory cytokine-stimulated hepatocytes. *Br. J. Pharm. Res.* 4, 2226–2244. doi: 10.9734/BJPR/2014/13301

Yabe, T., Tuchida, H., Kiyohara, H., Takeda, T., and Yamada, H. (2003). Induction of NGF synthesis in astrocytes by onjisaponins of *Polygala tenuifolia*, constituents of kampo (Japanese herbal) medicine, Ninjin-yoei-to. *Phytomed. Int. J. Phytother. Phytopharm.* 10, 106–114. doi: 10.1078/094471103321659799

17

Protective Effects of Total Glycoside from *Rehmannia glutinosa* Leaves on Diabetic Nephropathy Rats via Regulating the Metabolic Profiling and Modulating the TGF-β1 and Wnt/β-Catenin Signaling Pathway

Xinxin Dai, Shulan Su, Hongdie Cai, Dandan Wei, Hui Yan, Tianyao Zheng, Zhenhua Zhu, Er-xin Shang, Sheng Guo, Dawei Qian and Jin-ao Duan**

Jiangsu Collaborative Innovation Center of Chinese Medicinal Resources Industrialization, State Key Laboratory Cultivation Base for TCM Quality and Efficacy, Nanjing University of Chinese Medicine, Nanjing, China

***Correspondence:**
Shulan Su
sushulan1974@163.com
Jin-ao Duan
dja@njutcm.edu.cn

Rehmannia glutinosa Libosch (RG), is officially listed in the *Chinese Pharmacopoeia* and is widely used in China. The leaves of RG (LR) is an important vegetative organ of the plant. At present, the total glycosides of RG (TLR) were extracted from RG, and developed a national second class of new drugs to the Dihuangye total glycoside capsule (DTG). Additionally, DTG has the effect of nourishing yin and tonifying kidney, promoting blood circulation and blood cooling, and applicable to chronic glomerulonephritis mild to Qi and Yin Deficiency. Moreover, diabetic nephropathy (DN) rats model was induced by intraperitoneal injection of a small dose of streptozotocin (45 mg/kg) and high-fat diet and plus 5% glucose drinking water. Over 15 days, after oral administration TLR and DTG in DN rats, samples from serum, urine and kidney were collected for biochemical indicators measurements, pathological analysis, western blotting and metabolomics. Therefore, the analytical results of biochemical indicators, histopathological observations and western blotting showed that TLR and DTG exhibited a significant effect in renal protection. And 27 endogenous metabolites (12 in serum and 15 in urine) could be tentatively identified in the process of DN in rats using metabolomics method. Those endogenous metabolites were chiefly involved in sphingolipid metabolism; pentose, glucuronate interconversion; terpenoid backbone biosynthesis; purine metabolism and retinol metabolism. After drug intervention, these endogenous metabolites turned back to normal level some extent ($P < 0.05$). Furthermore, TLR and DTG prevent high glucose-induced glomerular mesangial cells (GMCs) by inhibiting TGF-β1 and Wnt/β-catenin signaling pathway, providing a powerful supports to develop a new therapeutic agent for DN. This study paved the way for further exploration of the pathogenesis of DN, early diagnosis and the evaluation of curative effect.

Keywords: total glycoside extracted from leaves of *Rehmannia*, Dihuangye total glycoside capsule, metabolomics, diabetic nephropathy, TGF-β1, Wnt/β-catenin signaling pathway

INTRODUCTION

Traditional Chinese medicine (TCM) with multi-components and multi-targets has been used in clinical for over 4000 years in China due to its efficacy and low side-effects (Yokozawa et al., 1986). RG, belonging to Scrophulariaceae family, is widely distributed in China, and its root tubers are commonly called "Dihuang" in China. So far large quantity of iridoids and phenylethanoid glycosides have been isolated from the root and leaves of RG, together with other types of active principles. "Dihuang" has the significant effects on cardiovascular diseases (Liu et al., 2011), neuroprotection (Cai et al., 2011), diabetes and its complications (Zhang et al., 2014), osteoporosis (Zhang Z. et al., 2013), and hyperlipidemia (Zhang R. et al., 2013). Currently, with the deep exploration of RG, the leaves of RG (LR) is gaining increased attention around the world. In order to find the possibility to be used as medicine, people are beginning to pay attention to the development and utilization of LR. At present, LR is officially listed in the *Beijing standard of Chinese herbal medicines*, and it has the effect of heat-clearing, promoting blood circulation, supplementing Qi and nourishing yin and tonifying kidney (Beijing Municipal Health Bureau, 1988). The total glycosides of RG (TLR) were extracted from RG. The major active components of DTG is the phenylethanoid glycosides, which is extracted from LR, and phenylethanoid glycosides are a class of natural glycosides containing hydroxyl groups, methoxy substituted phenethyl or cinnamoyl groups, usually containing β-glucose as the parent nucleus, and are widely present in dicotyledonous plants (Jiménez and Riguera, 1994). DTG can increased glomerular permeability and reduced glomerular hyperfiltration, thus reducing proteinuria and the protection of renal function (Shen et al., 2010).

Diabetic nephropathy (DN) is one of the most common microangiopathy in diabetic patients, and renal fibrosis is the main cause of death in patients with DN (Lv et al., 2015). At present, the clinical diagnosis of DN mainly depending on the urinary albumin excretion rate detection, however, urinary microalbumin content may be affected by many factors such as obesity, insulin resistance and there are limitations (Weir, 2007). Therefore, it is necessary to find an early diagnostic marker with high sensitivity and specificity. To the best of our knowledge, there is no unified theory about the pathogenesis of DN. The current research focuses on the aspects of glucose metabolism, lipid metabolism, oxidative stress (Oberg et al., 2004; Chen and Quilley, 2008; Balakumar et al., 2009), and so on. Studies have shown that Wnt/β-catenin signaling plays a prominent role in cell differentiation, adhesion, survival, and apoptosis and is involved in glomerular cell proliferation and renal fibrosis, which affected the occurrence and development of DN (Xiao et al., 2013).

Metabolomics, based on the dynamic changes of endogenous metabolites in organisms, revealing the overall physiological status in responding to pathophysiological stimuli or genetic, environmental, or lifestyle factors (Pereira and Chang, 2004), and it has been widely used in the diagnosis of diseases, marker screening and pathogenesis research as a kind of technical means to study the dynamic metabolism of biological organism or tissue cells in recent years (Odunsi et al., 2005; Hodavance et al., 2007; Hwang et al., 2010). Metabolomics is regarded as "biochemical phenotypes" of the whole functional state of organism, and can be real-time, sensitive and real to express the response and regulation of the overall functional state of the organism under various external factors (Nicholson and Lindon, 2008).

Therefore, this study parallel simultaneous analysis of DN rats and normal rats of serum and urine, markers of different metabolites, and to study the effect of DTG and TLR on DN by analyzing the regulation of different metabolites. Moreover, the high glucose-induced GMCs model *in vitro* evaluate the efficacy of DTG and TLR on DN by determination of TGF-β1, Wnt4 and β-catenin proteins expression levels.

MATERIALS AND METHODS

Chemicals and Instruments

UPLC-grade acetonitrile was purchased from Merck (Darmstadt, Germany), formic acid and STZ were purchased from Sigma-Aldrich (Sigma, St. Louis, MO, United States). HPLC-grade acteoside was purchased from the National Institutes for Food and Drug Control (Beijing, China) and the purity is above 98%. BUN reagent kit, LDL reagent kit, T-CHO reagent kit, TG reagent kit, Scr reagent kit, UP reagent kit, serum β2-microglobulin (β2-MG) reagent kit were bought from Nanjing Jiancheng Bioengineering Institute (Nanjing, China). Huangkui capsule was purchased from SZYY Group Pharmaceutical Limited; Irbesartan was purchased from Shenzhen Haibin Pharmaceutical Co., Ltd. DMEM and F12 were purchased from GIBCO, America; TGF-β1, Wnt4 and β-catenin first antibody were purchased from Abcam (Cambridge, United Kingdom). All other chemicals and reagents used in this study were of analytical grade and made in China.

Waters Acquity^{TM} Ultra Performance LC system (Waters, United States) equipped with a Quattro Micro MS spectrometer and a Waters Xevo TM G2 QTof MS (Waters MS Technologies, Manchester, NH, United States). Deionized water was purified on a Milli-Q system (Millipore, Bedford, MA, United States). Mass Lynx v4.1 workstation was adopted to analyze the data, and Ultra-high speed centrifuge at low temperature (Thermo Scientific, United Kingdom); DMI3000M microscope (Leica, Germany) were used.

Preparation of TLR and DTG

The plant material, LR were purchased from Henan farmers market, and identified by the Prof. Jin-Ao Duan (Department of Nanjing University of Chinese Medicine). Fresh LR were

Abbreviations: β2-MG, serum β2-microglobulin; BUN, serum urea nitrogen; C, control group; DHYH, TLR high dose group; DHYL, TLR low dose group; DN, diabetic nephropathy; DTG, Dihuangye total glycoside capsule; FBG, Fasting blood glucose; GMC, glomerular mesangial cells; HE, hematoxylin eosin; HK, Huangkui capsule group; JNH, DTG high dose group; JNL, DTG low dose group; LDL, low density lipoprotein; M, model group; MRHTG, Acteoside; RG, *Rehmannia glutinosa* Libosch; Scr, serum creatinine; STZ, streptozotocin; T-CHO, total cholesterol; TCM, Traditional Chinese medicine; TG, triglyceride; TLR, total glycoside extracted from leaves of *Rehmannia*; UP, urine protein; YX, Irbesartan group.

vacuum-dried in 80°C and ground into powder. The vacuum-dried LR (500 g) was extracted with 6 L 80% alcohol three times and 2 h each time with reflux extraction. In rotary evaporation instrument reduced pressure concentration, as TLR low dose oral solution. Concentrated on dose in the twice as high dose oral solution.

Before the experiment, the chemical of TLR and DTG were previously established by the UPLC-TQ-MS. And the main components of TLR identified mainly as catalpol, ajugol, and acteoside, the contents of above components were 0.6326%, 0.4105%, and 0.6833%, respectively. DTG were bought from Sichuan Meidakang Pharmaceutical Co., Ltd., the main component is acteoside, and the content of the acteoside in the DTG was 13.61%. The MRM chromatogram and structure of catalpol, ajugol and acteoside were presented in **Figure 1**. Moreover, we made the content of acteoside in TLR oral solution and DTG oral solution is consistent for rats.

Experimental Animals

All experiments were conducted with male Sprague–Dawley (SD) rats weighing 200–240 g purchased from Experimental animal center of Zhejiang Province (Zhejiang, China; Certificate no. SCXK 2014-0001). Animals were housed in cages with a constant humidity (ca. 60% ± 2%) and temperature (ca. 23 ± 2°C) and with a light/dark cycle of 12 h. The animals were underwent an adaptation period of 7 days, during which they were allowed unlimited access to chow and tap water.

After the 7-day acclimation period, animals were randomly divided into eight groups with 6 in each group: control group (normal saline, C), model group (normal saline, M), Huangkui capsule group (0.75 g/kg·d, HK), Irbesartan group (27 mg/kg·d, YX), TLR low dose group (4.3 g/kg·d, DHYL), TLR high dose group (7.2 g/kg·d, DHYH), DTG low dose group (216 mg/kg·d, JNL), DTG high dose group (360 mg/kg·d, JNH). Expect for control group rats, the rats in other groups were fed with high-fat diet (59% basic mice feed, 20% sugar, 18% lard, and 3% egg yolk) and 5% glucose water for 21 days, then, the rats were injected intraperitoneally with STZ (45 mg/kg) dissolved in 0.1 mol/L sodium citrate buffer (pH 4.5) to induce DN model. 72 h after the injection of STZ, rats with FBG levels of 16.7 mmol/L and above were considered to be in diabetic state and were used for the study. Moreover, in this study, Huangkui capsule and Irbesartan were selected as positive control drug. The animal dose of Huangkui capsule and Irbesartan were extrapolated from the human daily dose, using the body surface area normalization method. The formula for dose translation was as follows: human clinical equivalent dose of medicine × 70 × 0.018/0.2. The dose of JNL and JNH were three times and five times of the clinical equivalent dose, respectively. Moreover, TLR are about 20 times the corresponding dose of DTG. Then, the rats were given corresponding drug once a day by gastric gavage for 15 days, and the control group rats were given the same volume of saline at the same time. This study was carried out in accordance with the recommendations of the Institutional Animal Ethics Committee of Nanjing University of Chinese Medicine (Nanjing, China). The protocol was approved by the Institutional Animal Ethics Committee of Nanjing University of Chinese Medicine.

Sample Collection

During the experimental period, body weights were recorded at 3-days intervals, FBG levels were measured by a One Touch Ultra II blood glucose monitoring system (Life Scan, Milpitas, CA, United States) by tail vein at 3-days intervals (at 8 a.m). Prior to the experiments, rats were put individually in the

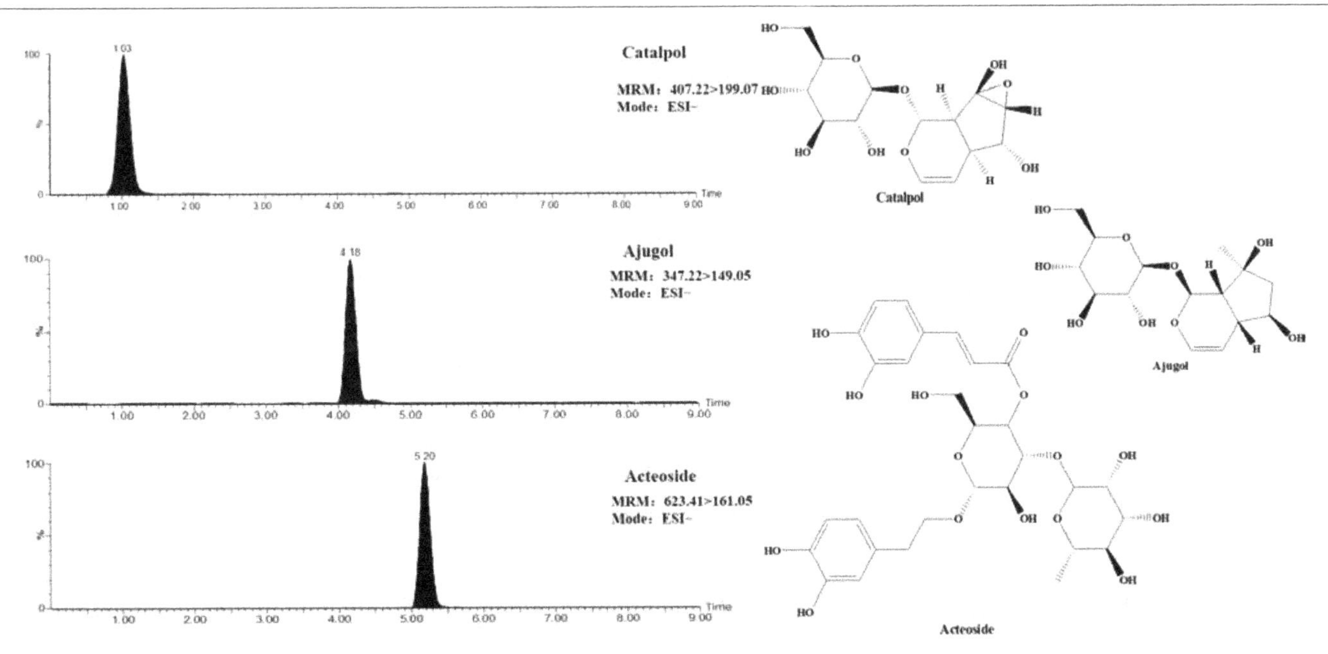

FIGURE 1 | MRM chromatogram and structure of catalpol, ajugol, and acteoside.

metabolism cages for 24-h urinary collection, all urine samples were immediately centrifugated at 3,000 rpm for 10 min after collection, and the supernatants were separated and stored at −80°C until analysis. At the end of study, rats were sacrificed under anesthesia by intraperitoneal injection of chloral hydrate (330 mg/kg body weight), and blood was collected for concentration of biochemical parameters and metabolomics study. Then, the blood samples were centrifugated at 3,000 rpm for 10 min, and the serum samples were separated and stored at −80°C until analysis. The right kidney was removed with one piece fixed with 10% neutral-buffered formalin for histologic examination. Renal cortex was isolated from the other piece and frozen in liquid nitrogen for western blotting analysis.

Biochemical Indicators Measurements, Pathological Analysis and Western Blotting

The therapeutic efficacy of TLR and DTG on DN rats was evaluated for the levels of UP in urine and FBG, LDL, T-CHO, TG, Scr, BUN and β2-MG in serum, which were detected followed by the description supplied by kits manufacturer. Part of the renal cortex were performed for HE staining in order to observe pathological changes in renal tissue, degrees of fibrosis tissue hyperplasia, structures of glomeruli and tubules through electron microscope (200×), and another part of the renal tissues samples were analyzed by western blotting for detecting the expression levels of Wnt4, β-catenin and TGF-β1 protein.

GMC Cells Culture

Glomerular mesangial cells were provided by Nanjing KeyGen Biotechnology Development Co., Ltd. The complete medium was low glucose DMEM with 10% FBS and 1% penicillin-streptomycin solution. The GMCs were cultured in 37°C, 5% CO_2 and saturated humidity. The GMCs were plated on 96-well plates, pretreated with DMEM low glucose (5 $mmol{\cdot}L^{-1}$), incubated at 37°C and 5% CO_2 for 6 h, and then were synchronized. The experimental groups were divided as follows: control group (C), which without intervention factor; model group (M), which cells were cultured in high glucose (30 $mmol{\cdot}L^{-1}$) DMEM solution; Acteoside (MRHTG) group (acteoside is stable in 0.1% DMSO in 24 h by analyzing its contents), TLR group (DHY) and DTG group (JN) at five dosages (5, 10, 25, 50, and 100 $\mu mol{\cdot}L^{-1}$), respectively. Cellular count was used to detect the number of cells in each group after incubation for 48 h, and then determined the total protein content of each group by BCA kit. The ratio of total cell protein/cell number was calculated and expressed as the total amount of protein (μg) contained in 10^3 cells as an indicator of GMCs hypertrophy. Moreover, these cells were prepared for the western blotting to examine the expression levels of TGF-β1, Wnt4 and β-catenin protein.

Sample Preparation and UPLC-QTOF/MS Analysis

All serum and urine samples were thawed at room temperature before preparation. The 300 μL acetonitrile was added to 100 μL serum samples to precipitated protein, and vigorously mixed for 60 s. The 100 μL acetonitrile was added to 100 μL urine samples to remove proteins and vigorously mixed for 30 s. All the samples were centrifuged at 13,000 rpm for 10 min at 4°C. Finally, the supernatant was injected to UPLC-QTOF/MS analysis.

Metabolites separation was performed using a Waters Acquity™ Ultra Performance LC system (Waters, United States) equipped with a Waters Xevo™ G2 Q/TOF-MS (Waters MS Technologies, Manchester, NH, United States). An aliquot of 2 μL of sample solution was injected on an Acquity UPLC BEH C_{18} (100 mm × 2.1 mm, 1.7 μm, Waters Corporation, Milford, CT, United States) at 35°C and the flowrate was 0.4 mL/min. The optimal mobile phase consisted of water (A) (containing 0.1% formic acid) and acetonitrile (B). The optimized UPLC elution conditions for serum were: 0 ∼ 3 min, 95% ∼ 55% A; 4 ∼ 13 min, 55% ∼ 5% A; 13 ∼ 14 min, 5% A. The optimized UPLC elution conditions for urine were: 0 ∼ 8 min, 95% ∼ 70% A; 8 ∼ 11 min, 70% ∼ 30% A; 11 ∼ 13 min, 30% ∼ 5% A; 13 ∼ 14 min, 5% A. The autosampler was maintained at 4°C.

Mass spectrometry was performed using a Xevo™ G2 QTof (Waters MS Technologies, Manchester, NH, United States), a quadrupole and orthogonal acceleration time-of- flight tandem mass spectrometer. Leucine-enkephalin was used as the lock mass generating an $[M+H]^+$ ion (*m/z* 556.2771) and $[M\text{-}H]^-$ ion (*m/z* 554.2615) in positive and negative modes, respectively. The concentration of Leucine-enkephalin 200 pg/mL and the infusion flow rate was 100 μL/min to ensure accuracy during the MS analysis via a syringe pump. Data were collected in centroid mode from 100 to 1000 *m/z*. For both positive and negative electrospray modes, the capillary and cone voltage were set at 3.0 kV and 30 V, respectively. The desolvation gas was set to 600 L/h at a temperature of 350°C, the cone gas was set to 50 L/h and the source temperature was set to 120°C. The data acquisition rate was set to 30 ms, with a 0.02 s interscan delay.

In addition, 10 serum (or urine) samples were randomly selected from each group and mixed together as the quality control (QC) samples, respectively. The QC sample was used to optimize the condition of UPLC-QTOF/MS, as it contained most information of whole samples. The QC samples were injected six times at the beginning of the running in order to condition or equilibrate the system and then every ten samples to further monitor the stability of the analysis. Every day, after the instrument was calibrated, the QC sample was firstly analyzed to test the stability of the instrument in order to ensure consistent performance of the system.

Metabolomics Data Processing and Analysis

All of the data acquisition and analyses of data were controlled by Waters MassLynx v4.1 software. The multivariate data matrix was analyzed by *EZ*info software 2.0 (Waters Corp., Milford, CT, United States). The main parameters include: retention time range 0 ∼ 14 min; mass ratio *m/z* 100 ∼ 1000, mass tolerance range 0.01 Da, peak intensity threshold 50,

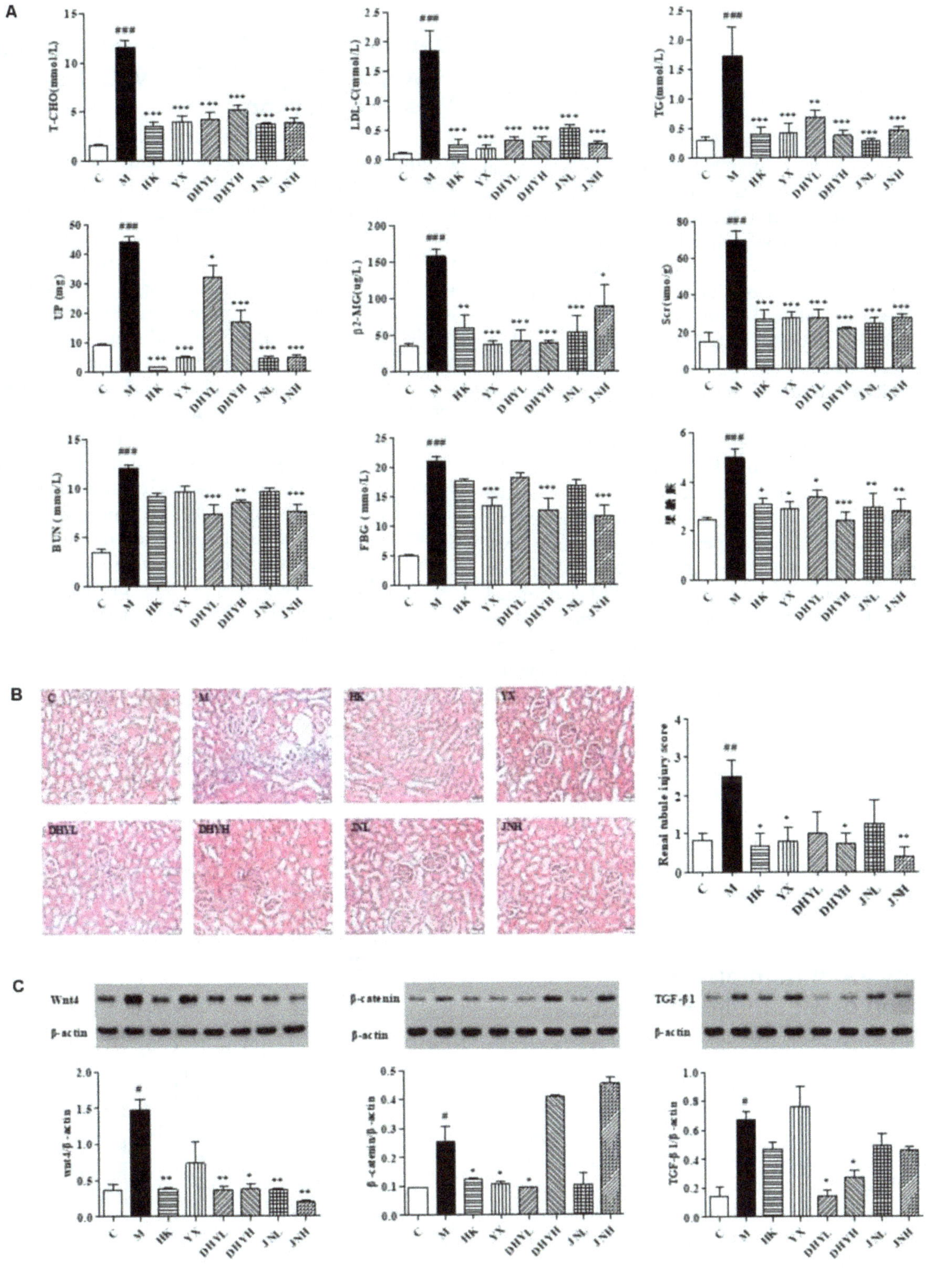

FIGURE 2 | Determination of biochemical indicators and analysis of renal pathological section and Western blotting among control group, model group and administered group. **(A)** Determination of FBG, LDL, T-CHO, TG, Scr, β2-MG in serum, and BUN, UP in urine. **(B)** HE staining of kidney biopsy (200×). **(C)** Western blotting analysis of renal tissues of control group, HK group, YX group, DHYL group, DHYH group, JNL group and JNH group. $^{\#}P < 0.05$, $^{\#\#}P < 0.01$, $^{\#\#\#}P < 0.001$: DN model group vs. control group; $^{*}P < 0.05$, $^{**}P < 0.01$, $^{***}P < 0.001$: after treatment by HK, YX, DHYL, DHYH, JNL and JNH vs. DN model group. Data were presented as the mean ± SE.

quality window 0.05 Da, retention time windows 0.20 min, automatic detection of 5% peak height and noise. The intensity of each ion was normalized with respect to the total ion count to generate a data matrix that consisted of the retention time, *m/z* value, and the normalized peak area.

The resultant data matrices were introduced to *EZinfo* 2.0 software for principal component analysis (PCA), partial least-squares-discriminant analysis (PLS-DA) and orthogonal projection to latent structures (OPLS-DA) analysis. From the OPLS-DA, various metabolites could be identified as being responsible for the separation between control group and model group and were therefore viewed as potential markers. Potential markers of interest were extracted from S-plots constructed following analysis with OPLS-DA, and variables that had significant contributions to discrimination between groups were subjected to further identification of the molecular formula.

The variable importance (VIP) in the projection value is a weighted sum of squares of the PLS weights, and the variables with VIP >1 were considered to be influential for the separation of samples in the score plots generated from OPLS-DA analysis. In all experiments, confidence level was set at 95% to determine the significance of difference ($P < 0.05$). Those variables were eventually selected as potential biomarkers. The PLS-DA score plots were described by the cross-validation parameter R^2Y and Q^2, which represents the total explained variation for the X matrix and the predictability of the model, respectively. Excellent models are obtained when the cumulative values of R^2Y and Q^2 are above 0.8. The relative distances between administration groups and control group from PLS-DA score plot was calculated with the average value (x-axis and y-axis) of all samples of the control group as the referenced point (Li et al., 2010). This quantitative value was used as an indicator of pharmacodynamic evaluation of metabolomics, and it solves the problem of lack of accurate and quantitative evaluation methods for many pharmacodynamics.

Metabolites Identification and Construction of Metabolic Pathway

Potential metabolites of DN selected were identified according to the determination of the accurate *m/z*, retention time, and typical MS/MS fragment and pattern of the potential biomarkers above, which were obtained in the positive and negative ion modes. The construction of metabolic pathway was performed with Metabo Analyst, which is a web-based tool for visualization of metabolomics[1] based on database source including the KEGG[2] and the HMDB[3] databases for searching. The retention time and typical MS/MS fragment and pattern had great avail to narrow the range of possible molecules.

[1] http://www.metaboanalyst.ca/faces/upload/PathUploadView.xhtmlpc

[2] http://www.genome.jp/kegg/

[3] http://www.hmdb.ca/

RESULTS

Determination of Biochemical Indicators, Histopathological Observations and Western Blotting

The analytical results of biochemical indicators were presented in **Figure 2A**. After 15 days of administration, the level of FBG, LDL, T-CHO, TG, Scr, BUN, β2-MG in serum, and UP in urine of DN rats increased significantly compared with that of control rats ($P < 0.05$ or $P < 0.01$ or $P < 0.001$). After treatment of HK (0.75 g/kg·d), YX (27 mg/kg·d), DHYL (4.3 g/kg·d), DHYH (7.2 g/kg·d), JNL (216 mg/kg·d), JNH (360 mg/kg·d), the levels of these indicators were nearly restored to normal. The results of the histological examination were consistent with the biochemical analysis (see **Figure 2B**). Compared with the control group, the DN model group showed renal tubular epithelial vacuolar degeneration, interstitial inflammatory cell infiltration, glomerular and tubular atrophy and interstitial fibrosis. Western blotting analysis (**Figure 2C**) showed the expression of Wnt4, β-catenin, TGF-β1 in renal tissue of control rats were significant from that in DN rats ($P < 0.05$). Compared with DN model group, the levels of creatinine, urea nitrogen, 24-h urinary protein and renal histopathology were significantly improved in the administration groups, and the expression levels of Wnt4, β-catenin and TGF-β1 protein was significantly decreased, especially TLR treatment.

Effect of TLR and DTG on GMCs Hypertrophy

As shown in **Figure 3**, high glucose increased the ratio of total protein to total cells in GMCs, resulting in cell hypertrophy,

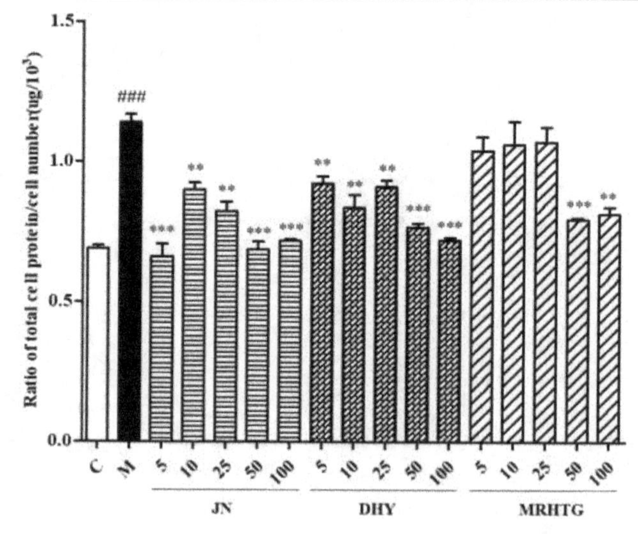

FIGURE 3 | Effects of DHY, JN, and MRHTG on hypertrophy of high glucose-induced GMCs. ###$P < 0.001$: model group vs. control group; **$P < 0.01$, ***$P < 0.001$: after treatment by DHY, JN, and MRHTG vs. model group. Data were presented as the mean ± SE.

whereas TLR, DTG and the major active ingredient acteoside (5, 10, 25, 50, and 100 μmol·L^{-1}), the ratio of total protein to total cell number decreased to a certain extent in a dose-dependent manner.

TGF-β1 and Wnt/β-Catenin Signaling Pathway on GMCs Treated With TLR and DTG

As shown in **Figure 4**, the protein expression levels of Wnt4, β-catenin and TGF-β1 were significantly increased in high glucose-induced GMCs ($P < 0.05$). The expression of Wnt4, β-catenin and TGF-β1 returned to the normal level after intervention of TLR and DTG, but there was no significant effect of the MRHTG group on the expression levels of Wnt4, β-catenin and TGF-β1.

Metabolomics Insights

QC samples Analysis

The relatively clustering of QC samples (**Figure 5A**) and relative standard deviations (RSD%) of ion intensity (**Table 1**) expound and prove the quality of QC data. The trend plot showing the variation of $t[1]$ over all observations (**Figure 5B**). The extracted ion chromatographic peaks of 10 ions were selected for method validation. The repeatability of method was evaluated by using six replicates of QC sample. This type of results demonstrated that the method had excellent repeatability and stability.

Multivariate Data Analysis

All the data containing the retention time, peak intensity and exact mass were imported in the MassLynx^{TM} software for multiple statistical analyses. The supervised OPLS-DA model, a pattern recognition approach, were established to separate serum or urine samples into two blocks between DN model group and control group. The supervised OPLS-DA with 100% sensitivity and no less than 95% specificity using a leave one out algorithm showed a better discrimination between the two groups (**Figures 6A1–A4**), which demonstrated that the DN model was built successfully. Based on these results, the OPLS-DA score plot (**Figures 6B1–B4**) were used to look for potential markers associated with DN progress. The R^2Y and Q^2 of PLS-DA model in positive and negative modes for serum and urine samples were suggested that the PLS-DA model was good to fitness and prediction.

The UPLC-QTOF/MS analysis platform provided the retention time and precise molecular mass within measurement errors (<5 ppm) as well as the fragments of corresponding production for the structural identification of metabolites. According to the precise molecular mass, predicted elemental composition was predicted and potential molecular formula could be searched out in Human Metabolome Database[4]. Twenty-seven endogenous metabolites (12 in serum and 15 in urine) were tentatively identified by comparing with authentic standards or based on the protocol detailed above method. The information about the detected endogenous metabolites was summarized in **Table 2**.

[4]http://www.hmdb.ca/

Changes of Relative Intensity of Endogenous Metabolites

In order to study the efficacy and action mechanism of TLR and DTG for treating DN disease, PLS-DA model analysis was built to obtain the changes during the control group, DN model group and administration group rats (**Figure 7**). The variations of metabolic profiling in serum and urine for administration group rats had the tendency to restore back to the levels of controls, especially TLR and DTG groups (**Table 3**). Furthermore, the relative quantities of 27 endogenous metabolites (12 in serum and 15 in urine) were ultimately identified by comparing with authentic standards or based on the protocol detailed above method. Twenty-four endogenous metabolites (except for taurochenodesoxycholic acid, chenodeoxycholic acid glycine conjugate and L-gulonolactone) in serum and urine significantly affected by TLR and DTG were restored back to a control-like level. The detailed information was showed in **Figure 8**.

Metabolic Pathway Analysis

The metabolic pathway was established by importing the potential metabolites into the web-based database MetPA. The pathway impact value calculated from pathway to topology analysis with MetPA above 0.1 was screened out as the potential target pathway. Here in **Figure 9**, for the five pathways, sphingolipid metabolism with the impact-value 0.31; pentose, glucuronate interconversion with the impact-value 0.27; terpenoid backbone biosynthesis with the impact-value 0.21; purine metabolism with the impact-value 0.15 and retinol metabolism with the impact-value 0.15 were filtered out as the most important metabolic pathways.

Correlation Analysis

Correlation networks is a useful tool to elucidate the relationship between biochemical indicators and potential biomarkers, providing supports for clinical diagnosis, medical treatment and pathophysiology research. Pearson correlation coefficient $r > 0.65$ and $r < -0.65$ separately represented for significant positive correlation and negative correlation (Cai et al., 2018). Here in **Figure 10**, BUN, UP, Scr, β2-MG positively correlated with ceramide (d18:1/12:0) ($r > 0.65$); and negatively correlated with sphingosine 1-phosphate and phytosphingosine ($r < -0.65$). Ceramide (d18:1/12:0), phytosphingosine and sphingosine 1-phosphate have been found and used to explain the sphingolipid metabolism. Therefore, BUN, UP, Scr, β2-MG closely related to sphingolipid metabolism.

DISCUSSION

The local and traditional uses of "Dihuang" are nourishing yin and tonifying kidney. The pharmacological studies stated that "Dihuang" possesses the significant effects on cardiovascular diseases, neuroprotection, diabetes and its complications, osteoporosis, and hyperlipidemia. Moreover, acteoside, as the main active component, was reportedly possesses widely

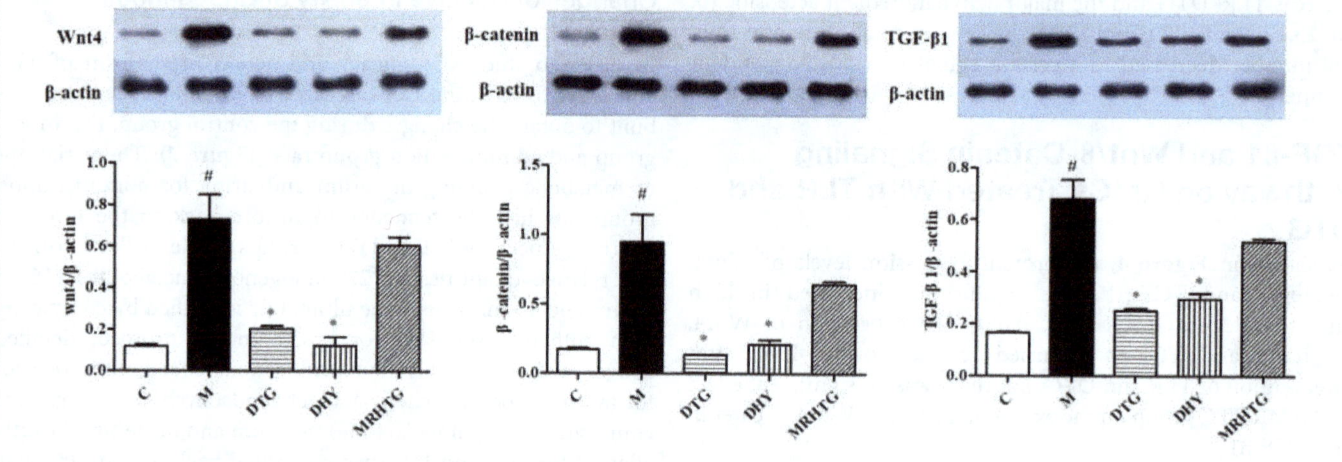

FIGURE 4 | Effects of DHY and JN on the expression of Wnt-4, β-catenin and TGF-β1 in GMCs. #P < 0.05: model group vs. control group; *P < 0.05: after treatment by DHY, JN, and MRHTG vs. model group. Data were presented as the mean ± SE.

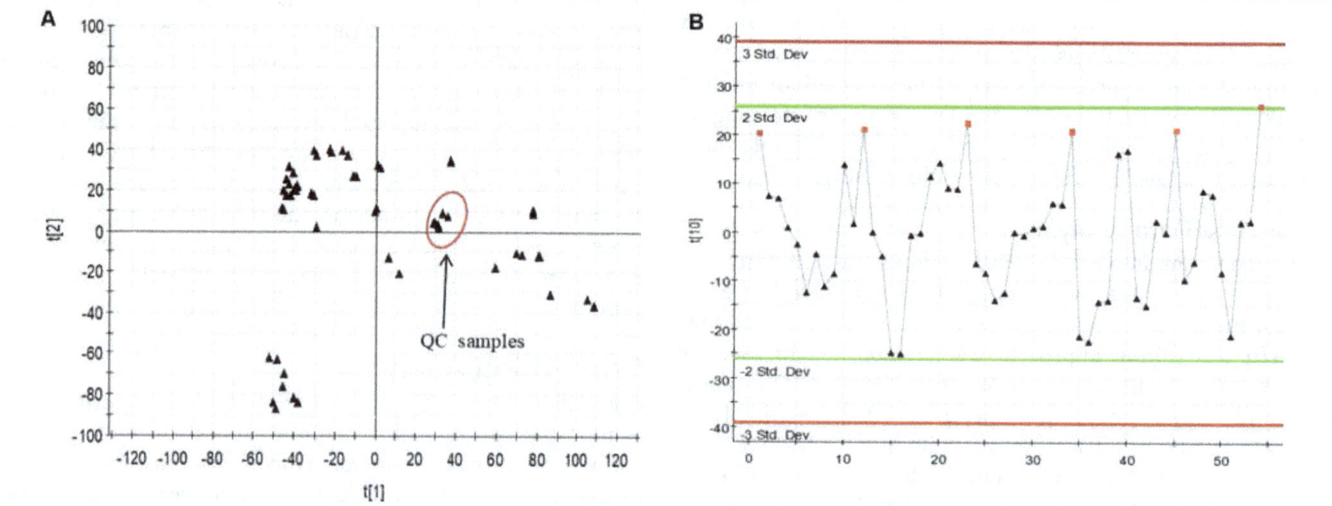

FIGURE 5 | Assessment of QC samples **(A)** PCA score plot (PC1 vs. PC2) of test samples and QC samples. **(B)** Trend plot showing the variation of *t*[1] over all observations. QC samples were colored as red boxes and test samples were colored as black triangle. *X*-axis numbers represented sample number (54 injections). *Y*-axis was arbitrary (3 SD).

TABLE 1 | Coefficient of variation of ion intensity of selected ions present in the QC samples covering the range of retention times.

T_R_*m/z* pairs	QC1	QC2	QC3	QC4	QC5	QC6	RSD%
1.11_136.0398	47.9838	49.0509	51.4734	49.2034	50.0331	52.3910	3.28
4.20_162.0556	95.4064	89.9217	92.6748	93.3017	95.6169	101.9378	4.29
6.27_170.0602	83.0727	85.1074	82.0747	83.6984	84.0937	73.3099	5.28
7.63_255.0649	51.3640	52.4464	48.6620	51.7397	52.9293	53.8687	3.45
10.09_149.0244	41.1500	42.0058	43.2755	41.8232	40.3977	43.2042	2.69
10.66_318.3001	48.3586	46.5870	45.4164	49.2801	44.6299	43.6165	4.73
2.84_179.0713	15.8304	16.2821	16.4652	15.2931	16.3969	15.1267	3.65
10.89_299.2012	20.8190	21.2219	21.8836	22.0706	21.5110	20.3967	2.99
4.48_146.0613	9.2522	10.0701	9.8090	8.8366	9.2831	8.9621	5.13
3.14_372.2377	26.8391	27.5472	29.8873	28.9075	26.5686	26.8156	4.85

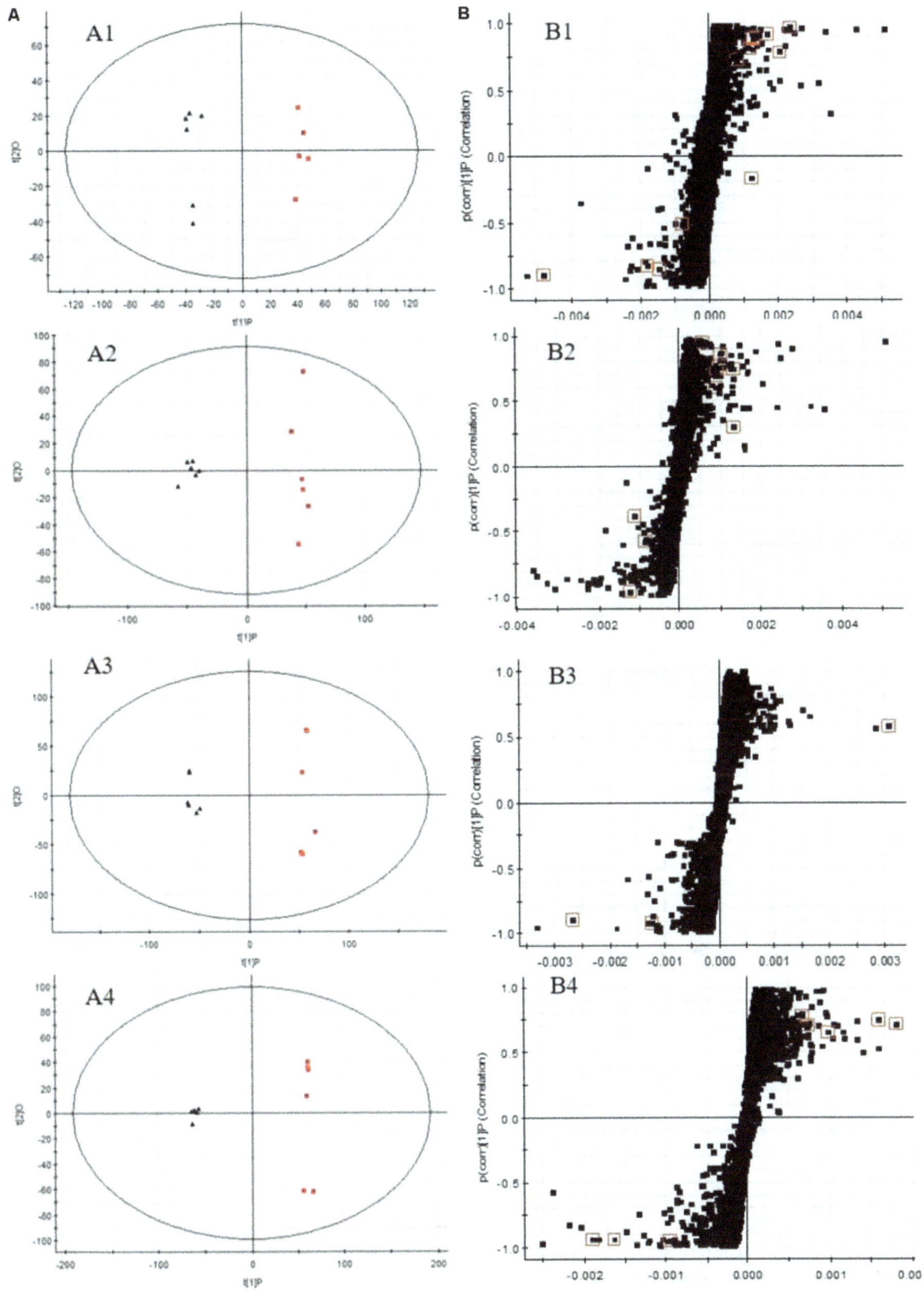

FIGURE 6 | OPLS-DA scores plots **(A)**, S-plot of OPLS-DA **(B)** for serum **(A1,A2,B1,B2)** and urine **(A3,A4,B3,B4)** samples of DN model group (red) vs. control group (black) in positive **(A1,B1,A3,B3)** and negative **(A2,B2,A4,B4)** ion mode. (**A1**, $R^2Y = 0.9920$, $Q^2 = 0.8994$; **A2**, $R^2Y = 0.9882$, $Q^2 = 0.9269$; **A3**, $R^2Y = 0.9932$, $Q^2 = 0.9363$; **A4**, $R^2Y = 0.9933$, $Q^2 = 0.9513$).

TABLE 2 | Potential metabolites selected and identified between DN model group and control group.

No.	T_R/min	*m/z*	Metabolites	VIP[a]	Trend[b]	HMDB	Source	Pathway
Sm1	1.70	146.0605	2-Keto-glutaramic acid	5.92	↓	01552	serum	Alanine, aspartate and glutamate metabolism
Sm 2	9.71	524.3721	Guanosine triphosphate	19.10	↓	01273	serum	Purine metabolism
Sm 3	4.01	353.2471	Thromboxane A2	3.73	↑	01452	serum	Arachidonic acid metabolism
Sm 4	8.24	522.3582	LysoPC(18:1(9Z))	14.38	↑	02815	serum	Glycerophospholipid metabolism
Sm 5	9.62	482.3251	Ceramide (d18:1/12:0)	4.42	↑	04947	serum	Sphingolipid metabolism
Sm 6	3.40	498.2887	Taurochenodesoxycholic acid	4.87	↓	00951	serum	Primary bile acid biosynthesis
Sm 7	6.15	378.2404	Sphingosine 1-phosphate	3.99	↓	00277	serum	Sphingolipid metabolism
Sm 8	6.98	504.3082	Thiamine triphosphate	4.04	↓	01512	serum	Thiamine metabolism
Sm 9	8.43	464.3147	Glycocholic acid	3.27	↓	00138	serum	Primary bile acid biosynthesis
Sm 10	10.28	301.2166	Retinyl ester	4.86	↓	03598	serum	Retinol metabolism
Sm 11	11.53	442.0717	Guanosine diphosphate	3.29	↓	01201	serum	Purine metabolism
Sm 12	4.93	448.3062	Chenodeoxycholic acid glycine conjugate	3.36	↑	00637	serum	Primary bile acid biosynthesis
Um 13	3.55	245.0116	Isopentenyl pyrophosphate	3.01	↑	01347	urine	Terpenoid backbone biosynthesis
Um 14	4.51	347.1695	Inosinic acid	5.76	↑	00175	urine	Purine metabolism
Um 15	2.81	173.9946	*N*-Acetyl-L-aspartic acid	3.63	↓	00812	urine	Alanine, aspartate and glutamate metabolism
Um 16	9.84	583.3128	Cholic acid glucuronide	4.77	↑	02577	urine	Pentose and glucuronate interconversions; Starch and sucrose metabolism
Um 17	3.70	300.0536	*N*-Acetyl-D-Glucosamine 6-Phosphate	5.78	↓	01062	urine	Amino sugar and nucleotide sugar metabolism
Um 18	7.57	343.0834	Thiamine monophosphate	6.59	↓	02666	urine	Thiamine metabolism
Um 19	9.30	253.1075	Galactosylglycerol	4.64	↓	06790	urine	Galactose metabolism
Um 20	1.11	136.0398	Adenine	11.10	↓	00034	urine	Purine metabolism
Um 21	4.20	162.0557	Aminoadipic acid	16.33	↓	04077	urine	Lysine degradation
Um 22	6.26	170.0603	Cysteic acid	7.40	↓	02757	urine	Taurine and hypotaurine metabolism
Um 23	7.63	255.065	5-L-Glutamyl-taurine	3.97	↓	04195	urine	Taurine and hypotaurine metabolism
Um 24	10.66	318.3002	Phytosphingosine	3.62	↓	04610	urine	Sphingolipid metabolism
Um 25	2.83	179.0713	L-Gulonolactone	3.40	↑	03466	urine	Ascorbate and aldarate metabolism
Um 26	4.47	146.0613	2-Keto-glutaramic acid	3.37	↑	01552	urine	Alanine, aspartate and glutamate metabolism
Um 27	10.09	149.0245	2-Oxo-4-methylthiobutanoic acid	8.94	↑	01553	urine	Cysteine and methionine metabolism

[a]Variable importance in the projection (VIP) values were obtained from cross-validated PLS-DA models with a threshold of 1. [b]Models vs. Controls: ↑ content increased; ↓ content decreased.

pharmacological activities, such as kidney protection, anti-oxidation, neuroprotection, liver protection, anti-cancer, and so on. But the action mechanisms still unclear completely. In our this study, the results *in vivo* showed that TLR and DTG can decrease 24-h urinary protein, serum creatine and blood urea nitrogen, alleviating the degree of renal interstitial fibrosis, reducing the expression of Wnt4, β-catenin and TGF-β1, played a role in renal protection. Moreover, the effect of the low dose group was more significant. Therefore, the optimal dose should be determined by further studies. Studies have shown that, the *in vivo* model of GMCs induced by high glucose simulates the pathophysiological changes of DN (Abboud, 2012). These *in vitro* results reveal that inhibitory effects of TLR and DTG on the hypertrophy and fibrosis of GMCs, and consistent with the *in vivo* results in this study. It is confirmed that the TLR and DTG had a better inhibiting effect on TGF-β1 and Wnt/β-catenin signaling pathway.

Notably, there are several distinct metabolic pathways in various stages of progress of DN. Ceramide (d18:1/12:0), phytosphingosine and sphingosine 1-phosphate have been found and used to explain the sphingolipid metabolism. Ceramides are one of the hydrolysis byproducts of sphingomyelin by the enzyme sphingomyelinase (sphingomyelin phosphorylcholine phosphohydrolase E.C.3.1.4.12) which has been identified in the subcellular fractions of human epidermis and many other

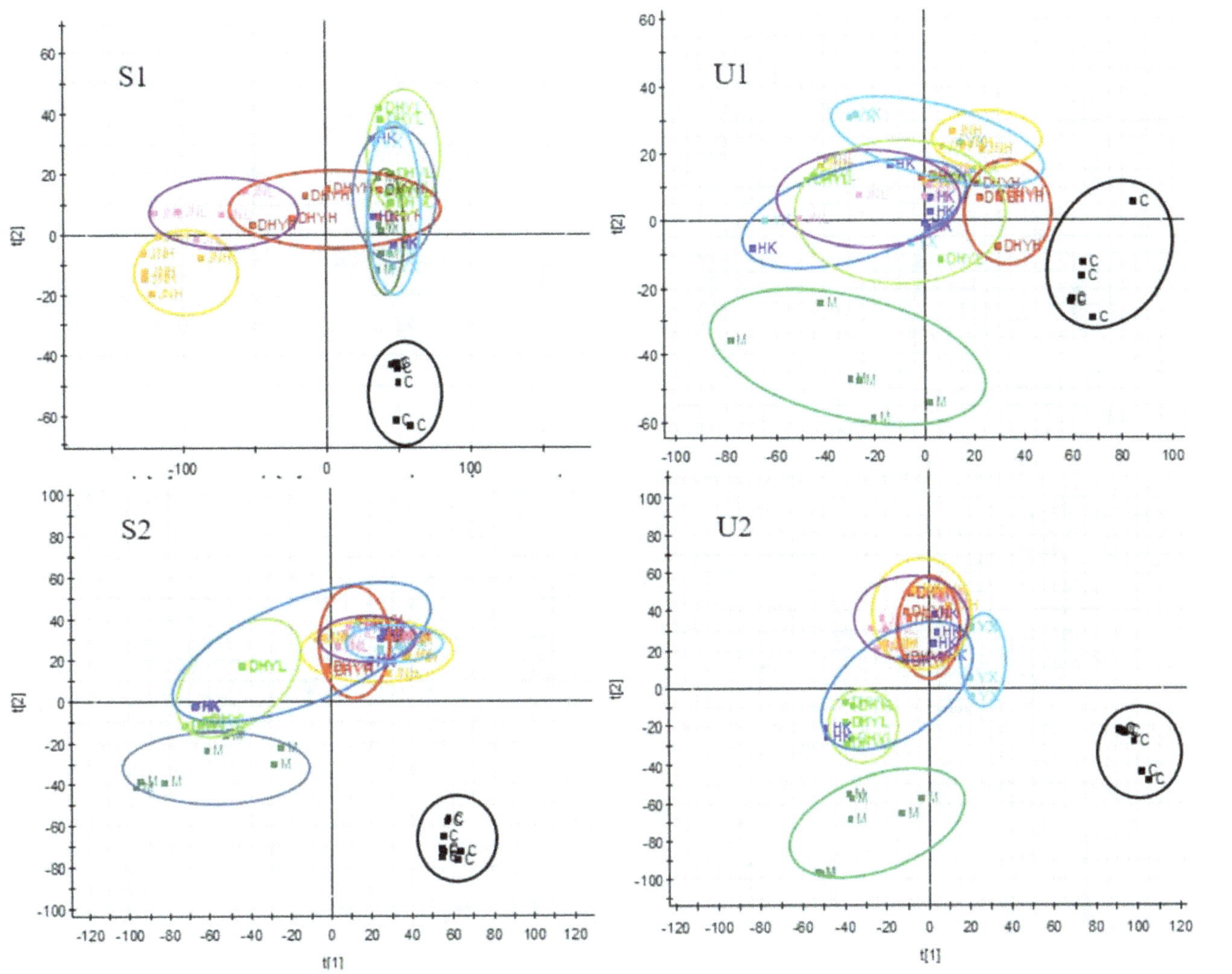

FIGURE 7 | PLS-DA scores plots for serum **(S1,S2)** and urine **(U1,U2)** samples from DN model rats and controls and administration group rats in positive and negative ion mode.

TABLE 3 | The relative distance between treatment groups and control group from the PLS-DA score plot (mean ± SE).

	Source	Serum		Urine	
	ESI	+	−	+	−
C	*X*-Axis	49.88	66.31	57.47	96.17
	Y-Axis	−50.77	−16.5	−68.63	−29.87
	M	50.51 ± 5.01	150.46 ± 5.75	126.77 ± 8.63	136.42 ± 7.81
	HK	44.61 ± 6.72	102.57 ± 10.46**	77.52 ± 19.3*	120.71 ± 7.86
	YX	35.66 ± 7.72	97.95 ± 11.71**	44.57 ± 2.21**	98.79 ± 6.56**
	DHYL	28.63 ± 4.41**	101.85 ± 9.7**	131.48 ± 7.32	135.53 ± 0.82
	DHYH	68.71 ± 11.11	75.37 ± 2.94**	53.11 ± 6.31**	124.65 ± 2.76
	JNL	144.12 ± 11.05	101.95 ± 8.87**	50.99 ± 4.71**	128.8 ± 3.41
	JNH	177.55 ± 6.24	79.26 ± 8.64**	51.4 ± 5.77**	125.71 ± 2.8

*Compared with model group, *$P < 0.05$, **$P < 0.01$.*

tissues (Summers, 2006). Besides, the accumulation of ceramide can cause many lipid metabolic diseases (Li et al., 2002), and some pathogen selectively alter metabolic pathways and promote the absorption of fat into ceramides. Studies have shown that high-fat diet for 3 weeks can significantly cause ceramide and sphingomyelin in the mouse liver and nucleus accumulation,

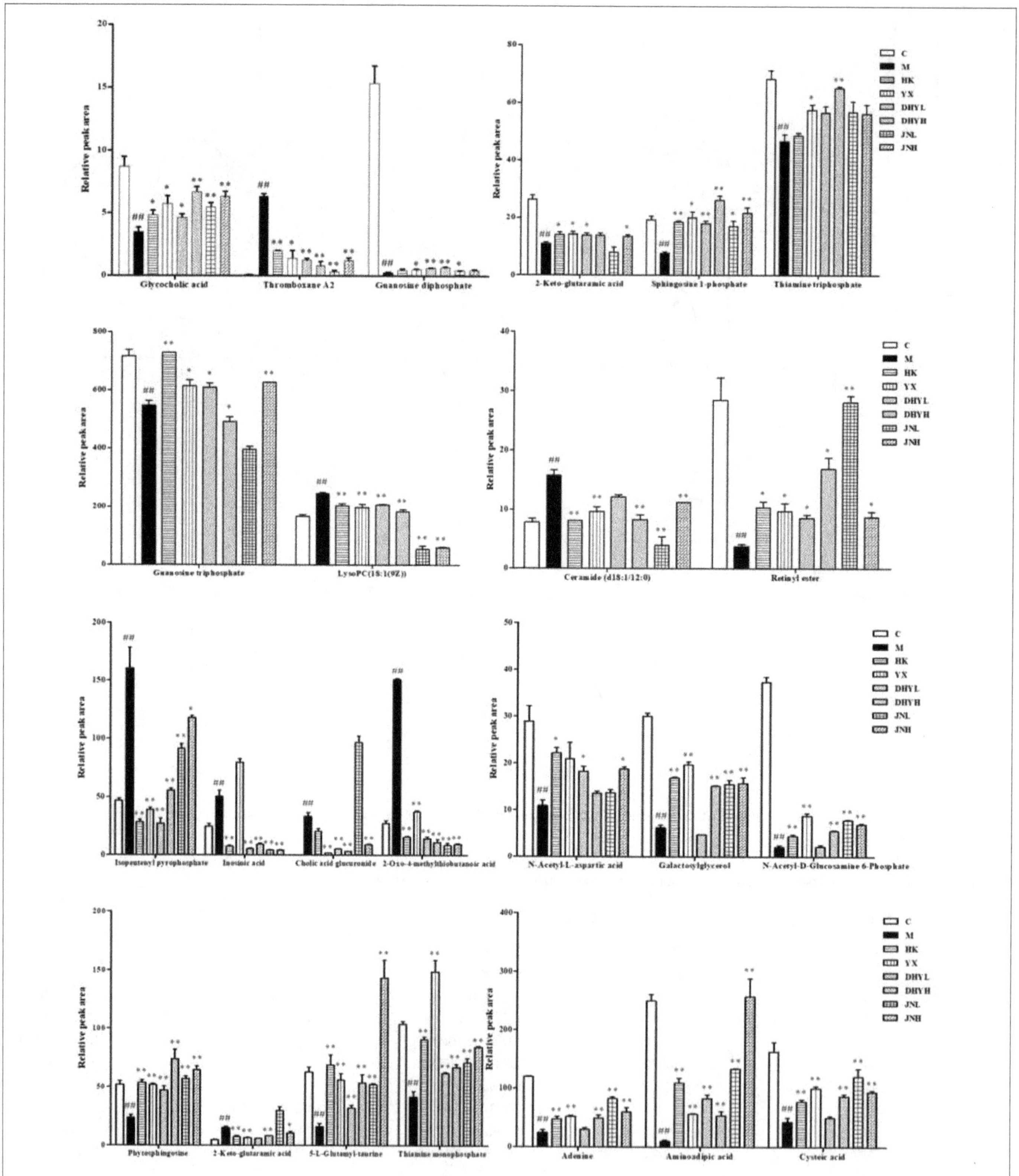

FIGURE 8 | Changes in the relative intensity of target metabolites identified by UPLC-QTOF/MS. A two tailed, parametric *t*-test was used to determine the significance of the change in relative intensity for each metabolite. Bars represent the mean relative metabolite concentration and standard deviations. $^{\#\#}P < 0.01$: model group vs. control group; $^{*}P < 0.05$, $^{**}P < 0.01$: after treatment by HK, YX, DHYL, DHYH, JNL, and JNH vs. model group. Data were presented as the mean ± SE.

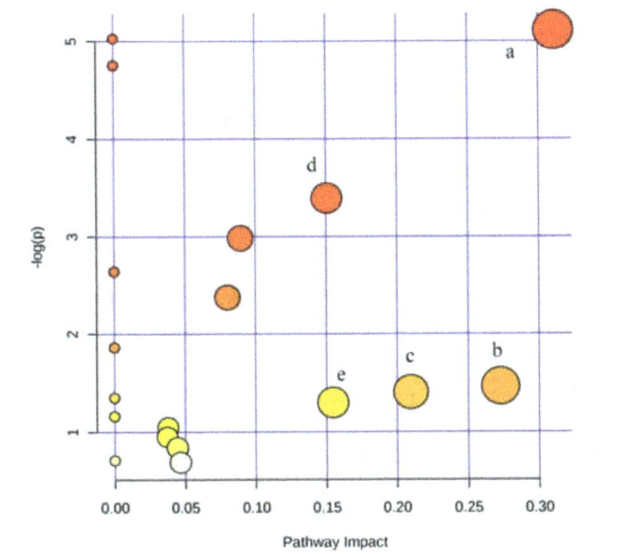

FIGURE 9 | Summary of pathway analysis of serum and urine samples of rats. (a) sphingolipid metabolism; (b) pentose and glucuronate interconversions; (c) terpenoid backbone biosynthesis; (d) purine metabolism; (e) retinol metabolism.

and ultimately make the liver browning and lead to fatty liver (Chocian et al., 2010). Scientists have recently demonstrated that inhibition and control of sphingolipid synthase contribute to the treatment of atherosclerosis, insulin resistance, diabetes and cardiomyopathy (Li et al., 2014). In DN, the content of ceramide increased significantly compared to normal rats and recovered to normal after administration of TLG and DTG. In recent years, studies have found that sphingosine 1-phosphate (S1P) can participate in the regulation of GMC growth and differentiation process (Spiegel and Kolesnick, 2002). Phytosphingosine is involved in diverse cell processes, including cell-cell interaction, cell proliferation, differentiation, and apoptosis. The contents of S1P and phytosphingosine decreased in DN, which was consistent with the injured of GMCs induced by DN. In addition, sphingolipid metabolic disorders may lead to cell death and are closely related to insulin-related diseases (Pang et al., 2008).

Cholic acid glucuronide has been found and used to explain the pentose and glucuronate interconversions. Cholic acid glucuronide is the glucuronidated metabolite of cholic acid, one of the four main acids produced by the liver where it is synthesized from cholesterol. Upon formation, the glucuronide is rapidly and effectively cleared from the circulation and excreted via urine (Little et al., 1985). In DN, the decreased amount of cholic acid glucuronide in urine indicated that the renal excretion was perturbed. Guanosine triphosphate, guanosine diphosphate, inosinic acid and adenine have been found and used to explain the purine metabolism. Inosinic acid is a purine nucleotide which has hypoxanthine as the base and one phosphate group esterified to the sugar moiety. The hypoxanthine in the purine metabolism oxidize to xanthine, adenosine monophosphate can degrade into uric acid and accumulate in the urine into uremic toxins, eventually leading to renal failure (Sánchez-Lozada et al., 2005; Seaman et al., 2008). Results suggested that these target

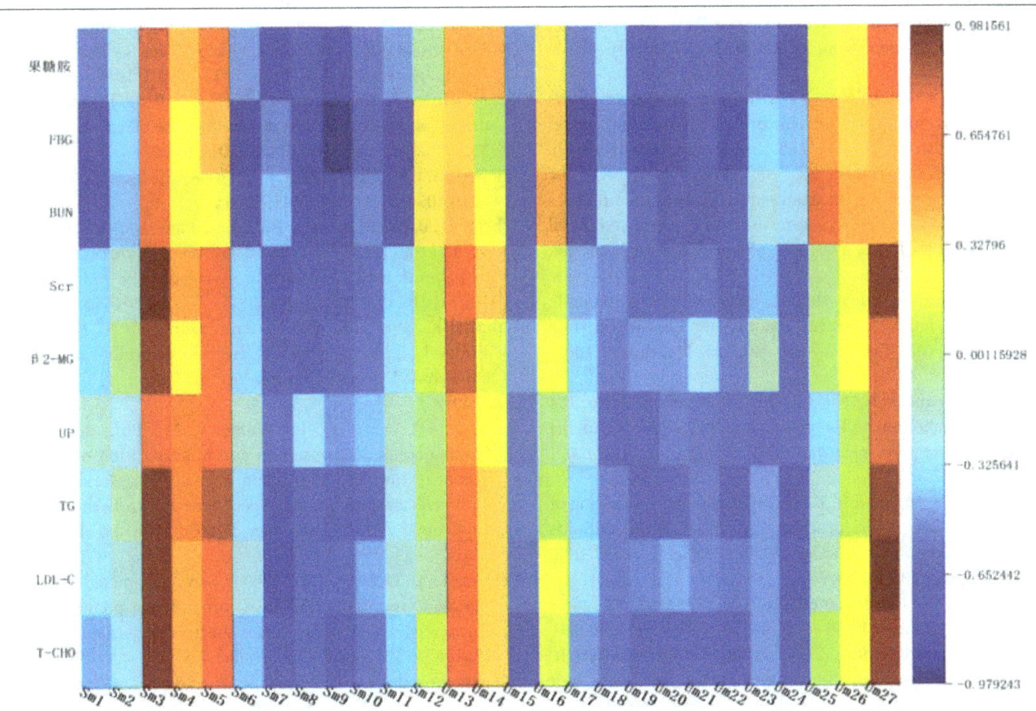

FIGURE 10 | Correlation heat-map between biochemical indicators and potential biomarkers.

pathways showed the marked perturbations over the time-course of the treatment and could contribute to the development of DN.

CONCLUSION

This study showed that TLR and DTG could prevent its occurrence and development of DN by combining biochemical and pathological indicators with metabolomics technology, and by assessing comprehensive curative effect. Through the application of metabolomics technology, 27 endogenous metabolites (12 in serum and 15 in urine) could be identified in the process of DN. After drug intervention, these markers varied to some extent ($P < 0.05$). The results showed that TLR and DTG played a significant role in regulating the expression levle of TGF-β1 protein in renal tissue and mesangial cells. Therefore, to further study the mechanism of TLR on TGF-β/Smad signaling pathway, it is necessary to systematically study the protective mechanism of TLR on DN. The study paved the way for further exploration of the pathogenesis of DN, early diagnosis and the evaluation of curative effect.

AUTHOR CONTRIBUTIONS

SS and J-aD designed the project. XD, HC, TZ, and HY performed the experiments. ZZ, E-xS, SG, DQ, and DW provided technology guidance. XD and SS wrote and modified the manuscript.

FUNDING

This work was supported by the National Natural Science Foundation of China (Nos. 81373889 and 81673533) and supported by program for excellent talents in school of pharmacy of Nanjing University of Chinese Medicine (15ZYXET-2). This work was also financially supported by Jiangsu Collaborative Innovation Center of Chinese Medicinal Resources Industrialization (No. ZDXM-1-10), Construction Project for Jiangsu Key Laboratory for High Technology of TCM Formulae Research (BM2010576), and a project funded by the Priority Academic Program Development of Jiangsu Higher Education Institutions (ysxk-2014).

REFERENCES

Abboud, H. E. (2012). Mesangial cell biology. *Exp. Cell Res.* 318, 979–985. doi: 10.1016/j.yexcr.2012.02.025

Balakumar, P., Arora, M. K., and Singh, M. (2009). Emerging role of PPAR ligands in the management of diabetic nephropathy. *Pharmacol. Res.* 60, 170–173. doi: 10.1016/j.phrs.2009.01.010

Beijing Municipal Health Bureau (1988). *Beijing Standard of Chinese Herbal Medicines*. Beijing: Capital Normal University press.

Cai, H. D., Su, S. L., Li, Y. H., Zeng, H. T., Zhu, Z. H., Guo, J. M., et al. (2018). *Salvia miltiorrhiza* protects adenine-induced chronic renal failure by regulating the metabolic profiling and modulating the NADPH oxidase/ROS/ERK and TGF-β/Smad signaling pathways. *J. Ethnopharmacol.* 212, 153–165. doi: 10.1016/j.jep.2017.09.021

Cai, Q. Y., Chen, X. S., Zhan, X. L., and Yao, Z. X. (2011). Protective effects of catalpol on oligodendrocyte death and myelin breakdown in a rat model of chronic cerebral hypoperfusion. *Neurosci. Lett.* 497, 22–26. doi: 10.1016/j.neulet.2011.04.013

Chen, Y. J., and Quilley, J. (2008). Fenofibrate treatment of diabetic rats reduces nitrosative stress, renal cyclooxygenase-2 expression, and enhanced renal prostaglandin release. *J. Pharmacol. Exp. Ther.* 324, 658–663. doi: 10.1124/jpet.107.129197

Chocian, G., Chabowski, A., Zendzian-Piotrowska, M., Harasim, E., Łukaszuk, B., and Górski, J. (2010). High fat diet induces ceramide and sphingomyelin formation in rat's liver nuclei. *Mol. Cell. Biochem.* 340, 125–131. doi: 10.1007/s11010-010-0409-6

Hodavance, M. S., Ralston, S. L., and Pelczer, I. (2007). Beyond blood sugar: the potential of NMR-based metabonomics for type 2 human diabetes, and the horse as a possible model. *Anal. Bioanal. Chem.* 387, 533–537. doi: 10.1007/s00216-006-0979-z

Hwang, G. S., Yang, J. Y., Ryudo, H., and Kwon, T. H. (2010). Metabolic profiling of kidney and urine in rats with lithium-induced nephrogenic diabetes insipidus by (1) H-NMR-based metabonomics. *Am. J. Physiol. Renal Physiol.* 298, F461–F470. doi: 10.1152/ajprenal.00389.2009

Jiménez, C., and Riguera, R. (1994). Phenylethanoid glycosides in plants: structure and biological activity. *Nat. Prod. Rep.* 11, 591–606. doi: 10.1039/NP9941100591

Li, H., Junk, P., Huwiler, A., Burkhardt, C., Wallerath, T., Pfeilschifter, J., et al. (2002). Dual effect of ceramide on human endothelial cells: induction of oxidative stress and transcriptional upregulation of endothelial nitric oxide synthase. *Circulation* 106, 2250–2256. doi: 10.1161/01.CIR.0000035650.05921.50

Li, W. X., Tang, Y. P., Guo, J. M., Shang, E.-X., Qian, Y. F., Wang, L. Y., et al. (2014). Comparative metabolomics analysis on hematopoietic functions of herb pair Gui-Xiong by ultra-high-performance liquid chromatography coupled to quadrupole time-of-flight mass spectrometry and pattern recognition approach. *J. Chromatogr. A* 1346, 49–56. doi: 10.1016/j.chroma.2014.04.042

Li, X., Becker, K. A., and Zhang, Y. (2010). Ceramide in redox signaling and cardiovascular diseases. *Cell Physiol. Biochem.* 26, 41–48. doi: 10.1159/000315104

Little, J. M., Chari, M. V., and Lester, R. (1985). Excretion of cholate glucuronide. *J. Lipid Res.* 26, 583–592.

Liu, C. L., Cheng, L., Kwok, H. F., Ko, C. H., Lau, T. W., Koon, C. M., et al. (2011). Bioassay-guided isolation of norviburtinal from the root of *Rehmannia glutinosa*, exhibited angiogenesis effect in zebrafish embryo model. *J. Ethnopharmacol.* 137, 1323–1327. doi: 10.1016/j.jep.2011.07.060

Lv, M., Chen, Z., Hu, G., and Qian, B. L. (2015). Therapeutic strategies of diabetic nephropathy: recent progress and future perspectives. *Drug Discov. Today* 20, 332–346. doi: 10.1016/j.drudis.2014.10.007

Nicholson, J. K., and Lindon, J. C. (2008). Systems biology: metabonomics. *Nature* 7216:1054. doi: 10.1038/4551054a

Oberg, B. P., McMenamin, E., Lucas, F. L., McMonagle, E., Morrow, J., Ikizler, T. A., et al. (2004). Increased prevalence of oxidant stress and inflammation in patients with moderate to severe chronic kidney disease. *Kidney Int.* 65, 1009–1016. doi: 10.1111/j.1523-1755.2004.00465.x

Odunsi, K., Wollman, R. M., Ambrosone, C. B., Hutson, A., McCann, S. E., Tammela, J., et al. (2005). Detection of epithelial ovarian cancer using 1H-NMR-based metabonomics. *Int. J. Cancer* 113, 782–788. doi: 10.1002/ijc.20651

Pang, L. Q., Liang, Q. L., Wang, Y. M., Ping, L., and Luo, G. A. (2008). Simultaneous determination and quantification of seven major phospholipid classes in human blood using normal-phase liquid chromatography coupled with electrospray mass spectrometry and the application in diabetes nephropathy. *J. Chromatogr. B* 869, 118–125. doi: 10.1016/j.jchromb.2008.05.027

Pereira, T., and Chang, S. W. (2004). Semi-automated quantification of ivermectin in rat and human plasma using protein precipitation and filtration with liquid chromatography/tandem mass spectrometry. *Rapid Commun. Mass Spectrom.* 18, 1265–1276. doi: 10.1002/rcm.1485

Sánchez-Lozada, L. G., Tapia, E. J., Avila, C. C., Avila-Casado, C., Soto, V., Nepomuceno, T., et al. (2005). Mild hyperuricemia induces vasoconstriction and maintains glomerular hypertension in normal and remnant kidney rats. *Kidney Int.* 67, 237–247. doi: 10.1111/j.1523-1755.2005.00074.x

Seaman, C., Moritz, J., Falkenstein, E., Van Dyke, K., and Klandorf, H. (2008). Inosine ameliorates the effects of hemin-induced oxidative stress in broilers. *Comp. Biochem. Physiol. A* 151, 670–675. doi: 10.1016/j.cbpa.2008.08.014

Shen, X., Li, D. F., Zong, G. Z., Wu, Z. L., and He, W. (2010). Effects of total saponins extracted from leaves of rehmannia on accelerated nephrotoxic nephritis induced by rabbit IgG in rat. *Chin. J. Exp. Tradit. Med. Form.* 16, 179–181.

Spiegel, S., and Kolesnick, R. (2002). Sphingosine 1-phosphate as a therapeutic agent. *Leukemia* 16, 1596–1602. doi: 10.1038/sj.leu.2402611

Summers, S. A. (2006). Ceramides in insulin resistance and lipotoxicity. *Prog. Lipid. Res.* 45, 42–72. doi: 10.1016/j.plipres.2005.11.002

Weir, M. R. (2007). Microalbuminuria and cardiovascular disease. *Clin. J. Am. Soc. Nephro.* 2, 581–590. doi: 10.2215/CJN.03190906

Xiao, L., Wang, M., Yang, S., Liu, F. Y., and Sun, L. (2013). A glimpse of the pathogenetic mechanisms of Wnt/β-catenin signaling in diabetic nephropathy. *Biomed. Res. Int.* 2013:987064. doi: 10.1155/2013/987064

Yokozawa, T., Suzuki, N., Oura, H., Nonaka, G., and Nishioka, I. (1986). Effect of extracts obtained from rhubarb in rats with chronic renal failure. *Chem. Pharm. Bull.* 34, 4718–4723. doi: 10.1248/cpb.34.4718

Zhang, R., Zhou, J., Li, M., Ma, H., Qiu, J., Luo, X., et al. (2014). Ameliorating effect and potential mechanism of *Rehmannia glutinosa* oligosaccharides on the impaired glucose metabolism in chronic stress rats fed with high-fat diet. *Phytomedicine* 21, 607–614. doi: 10.1016/j.phymed.2013.11.008

Zhang, R., Zhao, Y., Sun, Y., Lu, X., and Yang, X. (2013). Isolation, characterization, and hepatoprotective effects of the raffinose family oligosaccharides from *Rehmannia glutinosa* Libosch. *J. Agric. Food Chem.* 61, 7786–7793. doi: 10.1021/jf4018492

Zhang, Z., Meng, Y., Guo, Y., He, X., Liu, Q., Wang, X., et al. (2013). Rehmannia glutinosa polysaccharide induces maturation of murine bone marrow derived Dendritic cells (BMDCs). *Int. J. Biol. Macromol.* 54, 136–143. doi: 10.1016/j.ijbiomac.2012.12.005

18

Tricaproin Isolated from *Simarouba glauca* Inhibits the Growth of Human Colorectal Carcinoma Cell Lines by Targeting Class-1 Histone Deacetylases

Asha Jose[1], Motamari V. N. L. Chaitanya[2], Elango Kannan[3] and SubbaRao V. Madhunapantula[4*]*

[1] Department of Pharmacology, JSS College of Pharmacy, JSS Academy of Higher Education and Research, Udhagamandalam, India, [2] Department of Pharmacognosy and Phytopharmacy, JSS College of Pharmacy, Udhagamandalam, India, [3] Department of Pharmacology, JSS College of Pharmacy, Udhagamandalam, India, [4] Center of Excellence in Molecular Biology and Regenerative Medicine, JSS Medical College, JSS Academy of Higher Education and Research, Mysore, India

***Correspondence:**
SubbaRao V. Madhunapantula
madhunapantulas@yahoo.com;
mvsstsubbarao@jssuni.edu.in
Elango Kannan
elangokannanjsscpooty@hotmail.com

While anticancer properties of *Simarouba glauca* (SG, commonly known as Paradise tree) are well documented in ancient literature, the underlying mechanisms leading to cancer cell death begin to emerge very recently. The leaves of SG have been used as potential source of anticancer agents in traditional medicine. Recently attempts have been made to isolate anticancer agents from the leaves of SG using solvent extraction, which identified quassinoids as the molecules with tumoricidal activity. However, it is not known whether the anti-cancer potential of SG leaves is just because of quassinoids alone or any other phytochemicals also contribute for the potency of SG leaf extracts. Therefore, SG leaves were first extracted with hexane, chloroform, ethyl acetate, 70% ethanol, water and anti-cancer potential (for inhibiting colorectal cancer (CRC) cells HCT-116 and HCT-15 proliferation) determined using Sulforhodamine-B (SRB) assay. The chloroform fraction with maximal anticancer activity was further fractionated by activity-guided isolation procedure and structure of the most potent compound determined using spectral analysis. Analysis of the structural characterization data showed the presence of tricaproin (TCN). TCN inhibited CRC cells growth in a time- and dose dependent manner but not the normal cell line BEAS-2B. Mechanistically, TCN reduced oncogenic Class-I Histone deacetylases (HDACs) activity, followed by inducing apoptosis in cells. In conclusion, the anti-cancer potential of SG is in part due to the presence of TCN in the leaves.

Keywords: *Simarouba glauca*, laxmitaru, anti-cancer activity, tricaproin, sodium butyrate, histone deacetylases, apoptosis

INTRODUCTION

Simarouba glauca DC (*S. glauca, S.G)*, commonly known as laxmitaru and paradise tree, belongs to Simaroubaceae family (Govindaraju et al., 2009, NGPS). Parts of *S. glauca* plant have been used extensively in traditional medicine to treat cancers (Patil and Gaikwad, 2011). For example, decoction prepared using SG leaves has been reported to be effective in treating various cancers

(Rangarajan, 2003; Narendran, 2013). Supporting these traditional uses, preliminary studies by National Cancer Institute, United States demonstrated that alcoholic extracts of SG inhibited the growth of cancer cells even at a dose of 25 μg/ml.[1] Very recently, a study by Puranik et al. (2017) showed the anti-bladder cancer activity of ethanol extract using T-24 cell line. Similarly, a separate study isolating anticancer constituents using bio activity-guided fractionation of chloroform extract of *S. glauca* twigs reported the presence of six canthin-6-one type alkaloid derivatives – (1) canthin-6-one; (2) 2-methoxycanthin-6-one; (3) 9-methoxycanthin-6-one; (4) 2-hydroxycanthin-6-one; (5) 4,5-dimethoxycanthin-6-one; and (6) 4,5-dihydroxycanthin-6-one; a limonoid, melianodiol, an acyclic squalene-type triterpenoid, 14-deacetyleurylene, two coumarins – scopoletin and fraxidin, and two triglycerides – triolein and trilinolein. Further testing found that among these molecules, only canthin-6-one, 2-hydroxycanthin-6-one, limonoid and melianodiol could inhibit the growth of human cancer cell lines (Rivero-Cruz et al., 2005). Another study isolated scopoletin, canthin-6-one, canthine-6-one dimethoxy derivatives from wood extract and showed their potential to inhibit human breast cancer cell lines MCF-7 and SK-BR-3 at 2.0 μg/ml and 5.5 μg/ml respectively (Reynertson et al., 2011). In summary, all these studies conclude that the extracts of SG contain potential anticancer agents.

Histone deacetylases (HDACs) are key enzymes involved in chromatin re-modeling and oncogenic behavior of cells (Glozak and Seto, 2007). Deregulated HDACs promote cancer cell proliferation, prevent apoptosis and increase cell migration through the modulation of histone acetylation (Marks et al., 2000). Since histone acetylation helps in the packaging of DNA, removal of acetyl groups by HDACs is likely to increase chromatin tightening, which ultimately culminate in the down-regulation of tumor suppressor genes such as p53, Bax, Bad, p21 etc. (Mariadason, 2008). Therefore strategies that inhibit oncogenic HDACs have potential to become clinically viable drugs for treating cancers wherein HDAC plays an important role in the tumor development (Mottamal et al., 2015). For instance, US FDA approved the use of suberanilohydroxamic acid (SAHA) for treating cutaneous T-cell lymphoma in the year 2006 (Mottamal et al., 2015). Likewise, Belinostat and Panobinstat were also approved by US FDA for the treatment of peripheral T-cell lymphoma and multiple myeloma (Mottamal et al., 2015). Recently, studies from our laboratory have demonstrated the potential of HDAC inhibiting benzoic acid and cinnamic acid derivatives for treating carcinomas of colon and rectum (Anantharaju et al., 2016, 2017a,b). Although many studies have demonstrated the clinical utility of HDAC inhibitors, success of these agents as monotherapies is still a major concern (Kuendgen et al., 2006; Thurn et al., 2011). Hence, search for more potent HDAC inhibitors that work alone still continues. In this regard a separate study synthesized and tested the ability of a selenium containing HDAC inhibitor, known as SelSA (Gowda et al., 2012). SelSA showed much better HDAC inhibition compared to parent compound SAHA (Gowda et al., 2012). However, further development of this compound was not considered due to its toxicity in mice at higher doses (Gowda et al., 2012).

Short and medium-chain fatty acids, and lipids extracted from various plants are the major sources of potential anticancer agents (Hamburger et al., 1987; Selvaraj, 2017). Mechanistically, fatty acids and lipids inhibit HDACs thereby retard cancer cell growth (Waldecker et al., 2008). For example, sodium butyrate helps in the treatment of cancers by inhibiting class-I HDACs thereby sensitizing cancer cells to chemotherapeutic agents as well as radiation treatment (Sealy and Chalkley, 1978; Davie, 2003; Rada-Iglesias et al., 2007). Likewise, medium chain triglycerides and fatty acids are also known to inhibit oncogenic HDACs leading to apoptosis in cancer cells (Kuefer et al., 2004). Therefore, triglycerides containing short and medium chain (4–8 carbons) fatty acids are better anti-cancer agents (Fauser et al., 2013; Narayanan et al., 2015). Hence, SG leaves were extracted with solvents of low- and medium polarity, and anti-cancer potential tested for inhibiting colorectal carcinoma (CRC) cell lines expressing elevated HDAC activity. The chloroform extract, which exhibited potent anti-cancer activity, was further fractionated and a triaceyl glyceride containing hexanoic acid (Caproic acid) purified. The purified compound identified as "Tricaproin" (TCN) using GC-MS, FT-IR, ^{1}H and ^{13}C NMR. The pure TCN inhibited HDAC and cancer cell growth in a dose dependent manner. Mechanistically, HDAC inhibiting TCN induced apoptosis followed by cell growth arrest. In conclusion, results of this study demonstrate the purification of HDAC inhibiting TCN from SG leaves and showed that TCN induces CRC cells growth arrest. Additional studies are currently underway to determine the safety and efficacy of TCN in animals.

MATERIALS AND METHODS

Materials

Colorectal carcinoma cell lines HCT-116 and HCT-15 were procured from NCCS, Pune, Maharashtra, India. Human lung epithelial cell BEAS-2B was kindly provided by Dr. Rajeshkumar Thimmulappa, Associate Professor of Biochemistry, JSS Medical College. Cell culture reagents and disposables were from Life Technologies, Carlsbad, CA, United States and Tarson's India Limited, Kolkata, India, respectively. BSA was from Hi-Media, Mumbai, Maharashtra, India. Hexanoic acid and Sulforhodamine-B were from Sigma Chemical Company, St. Louis, MO, United States. Analytical grade n-Hexane, Chloroform, Ethyl acetate, Ethanol, Silica gel 60-120 and ALUGRAM-Xtra aluminum plate SIL G/UV 254 were from Loba Chemie, Mumbai, Maharashtra, India. Pierce BCA protein estimation kit [cat#: 23227] was from Thermo Fischer Scientific, Waltham, MA, United States. Lactate dehydrogenase activity assay kit [cat#: K730-500] was from BioVision, Milpitas, CA, United States. Histone deacetylase fluorometric (HDAC) kit [cat#:10011563] from Cayman, Ann Arbor, MI, United States. Acridine orange, ethidium bromide, sodium butyrate were from Sisco Research Laboratories Pvt., Ltd., Mumbai, Maharashtra,

[1] http://www.revalgo.com/blog/category/simarouba-glauca/

India. Accelrys Discovery Studio 4.1 software is from Biovia, San Diego, CA, United States (Available at JSS College of Pharmacy, Udhagamandalam, Tamil Nadu, India).

Methods

Preparation and Extraction of *S. glauca* Leaves

Fresh leaves from healthy, uninfected *Simarouba glauca* plant were collected from Palakkad district, Kerala, India. Plant taxonomist, Dr. N. Sasidharan, an Emeritus scientist from Kerala Forest Research Institute, Peechi, Thrissur, Kerala, India, has identified the plant. Leaves from taxonomically identified plants were processed as follows: (a) washing of leaves with tap water to remove dust and adherent materials; (b) rinsing with distilled water followed by drying under shade; (c) pulverization of completely dried leaves in to a fine powder using a sterile electric blender.

Sequential extraction of SG leaf powder

Hundred gram dried leaf powder was extracted successively in Soxhlet apparatus, using 500 ml Hexane (SGH), Chloroform (SGC), Ethyl acetate (SGEA), 70% aqueous Ethanol (SGE). Maceration was carried out for aqueous extraction (SGW). The solvent from each fraction was removed by evaporation at reduced pressure for 24 h; and the residue was frozen at −80°C for 48 h before lyophilization. Stock solution of each lyophilized sample was prepared by reconstituting 50mg material in 1.0 ml of 100% dimethyl sulfoxide (DMSO). The stock solutions were stored at 4°C until use.

Screening of Extracts for Anti-cancer Activity Using Colorectal Carcinoma Cell Lines HCT-116 and HCT-15

The anti-cancer activity of the crude samples was measured according to Madhunapantula et al. (2008). First, 5×10^3 cells, representing carcinomas of colon and rectum (HCT-116, HCT-15, in 100 μl DMEM) supplemented with 10% FBS, 5% penstrep, 5% glutamax were seeded in a 96-well plate. The cells were grown in a CO_2 incubator maintained at 37°C, 5% CO_2 and 95% relative humidity. After about 48 h, at which point all the wells were 60–70% confluent, the cells were exposed to increasing concentration of samples (dissolved in DMSO and diluted in DMEM-10% FBS medium) for 24, 48, and 72 h. Viability of cells was measured using sulforhodamine-B assay and the percentage growth inhibition calculated by comparing with vehicle DMSO treated cells.

Measurement of Cell Viability Using Sulforhodamine-B Assay (SRB Assay)

Viability of cells was measured using SRB assay as described by Skehan et al. (1990). Experimentally, cells were fixed in 1/4th volume of cold 50% (w/v) TCA for 1 h at 4°C. The media was removed and the wells washed with water (200 μl × 4 times) to remove TCA and serum proteins. The plates were dried, incubated with 100 μl 0.4% SRB for 20 min to stain the cellular proteins. Next, the wells were washed quickly with 1% acetic acid (200 μl × 4 times) to remove unbound SRB. The bound SRB was solubilized in 10.0 mM Tris base solution (100 μl/well) and the absorbance measured at 490 nm in a microplate reader.

Isolation of Tricaproin From the Most Potent Chloroform Extract

Preparation of fatty acid methyl esters (FAME)

Chloroform extract (3.5 g) was subjected to Silica Gel (60–120 mesh) column chromatography using chloroform as an eluant. Based on the TLC analysis, the chloroform fractions were pooled and evaporated to obtain a dried mass of 3.1 g. This dried mixture was refluxed using a mixture of methanol and acetyl chloride (95:5, 100 ml) for 4 h, to prepare FAME, and partitioned thrice using 450 ml of n-hexane containing 0.01% butylated hydroxytoluene (BHT) (A), 400 ml of ethyl acetate (B) and 300 ml of water (C). The pooled fractions were distilled under vacuum to obtain 0.9 g (A), 0.7 g (B) and 1.2 g (C) of dried material respectively from n-hexane (A), ethyl acetate (B) and water (C) solvents.

Enrichment of FAME using urea crystallization method

The obtained FAME was subjected to urea complexation to separate the saturated fatty acids from the polyunsaturated fatty acids as described by Jubie et al. (2015) with slight modification. In short, the obtained FAME (0.9 g, 0.7 g, 1.2 g) was treated with methanol (9.0 ml) and hot solution of urea (3.0 g at 60°C) and the mixture was heated (60°C for 30.0 min) to get a clear solution. It was then cooled at room temperature and stored at 0°C overnight. The material was further filtered to separate the crystals settled at the bottom. The filtrates were subjected to vacuum distillation, which yielded powdered samples designated as Fraction #1 (0.32 g), Fraction #2 (0.15 g), and Fraction #3 (0.62 g) respectively from fractions A, B, and C. The pale crystals obtained (2.0 g) were further refluxed with water (20 ml) using rota vapor at 50°C under pressure. The aqueous layer thus formed was partitioned with n-hexane (1:2). The collected *n*-hexane layer was subjected to vacuum distillation, which yielded: Fraction #4 (0.49 g) and Fraction #5 (0.51 g) from A and B, respectively. Fraction C produced a turbid aqueous layer, separation of which (same as above) yielded a 0.48 g oily product (Fraction #6).

Characterization and structural elucidation of Tricaproin (TCN)

Fraction #6, containing more pure tricaproin (as evidenced by gas chromatography-mass spectrometry (GC-MS), was selected for structural elucidation. The infra red (IR) spectra were recorded by fixed cell method with Schimadzu 8400S Fourier transformed infra red (FT-IR) spectrophotometer with a range of 4000–400cm^{-1}. The ^1H (1–11 ppm) and ^{13}C nuclear magnetic resonance (NMR) (10 – 220 ppm) spectra were recorded using Bruker Avance-II with $CDCl_3$ as solvent. GC-MS analysis was carried out using Thermo trace 1300 Gas chromatogram coupled with Thermo TSQ 8000 mass spectra using XCalibur 2.0SP1 with Foundation 2.0SP1 software. The injector temperature was 250°C and the column pressure was 100 kPa. Helium was used as the carrier gas (1.0 ml/min) and the injection volume was 1.0 μL. The temperature was set at 60°C for 2.0 min and increased to 280°C (10°C/min). Mass spectrometry conditions were as follows: ion source temperature – 230°C; electron energy – 70 eV; interface temperature – 250°C; quadrupole temperature –

150°C; mass scan range – 50–500 amu; detector – MS TSQ 8000.

Anti-cancer Activity and Selectivity of Tricaproin

The ability of tricaproin and hexanoic acid to inhibit carcinoma cells representing colon and rectum (HCT-116 and HCT-15) and non-cancerous human bronchial epithelium cell line (BEAS-2B) was carried out as detailed before. The cells were exposed to increasing concentration (7.8–1000 μM) of TCN and HA (dissolved in DMSO and diluted in DMEM-10% FBS medium) for 24, 48, and 72 h, and IC50 values calculated using GraphPad Prism software (2009) (Prism).

Comparative Assessment of the Binding Potential of Tricaproin to Sodium Butyrate Binding Site of HDACs Using Discovery Studio 4.1

Selection of HDAC structure from Protein Data Bank

The X-ray crystallographic structures of human HDAC1 with dimeric ELM2-SANT domain of MTA 1 from the NuRd complex (PDB ID-4BKX) having 482 aminoacids, HDAC2 consisting 367 aminoacids bound with *N*-(2-aminophenyl) benzamide (PDB ID-3MAX), HDAC3 complexed with a co-repressor inositol tetraphosphate with 376 aminoacid residues (PDB ID-4A69), HDAC 8 complexed with an inhibitor complex and having 388 aminoacids (PDB ID-2V5X), and HDAC4 complexed with hydroxamic acid inhibitor benzamide having 488 amino acids (PDB ID-2VQV) were retrieved from Protein data bank. The PDB files were cleaned and the hetero-atoms (HETATM) of the receptors were removed manually (Anantharaju et al., 2017a).

Generation of ligand data set

The structures of ligands-Tricaproin, Hexanoic acid, Sodium butyrate were obtained from PubChem compound database[2]. "Prepare ligand" module available in Discovery studio 4.1 was used for preparation of the ligands for removing duplicates, enumerating isomers and tautomers, and generating 3D conformations.

Active site analysis of HDACs structure

Possible binding sites of HDACs were identified by first defining the receptor molecule using binding site tools of Discovery Studio. Active sites were selected according to PDB site records. Total active sites were evaluated for their binding to ligands, which include the control sodium butyrate, with lowest C-Dock energies and selected the best active site for the further evaluation to identify the potent HDAC inhibitor (Anantharaju et al., 2017a).

Molecular docking using Discovery Studio 4.1

The docking of ligands in the receptor-binding site was performed using C-docker module available in Discovery studio 4.1. C-docker docks ligands using the validated CDOCKER algorithm, a grid based molecular docking method that uses CHARMm with CDOCKER. Briefly, initial ligand conformations were sampled using high temperature molecular dynamics, which include dynamics steps (1000) and dynamic target temperature (1000) and allowed to flex during the refinement. Next, the conformations were translated into binding site and candidate poses created using random rigid-body rotations. This was subjected for simulated annealing including heating steps (2000), heating target temperature (700), cooling steps (5000) and cooling target temperature (300). A final minimization with full potential is then used to refine the ligand poses. The binding mode for all ligands to human HDACs was investigated by CDOCKER protocol (Wu et al., 2003). Different poses of protein-ligand complex were obtained after docking process with their specific CDOCKER energy and CDOCKER interaction scores displayed in output file.

[2]https://pubchem.ncbi.nlm.nih.gov/

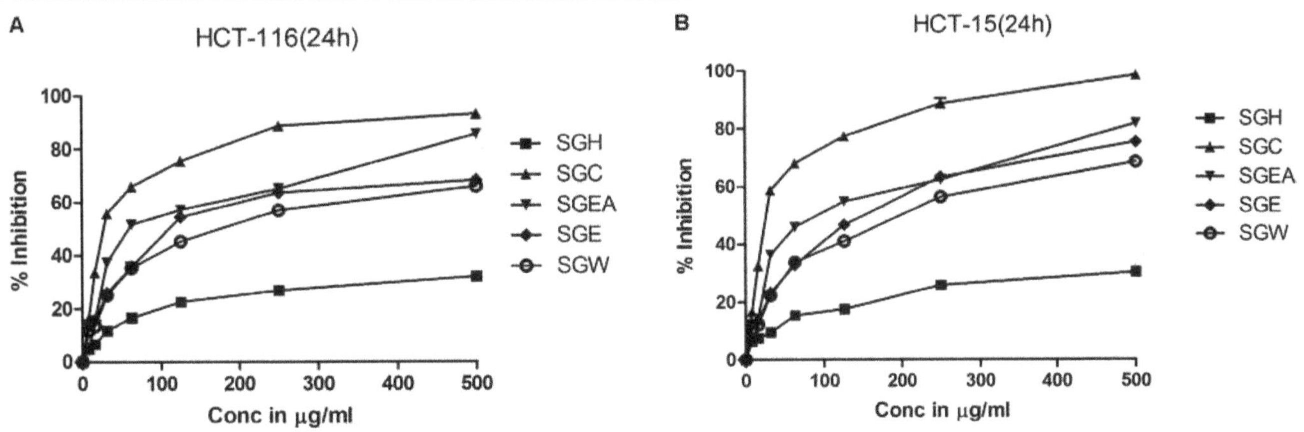

FIGURE 1 | Chloroform extract of SG (SGC), compared to other extracts, more effectively inhibit the viability of colorectal carcinoma cell lines: To screen and identify the most potent extract which can inhibit the growth of colorectal cancer cell lines, first, SG leaves were sequentially extracted with solvents of increasing polarity and tested for efficacy on HCT-116 **(A)** and HCT-15 **(B)** cell lines. Analysis of the data showed a significant growth reduction with increasing concentration of the extracts at 24 h of treatment. Among the extracts tested, chloroform extract showed much better cell proliferation inhibition indicating the presence of compounds that can inhibit the growth of colorectal carcinoma cells. The screening experiments were carried out thrice with at least 4 replicate wells in each experiment. The values represented are Mean ± SEM.

Assessment of HDAC Inhibitory Potential of Tricaproin

Histone deacetylase (HDAC) inhibitory potential of Tricaproin and Hexanoic acid was determined using the HDAC1 nuclear extract supplied in the kit (*Ex vivo* analysis; Histone deacetylase fluorometric (HDAC) assay kit (10011563) from Cayman, USA) as well as the nuclear extract collected from the CRC cells; HCT-116 and HCT-15 upon treatment with Tricaproin and Hexanoic acid (*In vitro* analysis). Details of the procedure can be obtained from the following link: https://www.caymanchem.com/pdfs/10011563.pdf.

Isolation of cellular nuclei and collection of nuclear extract

Isolation of nuclear fraction was performed as described in the kit[3]. In brief, 1×10^6 cells from control untreated, vehicle DMSO (1%) treated and Tricaproin and Hexanoic acid exposed flasks were collected by trypsinization, and centrifuged at 3000 rpm for 5.0 min. The pelleted cells were washed twice with PBS, and resuspended in 1.0 ml cold lysis buffer containing 10 mM Tris-HCl (pH 7.5), 10 mM NaCl, 15 mM $MgCl_2$, 250 mM Sucrose, 0.5% NP-40 and 0.1 mM EGTA. After vortexing for 10.0 s the cell suspension was incubated on ice for 15.0 min, centrifuged at 900 rpm for 10.0 min at 4°C with 4.0 ml of cold sucrose cushion. The pellet collected was washed using cold 10.0 mM Tris HCl (pH 7.5) and 10.0 mM NaCl, centrifuged at 900 rpm at 4°C for 10.0 min to obtain a fraction rich in nuclei.

[3]https://www.caymanchem.com/pdfs/10011563.pdf

Extraction of nuclear fraction

The fraction rich in nuclei was resuspended in 100.0 µl nuclear extraction buffer made up of 50 mM HEPES-KOH (pH 7.5), 420 mM NaCl, 0.5 mM Na_2EDTA, 0.1 mM EGTA, 10% Glycerol, and sonicated for 30.0 s. The mixture was incubated on ice for 30.0 min and centrifuged at 7000 rpm for 10 min. The supernatant containing crude nuclear extract was used for determination of HDAC activity. The protein content in the nuclear extract was estimated using BCA kit (Thermo Fischer, Waltham, MA, United States) as described below and extracts stored at −80°C until further use.

Estimation of total protein using BCA method

Total protein content in the nuclear extracts was determined using Pierce BCA kit from Thermo Fischer Scientific (Brown et al., 1989). A calibration graph was prepared by incubating increasing concentration of 25, 125, 250, 500, 750, 1000 and 1500 µg/ml bovine serum albumin (BSA, 10.0 µl) with 200 µl BCA reaction mixture containing of 50 parts of reagent A (made up of 0.8% sodium bicarbonate, 4% bicinchoninic acid and 0.16% sodium tartrate in 0.1 M sodium hydroxide) and 1 part of reagent B (made up of 4% cupric sulfate) at 37°C for 30.0 min, followed by measuring the absorbance at 562 nm using a multimode plate reader (PerkinElmer, Germany). Similarly suitably diluted test samples were also processed and concentration determined using the calibration curve.

HDAC inhibitory potential assessment using an ex vivo method

HDAC1 crude nuclear extract provided in the HDAC kit was used for determining the HDAC inhibitory potential of Tricaproin and Hexanoic acid. Experimentally, nuclear extracts containing 10 µg of protein is made up to 55 µl with assay buffer followed by addition of 5.0 µl fluoro-substrate to get 60 µl reaction volume. The reaction mixture was incubated for 30.0 min at 37°C. Appropriate experimental controls that include (a) no enzyme control with all components except the nuclear lysates; (b) a developer control consisting of fluorodeacetylated substrate instead of fluoro-substrate; (c) an inhibitor control with 5.0 µM of Tricostatin-A and 6, 12, 24 mM (HCT-116) and 20, 40, and 80 mM (HCT-15) sodium butyrate (a known HDAC Inhibitor); (d) TCN and CA of 75 µM (HCT-116) and 250 µM (HCT-15) and (e) a solvent control was also processed similarly. The

TABLE 1 | Percentage yield of crude extracts of *Simarouba glauca* leaves.

Extractant	Abbreviation	Percentage yield (gm/100 g of dried leaves of S.G)
Hexane	SGH	2.08 ± 0.15
Chloroform	SGC	3.53 ± 0.10
Ethyl acetate	SGEA	2.53 ± 0.12
70% Ethanol	SGE	8.54 ± 0.10
Water	SGW	5.51 ± 0.09

Table provides the percentage yield of Simarouba glauca extracts, which were prepared using solvents ranging from non-polar to polar. Extract prepared using hydro-alcohol (70% ethanol) provided maximum yield. The experiments were carried out at least three times and the values expressed as Mean ± SD.

TABLE 2 | IC50 value (µg/ml) of crude extracts of *Simarouba glauca* leaves on HCT-116 and HCT-15 colorectal carcinoma cells.

Extract	HCT-116			HCT-15		
	24 h	48 h	72h	24 h	48 h	72 h
SGH	ND[1]	ND	ND	ND	ND	ND
SGC	30.98 ± 0.33	23.63 ± 0.37	18.08 ± 0.17	29.37 ± 0.12	23.66 ± 0.64	18.15 ± 0.11
SGEA	78.86 ± 1.94	49.65 ± 1.96	45.84 ± 1.10	92.29 ± 2.05	46.87 ± 1.36	42.74 ± 0.79
SGE	129.67 ± 0.91	116.30 ± 3.20	82.27 ± 4.23	137.06 ± 3.23	117.46 ± 3.78	79.55 ± 1.65
SGW	169.16 ± 0.96	123.00 ± 4.47	98.69 ± 4.31	179.20 ± 3.29	129.13 ± 1.73	114.86 ± 2.78

Table represents the IC50 values of crude extracts on human colorectal carcinoma cell lines HCT-116 and HCT-15 at 24, 48, and 72h. Dose range of 7 to 500 µg/ml was tested and IC50 values were calculated. The chloroform extract showed a potent anti-colorectal cancer activity with an IC50 of 18 µg/ml at 72 h. These experiments were carried out three times with at least 4 replicate wells in each experiment. The values are expressed in Mean ± SEM. ND, not determined.

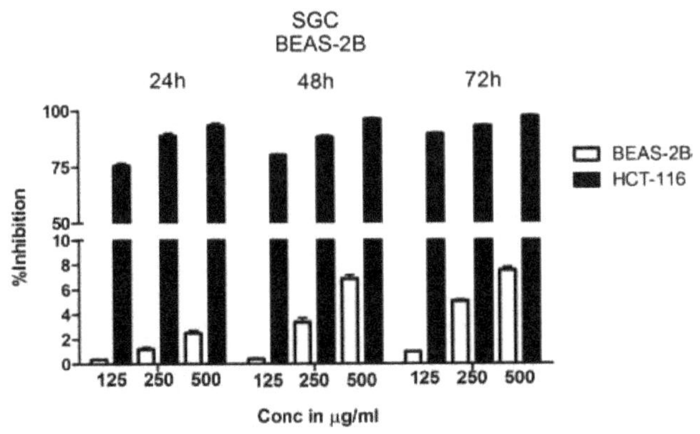

FIGURE 2 | Chloroform extract is selective to colorectal carcinoma cell line HCT-116 compared to normal lung epithelial cell line BEAS-2B. To determine the therapeutic index of chloroform extract, normal lung epithelial cell line BEAS-2B and colorectal carcinoma cell line HCT-116 were treated with increasing concentration of the extract for 24, 48, and 72 h. The number of viable cells determined using SRB and percentage inhibition calculated. Analysis of the data showed a significant difference in the efficacy of chloroform extract with HCT-116 cells more responsive to treatment compared to BEAS-2B, indicating the selectivity of chloroform fraction. The data shown is the Mean ± SEM of three independent experiments with 4 replicate wells in each experiment.

fluorescence was read in a kinetic mode after incubating for 15.0 min at room temperature with 15.0 μl of developer. The measurements were carried out at an excitation of 350 nm and emission of 450 nm.

HDAC inhibitory potential assessment using in vitro method

In vitro assessment of HDAC inhibitory potential was performed as described by Senawong et al. (2013) and Anantharaju et al. (2017a). In brief, 1×10^6 HCT-116 and HCT-15 cells were seeded in 10.0 ml of DMEM supplemented with 10% FBS in a 100 mm Petri plate. The exponentially growing HCT-116 and HCT-15 cells were treated with 7.8, 15.6, 31.2, 62.5, 125, and 250 μM TCN respectively for 48 h. Tricostatin A (5.0 μM), Sodium butyrate (6, 12, 24 mM for HCT-116) (20, 40, and 80 mM for HCT-15) were used as controls. The cells were trypsinized, and 10.0 μg of nuclear lysate was used for the determination of HDAC enzyme activity as detailed before.

Estimation of Intracellular Reactive Oxygen Species (ROS) in Colon Cancer Cells Treated With Tricaproin

Determination of ROS levels was performed according to Shailasree et al. (2015) with minor modifications (Shailasree et al., 2015; Anantharaju et al., 2017a). 0.5×10^4 HCT-116 and HCT-15 cells/well were seeded in a 96 well plate and allowed to grow in a carbon dioxide incubator maintained at 5% CO_2 and 37°C for 48 h. Then the exponentially proliferating cells were treated with 37.5, 75, 150 μM (for HCT-116) and 125, 250, 500 μM (for HCT-15) of TCN for 24 and 48 h. Traces of media in the cells were removed by washing with PBS. Then the cells were incubated with 10 μM of 2′, 7′-dichlorodihydrofluorescein diacetate (H2DCFDA, prepared in PBS) for 30.0 min and fluorescence intensity measured using a multimode plate reader operating at an excitation of 435 nm and emission of 520 nm.

Detection of Apoptosis by Acridine Orange and Ethidium Bromide Staining

Apoptosis detection by double staining using acridine orange and ethidium bromide was performed as detailed (Shailasree et al., 2015; Anantharaju et al., 2017a). Experimentally, 0.3×10^6 HCT-116 and HCT-15 cells were seeded in 6-well plates and exposed to increasing concentrations of TCN (37.5, 75, 150 μM) and Sodium butyrate (12 mM) on HCT-116 for about 48 h. The cells were trypsinized and mixed thoroughly to obtain a single cell suspension. The trypsin was neutralized by the addition of complete medium, and 20.0 μl cell suspension incubated with a mixture containing10.0 μl of 100.0 μg/ml each of ethidium bromide and acridine orange for 5.0 min. The cells were imaged using the fluorescence microscope using TRITC and FITC filters and later merged to obtain a combined image, which exhibited green and orange cells.

Confirmation of Apoptosis by Measuring Caspase-3 Activity

Activation of caspase-3 and 7 is the functional end point of apoptotic cascade and is an indicator of apoptosis induction in mammalian cells (Okada et al., 2016). The caspase-3/7 fluorescence assay kit was used to measure the caspase activity[4]. Experimentally, first, 1×10^4 HCT-116 and HCT-15 cells were treated with increasing concentrations of TCN at 37.5, 75, 150 μM (for HCT-116) and 125, 250, 500 μM (for HCT-15) for 48 h. Cells exposed to Sodium butyrate at 6, 12, 24 mM and 20, 40, 80 mM for HCT-116 and HCT-15 respectively served as positive control. The cells treated with 1% DMSO served as vehicle control. The plate was centrifuged at 560 rpm for 5.0 min. After aspirating the culture medium 200 μl of assay buffer was added and centrifuged at 560 rpm for 5.0 min. Hundred microliter of lysis buffer was then added and incubated on an orbital shaker at room temperature for 30.0 min followed by centrifugation at 560 rpm for 10.0 min. Ninety microliter of the supernatant from each well was then transferred to the corresponding well in a 96 well plate (black) and 10 μl of assay buffer was added. Hundred microliter of active caspase-3 positive control (1:500 in assay buffer) was added to the corresponding well. Further, the plate was incubated at 37°C for 30.0 min after adding 50 μl of substrate [combine100 μl of N-Ac-DEVD-N′-MC-R110, 400 μl DTT (1 M) assay reagent, 9.5 ml assay buffer] solution. The fluorescence intensity was measured using a multimode plate reader operating at an excitation of 485 nm and emission of 535 nm.

Statistical Analysis

All experiments were conducted in multiple replicates and the results were expressed as mean ±SEM. The results were subjected to one way ANOVA, followed by Tukey's *post hoc* test to analyze difference between experimental and control samples. A "*P*" value of < 0.05 was considered significant.

[4]https://www.caymanchem.com/product/10009135

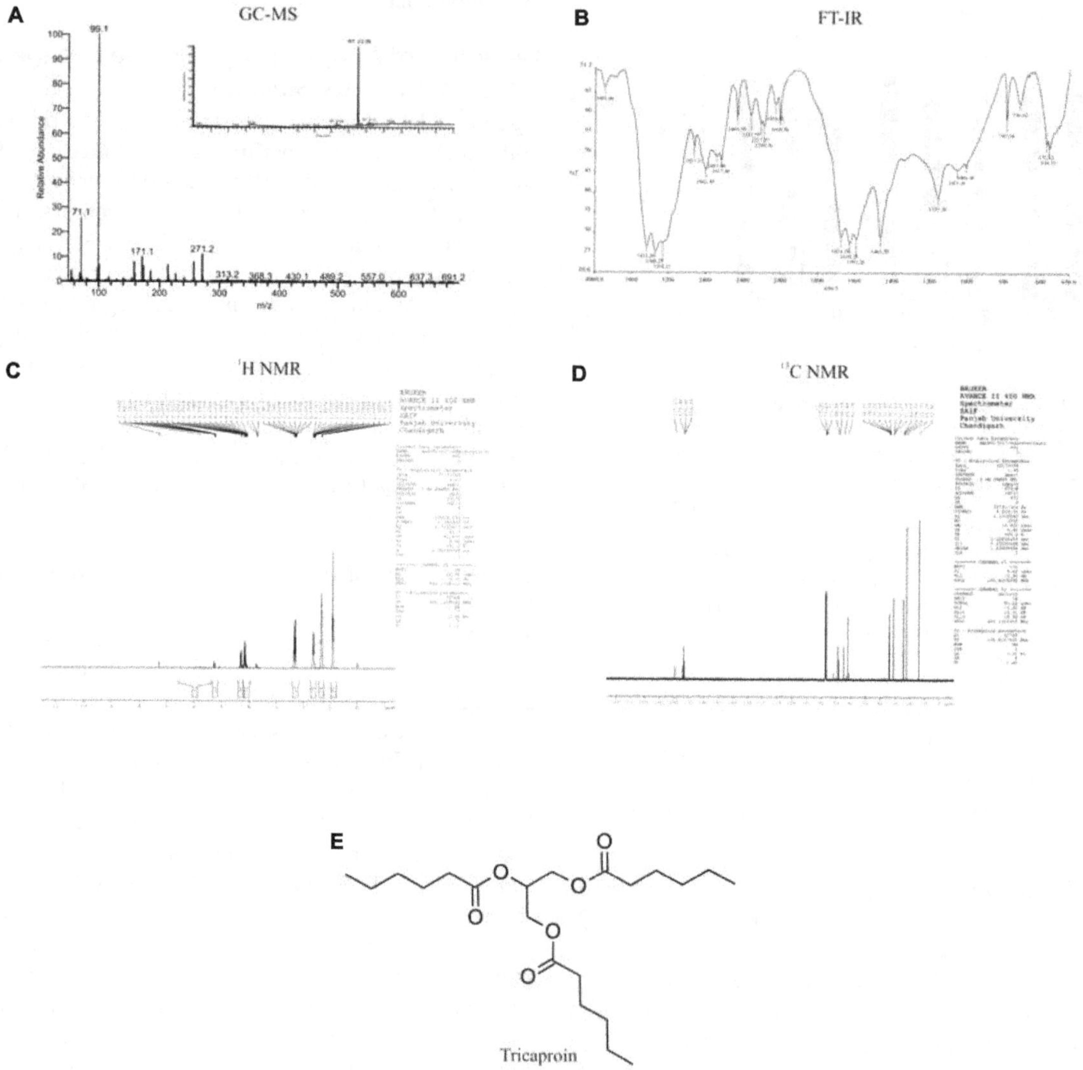

FIGURE 3 | Elucidation of the structure of purified compound: The pure compound obtained by the fractionation of chloroform extract was subjected for structural characterization using **(A)** GC-MS; **(B)** FT-IR; **(C)** ^{1}H-NMR; and **(D)** ^{13}C-NMR. Analysis of the data showed the presence of tricaproin **(E)**. Tricaproin is a triglyceride made up of 3 hexanoic (caproic) acid residues ester linked to the hydroxylic groups of glycerol.

All the graphs were generated using GraphPad Prism-5 software.

RESULTS

Fractionation of SG Leaves, Using Solvents, Yielded Extracts Containing Anti-cancer Agents With Good Therapeutic Index

To isolate the anti-cancer agents from *Simarouba glauca*, the leaves were successively extracted with n-hexane (SGH), chloroform (SGC), ethyl acetate (SGEA), hydroalcohol (70% ethanol; SGE) water (SGW) and anti-cancer potential in terms of CRC cells growth inhibition determined using SRB assay (**Figures 1A,B** and **Table 1**). Analysis of the data showed a dose- and time- dependent increase in the potency of each extract (**Figures 1A,B**, **Table 2**, and Supplementary Figures 1A–D). For instance, at 72 h of treatment of HCT-116 cells, the chloroform extract exhibited the most potent anti-cancer activity with an IC50 of ~18.0 μg/ml compared to ethyl acetate (IC50 ~45 μg/ml), hydroalcohol (IC50 ~80 μg/ml) and water (IC50 ~100.0 μg/ml) (Supplementary Figure 1B). However, the extract prepared using hexane had only minimal effect at all concentrations tested **(Figure 1A)**. For example, at 500 μg/ml concentration, only about 25% growth inhibition was observed at 24 h treatment **(Figure 1A)**. Extending the

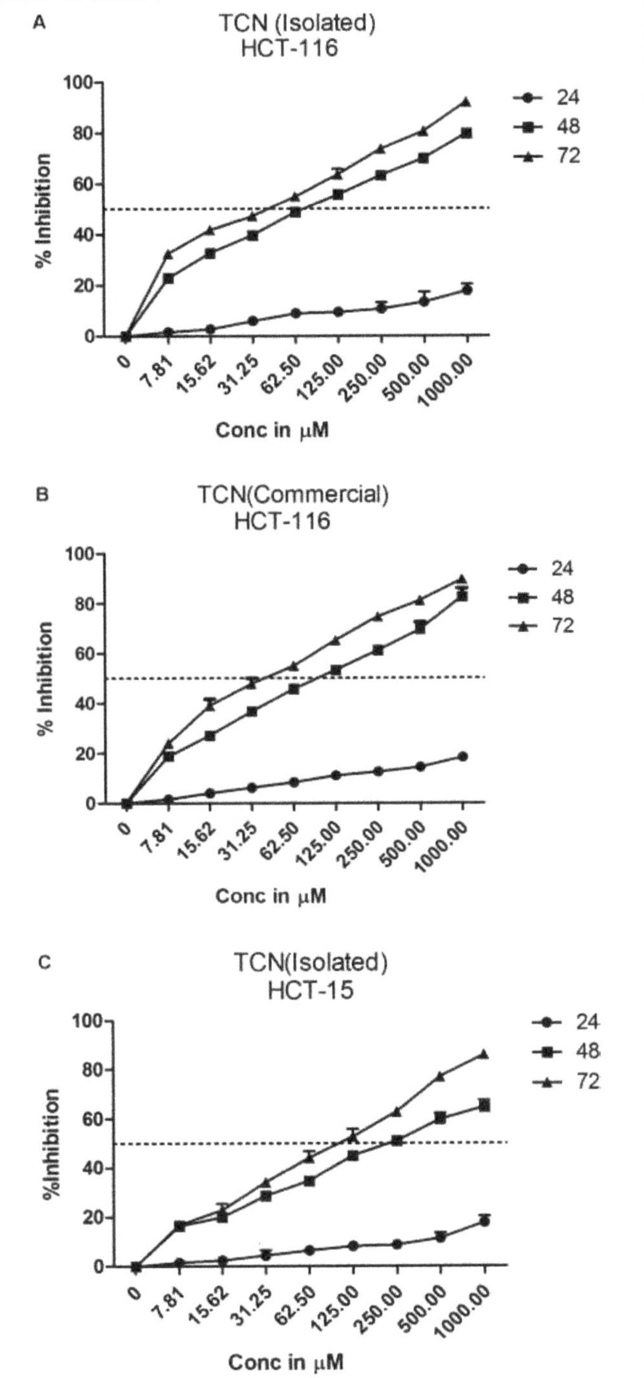

FIGURE 4 | Comparative assessment of commercially available tricaproin with that of the tricaproin purified from SG leaf. In order to determine whether the TCN purified from SG leaves has similar cytotoxic properties compared to commercially available TCN, colorectal carcinoma cells HCT-116 **(A,B)** and HCT-15 **(C)** were treated with increasing concentrations of TCN isolated (**A**: HCT-116 cell line and **C**: HCT-15 cell line) as well as TCN obtained from commercial sources for 24, 48, and 72 h. Percentage growth inhibition was calculated and the data compared between the two TCN molecules. Analysis of the data showed no much difference between the TCN isolated from SG leaves and the TCN obtained from commercial vendors. The data represented is the Mean ± SEM of three independent experiments.

treatment time for 48 and 72 h improved the efficacy marginally (**Table 2** and Supplementary Figures 1A,B). Similar trend was observed upon treatment of HCT-15 cells with crude extracts (**Figure 1B** and **Table 2**). The IC50 values were found to be in the order of SGC (~18 μg/ml), SGEA (~43 μg/ml), SGE (~80 μg/ml), SGW (~115 μg/ml) (**Table 2** and Supplementary Figures 1C,D).

Since chloroform extract showed better potency compared to other extracts, next, the selectivity was determined by comparing the percentage growth inhibition of normal bronchial epithelial cell line BEAS-2B with CRC cell line HCT-116 at 125 μg/ml, 250 μg/ml and 500 μg/ml concentrations treated for 24, 48, and 72 h. The chloroform extract showed much better selectivity to HCT-116 cell line compared to BEAS-2B cells (**Figure 2**). The selectivity is much better at lower concentrations compared to higher concentration (**Figure 2**). For example, at 24 h treatment with 125 μg/ml chloroform extract, only 0.38% growth inhibition was observed in BEAS-2B cells compared to 75% in case of HCT-116. However at 500 μg/ml concentration the % inhibition of BEAS-2B and HCT116 cells increased to ~2% and ~95% respectively (**Figure 2**). The selectivity of extract toward cancer cells decreased as the incubation time increases from 24 to 72 h, which is primarily due to increased growth retardation of even normal cells (**Figure 2**).

Purification and Characterization of Anti-cancer Agent Tricaproin From Chloroform Extract

Results of anti-cancer agent screening and selectivity data suggested the presence of potent anticancer agents with good safety profile in chloroform extract. Hence, the chloroform extract was further fractionated using silica gel column chromatography followed by preparation of fatty acid methyl esters as detailed in materials and methods (Supplementary Figure 2). This fractionation procedure yielded 6 fractions (Supplementary Table 1 and Supplementary Figure 3). Analysis of all these fractions by GC-MS (Electron ionization-Time of Flight (EI-TOF) showed that Fraction-6 with a yield of 0.24 g is pure compared to Fractions-1 to -5 (**Figure 3A** and Supplementary Tables 2–5). The fragment ions obtained (%intensity) are – 271 (20), 215 (5), 171 (5), 159 (10), 99 (100), 71 (50). Comparison of these fragment-ions with the mass spectral database suggested the presence of tricaproin ($C_{21}H_{38}O_6$) with a calculated molecular mass 386.529 g/mol. Next, Fraction-6 was subjected for further structural characterization using FT-IR (fixed cell method), ^{1}H NMR and ^{13}C NMR (**Figures 3B–D**). Analysis using FT-IR showed characteristic wavelength frequencies representing C-H stretching (2927 cm^{-1}), C-H bending (1465 cm^{-1}), C = O stretching (1674 cm^{-1}), C-O stretching (1155 and 1051 cm^{-1}) (**Figure 3B**). Analysis using 400 MHz ^{1}H NMR yielded additional structural details confirming the presence of - CH(COO)$_3$ (δ 5.5 s, 1H), -CH$_2$COO (δ 2.5–2.25 m, 6H), (CH$_2$)$_3$ (δ 1.70–1.60 m, 6H), -(CH$_2$-CH$_2$)$_3$ (1.50–1.20 m, 12H) (**Figure 3C**). Subsequent analysis using ^{13}C NMR (in CDCl$_3$-d6) yielded the following structural details: (a) presence of >C = O ester (173.91, 173.31, 172.85 δ ppm); (b) >C-O, -C-O- bonds 68.28, 65.00, 62.10 (δ ppm); (c) -C-C = O ester (34.14, 34.09, 34.04 δ ppm); (d) -CH_2 (33.99, 33.91, 31.23, 31.20, 31.16, 24.53, 24.50, 24.37, 22.24 δ ppm), and (e) -CH_3 (13.82 δ ppm) (**Figure 3D**). Taken together, these structural details confirmed the presence of a tricaproin in the pure fraction, which showed good anticancer activity (**Figure 3E**).

Tricaproin and Hexanoic Acid (Caproic Acid) Inhibit Colorectal Carcinoma Cells Growth *in Vitro*

Tricaproin is a molecule produced by the condensation of each of the hydroxylic groups of glycerol with hexanoic acid (also known as caproic acid) (**Figure 3E**). In order to determine and further confirm functionally that the Fraction-6 contain tricaproin, the cytotoxic potency of the commercially available tricaproin (procured from Sigma, St. Louis, MO, United States) was compared with the purified Fraction-6 on HCT-116 cells (**Figures 4A,B**). Analysis of the data showed similar growth inhibitory properties when tested on HCT-116 (**Figures 4A,B**). TCN was also tested on HCT-15 cell line, which yielded a dose and time dependent response (**Figure 4C**). Next, to check whether the monomeric hexanoic acid and glycerol exhibit anti-cancer activity, HCT-116 and HCT-15 cells were treated with increasing concentration of hexanoic acid and glycerol and viability determined using SRB at 24, 48, and 72 h (Supplementary Figures 4A–D). The data showed a significant growth reduction, which is similar to parent tricaproin, only with hexanoic acid treatment (Supplementary Figures 4A,B) but not with glycerol exposure (Supplementary Figures 4C,D). Therefore, the active molecule in tricaproin is hexanoic acid but not glycerol.

Selectivity of the TCN was tested against normal bronchial epithelial cell line BEAS-2B and CRC cell line HCT-116 at 250, 500, and 1000 μM concentrations treated for 24, 48, and 72 h. The compound exhibited more selectivity toward HCT-116 cell line compared to BEAS-2B cells (Supplementary Figure 5). For example, at 48 h treatment with 125 μg/ml TCN, only 1.4% growth inhibition was seen in BEAS-2B cells compared to 64% in case of HCT-116 cells (Supplementary Figure 5). Supporting the TCN cytotoxicity on cancer cell lines, analysis of lactate dehydrogenase released in to the cell culture media, an indicator of cell death, also showed that compound treatment induced death in colorectal cancer cells (Supplementary Figure 6).

Tricaproin and Hexanoic Acid Inhibit HDAC Activity More Potently Than Sodium Butyrate

Sodium butyrate (SB) is a known inhibitor of HDAC. Structurally, SB is shorter by two -CH_2 groups to hexanoic acid (Supplementary Figure 7). Since SB is known to inhibit HDAC activity, we have hypothesized that the hexanoic acid and tricaproin might also inhibit HDAC activity. To test this hypothesis, tricaproin, hexanoic acid and SB were first docked in to the sodium butyrate binding site of Class-I (HDACs −1, −2, −3, and −8) and Class-II HDAC (i.e., HDAC-4) and the binding energies compared (**Table 3** and **Figures 5A,B**). Analysis of the data showed a significant strong binding of TCN especially on HDAC 3 (**Figure 5B**), as evidenced by higher negative C-Docker energy as well as C-Docker interaction strength, compared to SB or Hexanoic acid to all HDACs evaluated (**Table 3**). The order of binding of TCN to Class-I HDACs is HDAC-3 > HDAC-2 > HDAC-1 > HDAC-8. Class-II HDAC, i.e., HDAC-4 showed the lowest C-Docker energy (**Table 3**). Therefore, *in silico* analysis showed better binding of TCN to Class-I HDACs compared to Class-II HDAC.

Since the *in silico* data showed better binding of TCN to Class-I HDACs, next, the ability of TCN to inhibit HDAC activity was determined by exposing HCT-116 and HCT-15 cells, which are known to contain elevated HDACs, to increasing concentrations of TCN for 48 h. Nuclear extract from the cells not exposed

TABLE 3 | Comparison of HDAC binding energies and key amino acid residues involved in the interactions of Tricaproin, Hexanoic acid, and Sodium butyrate.

Target	Compound	C Docker energy (Kcal/mol)	C Docker Interaction Energy (Kcal/mol)	Interacting residues
HDAC 1	SB	−24.701	−23.159	HIS 178, TYR 303, ASP 176, MET 30, LEU 139, CYS 151
	TCN	−52.499	−43.844	HIS 178, MET 30, LEU 139, CYS 151
	HA	−19.574	−19.992	TYR 303, MET 30, LEU 139, CYS 151
HDAC 2	SB	−25.158	−23.870	LYS (71 and 170), LEU 166
	TCN	−56.974	−45.540	LYS (71 and 170), LEU 166
	HA	−30.291	−29.548	LYS (71 and 170), LEU 169
HDAC 3	SB	−18.129	−17.151	HIS (135, 172), TYR 298, PHE 144, PHE 200
	TCN	−62.206	−55.954	HIS (134, 135, 172), GLY 143, CYS 145, LEU 133, PRO 23
	HA	−22.797	−20.664	HIS (134, 135, 172)
HDAC 8	SB	−16.799	−16.452	THR 105, TYR 154, ILE 108
	TCN	−49.471	−38.570	THR 105, GLU 106, SER 30, ALA 32, LEU 31
	HA	−8.049	−2.252	TRP 141, ILE 115, LEU 155
HDAC 4	SB	−40.117	−39.182	LYS 20, ARG (37 and 154), PHE 168
	TCN	−43.016	−30.362	LEU 299, HIS 198, PHE 227
	HA	−43.189	−41.172	LYS 20, ARG (154 and 37), PHE 168, TYR 332

Table: Comparative in silico analysis of the binding strengths of TCN to Class-I HDACs and Class-II HDAC.

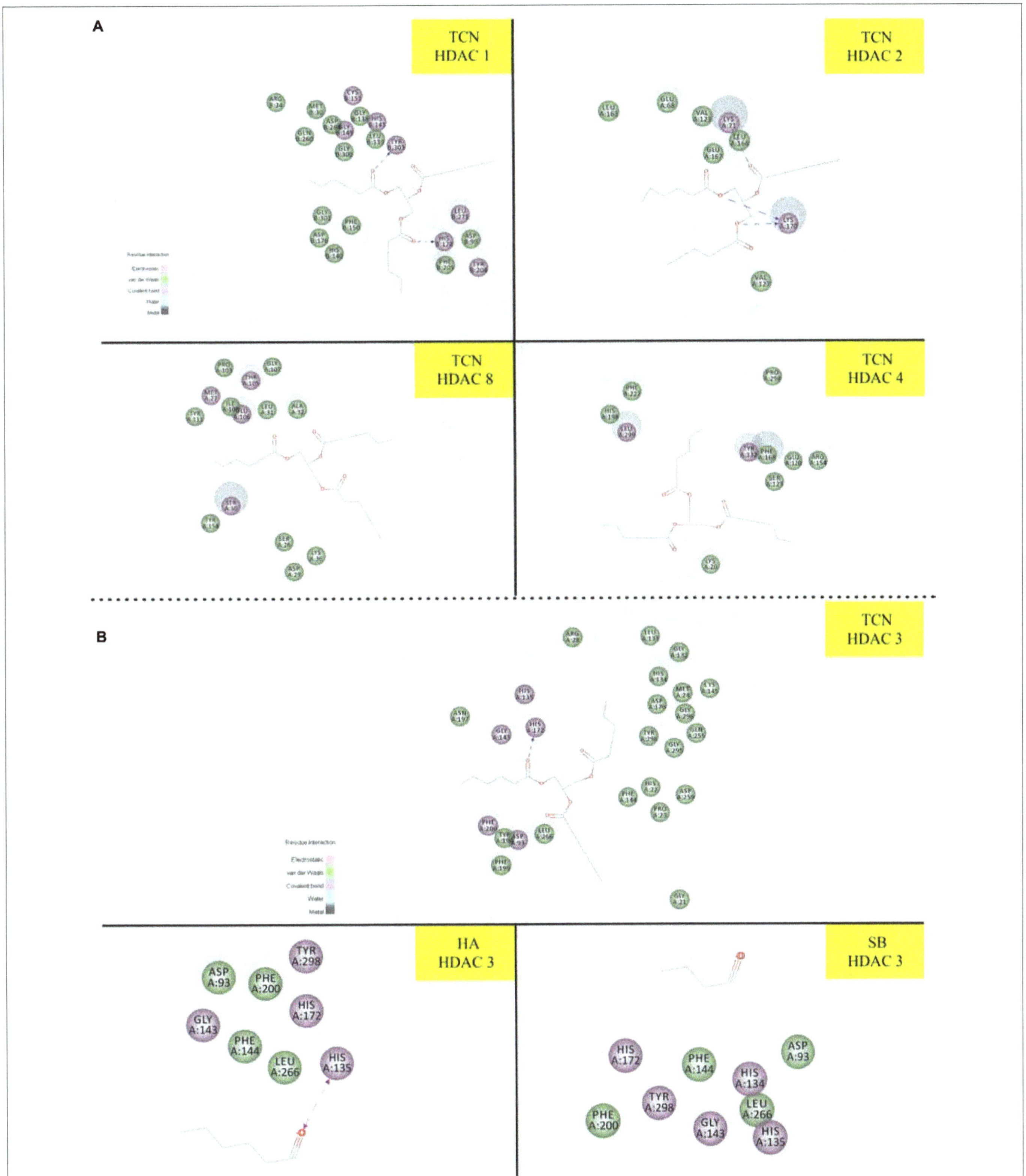

FIGURE 5 | Molecular docking studies demonstrating the ability of TCN to bind to Class-I HDACs: Since sodium butyrate is a known inhibitor of HDAC proteins, we have tested the ability of TCN to bind to sodium butyrate binding site of HDAC using Discovery software. As shown TCN binds to Class I HDACs 1, 2, 8 and Class II HDAC-4 **(A)**. Further analysis showed that TCN exhibited much better binding to HDAC-3 **(B)**. However, hexanoic acid and sodium butyrate exhibited poor binding to HDAC3 **(B)** indicating the selectivity of TCN toward HDAC3.

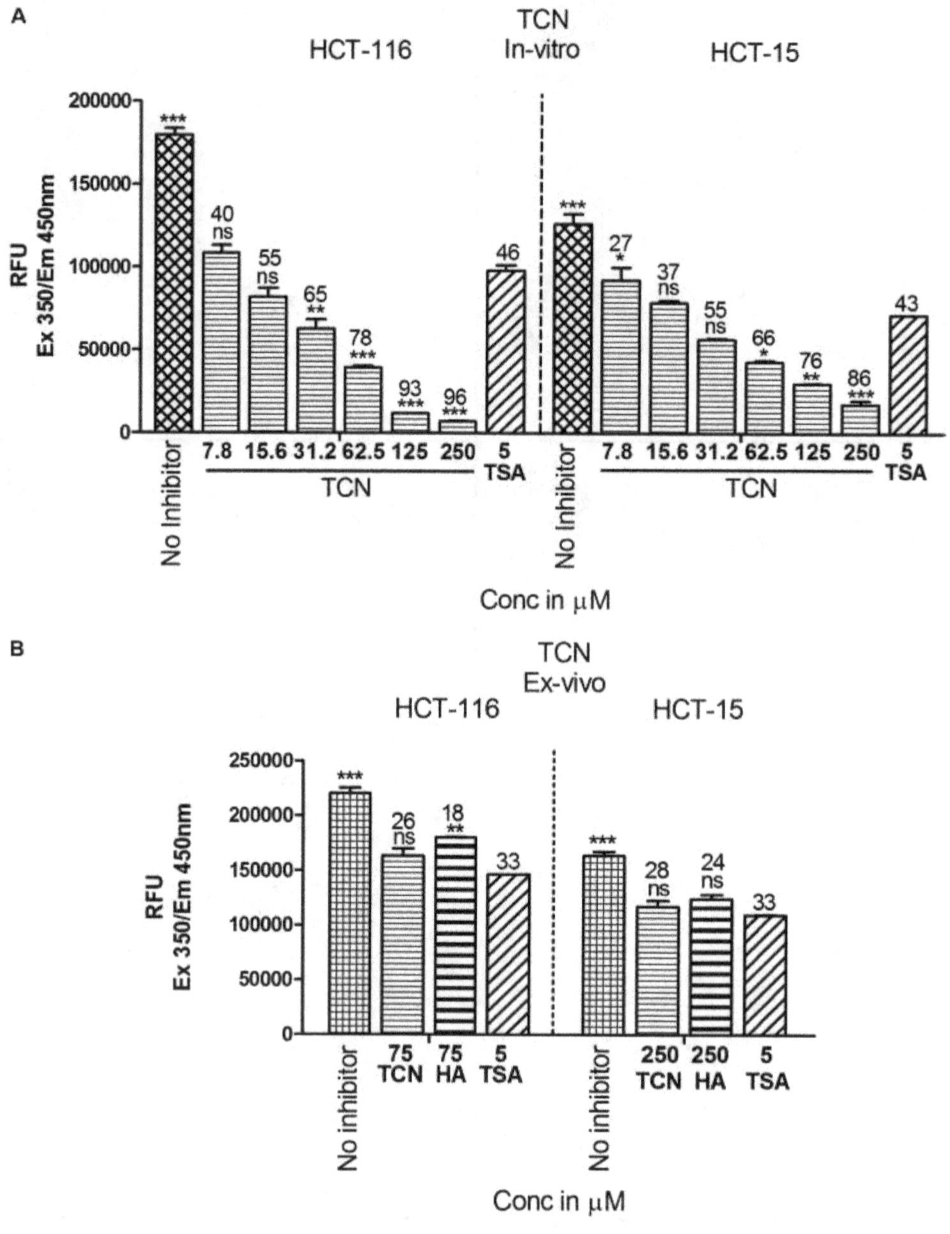

FIGURE 6 | TCN inhibited HDAC activity *in vitro*: Based on the *in silico* data, it is predicted that TCN binds to Class-I HDACs with more selectivity to HDAC3, which is likely the factor responsible for HDAC activity inhibition and cell growth retardation. To test whether this hypothesis, colorectal carcinoma cells were incubated with increasing concentration of TCN and nuclear and cytosolic fractions collected. HDAC activity compared to vehicle treated cells was assessed using a kit. Analysis of the data showed that TCN, indeed, inhibited HDAC activity *in vitro* when tested against HCT-116 and HCT-15 cells **(A)**. To further test the efficacy *ex vivo*, the nuclear extracts were isolated from HCT-116 and HCT-15 cells and treated with TCN at 75 and 250 μM concentration and percentage inhibition of HDAC activity calculated. HA and TSA were used as controls **(B)**. HDAC inhibition experiments were performed thrice with 3 replicates in each experiment and values expressed in Mean ± SEM.

to (untreated), or exposed to TCN or control TSA was isolated and HDAC activity measured as detailed in methods section (Senawong et al., 2013). A significant dose dependent decrease in HDAC activity was observed upon treatment of HCT-116 and HCT-15 cells (**Figure 6**). At 125.0 μM concentration, about 93 and 76% inhibition was observed, respectively, for HDACs isolated from HCT-116 and HCT-15 cell lines, confirming the *in silico* observations (**Figure 6A**). However, interestingly, when the TCN, HA and positive control TSA were incubated with nuclear extract collected from HCT-116 and HCT-15 cell lines, the percentage inhibition was significantly low (86% vs. 28% at 250 μM on HCT-15 cells, **Figure 6B**) compared to the *in vitro* experiments wherein cells were first exposed to the compounds, followed by assessing the HDAC activity in the nuclear extract (**Figure 6A**). To further test this interesting observation, HDAC1 (supplied as a control in HDAC kit)

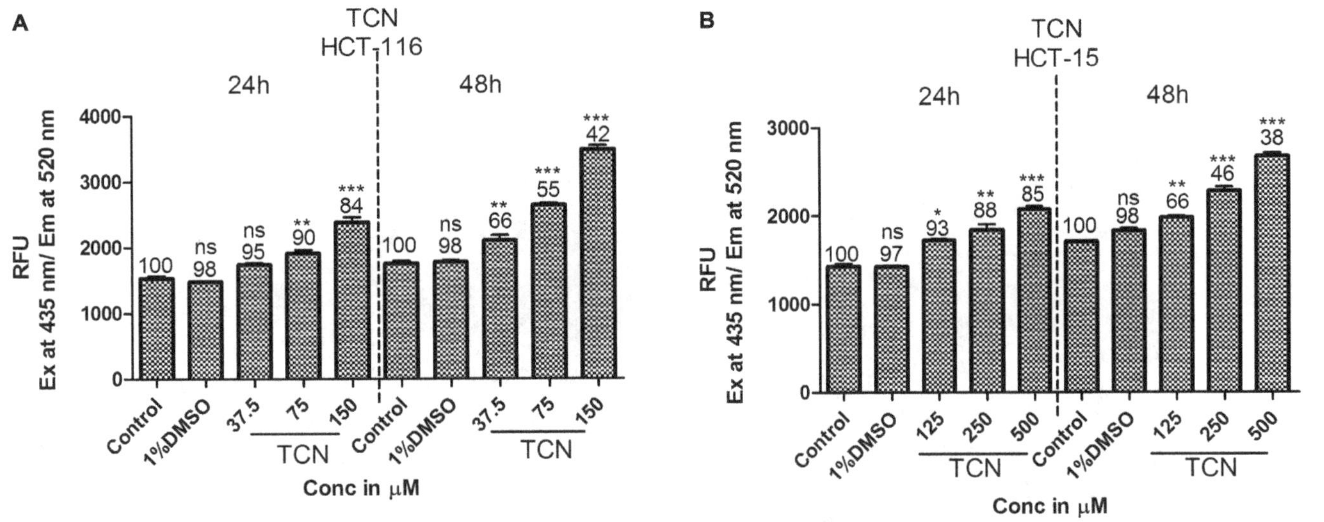

FIGURE 7 | HDAC inhibitor TCN enhances cellular ROS: HDAC inhibitors are known for their ability to induce cellular ROS. Hence, the ability of TCN to induce cellular ROS was measured using H2DCFDA procedure as detailed in materials and methods. As predicted, TCN induced cellular ROS thereby decreased the number of viable cells, especially at 48 h treatment on HCT-116 **(A)** and HCT-15 **(B)** cells. These experiments were carried out at least 3 times to check the reproducibility and the results expressed as Mean ± SEM.

was incubated with 250 μM TCN, 250 μM Hexanoic acid and 5.0 μM TSA and percentage inhibition compared to control vehicle exposed HDAC1 calculated. A non-significant 12 and 8% inhibition was observed, respectively with TCN and HA treatments (Supplementary Figure 8A). Even the positive controls TSA and SB exhibited similar reduction in percentage HDAC activity inhibition when tested using isolated nuclear extract or commercial HDAC1 (Supplementary Figures 8A–C)

Tricaproin Induced Reactive Oxygen Species in Colorectal Carcinoma Cells

HDAC is a known regulator of antioxidant enzymes super oxide dismutase (SOD), peroxidase and catalase in cells (Espinosa-Diez et al., 2015). Hence, accumulation of reactive oxygen species (ROS) is a characteristic features of HDAC inhibitors (Rosato et al., 2008). Furthermore, prior studies have demonstrated that HDAC inhibitors such as SAHA, SelSA, SB, benzoic acid and cinnamic acid derivatives induce cancer cells death by increasing the levels of ROS (Ruefli et al., 2001; Sanmartín et al., 2012; Anantharaju et al., 2017a; Salimi et al., 2017). Since, tricaproin also exhibited HDAC inhibitory activity, it is predicted that induction of CRC cells death due to tricaproin treatment might be due to elevated ROS levels. Therefore, to test this hypothesis, HCT-116 and HCT-15 cells were treated with increasing concentration of TCN and levels of ROS estimated as detailed in methods. As predicted, treatment of HCT-116 and HCT-15 cells with increasing concentrations of TCN significantly increased the reactive oxygen species at 24 and 48 h (**Figures 7A,B**). An about twofold increase in ROS was observed at 150.0 μM concentration in HCT-116 cell line at 48 h of treatment (**Figure 7A**). Similarly an about 1.6-fold increase in ROS was observed upon treatment of HCT-15 cells with 500.0 μM tricaproin (**Figure 7B**). The increase in ROS correlated directly with decrease in cell viability (Numbers on top of each bar).

Tricaproin Induced Apoptosis in Colorectal Carcinoma Cells

Increased ROS in a cell induces apoptosis thereby promote cell death (Simon et al., 2000). In order to determine whether TCN-treatment induced ROS also triggered apoptosis in HCT-116 and HCT-15 cells, the cells were stained with acridine orange and ethidium bromide, and the levels of caspase-3 (a marker for apoptosis) measured as detailed in materials and methods.

First, TCN treated and untreated HCT-116 cells (48 h) were stained with ethidium bromide and acridine orange to evaluate apoptosis. Theoretically, the cells undergoing apoptosis exhibit condensed chromatin and show orange-red color compared with the live cells that appear green when observed under fluorescence microscope. Analysis of photomicrographs showed significantly high orange and red stained cells when treated with TCN (**Figure 8A**). However, no such stained cells were observed in untreated or vehicle 1% DMSO treated cells (**Figure 8B**). The number of orange stained cells increased with increasing TCN concentration.

Induction of caspase-3/7 mediated apoptosis is a characteristic feature of HDAC inhibitors (Jasek et al., 2012; Okada et al., 2016). Therefore, the levels of caspase-3/7 were estimated using a fluorimetric Caspase-3/7 assay kit as detailed in materials and methods. A dose dependent increase in caspase-3 activity was observed upon exposing HCT-116 and HCT-15 cells to TCN as well as control compounds SB and hexanoic acid (**Figures 9A,B**). The efficacy of TCN and hexanoic acid for inducing caspase-3 activity is much higher compared to SB in both the cell lines (**Figure 9**). For example, at 0.038 mM concentration an about 1.6 and 1.5 fold increase in caspase-3 activity compared

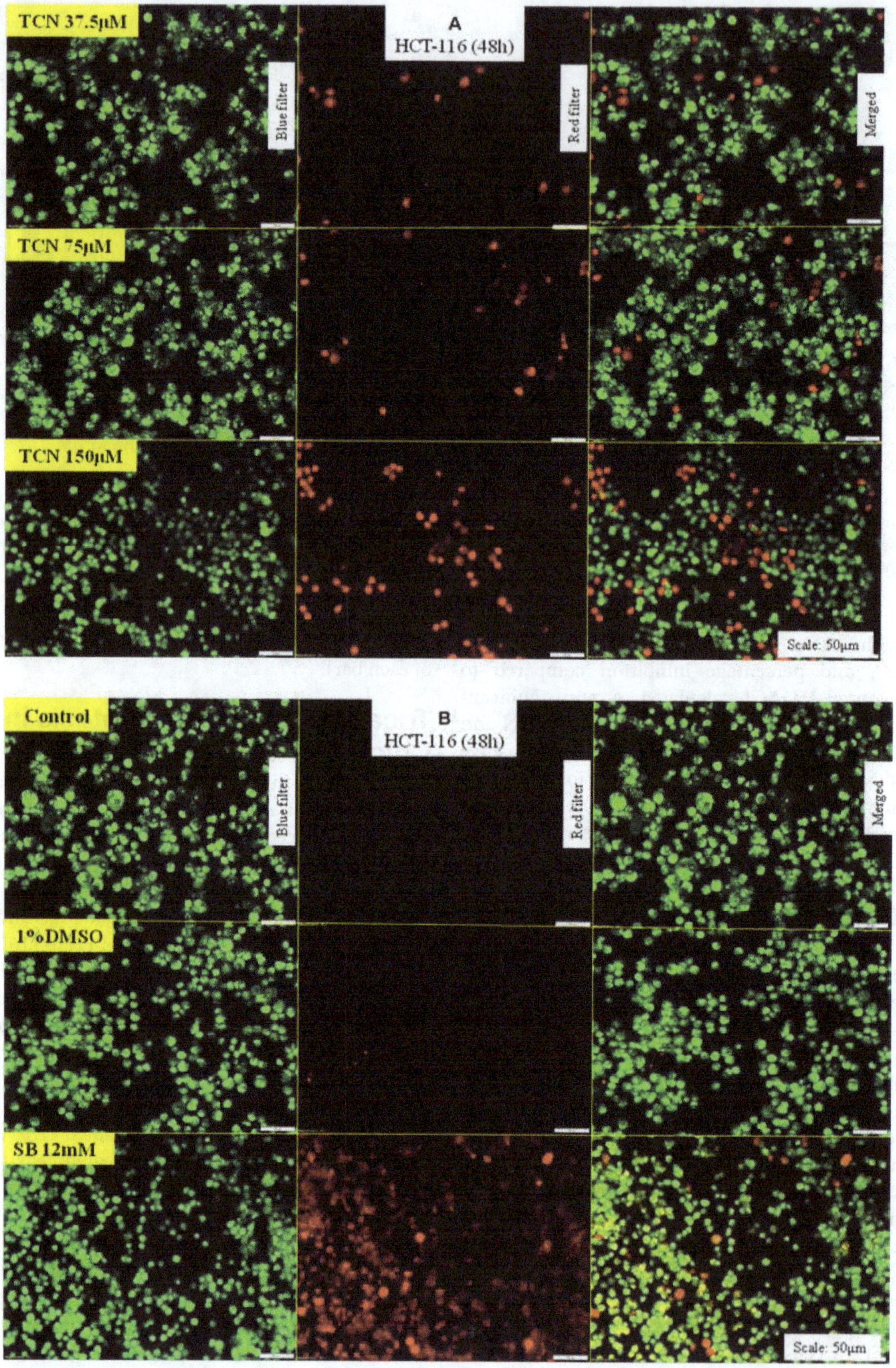

FIGURE 8 | TCN triggered apoptosis in HCT-116 cells: Acridine orange and ethidium bromide staining procedure helps to differentiate proliferating and apoptotic cells using a fluorescent microscope at a magnification of 20X. Since TCN inhibited cancer cells growth, now, the mechanistic basis for cell growth inhibition was assessed. As shown, treatment of colon cancer cells HCT-116 with TCN induced apoptosis as evidenced by the presence of condensed chromatin (orange stained cells) **(A)**. Untreated and vehicle treated cells exhibited no signs of apoptosis as there were no orange stained cells in these fields. The weak HDAC inhibitor sodium butyrate also induced apoptosis, but at 12 mM concentration **(B)**.

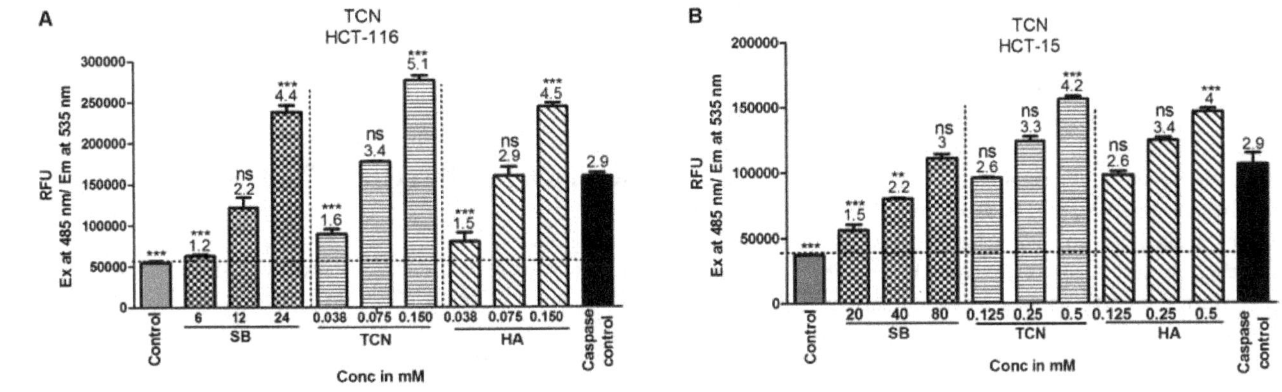

FIGURE 9 | TCN induced cell death is mediated by the induction of caspase-3 activity *in vitro*: Induction of caspases is one of the mechanisms often reported for anti-cancer agents. Therefore, to check whether TCN also triggers caspase-3 activity, HCT-116 **(A)** and HCT-15 **(B)** cells were treated with increasing concentrations of TCN for 48 h and cell lysates collected as detailed in materials and methods. The data showed induction of caspase-3 activity with increasing TCN concentration in both cell lines. The component hexanoic acid also induced apoptosis in these cell lines in a dose dependent fashion indicating that the effect could be due to short chain fatty acid hexanoic acid. Pure caspase-3, supplied in the kit, was used as positive control in this study. These experiments were carried out 3-times with 4 replicates in each experiment. The data represented is the Mean ± SEM.

to control DMSO treated cells was observed respectively with TCN and hexanoic acid treatment. However, even at 6.0 mM concentration of SB, only 1.2 fold increases in caspase-3 activity was observed. Similar trend was observed even in HCT-15 cell line (**Figures 9A,B**)

DISCUSSION

Evidences from traditional medicine reports and recent success with naturally occurring anti-cancer agents stimulated the scientific community to screen and identify potential phytochemicals for treating cancers (Shoeb, 2006). In addition, the advantages with natural products such as low-toxicity and easy availability also provided additional strength to anti-cancer agents screening research (Cragg and Newman, 2005; Shah et al., 2013). *Simarouba glauca*, a Simaroubaceae family plant, is a rich source of bitter substances with potential anti-cancer properties (Patil and Gaikwad, 2011). To date, not much is known about their anti-cancer potential. Moreover, it is also not known whether any other type of compounds (other than bitter substances) do present in SG leaf extracts (Puranik et al., 2017). Therefore, in this study, leaves of *Simarouba glauca* were extracted with solvents of increasing polarity and anti-cancer activity screen performed, which identified chloroform extract as a better source for compounds with potent anti-cancer activity (Rivero-Cruz et al., 2005; Puranik et al., 2017). Chloroform alone or in association with methanol (2:1) has been widely used to extract short chain fatty acids and triglyceride esters (King and Min, 1998). The chloroform extracted compound was identified as tricaproin (TCN) by structural analysis using GC-MS, FT-IR and ^{1}H and ^{13}C NMR (NIST, da Rocha et al., 2007, SDBS). TCN is an ester made up of three hexanoic acids ester linked to glycerol (da Rocha et al., 2007). Once enter in to cell, the tricaproin undergo hydrolysis to produce hexanoic acid and glycerol. Since short chain fatty acids such as butyrate (a weak inhibitor of HDAC) are known to inhibit HDAC, the ability of tricaproin and hexanoic acid were tested for their potency to reduce HDAC activity (Kuefer et al., 2004; Nande and Claudio, 2014). As predicted, TCN and hexanoic acid inhibited the HDAC activity and reduced cancer cell proliferation rates significantly compared to sodium butyrate. Further analysis showed that the glycerol moiety of tricaproin is not effective in reducing cell proliferation and HDAC activity, hence, the active component causing HDAC inhibition and cell death is hexanoic acid. Since, TCN is made up of 3 molecules of hexanoic acid, TCN is a preferred choice for delivering the active molecules compared to hexanoic acid as such.

Inhibition of HDAC is one of the viable strategies for inhibiting cancer cells growth (Glozak and Seto, 2007). Several *in vitro* and *in vivo* studies as well as clinical trials using HDAC inhibitors have demonstrated the potential use of these pharmacological agents for cancer therapy (Mottamal et al., 2015). Moreover, class-I HDACs have been shown to be over expressed in several carcinomas including colorectal cancers (Mariadason, 2008). Elevated HDACs promote cell proliferation, inhibit apoptosis and induce drug resistance in cancers (Glozak and Seto, 2007). Targeted inhibition of HDAC using naturally occurring pharmacological agents such as benzoic acid and cinnamic acid derivatives, and synthetic SelSA were demonstrated to retard CRC cells *in vitro* and in animals (Ruefli et al., 2001; Sanmartín et al., 2012; Gowda et al., 2012; Anantharaju et al., 2017a; Salimi et al., 2017). Whereas some of these inhibitors found successful in clinical trials for inhibiting AML and CML, other compounds have not shown promising results either due to poor efficacy or due to systemic toxicity (Mottamal et al., 2015). Therefore, several research groups continued their efforts to screen and identify HDAC inhibitors from natural sources (Anantharaju et al., 2017a). Tricaproin is one such naturally occurring inhibitor of HDAC. Mechanistically, tricaproin inhibited class-I HDACs, thereby increased the levels of apoptosis mediated by caspase-3. However, it is currently unknown whether any other proteins do have a role in the apoptosis induction. Several reports have shown the upregulation of p53, Bax and Bad upon HDAC inhibition (Richon et al., 2000; Sawa et al., 2001). Therefore, in the subsequent studies the effect of inhibiting HDAC using TCN will be evaluated further to assess the expression of tumor suppressor as well as oncogenic molecules. In addition, the future studies should focus on testing the efficacy of TCN for inhibiting tumor growth as well as metastasis in experimental animal models.

CONCLUSION

Results of our study report the purification and characterization of a Class-I HDAC inhibitor, tricaproin, from *Simarouba glauca*. Unlike sodium butyrate, a weak inhibitor of HDAC, TCN inhibited HDAC activity with more potency, hence, could be considered for further development.

Although the study showed thorough characterization of TCN, and initial testing of purified TCN in cell based assays, currently the study suffers from lack of in depth mechanistic based experiments. In summary, this is the first report demonstrating the purification and characterization of a lipid based HDAC inhibitor from *Simarouba glauca*

AUTHORS NOTE

This article is dedicated to Prof. M. N. Satishkumar, Professor of Pharmacology, JSS College of Pharmacy, Udhagamandalam, Tamil Nadu, India who breathed his last on 17th March 2015 after fighting against colorectal carcinoma.

AUTHOR CONTRIBUTIONS

AJ has performed the experiments, compiled the data, prepared tables and graphs. MC has performed the isolation and purification. EK and SM have assisted in designing, drafting, and editorial corrections of the manuscript.

ACKNOWLEDGMENTS

The authors are thankful to Department of Science and Technology, India for providing the INSPIRE Fellowship. The laboratory support extended by Center of Excellence in Molecular Biology and Regenerative Medicine is highly acknowledged. In addition, author AJ would like to acknowledge the DST-FIST funded Department of Biochemistry, JSS Medical College for providing an opportunity to work in CEMR laboratory. Further authors would like to acknowledge Punjab University for the characterization of the molecule. AJ would like to thank Mr. U. Jayaram, Research scholar, UGC-MAN (SRF) and Mr. Selvaraj Ayyamperumal, Research scholar, DBT-SRF from Department of Chemistry, JSS College of Pharmacy, Udhagamandalm, Tamil Nadu for assisting in the characterization and docking studies.

REFERENCES

Anantharaju, P. G., Gowda, P. C., Vimalambike, M. G., and Madhunapantula, S. V. (2016). An overview on the role of dietary phenolics for the treatment of cancers. *Nutr. J.* 15, 99–104. doi: 10.1186/s12937-016-0217-2

Anantharaju, P. G., Reddy, B. D., Padukudru, M. A., Kumari Chitturi, C. M., Vimalambike, M. G., and Madhunapantula, S. V. (2017a). Naturally occurring benzoic acid derivatives retard cancer cell growth by inhibiting histone deacetylases (HDAC). *Cancer Biol. Ther.* 18, 492–504. doi: 10.1080/15384047.2017.1324374

Anantharaju, P. G., Reddy, D. B., Padukudru, M. A., Kumari Chitturi, C. M., Vimalambike, M. G., and Madhunapantula, S. V. (2017b). Induction of colon and cervical cancer cell death by cinnamic acid derivatives is mediated through the inhibition of Histone Deacetylases (HDAC). *PLoS One* 12:e0186208. doi: 10.1371/journal.pone.0186208

Brown, R. E., Jarvis, K. L., and Hyland, K. J. (1989). Protein measurement using bicinchoninic acid: elimination of interfering substances. *Anal. Biochem.* 180, 136–139. doi: 10.1016/0003-2697(89)90101-2

Cragg, G. M., and Newman, D. J. (2005). Plants as a source of anti-cancer agents. *J. Ethnopharmacol.* 100, 72–79. doi: 10.1016/j.jep.2005.05.011

da Rocha, A. T., De Lima, M. R. F., Valentim, I. B., Pinheiro, D. M., and Sant'Ana, A. E. G. (2007). Chemical synthesis of tricaproin, trienantin and tricaprylin. *Int. J. Food Sci. Technol.* 42, 1504–1508. doi: 10.1111/j.1365-2621.2006.01376.x

Davie, J. R. (2003). Inhibition of histone deacetylase activity by butyrate. *J. Nutr.* 133, 2485S–2493S. doi: 10.1093/jn/133.7.2485S

Espinosa-Diez, C., Miguel, V., Mennerich, D., Kietzmann, T., Sánchez-Pérez, P., Cadenas, S., et al. (2015). Antioxidant responses and cellular adjustments to oxidative stress. *Redox Biol.* 6, 183–197. doi: 10.1016/j.redox.2015.07.008

Fauser, J., Matthews, G., Cummins, A., and Howarth, G. (2013). Induction of apoptosis by the medium-chain length fatty acid lauric acid in colon cancer cells due to induction of oxidative stress. *Chemotherapy* 59, 214–224. doi: 10.1159/000356067

Glozak, M., and Seto, E. (2007). Histone deacetylases and cancer. *Oncogene* 26, 5420–5432. doi: 10.1038/sj.onc.1210610

Govindaraju, K., Darukeshwara, J., and Srivastava, A. K. (2009). Studies on protein characteristics and toxic constituents of *Simarouba glauca* oilseed meal. *Food Chem. Toxicol.* 47, 1327–1332. doi: 10.1016/j.fct.2009.03.006

Gowda, R., Madhunapantula, S. V., Desai, D., Amin, S., and Robertson, G. P. (2012). Selenium-containing histone deacetylase inhibitors for melanoma management. *Cancer Biol. Ther.* 13, 756–765. doi: 10.4161/cbt.20558

GraphPad Prism software (2009). *R Package Version 5.0*. San Diego, CA: GraphPad Software Inc.

Hamburger, M., Handa, S. S., Cordell, G. A., Kinghorn, A. D., and Farnsworth, N. R. (1987). Plant anticancer agents, XLIII.(E, E)-7, 12-dioxo-octadeca-8, 10-dien-1-oic acid (ostopanic acid), a cytotoxic fatty acid from Ostodes paniculata. *J. Nat. Prod.* 50, 281–283. doi: 10.1021/np50050a036

Jasek, E., Lis, G. J., Jasińska, M., Jurkowska, H., and Litwin, J. A. (2012). Effect of histone deacetylase inhibitors trichostatin A and valproic acid on etoposide-induced apoptosis in leukemia cells. *Anticancer Res.* 32, 2791–2799.

Jubie, S., Dhanabal, S., and Chaitanya, M. (2015). Isolation of methyl gamma linolenate from spirulina platensis using flash chromatography and its apoptosis inducing effect. *BMC Complement. Altern. Med.* 15:263–270. doi: 10.1186/s12906-015-0771-8

King, J., and Min, D. (1998). Analysis of fatty acids. *Dev. Food Sci.* 39, 195–223. doi: 10.1016/S0167-4501(98)80010-1

Kuefer, R., Hofer, M., Altug, V., Zorn, C., Genze, F., Kunzi-Rapp, K., et al. (2004). Sodium butyrate and tributyrin induce in vivo growth inhibition and apoptosis in human prostate cancer. *Br. J. Cancer* 90, 535–541. doi: 10.1038/sj.bjc.6601510

Kuendgen, A., Schmid, M., Schlenk, R., Knipp, S., Hildebrandt, B., Steidl, C., et al. (2006). The histone deacetylase (HDAC) inhibitor valproic acid as monotherapy or in combination with all-trans retinoic acid in patients with acute myeloid leukemia. *Cancer* 106, 112–119. doi: 10.1002/cncr.21552

Madhunapantula, S. V., Desai, D., Sharma, A., Huh, S. J., Amin, S., and Robertson, G. P. (2008). PBISE, a novel selenium-containing drug for the treatment of malignant melanoma. *Mol. Cancer Ther.* 7, 1297–1308. doi: 10.1158/1535-7163.MCT-07-2267

Mariadason, J. M. (2008). HDACS and HDAC inhibitors in colon cancer. *Epigenetics* 3, 28–37. doi: 10.4161/epi.3.1.5736

Marks, P. A., Richon, V. M., and Rifkind, R. A. (2000). Histone deacetylase inhibitors: inducers of differentiation or apoptosis of transformed cells. *J. Natl. Cancer Inst.* 92, 1210–1216. doi: 10.1093/jnci/92.15.1210

Mottamal, M., Zheng, S., Huang, T. L., and Wang, G. (2015). Histone deacetylase inhibitors in clinical studies as templates for new anticancer agents. *Molecules* 20, 3898–3941. doi: 10.3390/molecules20033898

Nande, R., and Claudio, P. P. (2014). "Ultrasound contrast agents in cancer therapy," in *Cutting Edge Therapies for Cancer in the 21st Century*, eds P. P. Claudio and P. Vogiatzi (Bussum: Bentham Science Publisher), 425–512.

Narayanan, A., Baskaran, S. A., Amalaradjou, M. A. R., and Venkitanarayanan, K. (2015). Anticarcinogenic properties of medium chain fatty acids on human colorectal, skin and breast cancer cells *in vitro*. *Int. J. Mol. Sci.* 16, 5014–5027. doi: 10.3390/ijms16035014

Narendran, R. (2013). A tree of solace for cancer patients. *The New Indian Express*.

Okada, K., Hakata, S., Terashima, J., Gamou, T., Habano, W., and Ozawa, S. (2016). Combination of the histone deacetylase inhibitor depsipeptide and 5-fluorouracil upregulates major histocompatibility complex class II and p21 genes and activates caspase-3/7 in human colon cancer HCT-116 cells. *Oncol. Rep.* 36, 1875–1885. doi: 10.3892/or.2016.5008

Patil, M. S., and Gaikwad, D. (2011). A critical review on medicinally important oil yielding plant laxmitaru (*Simarouba glauca* DC.). *J. Pharm. Sci. Res.* 3, 1195–1213.

Puranik, S. I., Ghagane, S. C., Nerli, R. B., Jalalpure, S. S., and Hiremath, M. B. (2017). Evaluation of in vitro antioxidant and anticancer activity of *Simarouba glauca* leaf extracts on T-24 bladder cancer cell line. *Pharmacogn. J.* 9, 906–912. doi: 10.5530/pj.2017.6.142

Rada-Iglesias, A., Enroth, S., Ameur, A., Koch, C. M., Clelland, G. K., Respuela-Alonso, P., et al. (2007). Butyrate mediates decrease of histone acetylation centered on transcription start sites and down-regulation of associated genes. *Genome Res.* 17, 708–719. doi: 10.1101/gr.5540007

Rangarajan, A. D. (2003). 'Paradise tree' promises immense potential. *The Hindu*.

Reynertson, K. A., Charlson, M. E., and Gudas, L. J. (2011). Induction of murine embryonic stem cell differentiation by medicinal plant extracts. *Exp. Cell Res.* 317, 82–93. doi: 10.1016/j.yexcr.2010.10.010

Richon, V. M., Sandhoff, T. W., Rifkind, R. A., and Marks, P. A. (2000). Histone deacetylase inhibitor selectively induces p21wAF1 expression and gene-associated histone acetylation. *Proc. Natl. Acad. Sci. U.S.A.* 97, 10014–10019. doi: 10.1073/pnas.180316197

Rivero-Cruz, J. F., Lezutekong, R., Lobo-Echeverri, T., Ito, A., Mi, Q., Chai, H. B., et al. (2005). Cytotoxic constituents of the twigs of *Simarouba glauca* collected from a plot in Southern Florida. *Phytother. Res.* 19, 136–140. doi: 10.1073/pnas.180316197

Rosato, R. R., Almenara, J. A., Maggio, S. C., Coe, S., Atadja, P., Dent, P., et al. (2008). Role of histone deacetylase inhibitor-induced reactive oxygen species and DNA damage in LAQ-824/fludarabine antileukemic interactions. *Mol. Cancer Ther.* 7, 3285–3297. doi: 10.1158/1535-7163.MCT-08-0385

Ruefli, A. A., Ausserlechner, M. J., Bernhard, D., Sutton, V. R., Tainton, K. M., Kofler, R., et al. (2001). The histone deacetylase inhibitor and chemotherapeutic agent suberoylanilide hydroxamic acid (SAHA) induces a cell-death pathway characterized by cleavage of Bid and production of reactive oxygen species. *Proc. Natl. Acad. Sci. U.S.A.* 98, 10833–10838. doi: 10.1073/pnas.191208598

Salimi, V., Shahsavari, Z., Safizadeh, B., Hosseini, A., Khademian, N., and Tavakoli-Yaraki, M. (2017). Sodium butyrate promotes apoptosis in breast cancer cells through reactive oxygen species (ROS) formation and mitochondrial impairment. *Lipids Health Dis.* 16, 208–218. doi: 10.1186/s12944-017-0593-4

Sanmartín, C., Plano, D., Sharma, A. K., and Palop, J. A. (2012). Selenium compounds, apoptosis and other types of cell death: an overview for cancer therapy. *Int. J. Mol. Sci.* 13, 9649–9672. doi: 10.3390/ijms13089649

Sawa, H., Murakami, H., Ohshima, Y., Sugino, T., Nakajyo, T., Kisanuki, T., et al. (2001). Histone deacetylase inhibitors such as sodium butyrate and trichostatin A induce apoptosis through an increase of the bcl-2-related protein Bad. *Brain Tumor Pathol.* 18, 109–114. doi: 10.1007/BF02479423

Sealy, L., and Chalkley, R. (1978). The effect of sodium butyrate on histone modification. *Cell* 14, 115–121. doi: 10.1016/0092-8674(78)90306-9

Selvaraj, J. (2017). "Fatty acids and their analogues as anticancer agents," in *Biochemistry, Genetics And Molecular Biology*, ed. A. Catala (Rijeka: InTech), 1–18.

Senawong, T., Misuna, S., Khaopha, S., Nuchadomrong, S., Sawatsitang, P., Phaosiri, C., et al. (2013). Histone deacetylase (Hdac) inhibitory and antiproliferative activities of phenolic-rich extracts derived from the rhizome of Hydnophytum formicarum Jack.: sinapinic acid acts as Hdac inhibitor. *BMC Complement. Altern. Med.* 13:232–242. doi: 10.1186/1472-6882-13-232

Shah, U., Shah, R., Acharya, S., and Acharya, N. (2013). Novel anticancer agents from plant sources. *Chin. J. Nat. Med.* 11, 16–23. doi: 10.3724/SP.J.1009.2013.00016

Shailasree, S., Venkataramana, M., Niranjana, S., and Prakash, H. (2015). Cytotoxic effect of *p*-coumaric acid on neuroblastoma, N2a cell via generation of reactive oxygen species leading to dysfunction of mitochondria inducing apoptosis and autophagy. *Mol. Neurobiol.* 51, 119–130. doi: 10.1007/s12035-014-8700-2

Shoeb, M. (2006). Anticancer agents from medicinal plants. *Bangladesh J. Pharmacol.* 1, 35–41.

Simon, H.-U., Haj-Yehia, A., and Levi-Schaffer, F. (2000). Role of reactive oxygen species (Ros) in apoptosis induction. *Apoptosis* 5, 415–418. doi: 10.1023/A:1009616228304

Skehan, P., Storeng, R., Scudiero, D., Monks, A., Mcmahon, J., Vistica, D., et al. (1990). New colorimetric cytotoxicity assay for anticancer-drug screening. *J. Nat. Cancer Inst.* 82, 1107–1112. doi: 10.1093/jnci/82.13.1107

Thurn, K. T., Thomas, S., Moore, A., and Munster, P. N. (2011). Rational therapeutic combinations with histone deacetylase inhibitors for the treatment of cancer. *Future Oncol.* 7, 263–283. doi: 10.2217/fon.11.2

Waldecker, M., Kautenburger, T., Daumann, H., Busch, C., and Schrenk, D. (2008). Inhibition of histone-deacetylase activity by short-chain fatty acids and some polyphenol metabolites formed in the colon. *J. Nutr. Biochem.* 19, 587–593. doi: 10.1016/j.jnutbio.2007.08.002

Wu, G., Robertson, D. H., Brooks, C. L., and Vieth, M. (2003). Detailed analysis of grid-based molecular docking: a case study of Cdocker—A Charmm-based Md docking algorithm. *J. Comput. Chem.* 24, 1549–1562. doi: 10.1002/jcc.10306

19

Inhibition of Akt/mTOR/p70S6K Signaling Activity with Huangkui Capsule Alleviates the Early Glomerular Pathological Changes in Diabetic Nephropathy

Wei Wu[1,2†], Wei Hu[3†], Wen-Bei Han[1], Ying-Lu Liu[1,2], Yue Tu[4], Hai-Ming Yang[2], Qi-Jun Fang[2], Mo-Yi Zhou[2], Zi-Yue Wan[5], Ren-Mao Tang[6], Hai-Tao Tang[6‡] and Yi-Gang Wan[2*‡]*

[1] Department of Traditional Chinese Medicine, Nanjing Drum Tower Hospital Clinical College of Traditional Chinese and Western Medicine, Nanjing University of Chinese Medicine, Nanjng, China, [2] Department of Traditional Chinese Medicine, Nanjing Drum Tower Hospital, The Affiliated Hospital of Nanjing University Medical School, Nanjing, China, [3] Department of Pharmacy, Nanjing Drum Tower Hospital, The Affiliated Hospital of Nanjing University Medical School, Nanjing, China, [4] Department of TCM Health Preservation, Second Clinic Medical School, Nanjing University of Chinese Medicine, Nanjing, China, [5] Department of Social Work, Meiji Gakuin University, Tokyo, Japan, [6] Institute of Huanghui, Suzhong Pharmaceutical Group Co., Ltd., Taizhou, China

***Correspondence:**
Yi-Gang Wan
wyg68918@sina.com
Hai-Tao Tang
mtang@vip.sina.com

† These authors have contributed equally to this work.

‡ These corresponding authors have contributed equally to this work.

Huangkui capsule (HKC), a Chinese modern patent medicine extracted from *Abelmoschus manihot* (L.) medic, has been widely applied to clinical therapy in the early diabetic nephropathy (DN) patients. However, it remains elusive whether HKC can ameliorate the inchoate glomerular injuries in hyperglycemia. Recently the activation of phosphatidylinositol-3-kinase (PI3K)/serine-threonine kinase (Akt)/mammalian target of rapamycin (mTOR) signaling and its downstream regulator, 70-kDa ribosomal protein S6 kinase (p70S6K), play important roles in the early glomerular pathological changes of DN including glomerular hypertrophy, glomerular basement membrane (GBM) thickening and mild mesangial expansion. This study thereby aimed to clarify therapeutic effects of HKC during the initial phase of DN and its underlying mechanisms. Fifteen rats were randomly divided into 3 groups: the normal group, the model group and the HKC group. The early DN model rats were induced by unilateral nephrectomy combined with intraperitoneal injection of streptozotocin, and administered with either HKC suspension or vehicle after modeling and for a period of 4 weeks. Changes in the incipient glomerular lesions-related parameters in urine and blood were analyzed. Kidneys were isolated for histomorphometry, immunohistochemistry, immunofluorescence and Western blotting (WB) at sacrifice. *In vitro*, murine mesangial cells (MCs) were used to investigate inhibitory actions of hyperoside (HYP), a bioactive component of HKC, on cellular hypertrophy-associated signaling pathway by WB, compared with rapamycin (RAP). For the early DN model rats, HKC ameliorated micro-urinary albumin, body weight and serum albumin, but had no significant effects on renal function and liver enzymes; HKC improved renal shape, kidney weight and kidney hypertrophy index; HKC attenuated glomerular hypertrophy, GBM thickening and mild mesangial expansion; HKC inhibited the phosphorylation of

Akt, mTOR and p70S6K, and the protein over-expression of transforming growth factor-β1 in kidneys. *In vitro*, the phosphorylation of PI3K, Akt, mTOR and p70S6K in MCs induced by high-glucose was abrogated by treatment of HYP or RAP. On the whole, this study further demonstrated HKC safely and efficiently alleviates the early glomerular pathological changes of DN, likely by inhibiting Akt/mTOR/p70S6K signaling activity *in vivo* and *in vitro*, and provided the first evidence that HKC directly contributes to the prevention of the early DN.

Keywords: Huangkui capsule, hyperoside, diabetic nephropathy, glomerular hypertrophy, glomerular basement membrane thickening, mesangial expansion, Akt/mTOR/p70S6K signaling pathway

INTRODUCTION

The early diabetic nephropathy (DN) in both animal models and humans is characterized histologically by glomerular hypertrophy, glomerular basement membrane (GBM) thickening and mild mesangial expansion (Tervaert et al., 2010; Najafian et al., 2011). Since approximately 26 or 16.4% of the early DN patients in the United States (Afkarian et al., 2016) or in China (Liu, 2013) will progress to end-stage renal disease, the safe and effective therapeutic regiments for delaying the progression of DN are desired in clinic. However, so far, relatively little progress has been made in the treatment of the early DN patients (de Boer, 2017). Although angiotensin-converting enzyme inhibitors, angiotensin receptor blocker (Tuttle et al., 2014; Glassock, 2016) and some newly discovered drugs including glucagons-like peptide 1 agonists (Muskiet et al., 2017), dipeptidyl peptidase 4 inhibitors (Penno et al., 2016), sodium-glucose cotransporter 2 inhibitors (Zinman et al., 2015; Wanner et al., 2016) may help and treat the early DN patients by allowing tighter safer control of blood glucose level and by exerting beneficial direct effects on renal injuries, it is still unclear whether they can ameliorate the inchoate glomerular pathological changes including hypertrophic glomerulus, thickened GBM and mild mesangial expansion.

Mammalian target of rapamycin (mTOR) is a serine/threonine protein kinase, and its upstream signalings such as phosphatidylinositol-3-kinase (PI3K) and serine-threonine kinase (Akt) have been reported to regulate protein synthesis and cellular growth, specifically cellular hypertrophy (Yuan et al., 2011; Dibble and Cantley, 2015). PI3K/Akt/mTOR signaling pathway can directly regulate the functions of 70-kDa ribosomal protein S6 kinase (p70S6K) and eukaryotic initiation factor 4E-binding protein-1 (4EBP1), which are the important downstream regulators of ribosome protein synthesis, ribosome biogenesis, and mRNA translation initiation (Giasson and Meloche, 1995; Hall, 2016). Therefore, the activation of PI3K/Akt/mTOR signaling is thought to lead to an increase in the cellular capacity for protein synthesis and cellular hypertrophy. Sakaguchi et al. reported that rapamycin (RAP), a specific inhibitor of mTORC1 signaling, can attenuate renal enlargement and the enhanced phosphorylation of p70S6K in the kidneys of the early diabetic mice, suggesting the activation of PI3K/Akt/mTOR signaling and the phosphorylation level of p70S6K might play an important role in renal hypertrophy under hyperglycemia (Sakaguchi et al., 2006). Accordingly, targeting the activation of PI3K/Akt/mTOR signaling and the expression of phosphorylated p70S6K (p-p70S6K) in the kidneys could be therapeutic mechanisms for ameliorating the early glomerular lesions of DN.

Over the past 20 years, Huangkui capsule (HKC, the local name in China), a Chinese modern patent medicine extracted from *Abelmoschus manihot* (L.) medic (AM), has been approved by the China State Food and Drug Administration (Z19990040) for the conventional therapy of chronic glomerulonephritis (Guo et al., 2013; Zhang et al., 2014). HKC and its bioactive component hyperoside (HYP) can ameliorate proteinuria and renal dysfunction for patients and animal models with the early chronic kidney disease (CKD) (Chen et al., 2015; Ge et al., 2016). Recently, the increasing clinical evidences in China have been suggested that HKC at the safe and effective dose of 7.5 g/kg/day can reduce micro-urinary albumin (micro-UAlb) in the early DN patients and the IgA nephropathy patients (Liu et al., 2010; Li et al., 2017), and that its therapeutic action may be concerned with regulating transforming growth factor-β1 (TGF-β1) signaling *in vivo* (Tu et al., 2013), and inhibiting high-glucose (HG)-induced renal tubular epithelial-mesenchymal transition *in vitro* (Cai et al., 2017). In addition, our previous animal experiment as the first step revealed that, after the drug-intervention for 8 weeks, 2 g/kg/day dose of HKC can significantly attenuate the advanced renal fibrosis in the DN model rats induced by the unilateral nephrectomy combined with the intraperitoneal injection of streptozotocin

Abbreviations: Akt, serine-threonine kinase; Alb, serum albumin; ALT, alanine transaminase; α-SMA, α-smooth muscle actin; AM, *abelmoschus manihot* (L.) medic; AST, aspartate transaminase; BG, blood glucose; BUN, blood urea nitrogen; BW, body weight; CKD, chronic kidney disease; Col-I, collagen type I; DMSO, dimethylsulfoxide; DN, diabetic nephropathy; ECM, extracellular matrix; EM, electron microscopy; FN, fibronectin; 4EBP1, eukaryotic initiation factor 4E-binding protein-1; GAPDH, glyceraldehyde-3-phosphate dehydrogenase; GBM, glomerular basement membrane; GCP, glomerular cellular population; GV, glomerular volume; HFD, high-fat diet; HG, high-glucose; HKC, Huangkui capsule; HRP, horseradish peroxidase; HYP, hyperoside; HPLC, high performance liquid chromatography; IF, immunofluorescence; KHI, kidney hypertrophy index; KW, kidney weight; LM, light microscopy; MCs, mesangial cells; micro-UAlb, micro-urinary albumin; MNT, mannitol; mTOR, mammalian target of rapamycin; NLRC3, NOD-like receptor family CARD domain containing 3; p70S6K, 70-kDa ribosomal protein S6 kinase; PAS, periodic acid-Schiff; PB, phosphate buffer; PI, protease inhibitors; PI3K, phosphatidylinositol-3-kinase; RAP, rapamycin; Scr, serum creatinine; SDS, sodium dodecyl sulfate; SDS-PAGE, sodium dodecyl sulfate-polyacrylamide gel electrophoresis; STZ, streptozotocin; TGF-β1, transforming growth factor-β1; WB, Western blot.

(STZ) through regulating oxidative stress and p38 mitogen-activated protein kinase/Akt pathways (Mao et al., 2015). Despite these, up to present, there are still some important issues unresolved in the role of glomerular injuries in DN at the early stage treated by HKC, for instance, whether HKC can improve glomerular hypertrophy, GBM thickening and mild mesangial expansion by means of targeting PI3K/Akt/mTOR pathway and its signaling activity, and if yes, what are the underlying therapeutic mechanisms involved *in vivo* and *in vitro*.

Here, to address these issues, we designed the animal and cell experiments to verify these hypotheses that HKC at the dose of 2 g/kg/day may safely and efficiently alleviate the early glomerular pathological changes of the DN model rats, and inhibit the activation of PI3K/Akt/mTOR signaling pathway.

MATERIALS AND METHODS

HKC Preparation and Quality Control

HKC purchased from Suzhong Pharmaceutical Group Co., Ltd. (Taizhou, China) is composed by the extracts from AM. One capsule of HKC contains 0.5 g of AM. The extracted method and productive process of HKC are both subjected to strict quality control, and the main components are subjected to standardization (Trendafilova et al., 2011; Xue et al., 2011). In addition, HKC is not only manufactured as granules after dynamic cycle extraction and concentration by evaporating and spray drying, but also monitored for the absence of contaminants (heavy metals, pesticides, hormone and mycotoxins) prior to the formulation. In this study, HKC (the batch number: 2014062703) was dissolved in distilled water (HKC suspension) and stored at 4°C before use.

The quality of HKC was examined with fingerprint analysis by high performance liquid chromatography (HPLC) as our previous study (Mao et al., 2015). As shown in **Figure 1**, the known bioactive components including flavonoids like rutin ($C_{27}H_{30}O_{16}$; CAS: 153-18-4), hyperoside ($C_{21}H_{20}O_{12}$; CAS: 482-36-0), isoquercitrin ($C_{21}H_{20}O_{12}$; CAS: 482-35-9) and quercetin ($C_{15}H_{10}O_7$; CAS: 117-39-5) (**Figure 1A**) in 5 batches exhibited high stability.

Animals, Drugs and Reagents

All experiments were performed using the male Sprague-Dawley rats weighing from 200 to 220 g, purchased from Shanghai Jiesijie Experimental Animal Co., Ltd. [License No: SCXK (Shanghai) 2012-0006] and fed in the Experiment Animal Center of Nanjing Drum Tower Hospital, the Affiliated Hospital of Nanjing University Medical School. The surgical procedures and experimental protocol were approved by the Animal Ethics Committee of Nanjing University Medical School. HYP with the purity higher than 98% was purchased from Liangwei Biotechnology Co., Ltd. (Nanjing, China). STZ was purchased from Sigma-Aldrich (St. Louis, MO, USA). RAP and antibodies against Akt, phosphorylated Akt (p-Akt), p70S6K, p-p70S6K, mTOR, phosphorylated mTOR (p-mTOR), 4EBP1, phosphorylated 4EBP1 (p- 4EBP1), TGF-β1, Smad2, phosphorylated Smad2 (p-Smad2) and glyceraldehyde-3-phosphate dehydrogenase (GAPDH) were purchased from Cell Signaling Technology (Beverly, MA, USA). Antibody against nephrin was purchased from Abcam (Cambridge, UK). Antibodies against PI3K, phosphorylated PI3K (p-PI3K), proliferating cell nuclear antigen (PCNA) and horseradish peroxidase (HRP)-labeled IgG were purchased from Bioworld Technology (Louis Park, USA).

Animal Experimental Protocols

The animal experiment procedure is illustrated in **Figure 2**. All rats were fed by the high-fat diet (HFD) purchased from Shanghai SLAC Laboratory Animal Co., Ltd (Shanghai, China) for 4 weeks. The DN rat models were established as described in our previous studies (Mao et al., 2015). Fifteen rats were divided into 3 groups, 5 rats in the normal group, 5 rats in the model group and 5 rats in the HKC group. In clinic, HKC at a dose of 7.5 g/day is used to treat a patient weighting 60 kg (Chen et al., 2012, 2016), which is equivalent to 1 g/kg/day in the rats. Given that the dose of 1 g/kg/day is set as the middle one, 2 g/kg/day is identified as the high dose. Following the second injection of STZ, HKC suspension was given to the rats in the HKC group by gastric gavage once a day for 4 weeks, while the rats in the model group and the normal group were treated with 2 ml vehicle (distilled water). Four weeks after administration, all rats were anesthetized and sacrificed through cardiac puncture. Blood samples and kidneys were collected for detection of various indicators.

Rats' General Status and Biochemical Parameters

Energy level, diet, water intake, fur color and activities of the rats in each group were observed daily. Body weight (BW), blood glucose (BG) and micro-UAlb of the rats were detected respectively before and every 1 or 2 weeks after modeling. The right kidneys of rats in each group were removed and weighed after cardiac puncture. Kidney hypertrophy index (KHI) was calculated according to the method described by Lane et al. (1990), that is KHI = kidney weight (KW)/BW. At the end of week 4 after the drug-intervention, the rats were anesthetized and blood samples (5 ml) were drawn from the heart. The biochemical parameters including serum albumin (Alb), serum creatinine (Scr), blood urea nitrogen (BUN), serum alanine transaminase (ALT) and serum aspartate transaminase (AST) were detected, respectively.

Light Microscopy Examination

The tissue samples from renal cortex for light microscopy (LM) assessment were fixed with 10% neutral buffered formalin, embedded in paraffin, cut into 3-μm-thick sections and stained with the periodic acid-Schiff (PAS) or Masson reagent. Semiquantitative morphological studies of glomerular lesion were carried out by randomly selecting 20 full-sized glomeruli (80–100 μm) from each specimen. Glomerular cellular population (GCP) and glomerular volume (GV) were calculated with Image-Pro Plus 6.0 software (Media Cybernetic). Specifically, glomerular area was measured after glomerular capillary plexus profile was defined, and then GV was calculated in accordance with the method described by Lane et al. (1992),

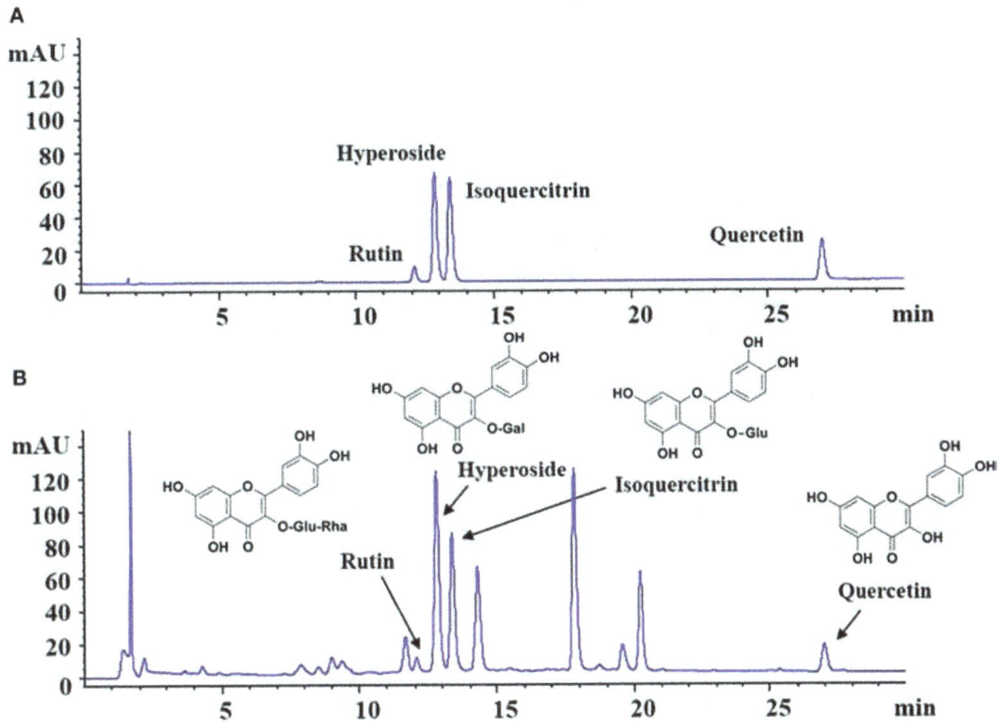

FIGURE 1 | Fingerprint analysis of HKC by HPLC. **(A)** The chromatograms of mixed standards. **(B)** The samples of HKC.

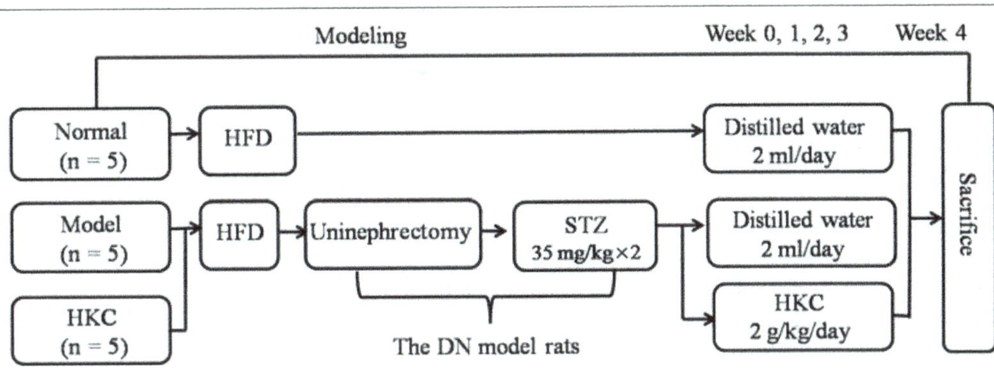

FIGURE 2 | Animal experimental procedure.

that is GV = area$^{1.5}$ × 0.75 + 0.21. The results were confirmed by the pathological professional doctor.

Electron Microscopy Investigation

The tissue samples from renal cortex for electron microscopy (EM) assessment were fixed in 2.5% glutaraldehyde in 0.1 mol/L phosphate buffer (PB) for several days at 4°C. After washing in PB and post-fixing in 1% OsO_4 for 2 h, the fixed material was dehydrated through an ethanolpropylene oxide series and embedded in Araldite M. The ultrathin sections were prepared and stained with uranyl acetate and lead citrate, and then, investigated and photographed under a JEM-1011 transmission electron microscope (JEOL, Tokyo, Japan). Three glomeruli were selected randomly from each section. On the basis of the method described by Haas (2009), GBM thickness was directly measured and calculated with Image-Pro Plus 6.0 software (Media Cybernetic). The results were confirmed by the pathological professional doctor.

Immunohistochemistry Assay

Collagen type I (Col-I) and fibronectin (FN) were detected in 3 μm thick paraffin-embedded renal sections. For immunostaining of Col-I and FN antibodies against-Col-I and FN (Serotec, Oxford, UK) were used, respectively. Quantitative analysis of Col-I and FN was performed in a blinded fashion and expressed as cells/glomerular cross section. The results were confirmed by the pathological professional doctor.

Immunofluorescence Assay

The tissue samples from renal cortex for immunofluorescence (IF) studies were snap-frozen in precooled n-hexane and stored at −70°C. Frozen sections were cut into 3 μm thick with a cryostat and stained with an antibody against α-smooth muscle actin (α-SMA) (IgG2a) (Sigma, St. Louis, MO, USA). Fluoresceine isothiocyanate-conjugated antibody against mouse IgG2a (Southern Biotechnology Associates, Birmingham, AL, USA) was used as a secondary antibody (DACO A/S). The degree of α-SMA staining was scored from 0 to 4 + in 10 randomly selected glomeruli according to the method described by Raij et al. (1984). The results were confirmed by the pathological professional doctor.

Western Blotting Analysis *in Vivo*

Western blot (WB) analysis was performed as previously described (Mao et al., 2015). Renal tissues from the rats were isolated with phosphate-buffered saline including protease inhibitors (PI) and sequentially solubilized with 1% Triton X-100, RIPA buffer [0.1% sodium dodecyl sulfate (SDS), 1% sodium deoxycholate, 1% Triton X-100, 0.15 mol/L NaCl, and 0.01 mol/L ethylenediaminetetraacetic acid in 0.025 mol/L Tris-HCl, pH 7.2] with PI, and separated into Triton X-100-soluble (T), RIPA-soluble (R) and RIPA-insoluble (S) fractions. The RIPAI-insoluble fraction was solubilized with sodium dodecyl sulfate-polyacrylamide gel electrophoresis (SDS-PAGE) sample buffer (2% SDS, 10% glycerol and 5% 2-mercaproethanol in 0.0625 mol/L Tris-HCl, pH 6.8) (S fractions). Equal amounts of these sequentially solubilized fractions were subjected to SDS-PAGE with 7.5 or 10% acrylamide gel, and transferred onto a polyvinylidene fluoride membrane (Bio-Rad, Hercules, CA, USA) by electrophoretic trans-blotting for 30 min using Trans-Blot SD (Bio-Rad). After blocking with BSA, the strips of membrane were exposed to anti-PI3K, p-PI3K, Akt, p-Akt, mTOR, p-mTOR, p70S6K, p-p70S6K, 4EBP1, p-4EBP1, TGF-β1, Smad2, p-Smad2, nephrin, and GAPDH antibodies, respectively. They were washed and incubated with peroxidase-conjugated secondary antibodies for 1 h at room temperature. The bands were visualized by employing an alkaline phosphatase chromogen kit (5-bromo-4-chloro-3-indolil phosphate p-toluidine salt/nitro blue tetrazolium; Biomedica, AG, Staad, Switzerland). The density of the positive bands was quantitated by Densitograph (ATTO, Tokyo, Japan). The ratio of the densitometric signal of the molecules examined to that of GAPDH was determined. The data are shown as ratios relative to control findings and expressed as mean ± S.E. of 3 independent experiments.

Mesangial Cell Culture and Treatment

Murine mesangial cells (MCs) were kindly provided by Dr. Jian Yao (University of Yamanashi, Chuo, Japan) and cultured as described previously (Zhang et al., 2016). Briefly, MCs were cultured in RPMI-1640 medium supplemented with 10% heat-inactivated low endotoxin fetal bovine serum, penicillin/streptomycin and HEPES (GIBCO, California, USA) at 37°C in a humidified atmosphere containing 95% air and 5% CO_2. MCs were treated with normal glucose (Normal, 5.5 mmol/L D-glucose) as control group, mannitol (MNT, 24.5 mmol/L MNT) as osmotic pressure control group, dimethylsulfoxide (DMSO, 0.1% DMSO) as DMSO control group and HG (30 mmol/L D-glucose) without or with HYP at the dose of 5 or 15 μg/ml and RAP at the dose of 20 nmol/L for 24, 48, or 72 h. Here, the low dose of HYP (5 μg/ml) and the high dose of HYP (15 μg/ml) were determined by the reference of Zhang et al. (2016). As HYP was dissolved in 0.1% DMSO, a similar volume of DMSO was added to DMSO control group.

Cell Viability Assessment

MCs were cultured in 96-well microplates at a density of 5,000 cells/well. Twenty-four hours after cultivation, MCs were serum starved and treated with the different concentrations of HYP at 5, 10, 15, and 20 μg/ml or RAP at 10, 15, 20, and 25 nmol/L. After the exposure to drugs for 72 h, the cytotoxicity assay was performed using Cell Counting Kit-8 (CCK-8, Beyotime Institute of Biotechnology, Shanghai, China). The optical density (OD), the absorbance value at 450 nm, was read using a 96-well plate reader (BioTek, VT, USA), and the OD absorbance was proportional to the vitality of cells.

Western Blot Analysis *in Vitro*

MCs were treated in the different groups for 24, 48, or 72 h, respectively. After the treatment, cell lysates were separated by gel electrophoresis and blotted with antibodies against PI3K, p-PI3K, Akt, p-Akt, mTOR, p-mTOR, p70S6K, p-p70S6K, and GAPDH. The secondary antibody was HRP-conjugated anti-rabbit IgG antibody. WB analysis for cells was carried out according to our previous protocols (Tu et al., 2017).

Statistics Analysis

The differences among groups were analyzed by one-way analysis of variance (ANOVA), and LSD method was used for multiple comparison. Qualitative data were analyzed using Fisher's exact test as indicated. $P < 0.05$ was considered statistically significant.

RESULTS

HKC Ameliorates General Condition and Biochemical Parameters of the Early DN Model Rats

Throughout the experiment, the general status, micro-UAlb and BG of the normal group rats did not change significantly, while BW continued to rise. After modeling successfully, the rats both in the model group and the HKC group showed increased diet, water intake and urine volume, but low activity, dull fur and BW loss in different degrees. In which, the changes of the model group rats were particularly obvious. Compared with the normal group rats, BW of the model group rats rose slowly, but BG increased significantly and maintained above 16.7 mmol/L, moreover, micro-UAlb went up obviously (more than 20 mg/L), and the difference was statistically significant ($P < 0.05$). After HKC treatment for 4 weeks, micro-UAlb of the HKC group rats decreased, and compared with that of the model group rats, the difference was statistically significant ($P < 0.05$). At the end of 3 and 4 weeks after HKC treatment, BW of the HKC group rats increased, and compared with that of the model group rats, the difference was statistically significant ($P < 0.05$). However, HKC had no obvious effect on BG of the model group rats (**Figures 3A,B**).

Next, we investigated the effects of HKC on serum biochemical parameters in the 3 rat groups. As shown in **Figure 3**, Alb, Scr, BUN, ALT, AST of the normal group rats always kept at the normal levels during the whole experiment. After modeling successfully, Alb of the model group rats decreased gradually, while Scr and BUN increased slightly. At the end of 4 weeks after modeling, compared with those of the normal group rats, the differences were statistically significant ($P < 0.01$). After HKC treatment for 4 weeks, Alb of the HKC group rats increased significantly, and compared with that of the model group rats, the difference was statistically significant ($P < 0.05$). However, there were no obvious changes in Scr and BUN of the HKC group rats. In addition to these, the major liver enzymes including ALT and AST remained unchanged among the 3 rat groups (**Figures 3D–H**).

These results indicated that HKC could ameliorate micro-UAlb, BW and Alb of the early DN model rats, but had no significant effects on renal function and liver enzymes.

HKC Improves Renal Enlargement of the Early DN Model Rats

As shown in **Figure 4**, at the end of 4 weeks after modeling, renal shape, KHI and KW of the normal group rats were normal, while the kidneys of the model group rats significantly swelled and over-weighted. After HKC treatment for 4 weeks, renal shape KHI and KW of the HKC group rats were obviously improved, and compared with those of the model group rats, the differences were statistically significant ($P < 0.05$). Moreover, KHI decreased obviously, and compared with that of the model group rats, the difference was statistically significant ($P < 0.01$) (**Figures 4A–C**).

These results indicated that HKC could ameliorate renal shape, KW and KHI of the early DN model rats.

HKC Attenuates Glomerular Pathological Changes of the Early DN Model Rats

Firstly, we investigated the effects of HKC on glomerular form, glomerular volume, mesangial matrix and GCP in the 3 rat groups. As shown in **Figure 5**, at the end of 4 weeks after modeling, upon the observation under LM, the entire and clear glomerular structure and open glomerular capillary loops were seen in the normal group rats. By contrast, hypertrophic glomerular form, increased glomerular volume and GCP and mild mesangial matrix expansion of the model group rats were found respectively, and the differences were statistically significant ($P < 0.01$). After HKC treatment for 4 weeks, the early glomerular pathological changes of the HKC group rats were improved significantly, and compared with those of the model group rats, the differences were statistically significant ($P < 0.01$ or $P < 0.05$) (**Figures 5A–D**). Here, notably, neither Masson-staining of collagen nor immunostainings of Col-I and FN (**Figures 6A–C**) was detected obviously in glomeruli of the 3 rat groups.

Then, we observed the effects of HKC on the fluorescence staining of α-SMA in glomeruli and the protein expression of PCNA in the kidneys of the 3 rat groups. PCNA and α-SMA are the acknowledged markers of mesangial cell proliferation. At the end of 4 weeks after modeling, the normal group rats had weak expressions of α-SMA in glomeruli and PCNA in the kidneys. By contrast, the extent of α-SMA fluorescence staining in glomerulai and the level of PCNA protein expression in the kidneys of the model group rats increased significantly, and the differences were statistically significant ($P < 0.01$). After HKC treatment for 4 weeks, the expressions of α-SMA in glomeruli and PCNA in the kidneys of the HKC group rats were decreased significantly, and compared with those of the model group rats, the differences were statistically significant ($P < 0.01$) (**Figure 7**).

Thirdly, we examined the effects of HKC on GBM thickness, foot process form and nephrin protein expression in the kidneys of the 3 rat groups. As shown in **Figure 8**, at the end of 4 weeks after modeling, the thickness of GBM, the form of foot process and the protein expression level of nephrin in the kidneys of the normal group rats did not change. By contrast, GBM thickening and foot process loss and effacement were detected in the model group rats, thereinto, GBM thickening is obvious, and compared with that of the normal group rats, the difference was statistically significant ($P < 0.05$). Here, it is noted that the protein expression of nephrin in the kidneys of the 3 rat groups remained unchanged. After HKC treatment for 4 weeks, GBM thickening of the HKC group rats decreased, and compared with that of the model group rats, the difference was statistically significant ($P < 0.05$). However, unfortunately, the significant improvement in foot process loss and effacement and nephrin protein expression in the kidneys of the HKC group rats was not found.

These results indicated that HKC could ameliorate glomerular pathological changes of the early DN model rats, such as glomerular hypertrophy, GBM thickening and mild mesangial expansion.

HKC Inhibits Activation of mTOR Signaling by PI3K/Akt Pathway, Not by TGF-β1/Smad2 Pathway in the Kidneys of the Early DN Model Rats

PI3K/Akt/mTOR and TGF-β1/Smad2 signaling pathways play the different roles in the progression of DN. The key signaling molecules of PI3K/Akt/mTOR and TGF-β1/Smad2 pathways include p-PI3K (Tyr458), p-Akt (Ser473), p-mTOR (Ser2448), p-p70S6K (Thr389), p-4EBP1 (Thr37/46), TGF-β1 and p-Smad2 (Ser465/467). At the end of 4 weeks after modeling, there was no significant change in p-PI3K protein expression level among the 3 rat groups (**Figure 9A**), but the protein expression levels of p-Akt, p-mTOR, p-p70S6K, p-4EBP1, TGF-β1 and p-Smad2 in the kidneys of the model group rats were up-regulated significantly, and compared with those of the normal group rats, the differences were statistically significant ($P <$

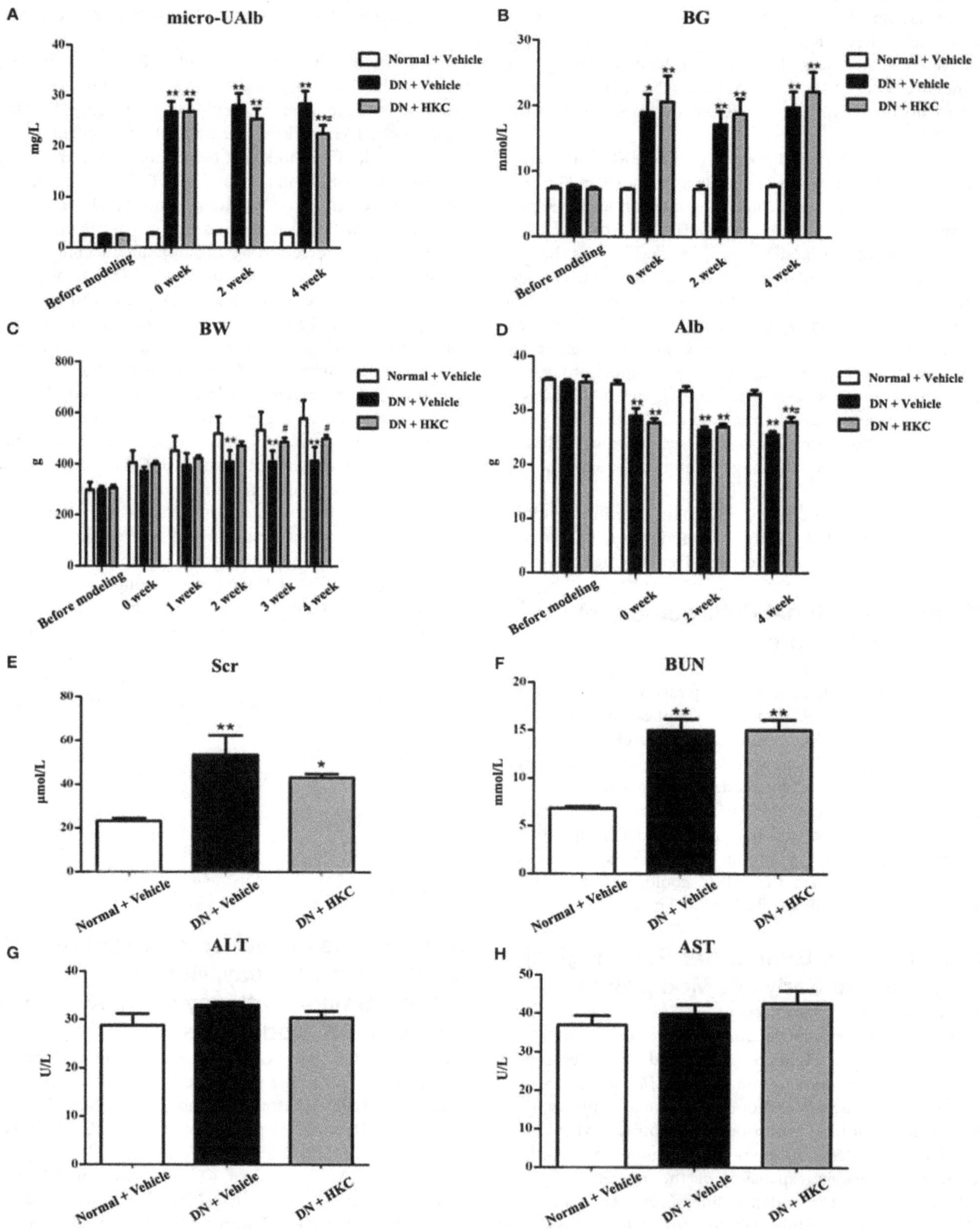

FIGURE 3 | Effects of HKC on micro-UAlb **(A)**, BG **(B)**, BW **(C)**, Alb **(D)**, Scr **(E)**, BUN **(F)**, ALT **(G)**, and AST **(H)** of the early DN model rats. The data are expressed as mean ± S.E. $^{*}P < 0.05$, $^{**}P < 0.01$ vs. the normal group; $^{\#}P < 0.05$ vs. the model group.

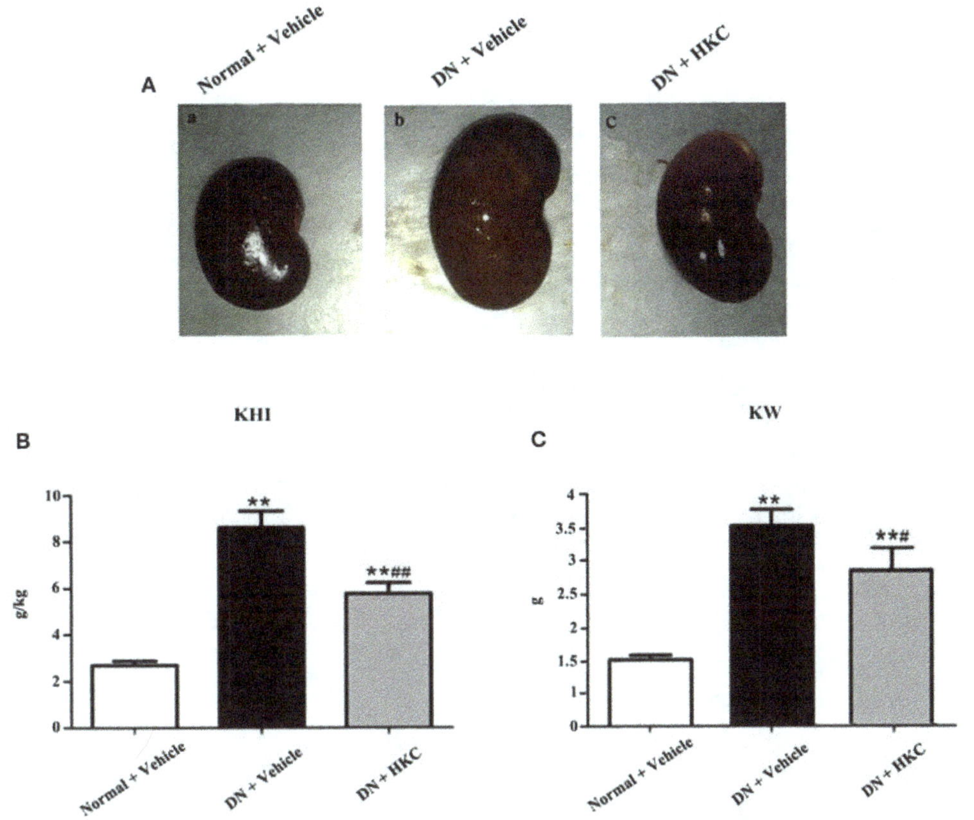

FIGURE 4 | Effects of HKC on renal shape **(A)**, KHI **(B)**, and KW **(C)** of the early DN model rats. The data are expressed as mean ± S.E. $^{**}P < 0.01$ vs. the normal group; $^{\#}P < 0.05$, $^{\#\#}P < 0.01$ vs. the model group.

0.01) (**Figures 9B–G**). After HKC treatment for 4 weeks, the protein expression levels of p-Akt, p-mTOR, p-p70S6K, and TGF-β1 in the kidneys of the HKC group rats were down-regulated significantly, and compared with those of the model group rats, the differences were statistically significant ($P < 0.01$) (**Figures 9B–D**). Despite this, the protein expressions of p-Smad2 and p-4EBP1 in the kidneys of the HKC group rats and the model group rats remained unchanged within 4 weeks after vehicle or drug-intervention (**Figures 9E,G**).

These results indicated that HKC could inhibit the protein over-expressions of p-Akt, p-mTOR, p-p70S6K, and TGF-β1 in the kidneys of the early DN model rats, but had no significant effect on the protein expressions of p-PI3K, p-Smad2, and p-4EBP1.

Hyperoside Abrogates Phosphorylation of PI3K, Akt, mTOR and p70S6K Induced by High-Glucose in the Cultured Mesangial Cells *in Vitro*

Prior to the formal cellar experiments, the cytotoxicity of HYP and RAP on the cultured MCs was analyzed using CCK-8. As shown in **Figure 10**, the cell viabilities were significantly decreased under the highest concentrations of HYP at 20 μg/ml (**Figure 10A**) and RAP at 25 nmol/L (**Figure 10B**) compared with the 15 μg/ml dose of HYP and the 20 nmol/L dose of RAP, respectively. According to these results, the suitable doses of HYP (5 and 15 μg/ml) and RAP (20 nmol/L) were selected respectively. Coincidentally, these drug concentrations were similar to the report of Zhang et al. (2016). To confirm further whether HG affects the phosphorylation of PI3K, Akt, mTOR, and p70S6K *in vitro*, we tested the protein expressions of PI3K, p-PI3K, Akt, p-Akt, mTOR, p-mTOR, p70S6K, and p-p70S6K in the cultured MCs treated with HG at 24, 48, and 72 h, compared with the treatment of MNT or DMSO. The results showed that HG increased the protein expressions of p-PI3K, p-Akt, p-mTOR, and p-p70S6K in the cultured MCs in a time-dependent manner, suggesting HG could induce the phosphorylation of PI3K, Akt, mTOR, and p70S6K *in vitro* (**Figures 11A–D**). In addition, it is noted that the treatment with HYP at the different doses and RAP (mTORC1 inhibitor) at 72 h significantly down-regulated HG-induced changes in the protein expressions of p-PI3K, p-Akt, p-mTOR, and p-p70S6K in the cultured MCs, compared with the treatment of HG (**Figures 11E–H**). In which, the suppressive effect of H-HYP (15 μg/ml) on the phosphorylation of p70S6K was better than RAP, and the difference was statistically significant ($P < 0.01$). Whereas, the repressive actions of RAP on the phosphorylation of Akt and mTOR were better than H-HYP, and the differences were statistically significant ($P < 0.01$).

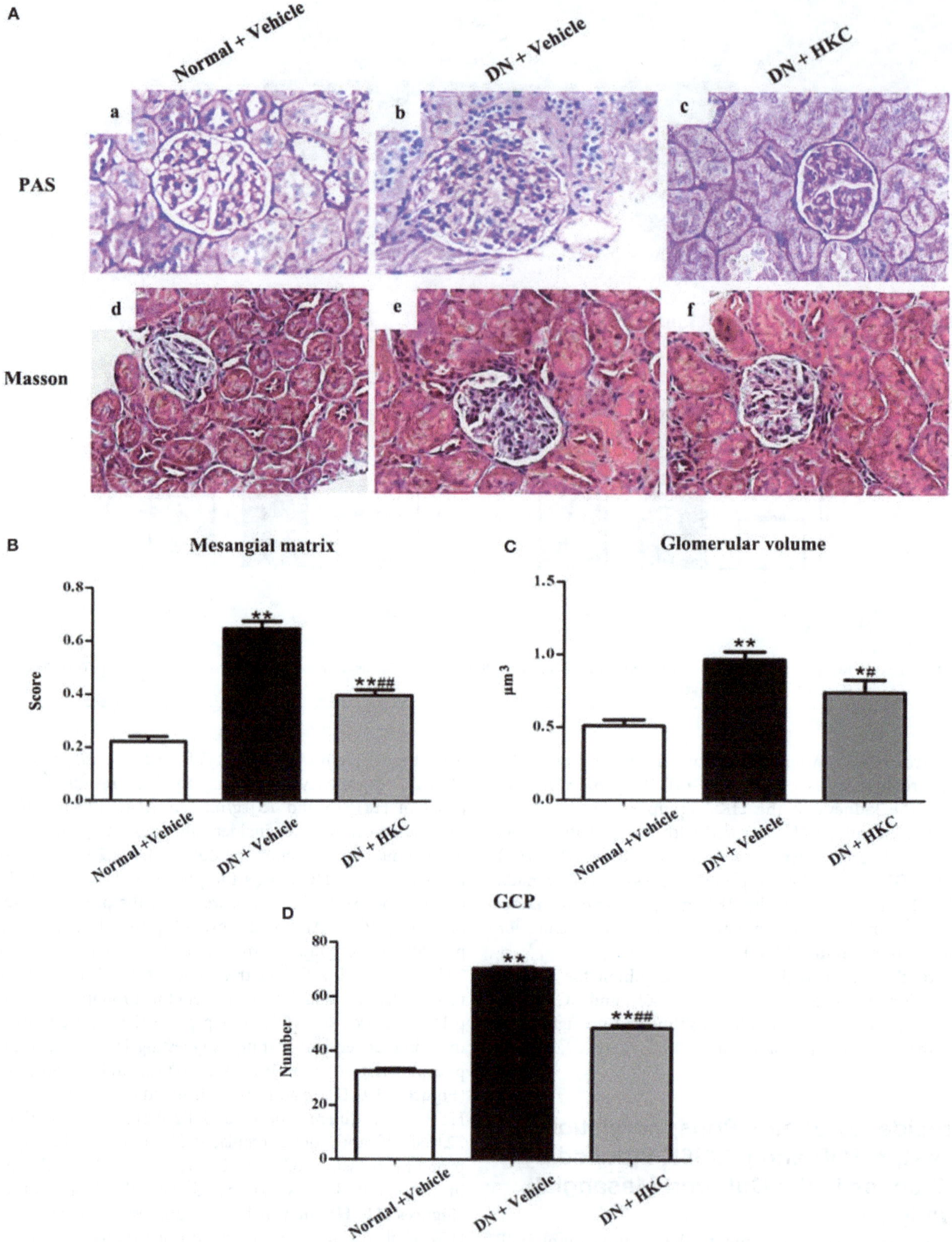

FIGURE 5 | Effects of HKC on glomerular pathological changes of the early DN model rats. **(A)** Light microscopy; **(B)** Mesangial matrix score; **(C)** Glomerilar volume; **(D)** GCP; **(a–c)**: PAS staining × 400, **(d–f)**: Masson staining × 400. The data are expressed as mean ± S.E. *$P < 0.05$, **$P < 0.01$ vs. the normal group; #$P < 0.05$, ##$P < 0.01$ vs. the model group.

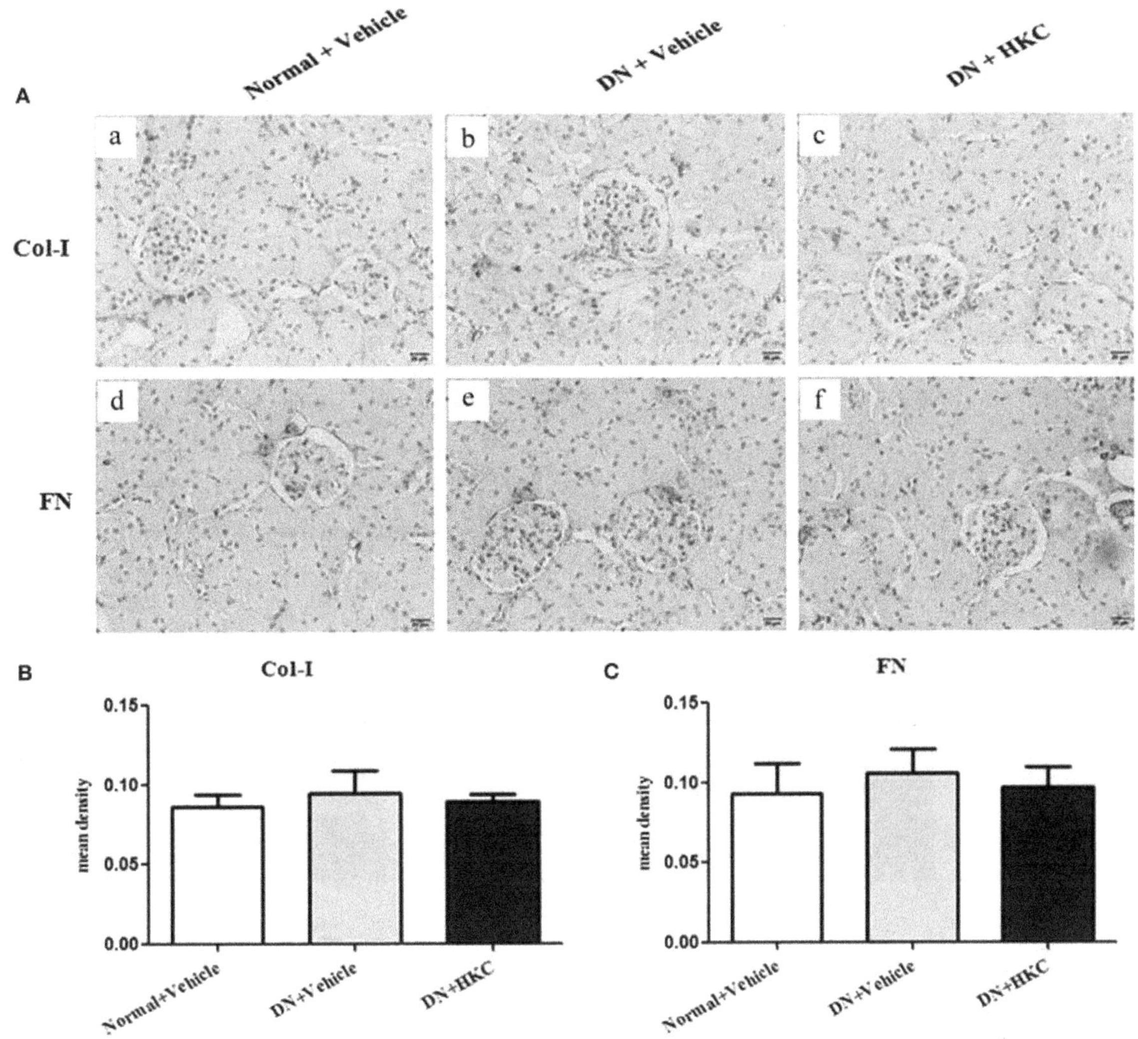

FIGURE 6 | Effects of HKC on Col-I and FN immunohistochemical stainings in the kidneys of the early DN model rats. **(A)** Col-I **(a–c)** and FN **(d–f)** immunohistochemical staining in glomeruli (× 400); **(B)** Mean density of Col-I immunohistochemical staining; **(C)** Mean density of FN immunohistochemical staining. The data are expressed as mean ± S.E.

These results indicated that HYP, different from RAP, could inhibit the phosphorylation of PI3K, Akt, mTOR, and p70S6K induced by HG in the cultured mesangial cells *in vitro*.

DISCUSSION

In the present study, using a modified DN rat model and the murine MCs, we emphatically demonstrated that HKC at the safe and effective dose of 2 g/kg/day can not only improve micro-UAlb and renal enlargement but also alleviate the early glomerular pathological changes including glomerular hypertrophy, GBM thickening and mild mesangial expansion, and that, more importantly, these ameliorative effects are closely related with the inhibition of Akt/mTOR/p70S6K signaling activity *in vivo* and *in vitro*.

A well-defined sequence of glomerular injuries in the early DN has been identified (Tervaert et al., 2010). The histologically characteristics of DN in both animal models and humans are 3 lesions, namely hypertrophic glomerulus, thickened GBM and mild mesangial expansion. In which, glomeruli may show only hypertrophy or be of normal size without any lesions in the earliest stage. GBM thickening is due to the increased accumulation of mesangial expansion, and progresses with the increased duration of diabetes (Najafian et al., 2011). For these reasons, in this study, we firstly tried to establish the useful and early DN rat model by unilateral nephrectomy combined with STZ intraperitoneal injections with the low doses of 35 mg/kg BW for twice at 72 h-interval. Our results showed that, these DN model rats were well-replicated hyperglycemia (more than 16.7 mmol/L), micro-UAlb (more than 20 mg/L), renal enlargement and the early glomerular pathological changes such

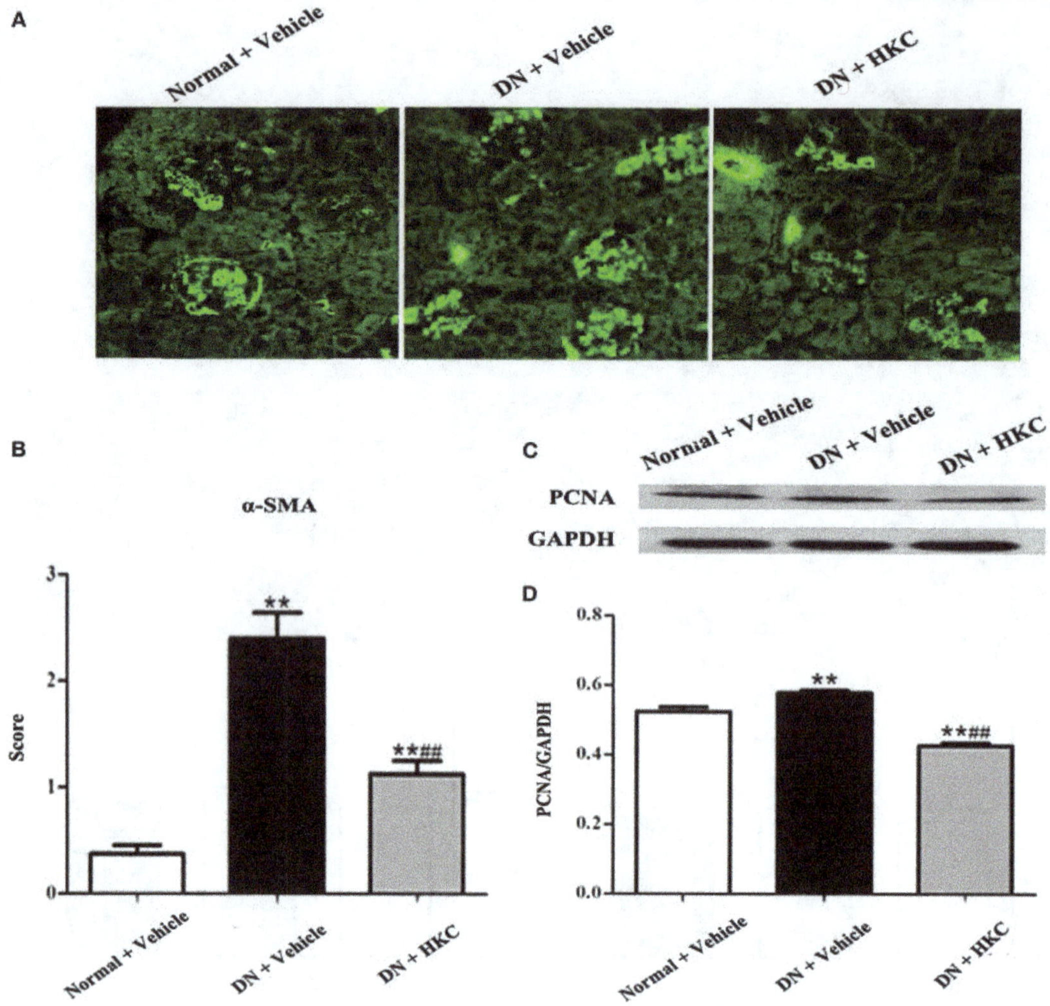

FIGURE 7 | Effects of HKC on α-SMA fluorescence staining in glomeruli and PCNA protein expression in the kidneys of the early DN model rats. **(A,B)** α-SMA fluorescence staining in glomeruli (× 400) and its score, **(C,D)** WB analysis (upon) for PCNA protein expression in the kidney, with the quantification (below). The data are expressed as mean ± S.E. $^{**}P < 0.01$ vs. the normal group; $^{\#\#}P < 0.01$ vs. the model group.

as hypertrophic glomerulus, thickened GBM and mild mesangial expansion within 4 weeks after modeling. Furthermore, it is noteworthy that most of the DN model rats did not exhibit a mass of proteinuria, renal dysfunction and the typical glomerular sclerosis marked by the severe collagen accumulation and the significant stainings of FN and Col-I in glomeruli, which are the recognized glomerular damaged features in the middle and advanced stages of DN. Whereupon, we considered that this modified DN rat model should be helpful in unraveling the early glomerular injuries and finding the novel therapeutic drugs in human DN.

In our previous studies, we described that HKC, a Chinese modern patent medicine in the long-time clinical practice (Zhang et al., 2014; Chen et al., 2015, 2016), with the dose of 2 g/kg/day is renoprotective via attenuating the advanced renal fibrosis after the drug administration for 8 weeks in the DN rat model (Mao et al., 2015). By comparison, in the present study, on the basis of the inchoate glomerular damaged animal model induced by unilateral nephrectomy and STZ injections, we further expounded whether HKC could improve the early glomerular pathological changes within 4 weeks after modeling. Our data indicated that HKC significantly ameliorated renal shape, KW and KHI, and improved hypertrophic glomerular form, increased glomerular volume and GCP and mild mesangial matrix expansion of the early DN model rats. In addition to these, HKC decreased the fluorescence staining of α-SMA in glomeruli and the protein expression of PCNA in the kidneys, which are the acknowledged markers of mesangial cell proliferation leading to glomerular hypertrophy in the early stage of DN (Hall et al., 1990; Cheng et al., 2014). Thus, we confirmed that HKC at the dose of 2 g/kg/day could attenuate glomerular hypertrophy *in vivo*, which is one of the main glomerular pathological characteristics of the early DN.

To our knowledge, GBM thickening is another characteristic pathological change in type 1 and type 2 DN and increases with the duration of the disease (White and Bilous, 2000). GBM

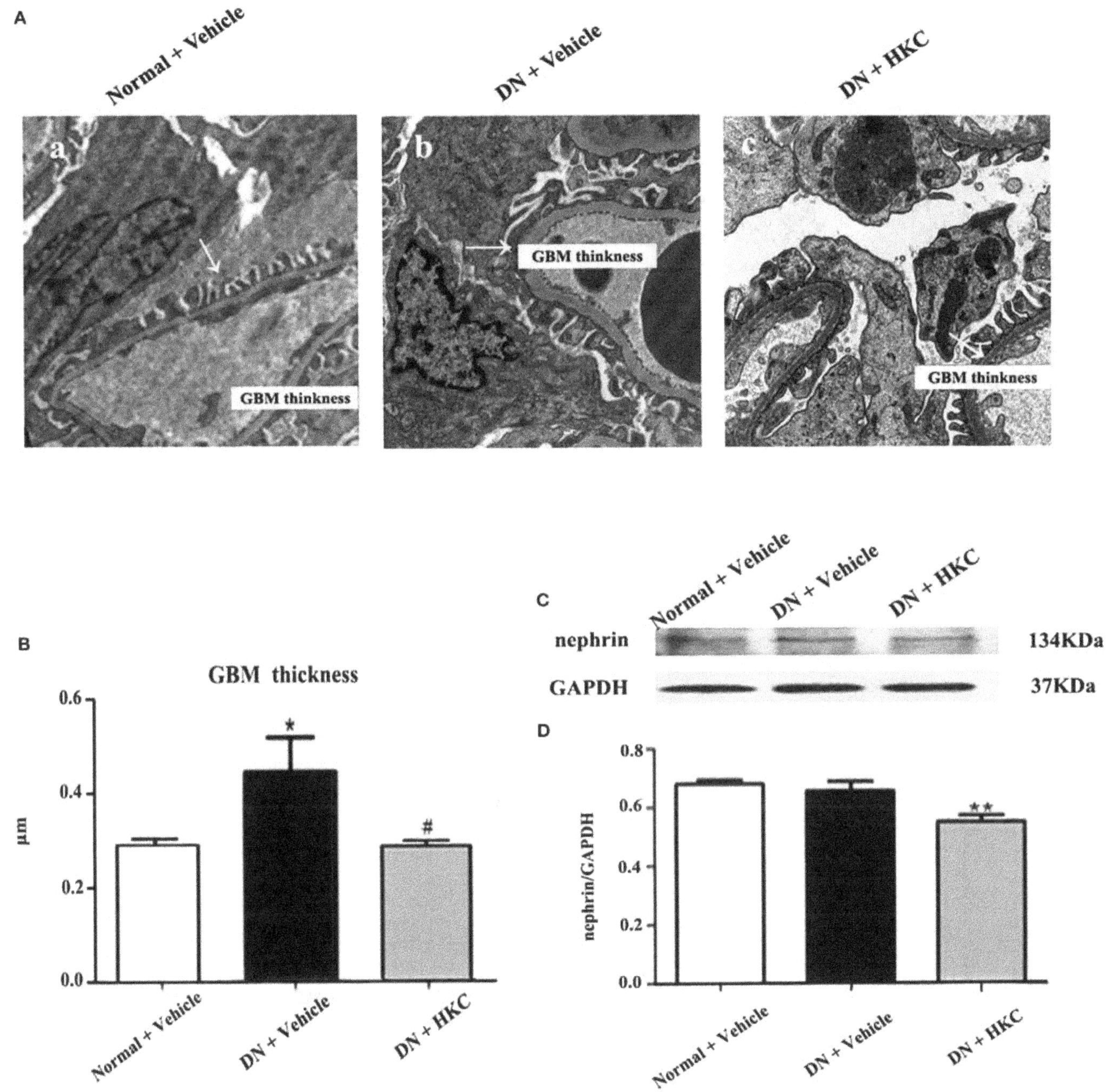

FIGURE 8 | Effects of HKC on GBM thickness, foot process form and nephrin protein expression in the kidneys of the early DN model rats. **(A)** Foot process ultrastructure (× 1,700); **(B)** GBM thickness; **(C,D)** WB analysis (upon) for nephrin protein expression in the kidney, with the quantification (below). The data are expressed as mean ± S.E. **P* < 0.05, ***P* < 0.01 vs. the normal group; #*P* < 0.05 vs. the model group.

thickening is a consequence of mesangial matrix expansion, with the increased deposition of normal mesangial matrix components such as Col-I and FN. Such accumulations result from the increased production of these proteins, their decreased degradation, or a combination of the two (Kim et al., 1991). In this study, we found that GBM thickening and mild mesangial expansion, as well as the ultrastructural changes of podocyte such as foot process loss and effacement were detected respectively in the early DN model rats, and ameliorated distinctly after HKC treatment for 4 weeks, at the same time, micro-UAlb of the DN model rats also decreased in a different degree. Interestingly, similar to our finding, An et al. (2017) reported recently that the pre-treatment of HYP, a bioactive component of HKC, prevents GBM damage in DN by inhibiting podocyte heparanase expression. Therefore, we had reasons to believe that HKC at the dose of 2 g/kg/day and its bioactive component

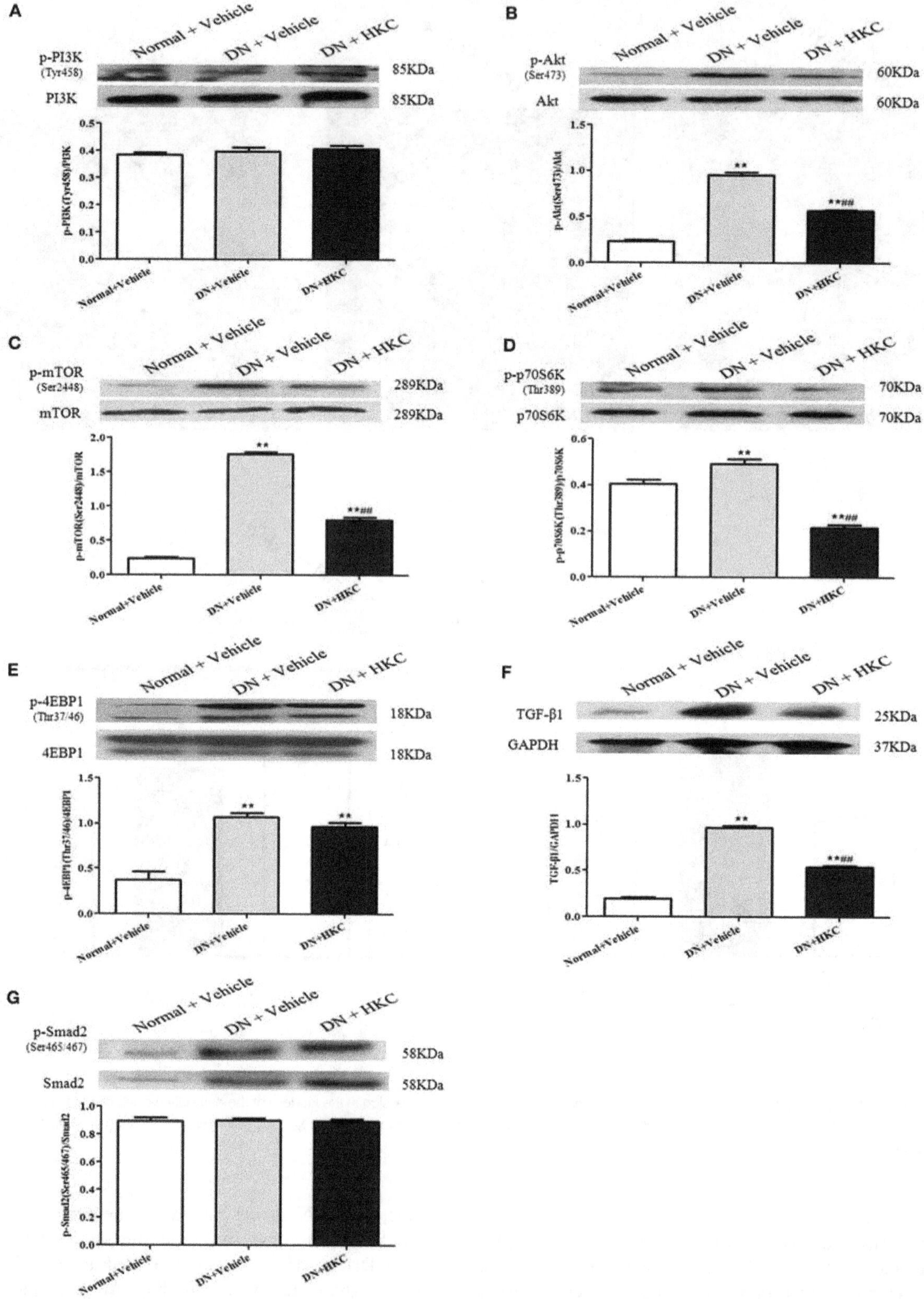

FIGURE 9 | Effects of HKC on the key signaling molecules of PI3K/Akt/mTOR and TGF-β1/Smad2 signaling pathways in the kidneys of the early DN model rats. **(A–E)** WB analysis (upon) for the protein expressions of PI3K, p-PI3K, Akt, p-Akt, mTOR, p-mTOR, p70S6K, p-p70S6K, 4EBP1, and p-4EBP1, with the quantification (below); **(F,G)** WB analysis (upon) for the protein expressions of TGF-β1, Smad, p-Smad2 and GAPDH, with the quantification (below). The data are expressed as mean ± S.E. $^{**}P < 0.01$ vs. the normal group; $^{\#\#}P < 0.01$ vs. the model group.

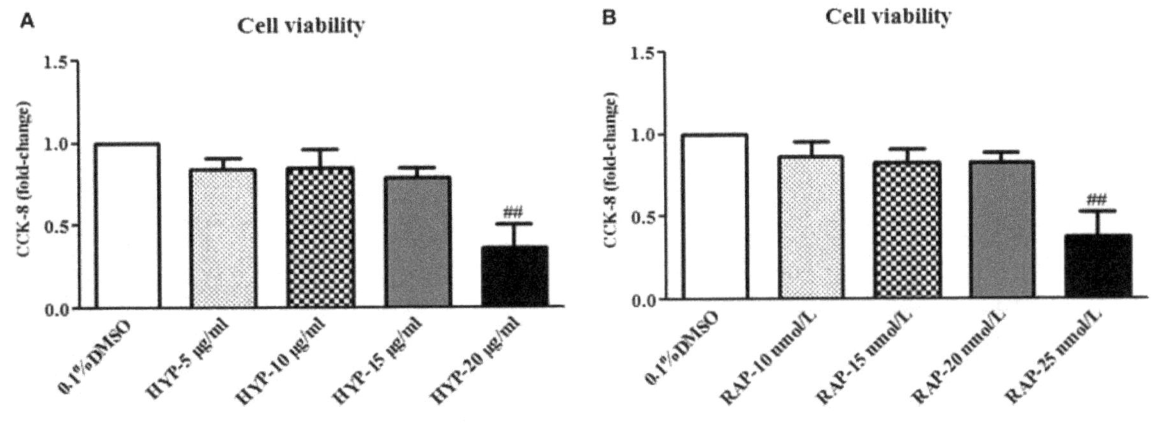

FIGURE 10 | The cell viability in the cultured mesangial cells. **(A)** The MCs were exposed to 0.1% DMSO and HYP at 5, 10, 15, and 20 μg/ml for 72 h; **(B)** The MCs were exposed to 0.1% DMSO and RAP at 10, 15, 20, and 25 nmol/L for 72 h. The data are expressed as mean ± S.E. ##$P < 0.01$ vs. the treatment of HYP at 15 μg/ml or RAP at 20 nmol/L.

could alleviate glomerular pathological changes of the early DN model rats.

Animal and clinical studies have reported the roles for PI3K/Akt/mTOR and TGF-β1/Smad2 signaling pathways in the early stage of DN, and the blockade of these pathways slows the progression and development of DN (Gangadharan-Komala et al., 2016; Li et al., 2016). Sakaguchi et al. (2006) reported that mTOR signaling is activated in the early DN model mice and the cultured mouse proximal tubule cells, and that mTOR signaling causes renal enlargement and glomerular hypertrophy through regulating the phosphorylation of p70S6K. Nagai et al. (2005) also reported that the activated PI3K/Akt/mTOR signaling and the enhanced p-p70S6K expression are detected in glomeruli in diabetes-induced by STZ injection. In addition, Lu et al. (2015) reported that the extract of *Ginkgo biloba* leaves (GbE) prevents renal fibrosis in rats with DN-induced by STZ injection, which is most likely to be associated with its abilities to inhibit Akt/mTOR signaling pathway. Hence, we proposed that regulating the activation of PI3K/Akt/mTOR and/or TGF-β1/Smad2 pathways in this DN rat model is a successful way to identify the therapeutic mechanisms *in vivo* of HKC on attenuating the early glomerular pathological changes. Our data clearly indicated that the increased protein expressions of p-Akt (Ser473), p-mTOR (Ser2448), p-p70S6K (Thr389), p-4EBP1 (Thr37/46), TGF-β1 and p-Smad2 in the kidneys were obviously revealed in the DN model rats, in the meantime, concomitant with the appearance of glomerular pathological changes including glomerular hypertrophy, GBM thickening and mild mesangial expansion. These results forcefully suggested that Akt/mTOR and TGF-β1/Smad2 signaling pathways are activated in this DN rat model, and there is a strong causality *in vivo* between the key signaling molecular expressions in these signaling pathways and the early glomerular injuries. More importantly, we also found that HKC simultaneously inhibited the activation of Akt/mTOR pathway as well as the protein expression of p-p70S6K in the kidneys of the DN model rats within 4 weeks. By contrast, the protein expressions of p-Smad2 as a key signaling molecule of TGF-β1/Smad2 pathway and p-4EBP1 as a downstream target of mTOR in the kidneys remained unchanged after HKC treatment. Here, without using the mTOR inhibitor, it is puzzling why the activation of 4EBP1 was not affected after the treatment with HKC. On the whole, using an intravital DN rat model, we suggested that HKC *in vivo* at the dose of 2 g/kg/day could only inhibit the activation of Akt/mTOR signaling and the phosphorylation level of p70S6K in the kidneys. Interestingly, consistent with the *in vivo* results basically, based on the murine MCs, we preliminarily confirmed the given doses of HYP, a bioactive component of HKC, could also inhibit the activation of PI3K/Akt/mTOR/p70S6K signaling axis induced by HG *in vitro*, which is a little bit different from RAP (mTORC1 inhibitor). Recently NOD-like receptor family CARD domain containing 3 (NLRC3) has been identified as the upstream negative molecule in PI3K/Akt/mTOR signaling axis to inhibit the activation of PI3K, Akt and mTOR in cancer (Karki et al., 2016). If so in the kidneys under the HG status, we boldly hypothesize HKC or HYP at the upstream can inhibit NLRC3 to regulate PI3K/Akt/mTOR signaling axis. Further detailed analyses *in vitro* and *in vivo* of NLRC3 are needed to address this hypothesis.

Finally, we need to bring up 2 additional points. First, HKC, a natural anti-nephritic phytomedicine, did not lower hyperglycemia in this DN rat model. We unavoidably thought of the cause-and-effect of relationship between hyperglycemia and the early glomerular pathological changes. Some studies have showed that GBM thickening and glomerular hypertrophy are described as a "pre-diabetic" lesion (Mac-Moune-Lai et al., 2004). We thereby believed that HKC has the renoprotective action, completely independent of lowering hyperglycemia. Second, 2 g/kg/day dose of HKC has been proved effective in attenuating the advanced renal fibrosis in the DN model rats (Mao et al., 2015). To exclude the side effects of HKC at such high dose on hepatic damage in this DN rat model, we emphatically compared

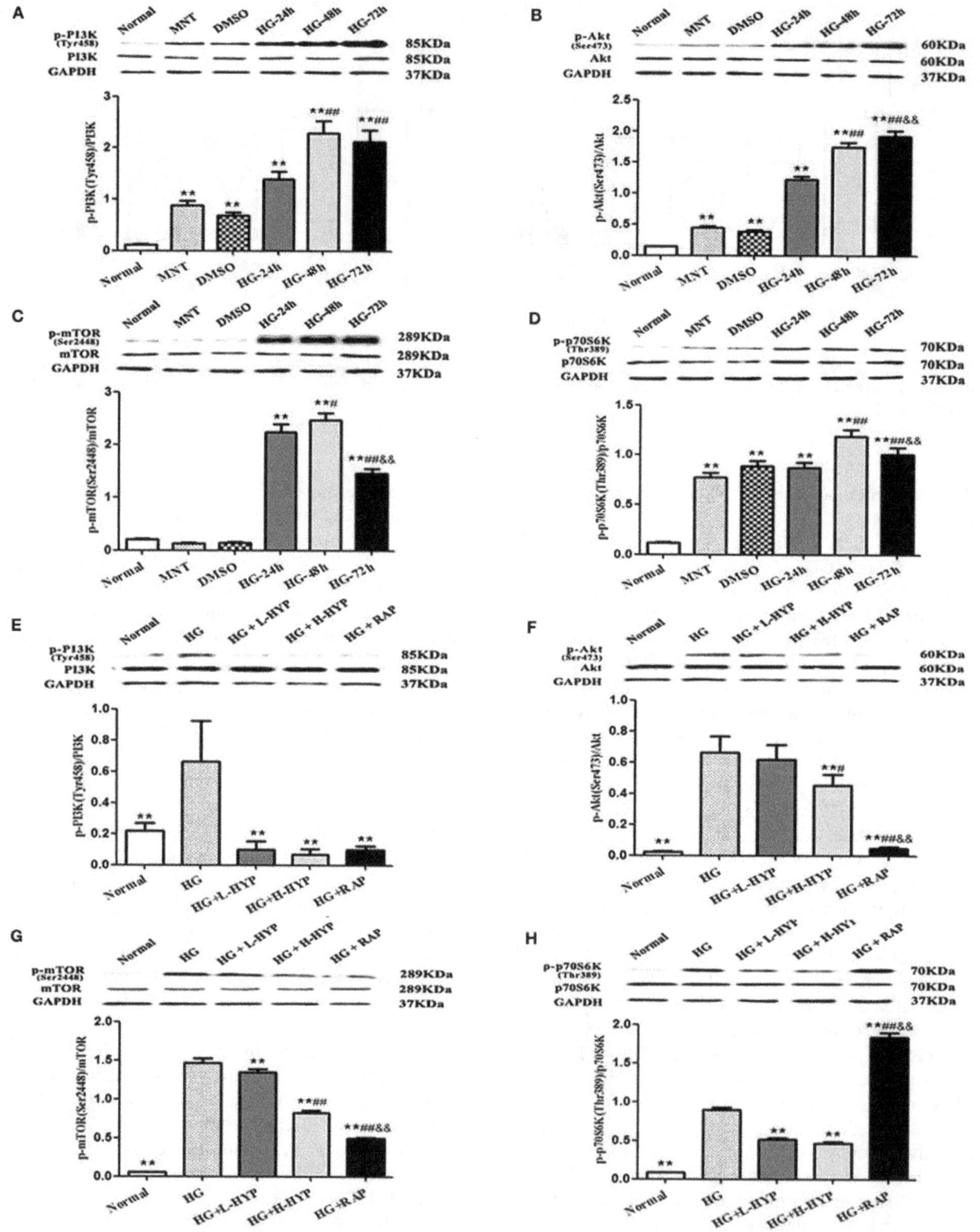

FIGURE 11 | Effects of HYP on the phosphorylation of PI3K, Akt, mTOR, and p70S6K induced by HG in the cultured mesangial cells *in vitro*. **(A–D)** WB analysis (upon) for the protein expressions of PI3K, p-PI3K, Akt, p-Akt, mTOR, p-mTOR, p70S6K, and p-p70S6K treated with normal glucose (Normal), MNT, DMSO and HG at 24, 48, and 72 h, respectively, with the quantification (below); **(E–H)** WB analysis (upon) for the protein expressions of PI3K, p-PI3K, Akt, p-Akt, mTOR, p-mTOR, p70S6K, and p-p70S6K after the treatment with normal glucose, HG, L-HYP, H-HYP, and RAP at 72 h, respectively, with the quantification (below). The data are expressed as mean ± S.E. **(A–D)** $^{**}P < 0.01$ vs. the normal glucose (Normal) group; $^{\#}P < 0.05$, $^{\#\#}P < 0.01$ vs. the HG-24 h group; $^{\&\&}P < 0.01$ vs. the HG-48 h group. **(E–H)** $^{**}P < 0.01$ vs. the HG group; $^{\#}P < 0.05$, $^{\#\#}P < 0.01$ vs. the HG+L-HYP group; $^{\&\&}P < 0.01$ vs. the HG+H-HYP group.

the levels of serum ALT and AST in 3 group rats. Our results revealed that serum ALT and AST in each group had no obvious changes, suggesting HKC at the dose of 2 g/kg/day has no negative effect on liver function *in vivo*.

In conclusion, the results of this report further demonstrated that HKC at the safe and effective dose of 2 g/kg/day can alleviate the early glomerular pathological changes of the DN model rats including glomerular hypertrophy, GBM thickening and mild mesangial expansion, likely by the inhibition of Akt/mTOR/p70S6K signaling activity *in vivo* and *in vitro*. This study provided the first evidence that HKC directly contributes to the prevention of the early DN.

AUTHOR CONTRIBUTIONS

Y-GW and H-TT provided the conception and design of research. WW, WH, W-BH, Y-LL, YT, H-MY, Q-JF, M-YZ, and Z-YW performed the experiments; WW and WH analyzed the data and interpreted the results of experiments; WW prepared the figures; WW and WH drafted the manuscript; Y-GW, H-TT, and R-MT edited and revised the manuscript; WW and Y-GW approved the final version of manuscript.

FUNDING

This study was supported by 3 grants from the National Natural Science Foundation of China (81573903, 81603675, and 81374030) to Y-GW and YT, and a grant from Nanjing Medical Science and Technique Development Foundation (QRX17042) to WW.

ACKNOWLEDGMENTS

The authors thank Dr. Xun-Yang Luo and Dr. Le Zhang (Department of Laboratory Medicine, Nanjing Drum Tower Hospital, The Affiliated Hospital of Nanjing University Medicine School, Nanjing, China) for their technical assistance and instructions. The authors also thank Prof. Jian Yao (Division of Molecular Signaling, Department of Advanced Biomedical Research, Interdisciplinary Graduate School of Medicine and Engineering, University of Yamanashi, Yamanashi, Japan) and Prof. Yan Chen (Key Laboratory of New Drug Delivery System of Chinese Meteria Medica, Jiangsu Provincial Academy of Chinese Medicine, Nanjing, China) for their helpful discussions and technical assistance.

REFERENCES

Afkarian, M., Zelnick, L. R., Hall, Y. N., Heagerty, P. J., Tuttle, K., Weiss, N. S., et al. (2016). Clinical manifestations of kidney disease among US adults with diabetes, 1988-2014. *JAMA* 316, 602–610. doi: 10.1001/jama.2016.10924

An, X., Zhang, L., Yuan, Y., Wang, B., Yao, Q., Li, L., et al. (2017). Hyperoside pre-treatment prevents glomerular basement membrane damage in diabetic nephropathy by inhibiting podocyte heparanase expression. *Sci. Rep.* 7:6413. doi: 10.1038/s41598-017-06844-2

Cai, H. D., Su, S. L., Qian, D. W., Guo, S., Tao, W. W., Cong, X. D., et al. (2017). Renal protective effect and action mechanism of Huangkui capsule and its main five flavonoids. *J. Ethnopharmacol.* 206, 152–159. doi: 10.1016/j.jep.2017.02.046

Chen, P., Wan, Y. G., Wang, C. J., Zhao, Q., Wei, Q. X., Tu, Y., et al. (2012). Mechanisms and effects of *Abelmoschus manihot* preparations in treating chronic kidney disease. *China J. Chin. Mater. Medica. (Zhongguo Zhong Yao Za Zhi)* 37, 2252–2256 (in Chinese).

Chen, Y., Cai, G., Sun, X., and Chen, X. (2016). Treatment of chronic kidney disease using a traditional Chinese medicine, Flos Abelmoschus manihot (Linnaeus) Medicus (Malvaceae). *Clin. Exp. Pharmacol. Physiol.* 43, 145–148. doi: 10.1111/1440-1681.12528

Chen, Y. Z., Gong, Z. X., Cai, G. Y., Gao, Q., Chen, X. M., Tang, L., et al. (2015). Efficacy and safety of Flos *Abelmoschus manihot* (Malvaceae) on type 2 diabetic nephropathy: A systematic review. *Chin. J. Integr. Med.* 21, 464–472. doi: 10.1007/s11655-014-1891-6

Cheng, H., Chen, C., Wang, S., Ding, G., and Shi, M. (2014). The effects of urokinase-type plasminogen activator (uPA) on cell proliferation and phenotypic transformation of rat mesangial cells induced by high glucose. *Diabetes Res. Clin. Pract.* 103, 489–495. doi: 10.1016/j.diabres.2013.11.016

de Boer, I. H. (2017). A new chapter for diabetic kidney disease. *N. Engl. J. Med.* 377, 885–887. doi: 10.1056/NEJMe1708949

Dibble, C. C., and Cantley, L. C. (2015). Regulation of mTORC1 by PI3K signaling. *Trends. Cell. Biol.* 25, 545–555. doi: 10.1016/j.tcb.2015.06.002

Gangadharan-Komala, M., Gross, S., Zaky, A., Pollock, C., and Panchapakesan, U. (2016). Saxagliptin reduces renal tubulointerstitial inflammation, hypertrophy and fibrosis in diabetes. *Nephrology* 21, 423–431. doi: 10.1111/nep.12618

Ge, J., Miao, J. J., Sun, X. Y., and Yu, J. Y. (2016). Huangkui capsule, an extract from *Abelmoschus manihot* (L.) medic, improves diabetic nephropathy via activating peroxisome proliferator-activated receptor (PPAR)-α/γ and attenuating endoplasmic reticulum stress in rats. *J. Ethnopharmacol.* 189, 238–249. doi: 10.1016/j.jep.2016.05.033

Giasson, E., and Meloche, S. (1995). Role of p70 S6 protein kinase in angiotensin II-induced protein synthesis in vascular smooth muscle cells. *J. Biol. Chem.* 270, 5225–5231. doi: 10.1074/jbc.270.10.5225

Glassock, R. J. (2016). Control of albuminuria in overt diabetic nephropathy durability counts. *Nephrol. Dial. Transplant.* 31, 1371–1373. doi: 10.1093/ndt/gfv462

Guo, J. M., Lin, P., Lu, Y. W., Duan, J. A., Shang, E. X., Qian, D. W., et al. (2013). Investigation of *in vivo* metabolic profile of *Abelmoschus Manihot* based on pattern recognition analysis. *J. Ethnopharmacol.* 148, 297–304. doi: 10.1016/j.jep.2013.04.029

Haas, M. (2009). Alport syndrome and thin glomerular basement membrane nephropathy: a practical approach to diagnosis. *Arch. Pathol. Lab. Med.* 133, 224–232. doi: 10.1043/1543-2165-133.2.224

Hall, M. N. (2016). TOR and paradigm change: cell growth is controlled. *Mol. Biol. Cell.* 15, 2804–2806. doi: 10.1091/mbc.E15-05-0311

Hall, P. A., Levison, D. A., Woods, A. L., Yu, C. C., Kellock, D. B., Watkins, J. A., et al. (1990). Proliferating cell nuclear antigen (PCNA) immunolocalization in paraffin sections: an index of cell proliferation with evidence of deregulated expression in some neoplasms. *J. Pathol.* 162, 285–294. doi: 10.1002/path.1711620403

Karki, R., Man, S. M., Malireddi, R. K., Kesavardhana, S., Zhu, Q., Burton, A. R., et al. (2016). NLRC3 is an inhibitory sensor of PI3K-mTOR pathways in cancer. *Nature.* doi: 10.1038/nature 20597. [Epub ahead of print].

Kim, Y., Kleppel, M. M., Butkowski, R., Mauer, S. M., Wieslander, J., and Michael, A. F. (1991). Differential expression of basement membrane collagen chains in diabetic nephropathy. *Am. J. Pathol.* 138, 413–420.

Lane, P. H., Steffes, M. W., and Mauer, S. M. (1990). Renal histologic changes in diabetes mellitus. *Semin. Nephrol.* 10, 254–259.

Lane, P. H., Steffes, M. W., and Mauer, S. M. (1992). Estimation of glomerular volume: a comparison of four methods. *Kidney. Int.* 41, 1085–1089. doi: 10.1038/ki.1992.165

Li, D., Lu, Z., Xu, Z., Ji, J., Zheng, Z., Lin, S., et al. (2016). Spironolactone promotes autophagy via inhibiting PI3K/AKT/mTOR signalling pathway and reduce adhesive capacity damage in podocytes under mechanical stress. *Biosci. Rep.* 36:e00355. doi: 10.1042/BSR20160086

Li, P., Chen, Y. Z., Lin, H. L., Ni, Z. H., Zhan, Y. L., Wang, R., et al. (2017). *Abelmoschus manihot*-a traditional Chinese medicine versus losartan potassium for treating IgA nephropathy: study protocol for a randomized controlled trial. *Trials* 18:170. doi: 10.1186/s13063-016-1774-6

Liu, H., Zhong, L. Y., and Li, R. H. (2010). Observation of effect and investigation of mechanism of Huangkui capsule for the treatment of diabetic nephropathy. *Chin. J. Integr. Tradit. West. Nephrol.* 7, 633–634.

Liu, Z. H. (2013). Nephrology in China. *Nat. Rev. Nephrol.* 9, 523–528. doi: 10.1038/nrneph.2013.146

Lu, Q., Zuo, W. Z., Ji, X. J., Zhou, Y. X., Liu, Y. Q., Yao, X. Q., et al. (2015). Ethanolic *Ginkgo biloba* leaf extract prevents renal fibrosis through Akt/mTOR signaling in diabetic nephropathy. *Phytomedicine* 22, 1071–1078. doi: 10.1016/j.phymed.2015.08.010

Mac-Moune-Lai, F., Szeto, C. C., Choi, P. C., Ho, K. K., Tang, N. L., Chow, K. M., et al. (2004). Isolate diffuse thickening of glomerular capillary basement membrane: a renal lesion in prediabetes?. *Mod. Pathol.* 17, 1506–1512. doi: 10.1038/modpathol.3800219

Mao, Z. M., Shen, S. M., Wan, Y. G., Sun, W., Chen, H. L., Huang, M. M., et al. (2015). Huangkui capsule attenuates renal fibrosis in diabetic nephropathy rats through regulating oxidative stress and p38MAPK/Akt pathways, compared to α-lipoic acid. *J. Ethnopharmacol.* 173, 256–265. doi: 10.1016/j.jep.2015.07.036

Muskiet, M. H. A., Tonneijck, L., Smits, M. M., van-Baar, M. J. B., Kramer, M. H. H., Hoorn, E. J., et al. (2017). GLP-1 and the kidney: from physiology to pharmacology and outcomes in diabetes. *Nat. Rev. Nephrol.* 13, 605–628. doi: 10.1038/nrneph.2017.123

Nagai, K., Matsubara, T., Mima, A., Sumi, E., Kanamori, H., Iehara, N., et al. (2005). Gas6 induces Akt/mTOR-mediated mesangial hypertrophy in diabetic nephropathy. *Kidney. Int.* 68, 552–561. doi: 10.1111/j.1523-1755.2005.00433.x

Najafian, B., Alpers, C. E., and Fogo, A. B. (2011). Pathology of human diabetic nephropathy. *Contrib. Nephrol.* 170, 36–47. doi: 10.1159/000324942

Penno, G., Garofolo, M., and Del-Prato, S. (2016). Dipeptidyl peptidase-4 inhibition in chronic kidney disease and potential for protection against diabetes-related renal injury. *Nutr. Metab. Cardiovasc. Dis.* 26, 361–373. doi: 10.1016/j.numecd.2016.01.001

Raij, L., Azar, S., and Keane, W. (1984). Mesangial immune injury, hypertension, and progressive glomerular damage in Dahl rats. *Kidney. Int.* 26, 137–143. doi: 10.1038/ki.1984.147

Sakaguchi, M., Isono, M., Isshiki, K., Sugimoto, T., Koya, D., and Kashiwagi, A. (2006). Inhibition of mTOR signaling with rapamycin attenuates renal hypertrophy in the early diabetic mice. *Biochem. Biophys. Res. Commun.* 340, 296–301. doi: 10.1016/j.bbrc.2005.12.012

Tervaert, T. W., Mooyaart, A. L., Amann, K., Cohen, A. H., Cook, H. T., Drachenberg, C. B., et al. (2010). Pathologic classification of diabetic nephropathy. *J. Am. Soc. Nephrol.* 21, 556–563. doi: 10.1681/ASN.2010010010

Trendafilova, A., Todorova, M., Nikolova, M., Gavrilova, A., and Vitkova, A. (2011). Flavonoid constituents and free radical scavenging activity of *Alchemilla mollis*. *Nat. Prod. Commun.* 6, 1851–1854.

Tu, Y., Gu, L., Chen, D., Wu, W., Liu, H., Hu, H., et al. (2017). Rhein inhibits autophagy in rat renal tubular cells by regulation of AMPK/mTOR signaling. *Sci. Rep.* 7:43790. doi: 10.1038/srep43790

Tu, Y., Sun, W., Wan, Y. G., Che, X. Y., Pu, H. P., Yin, X. J., et al. (2013). Huangkui capsule, an extract from *Abelmoschus manihot* (L.) medic, ameliorates adriamycin-induced renal inflammation and glomerular injury via inhibiting p38MAPK signaling pathway activity in rats. *J. Ethnopharmacol.* 147, 311–320. doi: 10.1016/j.jep.2013.03.006

Tuttle, K. R., Bakris, G. L., Bilous, R. W., Chiang, J. L., de-Boer, I. H., Goldstein-Fuchs, J., et al. (2014). Diabetic kidney disease: a report from an ADA Consensus Conference. *Diabetes Care* 37, 2864–2883. doi: 10.2337/dc14-1296

Wanner, C., Inzucchi, S. E., Lachin, J. M., Fitchett, D., von-Eynatten, M., Mattheus, M., et al. (2016). Empagliflozin and progression of kidney disease in type 2 diabetes. *N. Engl. J. Med.* 375, 323–334. doi: 10.1056/NEJMoa1515920

White, K. E., and Bilous, R. W. (2000). Type 2 diabetic patients with nephropathy show structural-functional relationships that are similar to type 1 disease. *J. Am. Soc. Nephrol.* 11, 1667–1673.

Xue, C. F., Guo, J. M., Qian, D. W., Duan, J. A., Shang, E. X., Shu, Y., et al. (2011). Identification of the potential active components of *Abelmoschus manihot* in rat blood and kidney tissue by microdialysis combined with ultra-performance liquid chromatography/quadrupole time-of-flight mass spectrometry. *J. Chromatogr. B Anal. Technol. Biomed. Life. Sci.* 879, 317–325. doi: 10.1016/j.jchromb.2010.12.016

Yuan, T. L., Wulf, G., Burga, L., and Cantley, L. C. (2011). Cell-to-cell variability in PI3K protein level regulates PI3K-AKT pathway activity in cell populations. *Curr. Biol.* 21, 173–183. doi: 10.1016/j.cub.2010.12.047

Zhang, L., He, S., Yang, F., Yu, H., Xie, W., Dai, Q., et al. (2016). Hyperoside ameliorates glomerulosclerosis in diabetic nephropathy by downregulating miR-21. *Can. J. Physiol. Pharmacol.* 94, 1249–1256. doi: 10.1139/cjpp-2016-0066

Zhang, L., Li, P., Xing, C. Y., Zhao, J. Y., He, Y. N., Wang, J. Q., et al. (2014). Efficacy and safety of *Abelmoschus manihot* for primary glomerular disease: a prospective, multicenter randomized controlled clinical trial. *Am. J. Kidney. Dis.* 64, 57–65. doi: 10.1053/j.ajkd.2014.01.431

Zinman, B., Wanner, C., Lachin, J. M., Fitchett, D., Bluhmki, E., Hantel, S., et al. (2015). Empagliflozin, cardiovascular outcomes, and mortality in type 2 diabetes. *N. Engl. J. Med.* 373, 2117–2128. doi: 10.1056/NEJMoa1504720

20

Identification of Steroidogenic Components Derived from *Gardenia jasminoides* Ellis Potentially Useful for Treating Postmenopausal Syndrome

Xueyu Wang[1], Guo-Cai Wang[2], Jianhui Rong[1], Shi Wei Wang[1], Tzi Bun Ng[3], Yan Bo Zhang[1], Kai Fai Lee[4], Lin Zheng[1], Hei-Kiu Wong[1], Ken Kin Lam Yung[5] and Stephen Cho Wing Sze[5]**

[1] School of Chinese Medicine, LKS Faculty of Medicine, The University of Hong Kong, Hong Kong, China, [2] Institute of Traditional Chinese Medicine and Natural Products, College of Pharmacy, Jinan University, Guangzhou, China, [3] School of Biomedical Sciences, Faculty of Medicine, The Chinese University of Hong Kong, Hong Kong, China, [4] Department of Obstetrics and Gynaecology, LKS Faculty of Medicine, The University of Hong Kong, Hong Kong, China, [5] Department of Biology, Faculty of Science, Hong Kong Baptist University, Hong Kong, China

***Correspondence:**
Ken Kin Lam Yung
kklyung@hkbu.edu.hk
Stephen Cho Wing Sze
scwsze@hkbu.edu.hk

Estrogen-stimulating principles have been demonstrated to relieve postmenopausal syndrome effectively. *Gardenia jasminoides* Ellis (GJE) is an herbal medicine possessing multiple pharmacological effects on human health with low toxicity. However, the therapeutic effects of GJE on the management of postmenopausal syndrome and its mechanism of action have not been fully elucidated. In this study, network pharmacology-based approaches were employed to examine steroidogenesis under the influence of GJE. In addition, the possibility of toxicity of GJE was ruled out and four probable active compounds were predicted. In parallel, a chromatographic fraction of GJE with estrogen-stimulating effect was identified and nine major compounds were isolated from this active fraction. Among the nine compounds, four of them were identified by network pharmacology, validating the use of network pharmacology to predict active compounds. Then the phenotypic approaches were utilized to verify that rutin, chlorogenic acid (CGA) and geniposidic acid (GA) exerted an estrogen-stimulating effect on ovarian granulosa cells. Furthermore, the results of target-based approaches indicated that rutin, CGA, and GA could up-regulate the FSHR-aromatase pathway in ovarian granulosa cells. The stimulation of estrogen production by rat ovarian granulosa cells under the influence of the three compounds underwent a decline when the follicle-stimulating hormone receptor (FSHR) was blocked by antibodies against the receptor, indicating the involvement of FSHR in the estradiol-stimulating activity of the three compounds. The effects of the three compounds on estrogen biosynthesis- related gene expression level were further confirmed by Western blot assay. Importantly, the MTT results showed that exposure of breast cancer cells to the three compounds resulted in reduction of cell viability, demonstrating the cytotoxicity of the three compounds. Collectively, rutin, chlorogenic acid and geniposidic acid may contribute to the therapeutic potential of GJE for the treatment of postmenopausal syndrome.

Keywords: estrogen, *Gardenia jasminoides* Ellis, menopause, network pharmacology, ovarian granulosa cells

INTRODUCTION

Natural menopause is classified as permanent cessation of menstruation, induced by ovarian follicular failure and ovarian hormone instability (Burger et al., 2007). Due to a global population aging, there will be one billion women over the age of 60 years by the year 2050 (Hoga et al., 2015). Currently, more than 50% of women in the world are afflicted with postmenopausal syndrome at the climacteric stage (Su et al., 2013; Dalal and Agarwal, 2015). It is widely accepted that estrogen deprivation plays an important role in the postmenopausal syndrome (World Health Organization, 1996; Greendale et al., 1998; Constantine and Pickar, 2003). In the climacteric period, the decline of estrogen may induce depression (Kaufert et al., 1992; Avis et al., 1994; Al-Safi and Santoro, 2014; Citraro et al., 2015), memory loss (Devi et al., 2005; Weber and Mapstone, 2009), bone resorption (Hernandez et al., 2003; Society, 2006), metabolic syndrome (Carr, 2003; Janssen et al., 2008), and colorectal cancer (Al-Azzawi and Wahab, 2002; Barzi et al., 2013). The physiological problems caused by estrogen deficiency adversely influence the quality of life of modern people and have become a substantial public health burden. To relieve the reduced level of estrogen, women in climacterium usually opt to undergo hormone replacement therapy (HRT) (Barnabei et al., 2002). However, a WHO study has established that HRT can significantly heighten the risk of endometrial cancer, breast cancer and gallbladder diseases in climacteric women (Nelson et al., 2002; Davey, 2013; Chuffa et al., 2016). In addition, HRT is usually accompanied by considerable untoward side effects, including vaginal bleeding, genital irritation and headache (Clarke et al., 2002). Therefore, a safe and effective treatment of postmenopausal syndrome is necessitated.

As an alternative therapy for postmenopausal syndrome, herbal medicine has a long history of a thousand years and a wide range of applications for improving women's health (Johnston, 1997; Feng and Cao, 2010). In the US, over 80% of the physicians suggest that their patients alleviate postmenopausal syndrome with herbal medicine (Meisler, 2003). In China and other Asian countries, herbal medicine has been extensively and chronically deployed to alleviate postmenopausal syndrome, due to its well-known safety and efficacy (Scheid, 2007; Liu et al., 2008; Chen et al., 2010; Scheid et al., 2010). Among the selected herbal medicine, *Gardenia jasminoides* Ellis (GJE) is a potential candidate for the treatment of gynecological disorders (Yang et al., 2016). GJE has a wide range of pharmacological effects, including anti-allergy (Sung et al., 2014), anti-oxidative, anti-atherosclerotic, anti-platelet aggregating, anti-hypertensive activities, and so on (Liu et al., 2013). Nevertheless, the effects of GJE on the management of climacterium have rarely been reported. Recently, several studies reported that the fractions of GJE and the major compounds in GJE could display antidepressant activities in rodent models (Cai et al., 2015; Zhang et al., 2015; Ren et al., 2016; Wang et al., 2016). Additionally, previous studies indicated that GJE and its active components could improve memory and learning ability, and protect the neurons in animals with brain injury (Sheng et al., 2006; Chen et al., 2015; Zhang et al., 2016). Genipin, a major phytoconstituent of GJE, is a candidate for the treatment of osteoporosis (Hoon Lee et al., 2014). GJE was also able to attenuate metabolic syndrome with a combination of other herbal drugs in estrogen-deficient rats (Yang et al., 2016). Moreover, the components of GJE exerted suppressive effects on colon cancer cells and breast cancer cells (Kim et al., 2012; Oliveira et al., 2017). Gardenia oil also augmented plasma estradiol levels (Li et al., 2013). Collectively, GJE can be regarded as a promising candidate for the treatment of estrogen deprivation. However, neither systematic mechanistic studies of GJE related to estrogen deprivation nor the estrogen-stimulating effects of GJE have been reported. Hence, it was hypothesized that there are several active compounds derived from GJE that are endowed with the ability of stimulating estrogen biosynthesis in ovarian granulosa cells.

In this study, network and systemic pharmacological analysis was used to identify the therapeutic role of GJE in the treatment of postmenopausal syndrome and in the prevention of the risks of HRT. Firstly, the possible bioactive compounds of GJE were predicted by network pharmacology. Afterwards, the fractions of GJE were isolated by HPLC and the bioactive fraction of GJE that could be adopted to treat postmenopausal syndrome was explored by using the estradiol assay. The major components were then extracted from the bioactive fraction and converged with the probable active ingredients predicted by network pharmacology. Among these components, phenotypic (based on the estradiol assay) and target-based (based on the molecular docking analysis, Western blot assay and FSHR inhibition assay) drug-screening principles were applied to screen bioactive compounds with estrogen-stimulating effects (Hughes et al., 2011; Lu et al., 2016). Breast cancer cells were also used to pre-evaluate the cancer risk of GJE active ingredients. The workflow to explore the bioactive compounds is illustrated in **Figure 1**. Results obtained from this study disclose the estrogen-stimulating action of GJE, which further supports the clinical use of GJE to attenuate postmenopausal syndrome.

METHODS

Network Pharmacology

For the identification of chemicals, the constituent components of GJE can be found in TCMSP (Traditional Chinese Medicine Systems Pharmacology) database (http://lsp.nwu.edu.cn/tcmsp.php), TCM Database@Taiwan (http://tcm.cmu.edu.tw/) and TCMID (Traditional Chinese Medicines Integrated Database, http://www.megabionet.org/tcmid/) (Wang et al., 2015). Subsequently, TCMSP database was used to screen the compounds based on DL (drug-likeness) values. Only ingredients with a DL value higher than 0.18 can be retained as candidate compounds (Xiang et al., 2016; Mao et al., 2017). For the identification of GJE associated proteins and genes, STITCH ("search tool for interactions of chemicals") database 4.0 (http://stitch.embl.de/) was used to explore the compound-protein interactions of GJE. In addition, CTD (comparative toxicogenomics database, http://ctd.mdibl.org/) was searched to ascertain the compound-gene interactions of GJE (Mattingly et al., 2003; Kuhn et al., 2008). In STITCH and CTD database, confidence score and gene frequency indicate the strength of

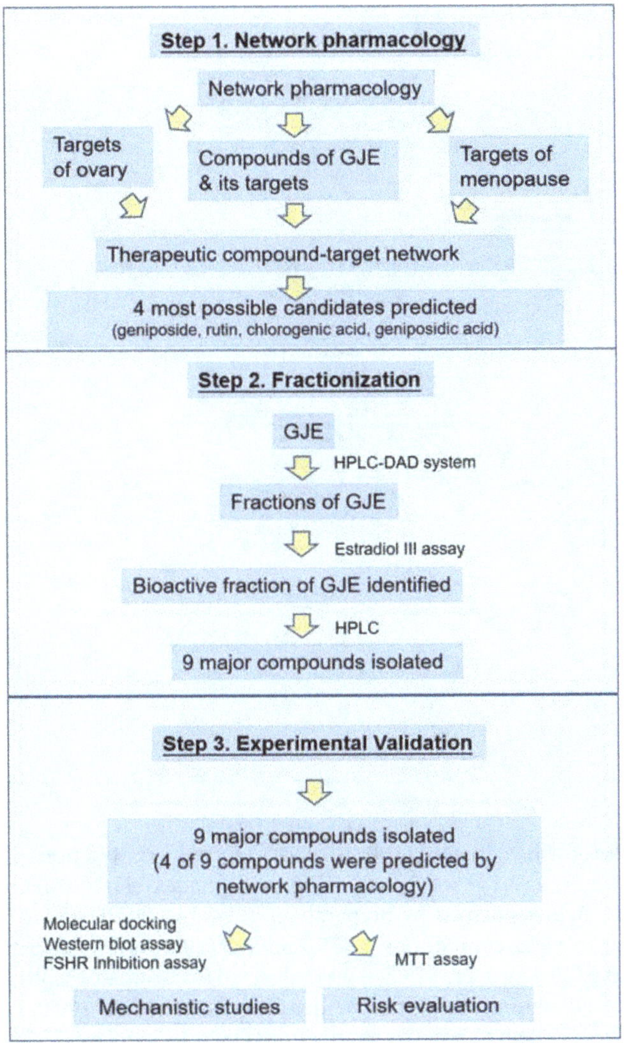

FIGURE 1 | Process overview.

the chemical-target interaction. Therefore, only proteins with a chemical-protein interaction confidence score $\geq$0.9 (highest confidence) and genes with gene frequency $\geq$1.84 (average of gene frequency) were chosen (Wang et al., 2015). TCMSP database was also used to investigate the targets related to the compounds of GJE. For the therapeutic compound target network, the targets related to menopause can be found with the key word "menopause" or "climacteric" at TTD (Therapeutic Target Database, http://bidd.nus.edu.sg/group/cjttd/), DrugBank database (https://www.drugbank.ca/) and GeneCards database (http://www.genecards.org/). Then OKdb (Ovarian Kaleidoscope Database, http://okdb.appliedbioinfo.net/) was used to identify gene expression in the human ovary. The ingredients of GJE that can target genes associated with both menopause and the ovary could be selected. For the enrichment analysis, in order to search the significant pathway and tissue specificity, JEPETTO (http://apps.cytoscape.org/apps/jepetto) with the KEGG database and Funrich (http://www.funrich.org/) with COSMIC database were utilized to identify and analyze the significant pathway and tissue specificity of GJE components, respectively (Winterhalter et al., 2014; Wang et al., 2015). Among the numerous compounds of GJE that can target genes related to both menopause and the ovaries, several bioactive molecules were selected for the validation of the basic experiment. To search for three or four potent pharmaceutical ingredients of GJE, the screening of blood-brain barrier (BBB) and the AlogP value was proposed. It demonstrated that BBB is critical for measuring the capacity of compounds entering the CNS (central nervous system) (Tattersall et al., 1975) and AlogP indicates hydrophobicity of the molecule (Ghose et al., 1988). Therefore, only GJE compounds with BBB < -0.3 (non-penetrating) and AlogP ≤ 5 can be chosen as the potential drug candidates (Ru et al., 2014; Kotapalli et al., 2015). Several compounds with a relatively higher DL value were then selected. A high DL value indicates a high drug-like property of bioactive compounds as therapeutic agents (Ru et al., 2014). The workflow of the network pharmacology study of GJE is presented in **Figure 2** and **Table S1**.

Extraction and Isolation of GJE Bioactive Fraction

Sample Preparation

GJE was dried and ground into a powder form, followed by extraction using 80% ethanol. After that, GJE was concentrated and extracted with different solvents, including ethanol, petroleum ether, ethyl acetate, n-butanol and water (**Figure S1**). The yields of several fractions were as follows: (1) Ethanol fraction: 12.2 (g/100 g); (2) Petroleum fraction: 4.4 (g/100 g); (3) Ethyl acetate fraction: 10 (g/100 g); (4) N-butanol fraction: 3.01 (g/100 g); and (5) Water fraction: 12.02 (g/100 g).

HPLC Analysis

HPLC analysis was performed with an HPLC equipment (Water 996 Photodiode Array Detector, Water 717 Plus AutoSampler, Water 600s Controller, Water 626 Pump, Millennium system). A C18 column (4.6 × 250 mm, 5 μm) was employed with the mobile phase of 0.2% phosphoric acid: acetonitrile (15:85) and a flow velocity at 1.0 mL/min at room temperature. Chromatograms were detected at 240 nm using a DAD detector. A standard solution of geniposide (2.1 mg) dissolved in 2 mL methanol was prepared and serially diluted to form different concentrations (0.5, 0.25, 0.125, and 0.0625 mg/mL). The sample solution was diluted 1:10 in methanol.

Isolation and Structure Elucidation of Major Compounds From EA-Fraction of GJE

Experimental Materials and Procedures

NMR spectra were scanned using a Bruker AV-500 spectrometer with TMS as the internal standard. HRESIMS data were determined using an Agilent 6210 ESI/TOF mass spectrometer. For column chromatography (CC), ODS (50 μm, YMC, Kyoto, Japan), silica gel (200–300 mesh, Qingdao Marine Chemical Plant, Qingdao, P. R. China), and Sephadex LH-20

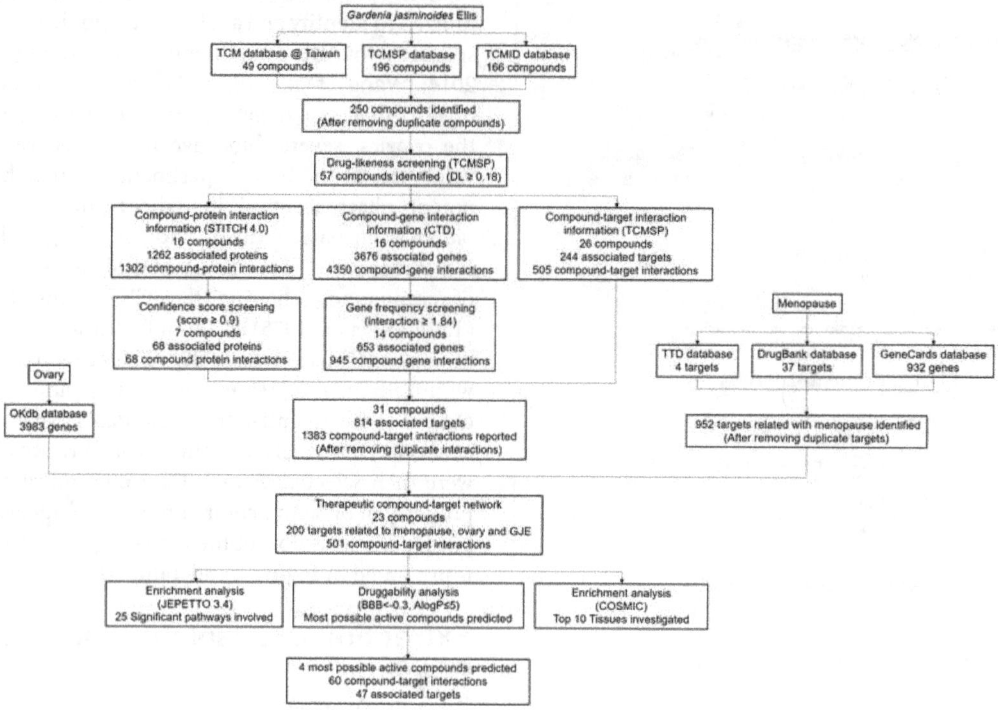

FIGURE 2 | The workflow of network pharmacology study of GJE.

(Pharmacia Biotech, Uppsala, Sweden) were used. Thin-layer chromatography (TLC) was carried out by using silica gel GF_{254} plates (Yantai Chemical Industry Research Institute, Yantai, China). Analytical HPLC was performed with A Waters system (e2695 Separations Module, 2998 Photodiode Array Detector) and a Cosmosil C_{18} analytical column (5 μm, 4.6 × 250 mm). An Agilent 1100 LC series with a diode array detector (DAD) using a preparative Cosmosil C18 column (20 × 250 mm, 5 μm) was applied for preparative HPLC. HPLC separations were performed using a COSMOSIL C_{18} preparative column (5 μm, 20 × 250 mm). All chemical reagents were purchased from Tianjin Damao Chemical Company (Tianjin, P. R. China).

Plant Material

The dried fruits of *Gardenia jasminoides* Ellis were collected in Guangdong Province of China in August 2015 and authenticated by Professor Guang-Xiong Zhou (Jinan University, Guangzhou, China). A voucher specimen (20150810) was deposited in the Institute of Traditional Chinese Medicine & Natural Products, Jinan University.

Extraction and Isolation

The air-dried fruits of GJE (1 kg) were crushed into powder and extracted three times with 80% ethanol at room temperature. The solvent was removed with a rotary evaporator under reduced pressure to get a residue, which was suspended in water and then partitioned by using petroleum ether, ethyl acetate and *n*-butanol, successively. The ethyl acetate extract (49 g) was chromatographed on a silica gel column which was eluted with chloroform/methanol (100:0–0:1, *v*/*v*) to yield six fractions (Fr. 1–6). Fr. 3 (7.1 g) was fractionated on Sephadex LH-20 (MeOH) and further purified by preparative HPLC (MeOH/H_2O, 50:50, *v*/*v*) to yield compounds **1** (35.7 mg), **2** (20.9 mg), **4** (18.6 mg) and **6** (20.2 mg). Fr. 5 (5.5 g) was subjected to chromatography on an ODS column using the methanol/water (40:60, to 100:0, *v*/*v*) solvent system to give five subfractions (Fr. 5.1–5.5). Fr. 5.2 (0.5 g) was purified by preparative HPLC (MeOH/H_2O, 35:65, *v*/*v*) to yield compounds **7** (12.3 mg), **8** (18.2 mg), and **9** (23.1 mg). Fr. 5.3 (1.1 g) was separated by preparative HPLC (MeOH/H_2O, 35:65, *v*/*v*) to yield compound **5** (9.8 mg). Compound **3** (19.0 mg) was obtained by chromatography of Fr. 1 (2.5 g) on Sephadex LH-20 (MeOH/$CHCl_3$, 1:1, *v*/*v*). The extracted compounds were dissolved in dimethyl sulfoxide (DMSO) and stored at −20°C for further study.

Primary Ovarian Granulosa Cell Culture and Estradiol Assay

Female Sprague Dawley rats (21–22 days old) purchased from the Laboratory Animal Unit, the University of Hong Kong, received 15 IU pregnant mare serum gonadotropin (PMSG) by intraperitoneal injection. After 48 h, the animals were sacrificed and the ovaries were excised. The experiment had been approved by the Committee on the Use of Live Animals in Teaching and Research (CULATR Ref. 2100-10, 3203-14) of Li Ka Shing Faculty of Medicine, the University of Hong Kong. Granulosa cells were obtained by using a 25G needle to puncture the ovarian granulosa layer and collected by centrifugation at 201 force-G for

5 min. The granulosa cells in serum-free DME/F12 1:1 medium (Thermo Scientific, USA) supplemented with 0.1% bovine serum albumin (Sigma-Aldrich, USA), 1% penicillin-streptomycin (Sigma-Aldrich, USA), and 1 μg/mL insulin (Sigma-Aldrich, USA) were seeded at a density of 2×10^4 cells/well in a 48-well plate and were incubated at 37°C in 5% CO_2 in an atmosphere for 2 h. Afterwards, the vehicle or different concentrations of GJE fractions (0.001%, 0.01%, 0.1%, 1%) or GJE components (10, 100 μM) were added to granulosa cells for 12 h. After that, the 17β-estradiol concentration in the cell culture medium was measured using an electro-chemiluminescence immunoassay (Elecsys, 2010, Roche Diagnostics, Basel, Switzerland) with a 17β-estradiol II kit (Roche Diagnostics, Switzerland) in a single batch. In order to explore whether GJE active components could bind to FSHR on FSHR-attenuated ovarian granulosa cells, ovarian granulosa cells were pretreated with FSHR (2 μg/mL, #sc13935; Santa Cruz, CA) for 0.5 h. After incubation with FSHR, granulosa cells were treated with GJE active compounds (100 μM) for 12 h (Wong et al., 2015).

Western Blot

Proteins were extracted from rat ovarian granulosa cells, washed with HBSS and then lysed with RIPA buffer (Sigma-Aldrich, USA) containing protease inhibitors (Roche, Germany) for 30 min. The Bradford assay was used to determine the protein concentration. Equal amounts of total protein (15 μg) were loaded, separated on SDS-PAGE, transferred to a nitrocellulose membrane, and then immunoblotted with the appropriate antibody: ERα (#04-820, Millipore), ERβ (#92731, Millipore), FSHR (#sc13935; Santa Cruz, CA) StAR (#sc25806, Santa Cruz, CA), aromatase (#14245, Santa Cruz, CA), β-actin (13E5, Cell Signaling Technology), GADPH (#sc48116, cell signaling). ECL detection kit (GE, health care) was used to visualize the protein and Quality One software (Bio-Rad) was applied to quantify the intensities.

Cell Viability Assay

The cytotoxic effects of the active compounds of GJE on the cell viability of estrogen-responsive MCF-7 breast cancer cells were determined by employing the 3-(4,5-dimethylthiazol-2-yl)-2,5-diphenyltetrazolium bromide (MTT) assay. MCF-7 cells were serum-starved at a density of 5,000 cells/well in 96-well culture plates for 12 h. MCF-7 cells were then treated with either vehicle or various concentrations of the active compounds of GJE and with or without co-treatment with 17β-estradiol (Sigma-Aldrich, USA) for 48 h. At the end of the incubation, 100 μL MTT solution (0.5 mg/mL) (Sigma-Aldrich, USA) was added to each well followed by incubation for an additional 4 h. Afterwards, the formazan crystals formed were dissolved in 100 μL DMSO. Absorbance of the content of each well was detected with a microplate reader (Bio-rad, USA) at 595 nm.

Molecular Docking Analysis

As an increasingly important tool for structural molecular biology, molecular docking can identify binding modes and predict binding affinity of molecules that fit together. In our study, molecular docking (semi-flexible) was performed using AutoDock Vina 1.1.2 software to investigate intermolecular interactions between the ligands and target proteins. The 3D structural information on FSHR and aromatase was retrieved from the Protein Data Bank (PDB; PDB id of FSHR: 4AY9; PDB id of aromatase: 3EQM). The structure visualization used for molecular docking was done with PyMol. The CIDs of rutin, CGA and GA were 5280805, 1794427 and 443354, respectively. The ligand binding energy with target protein was predicted by the free binding energy implemented in AutoDock Vina software.

Statistical Analysis

Statistical analysis was performed using the GraphPad Prism version 5.0. All data are shown as mean ± standard error of mean (SEM) from at least three independent experiments. The intensities of bands detected in Western blotting were normalized with the internal control β-actin. Differences in the mean values of two groups were tested with unpaired t-test. A p-value below 0.05 was regarded as statistically significant.

RESULTS

Bioactive Constituents in GJE Were Predicted by the Network Pharmacology

There were 196 phytochemicals reported in GJE by TCMSP database, 49 phytochemicals reported in GJE by TCM database @ Taiwan and 166 phytochemicals reported in GJE by TCMID database. After the removal of duplicates, totally 250 compounds were identified in GJE. Among the 250 compounds, there were 57 compounds with a DL value higher than 0.18. There were 16 compounds with 1,302 compound-protein interactions, and 68 compound-protein interactions with confidence score exceeding 0.9 were selected. In addition, there were 16 compounds explored to have 4,350 compound-gene interactions, and 653 genes with frequency exceeding 1.84 were chosen. Simultaneously, there were 26 compounds with 505 compound-target interactions reported from the TCMSP database. After the deletion of duplicate interactions, there were 31 compounds with totally 1,383 compound-target interactions declared. Afterwards, proteins that were potential therapeutic targets of menopause and the ovary were elucidated. There were 4 targets in menopause reported by TTD database, 37 targets in menopause reported by DrugBank database, and 932 genes in menopause reported by GeneCards database. Following the removal of duplicates, totally 952 targets were identified in menopause. Moreover, there were 3,983 genes in the ovary reported by Okdb database. Collectively, the integrated compound-target network was established (**Figure 4**), based on the association between molecules of GJE and targets shared by menopause and the ovary (**Figure 3A**). Collectively, there were 23 ingredients of GJE that can possess interactions of 200 targets shared by menopause and the ovary (**Table S1**). In JEPETTO, pathways with an XD-score higher than 0.36 were considered as significant pathways. With the enrichment analysis completed, there were 25 significant pathways (**Table S2**), especially including the steroid hormone biosynthesis pathway reported (**Figure 3C**), which indicated a strong association between GJE and steroidogenesis. As shown in **Figure 3B**, the ovary was the major tissue that bioactive

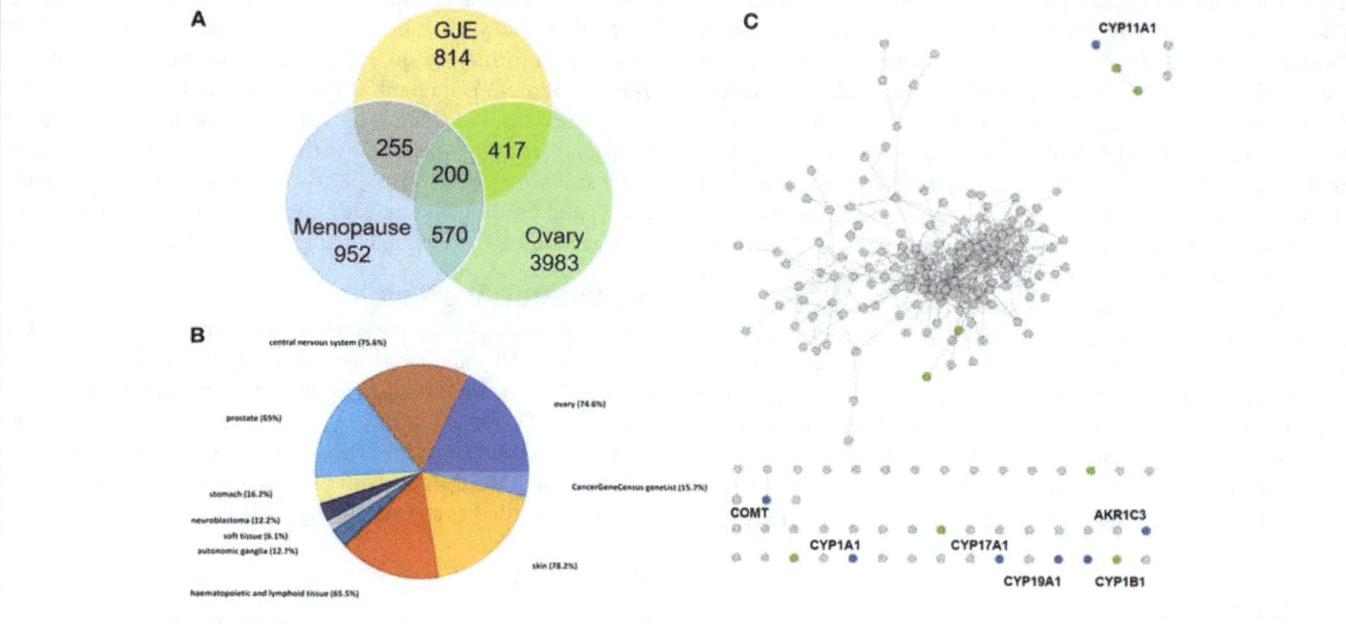

FIGURE 3 | Steroidogenesis under influence of GJE was predicted by network pharmacology. **(A)** The Venn diagram of targets from the ovaries, menopause and GJE regulated. **(B)** The pie chart of tissue specificity of bioactive compounds in GJE. **(C)** Chemical-protein interactions related to steroid hormone biosynthesis pathways. "gray dots" represent genes in the target set, "green dots" represent genes associated with steroid biosynthesis pathway, "blue dots" represent the overlap between the related pathway and the input protein set.

compounds of GJE would target on, indicating tissue specificity of the GJE components. Druggability assay was conducted to evaluate several bioactive compounds with regard to BBB, AlogP, and DL value. Firstly, the potential candidate is described as an ingredient with BBB < -0.3 and AlogP ≤ 5 (Ru et al., 2014; Kotapalli et al., 2015). **Table 1** ranks in the order of DL, and the top five compounds with relative high DL values are considered to be more effective candidates with a relatively more desirable drug-like property for regulating the disorder. Among these five ingredients, possible estrogenic effects have been declaimed in chlorogenic acid (CGA), geniposide, and geniposidic acid (GA) (An et al., 2016). Additionally, like 17β-estradiol, rutin can slow down the rate of bone resorption (Horcajada-Molteni et al., 2000; Rassi et al., 2005). However, there are no reports on estrogen-related activities in hirsutrin. Therefore, hirsutrin was excluded and the remaining four compounds (rutin, geniposide, CGA, and GA) were chosen as potential therapeutic agents of menopause for further investigation.

HPLC-DAD System

The Calibration Curves and Linearity

As shown in **Figure 5** and **Figure S2**, the regression equation of standard constituents is Area = 85.36C-164.88. The standard constituents showed a good linearity ($R^2 = 0.999643$) with the linear range being 62.5~1,000 μg/mL.

Precision

For the precision test, 10 μL sample solution was injected into the HPLC system 3 times. The chromatogram was recorded and the peak area of geniposide was measured. The relative standard deviations (RSD) value was found to be 3.02% (**Table S3**).

Stability, Recovery, and Content of Geniposide Measurement

For the stability test, 10 μL sample solution was injected into the HPLC system at 0, 1, and 4 h. The chromatogram was recorded and the peak area of geniposide was measured. As shown in **Table S4**, the RSD of peak area of sample solution was 3.25% ($n = 3$), which indicates that the contents of analytes were stable within 4 h. Then the sample solution at various concentrations was added, and the range of average recovery was between 96.2 and 101% (**Table S5**). For the measurement of geniposide content, 10 μL sample solution was injected into the HPLC system 3 times. The chromatogram was recorded (**Table 2**, **Figure 6**, and **Figure S3**).

Identification of Bioactive Fraction in GJE

To identify the bioactive fraction of GJE that can stimulate estradiol, the estradiol levels in cell culture medium of rat granulosa cells treated with various GJE fractions were measured. Among the various GJE fractions, the estrogen level of ethyl acetate fraction (1%) group was the highest (**Figure 7**), which indicated that the ethyl acetate fraction of GJE (GJE-EA) significantly stimulated estrogen synthesis *in vitro*. The effect of GJE-EA on CYP19 and FSHR expression *in vitro* was then examined by Western blot assays. Rat granulosa cells were treated with either vehicle or different GJE fractions for 12 h. The GJE-EA (1%) significantly increased the expression levels of CYP19 and FSHR compared with the vehicle control group (**Figure S4**),

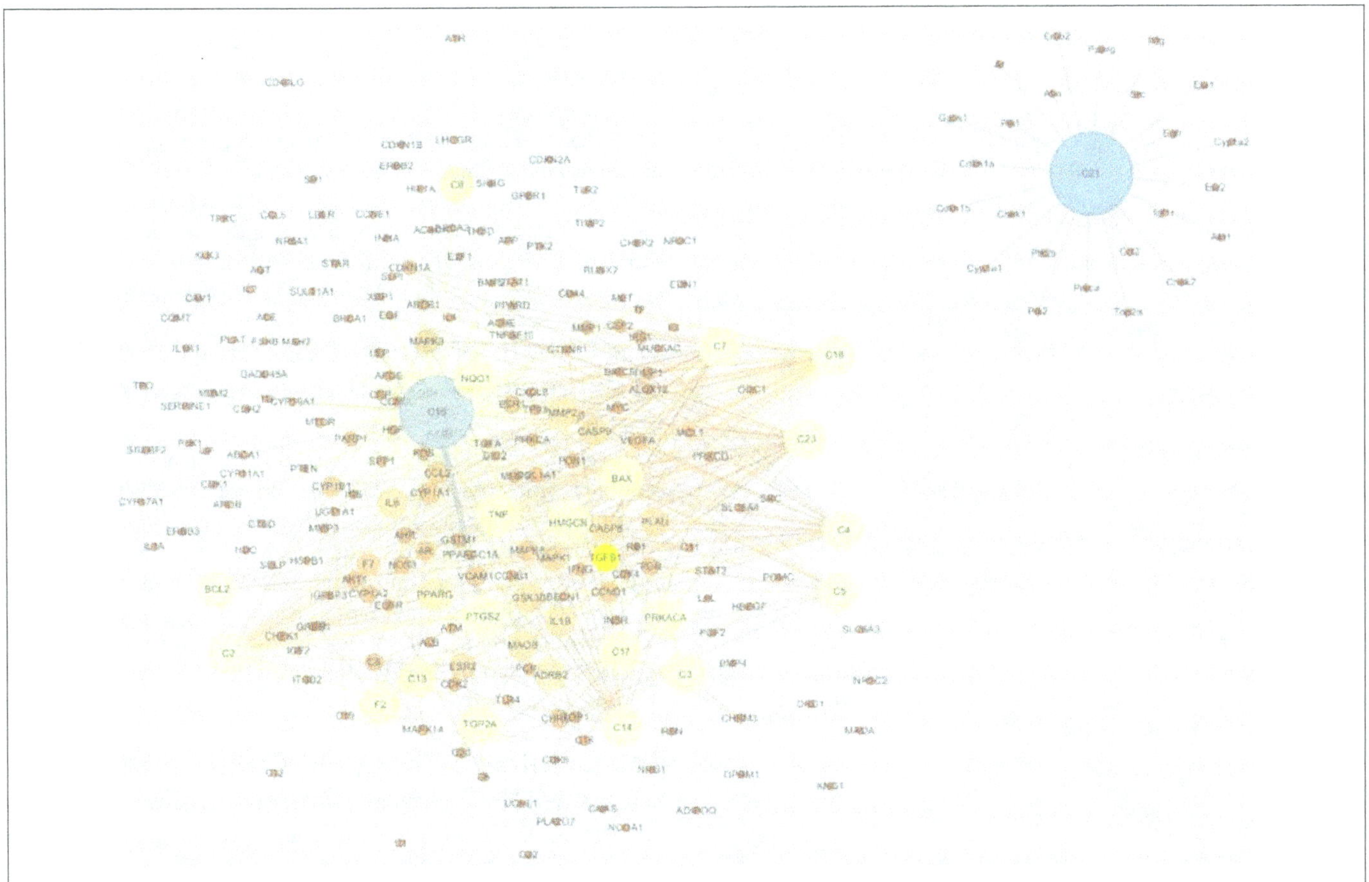

FIGURE 4 | Therapeutic compound-target network of menopause and GJE. The size of nodes and edges is proportional to its value. The color brightness of the nodes is inversely related with its value. In other words, the value of the node is the highest when the color is blue, and the value of the node is the lowest when the color is red.

which suggested that the ethyl acetate fraction of GJE afforded stimulation of estradiol biosynthesis probably by up-regulation of the FSHR-aromatase pathway.

Identification of the Major Components of GJE-EA Fraction

Nine compounds (1–9) (**Figure 8**) were isolated from the GJE-EA fraction. Their structures were identified as geniposide (Tsai et al., 2002), (1) rutin (2) (Su et al., 2014), ursolic acid (3) (Pieroni et al., 2011), liquiritoside (4) (Liu et al., 2005), CGA (5) (Peng et al., 2000), GA (6) (El Bitar et al., 2004), 3,5-O-dicaffeoylquinic acid (7) (Peng et al., 2000), 3,5-O-dicaffeoylquinic acid methyl ester (8) (Peng et al., 2000), and 3,4-O-dicaffeoylquinic acid (9) (Chen et al., 2014) by comparison of their spectral data with those reported in the literature.

Determination of Bioactive Components in GJE With Estradiol Biosynthesis Stimulating Effect

The 9 compounds from GJE-EA were identified with 4 of them predicted using network pharmacology. To identify the active compounds from the 9 compounds with estradiol-stimulating ability, the estradiol levels in ovarian granulosa cells were determined. After 12 h of treatment with the compounds isolated from GJE-EA, production of estradiol in rat ovarian granulosa cells was determined. As shown in **Figure 9**, rutin, CGA, GA, and 3,5-O-dicaffeoylquinic acid also enhanced steroidogenesis *in vitro*. However, the estrogen stimulating effect of 3,5-O-dicaffeoylquinic acid was not predicted by network pharmacology. Thus, rutin, CGA, and GA probably contributed to the stimulatory effect of GJE on estradiol biosynthesis in rat ovarian granulosa cells.

Molecular Docking of Rutin, CGA, and GA With FSHR and Aromatase

Estrogen can be produced by the target of classical FSHR-aromatase pathway (Simpson et al., 1994; Hunzicker-Dunn and Maizels, 2006; Luo and Wiltbank, 2006).To determine whether rutin, CGA, and GA could activate FSHR and aromatase, molecular docking studies were performed to predict the binding energies between 3D structure of ligands and FSHR; ligand and aromatase, respectively.

TABLE 1 | Twenty-three compounds derived from GJE that can target genes associated with both menopause and the ovary.

Rank	Ingredient name	DL	BBB	BBB
C1	Hirsutrin	0.77	−2.31	−0.59
C2	Rutin	0.68	−2.75	−1.45
C3	Geniposide	0.44	−2.61	−2.25
C4	Genioisidic acid	0.41	−2.63	−2.5
C5	Chlorogenic acid	0.33	−1.71	−0.42
C6	Quercetin	0.28	−0.77	1.5
C7	3-Methylkempferol	0.26	−0.49	1.84
C8	Crocetin	0.26	−0.83	4.58
C9	Kaempferol	0.24	−0.55	1.77
C10	Genistein	0.21	−0.4	2.07
C11	Oleanolic acid	0.76	0.07	6.42
C12	Stigmasterol	0.76	1	7.64
C13	Ursolic acid	0.75	0.07	6.47
C14	Beta-sitosterol	0.75	0.99	8.08
C15	Syringaresinol	0.72	−0.03	2.1
C16	Sudan III	0.59	0.1	7.21
C17	Lutein	0.55	−0.99	9.47
C18	Artemisetin	0.48	−0.09	2.31
C19	5-hydroxy-7-methoxy-2-(3,4,5-trimethoxyphenyl)chromone	0.41	−0.21	2.8
C20	Isoimperatorin	0.23	0.66	3.65
C21	Ammidin	0.22	0.92	3.65
C22	Mandenol	0.19	1.14	6.99
C23	Chrysin	0.18	0.01	2.6

Compounds are listed in the order of DL. C1 to C10 which satisfied the conditions of BBB < -0.3 and AlogP < 5.

The estimated free energy of binding with FSHR for rutin was −8.7 kcal/mol, for CGA was −7.8 kcal/mol, for GA was −7.1 kcal/mol (**Figure 10A**); aromatase for rutin was −0.8 kcal/mol, for CGA was −8.5 kcal/mol and for GA was −7.3 kcal/mol (**Figure 10A**), which revealed that all compounds can bind with FSHR and aromatase. The results of in silico docking analysis revealed the optimal binding conformation of the FSHR-rutin complexes (**Figure 10B**), FSHR-CGA complexes (**Figure 10C**), FSHR-GA complexes (**Figure 10D**), respectively; aromatase-rutin complexes (**Figure 10E**), aromatase-CGA complexes (**Figure 10F**) and aromatase-GA complexes, respectively (**Figure 10G**).

Effects of Rutin, CGA, and GA on FSHR-Attenuated Ovarian Granulosa Cells and StAR-FSHR-aromatase Pathway

To investigate the mechanism of action of the estrogen-stimulating effect of rutin, CGA, and GA, Western blotting assay was performed to detect the changes in expression level of steroidogenic acute regulatory protein (StAR), CYP19 and FSHR in ovarian granulosa cells treated with either vehicle or different concentrations of rutin, CGA, and GA, respectively. To clarify whether the estradiol-stimulating effects of rutin, CGA, and GA are mediated by FSHR in ovarian granulosa cells, the FSHR antibody was used. In the FSHR-attenuated ovarian granulosa cell model, the estrogen-stimulating effects of rutin, CGA, and GA were abolished, indicating the involvement of FSHR in the effects of ruin, CGA, and GA on estradiol biosynthesis (**Figure 11B**). StAR mediates the progressive uptake of cholesterol, which works as a raw material for estrogen synthesis (Papadopoulos and Miller, 2012). Western blot results showed that rutin and CGA significantly up-regulated FSHR expression (**Figure 11A**); all ligands markedly increased the expression levels of both StAR and CYP19 (**Figures 11C,D**).

The Effects of Rutin, CGA, and GA on Level of Expression of Estrogen Receptors α and β

To investigate the role of ER status on the estrogen-stimulating action of rutin, CGA, and GA, western blot analysis was used to confirm the expression of estrogen receptor α (ERα) and estrogen receptor β (ERβ). Rutin had no discernible effect on ERα expression level but significantly increased the protein expression levels of ERβ in granulosa cells after 12 h of treatment; CGA significantly activated ERβ expression and inhibited ERα expression; while GA markedly suppressed the expression of ERα (**Figures 12A,B**).

The Cytotoxic Effects of Rutin, CGA, and GA on MCF-7 Breast Cancer Cells

The effects of GJE bioactive compounds (rutin, CGA, and GA) on cell proliferation of MCF-7 breast cancer cells, whose growth is positively associated with estrogen level, were investigated with MTT assay. The cell viability curves indicated that the viability of MCF-7 breast cancer cells decreased, both in the presence and in the absence of 1×10^{-7}M 17β-estradiol after treatment for 48 h with rutin, CGA, and GA, respectively (**Figure 13**).

DISCUSSION

As a hallmark of menopause, estrogen depletion can be effectively regulated by targeting 17β-estradiol level via estrogen biosynthesis (Pollow et al., 2015). GJE was traditionally adopted to improve women's health in Asia (Yang et al., 2016). Recent evidence also suggests that GJE or its active constituents have diverse functions such as anti-depressant (Cai et al., 2015; Zhang et al., 2015; Ren et al., 2016; Wang et al., 2016), anti-cancer, anti-oxidant, and neuroprotective activities (Phatak, 2015). However, whether or not GJE can relieve estrogen depletion, the identities of its active compounds as well as its mechanism of action remain poorly understood. Here, network pharmacology was conducted to elucidate the association between GJE and steroid biosynthesis pathway and predict the most likely active ingredients in GJE (**Figure 2**, **Table 1**). Then the HPLC-DAD system was used to isolate several fractions from GJE (**Figure S1**). The active fraction of GJE and its major compounds were also investigated. With the combination of the major compounds from the active fraction and possible active ingredients from network pharmacology, phenotypic (estrogen-stimulating effect) and target-based (aromatase/FSHR/StAR/ERα/ERβ) methods

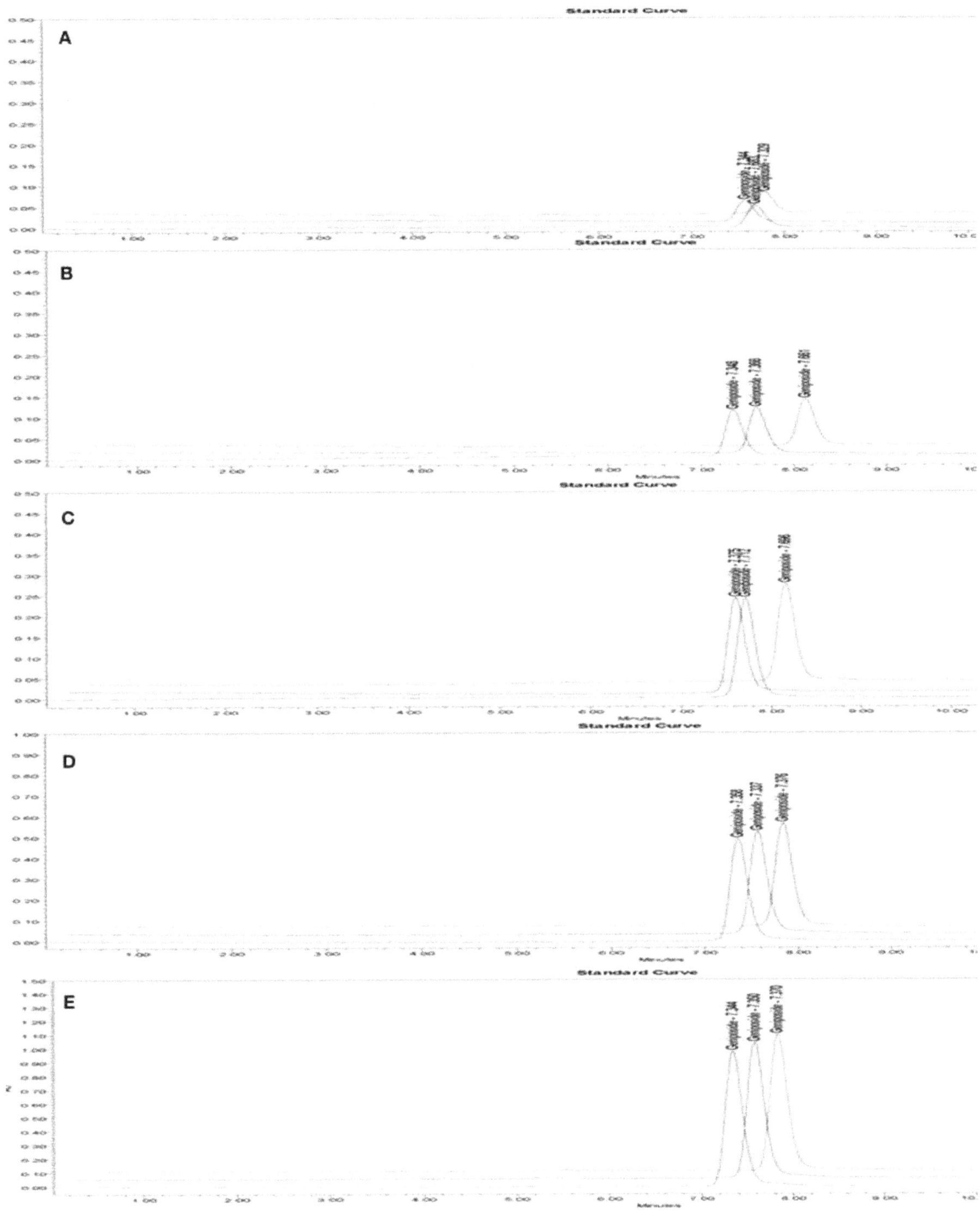

FIGURE 5 | HPLC chromatogram of geniposide in standard solution with different geniposide concentrations. Time (min) as unit of Y-axis and chromatographic profiles are reported at 240 nm. The concentration of standard solution was 0.0625 mg/mL **(A)**, 0.125 mg/mL **(B)**, 0.25 mg/mL **(C)**, 0.5 mg/mL **(D)**, 1 mg/mL **(E)**.

were used to find the active components of GJE (Lu et al., 2016). Phenotypic approaches play a crucial role in drug discovery because data from the large-scale drug screening and target-based approaches suggest the relationships between a potential new drug and its molecular targets (Gilbert, 2013; Swamidass et al., 2014). Finally, the bioactive compounds of GJE that could stimulate the biosynthesis of ovarian estradiol was reported (**Figure 1**).

Network pharmacology works as a proximal tool for the investigation of ingredients in Traditional Chinese Medicine (TCM) nowadays (Hopkins, 2008; Huang et al., 2013; Wang et al., 2013; Zhang et al., 2013). In the current study, TCM network

TABLE 2 | The concentrations of geniposide in different fractions derived from GJE.

	Concentration of geniposide (μg/mL)	Average (μg/mL)
Petroleum fraction	83.256 89.184 87.020	86.486
Ethyl acetate fraction	407.739 425.260 402.376	411.792
N-butanol fraction	473.618 489.030 483.501	482.050
Water fraction	46.203 45.061 45.574	45.613
Ethanol fraction	298.965 312.941 317.288	309.732

pharmacology approaches were used to establish the therapeutic compound-target interaction network (Shao and Zhang, 2013). It was shown that the combination of GJE and other herbal medicine can attenuate menopausal symptoms (Chen et al., 2003). In accordance with previous studies, there were 200 targets shared by menopause, the ovary and 23 compounds of GJE, which signifies a therapeutic role of GJE for treating postmenopausal syndrome (**Table 1, Table S1**, and **Figures 3A, 4**). Moreover, steroid hormone biosynthetic pathway was the pathway most significantly related to GJE (**Table S2, Figure 3B**). The pathway was used to present the effects of GJE on estrogen production. The tissue specificity assay has confirmed that the ovary worked as the main organ targeted by GJE compounds (**Figure 3C**). Importantly, four possible bioactive compounds of GJE, including rutin, geniposide, GA, and CGA were identified with the druggability assay.

There were five fractions of GJE isolated by the HPLC-DAD system. Our results showed that the RSD value was smaller than 5% and the recovery value was not less than 95%, which demonstrated that the conditions used in the quantitative analysis met the standard (**Tables S3–S5**). Additionally, the HPLC chromatograms of geniposide from the different extracts of GJE showed that the concentration of geniposide in the N-butanol fraction was the highest, followed successively by the ethyl acetate fraction, ethanol fraction, petroleum fraction and water fraction (**Table 2, Figures 5, 6**, and **Figure S3**). Among the five fractions of GJE, GJE-EA was identified to be the fraction that most significantly increased estradiol production in ovarian granulosa cells (**Figure 7**). Aromatase, encoded by gene CYP19, catalyzes the process of estrogen biosynthesis in ovarian granulosa cells (Luo and Wiltbank, 2006). When women experience menopause, the activity of aromatase decreases abruptly (Sze et al., 2009). It was demonstrated that CYP19 can be activated by upregulation of follicle-stimulating hormone receptor (FSHR) (Simpson et al., 1994). Importantly, it has been reported that the activation of FSHR can mediate estrogen production in ovarian granulosa cells (Hunzicker-Dunn and Maizels, 2006). Therefore, estrogen production can be promoted by activation of the FSHR-aromatase pathway. The results of Western blot showed that the protein levels of both FSHR and aromatase were increased significantly in ovarian granulosa cells treated with 0.1% GJE-EA (**Figure S4**).

Nine major compounds from GJE-EA were then isolated (**Figure 8**) and four of the nine compounds were predicted by network pharmacology. The phenotypic approach was then utilized to screen the steroidogenic ability of the probable active compounds. It was found that rutin, CGA, and GA displayed estrogen-stimulating activities (**Figure 9**). Importantly, treatment with GJE-derived compounds resulted in higher estrogen levels in ovarian granulosa cells than that induced by the three bioactive compounds alone and that the combination treatment may, at least partly, explain the principle of estrogen stimulating effect of GJE extract alone. Numerous *in vivo* and *in vitro* studies suggest that rutin, CGA, and GA possess multiple biological functions and various pharmacological activities, such as anti-cancer, anti-osteoporotic and neuroprotective properties. For the suppression of breast cancer, rutin reduced proliferation and induced apoptosis in MCF-7 breast cancer cells (Kamaludin et al., 2013; Kamaludin, 2015). CGA reduced viability of estrogen-independent DA-MB-435 breast cancer cells but not normal MCF-10A cells (Noratto et al., 2009). Although there is little information about the anti-cancer activity of GA, GA had a potential inhibitory effect on tumor growth (Hsu et al., 1997). For the inhibition of bone loss, rutin inhibited osteopenia through suppressing bone resorption and enhancing osteoblastic activity in ovariectomized (Ovx) rats (Horcajada-Molteni et al., 2000); CGA prevented the decrease of mineralization and promoted the increase the mechanical properties and thus inhibited bone loss in Ovx animals (Folwarczna et al., 2015; Zhou et al., 2016); GA promoted osteogenesis by increasing the proliferation of osteoblasts and inhibited osteolysis by decreasing the proliferation of osteoclasts (Ha et al., 2003). For the promotion of neuron regeneration, rutin was reported to prevent spatial and emotional memory impairment (Qu et al., 2014; Ramalingayya et al., 2016); CGA supplementation could interfere in neurological degeneration (Heitman and Ingram, 2017); Though less evidence indicates a direct connection of GA with cognitive improving activities, GA is the main component of Tong Luo Jiu Nao, which was shown to prevent neuronal damage and improve learning and memory (Liu et al., 2011, 2013). It is accepted that long-term use of HT can elevate the risk of breast cancer in menopausal women (Colditz, 1998). In addition, osteoporosis and cognitive decline are the major menopausal symptoms caused by estrogen deprivation in postmenopausal women (Lufkin et al., 1992; Prelevic and Jacobs, 1997; Miller et al., 2013; Lobo et al., 2014). Therefore, the abovementioned evidence may contribute to the therapeutic role and safety of rutin, CGA, and GA in the management of postmenopausal syndrome.

In this study, in order to gain an insight into the likely molecular basis of the estrogen stimulating effect of rutin, CGA,

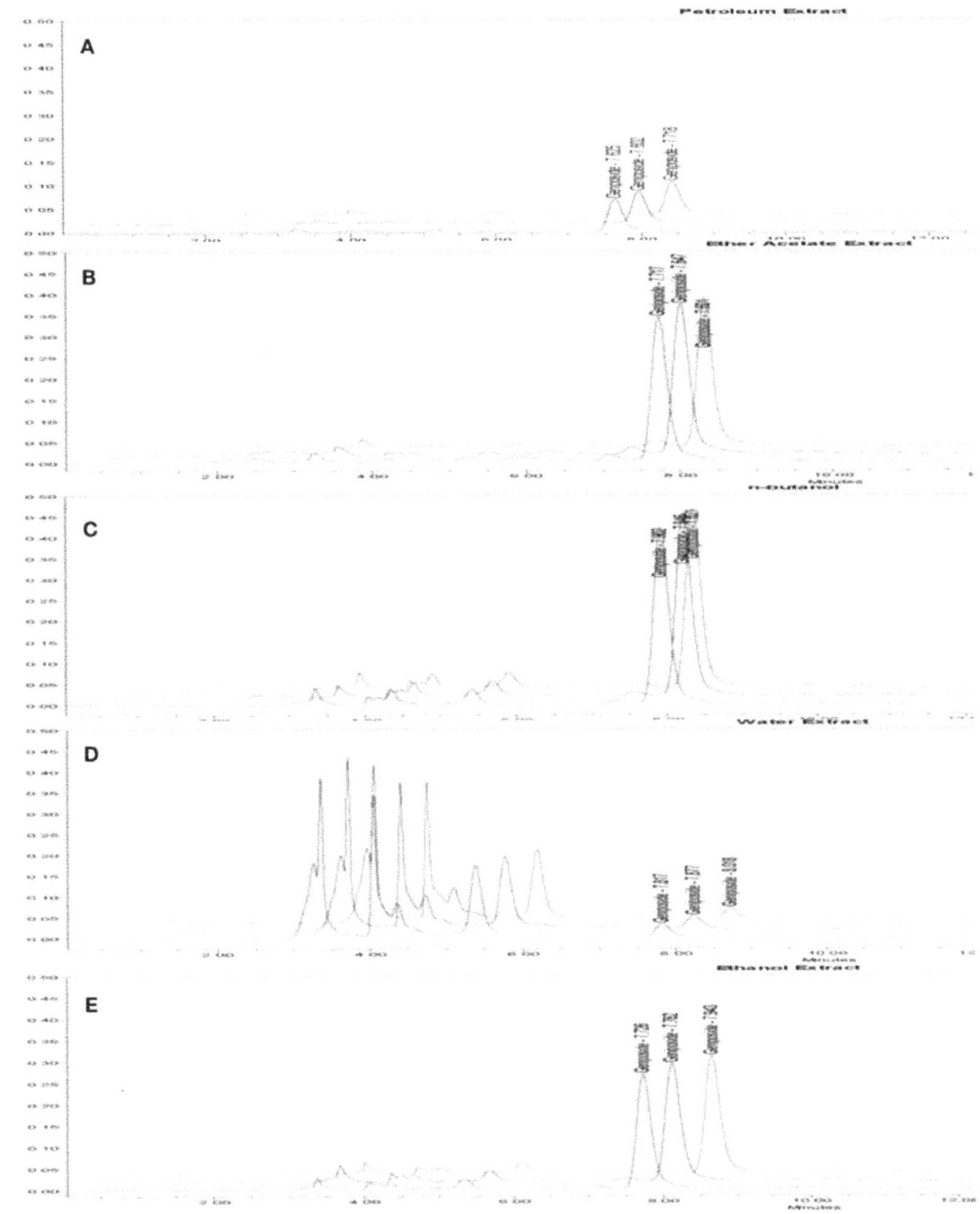

FIGURE 6 | HPLC chromatogram of geniposide from different fractions derived from GJE. Time (min) as unit of Y-axis and chromatographic profiles are reported at 240 nm. The contents of geniposide are shown in petroleum fraction **(A)**, Ethyl acetate fraction **(B)**, N-butanol fraction **(C)**, Water fraction **(D)**, Ethanol fraction **(E)**.

and GA, molecular docking analysis was used to predict the binding mode of rutin, CGA, and GA with FSHR and aromatase, respectively (**Figure 10**). Western blotting assay was used to validate the effects of rutin, CGA, and GA at the protein expression levels of FSHR and CYP19 *in vitro*. Results showed that rutin and CGA were able to increase the expression of FSHR and all compounds were able to increase the expression level of CYP19 in ovarian granulosa cells (**Figures 11A,C**). Then the FSHR involvement in the estrogen-stimulating effects of rutin, CGA, and GA was also detected. It was found that the estrogen-stimulating effects brought about by rutin, CGA, and GA were attenuated when the FSHR on ovarian granulosa cells were blocked by antibodies (**Figure 11B**). Apart from FSHR and aromatase, steroidogenic acute regulatory protein (StAR) also plays an essential role in estradiol biosynthesis, due to the fact that StAR can regulate the uptake of cholesterol into the mitochondria of theca cells, which is the raw material for estradiol biosynthesis (Papadopoulos and Miller, 2012). In this study, the expression level of StAR in ovarian granulosa cells was further tested. All three compounds were found to

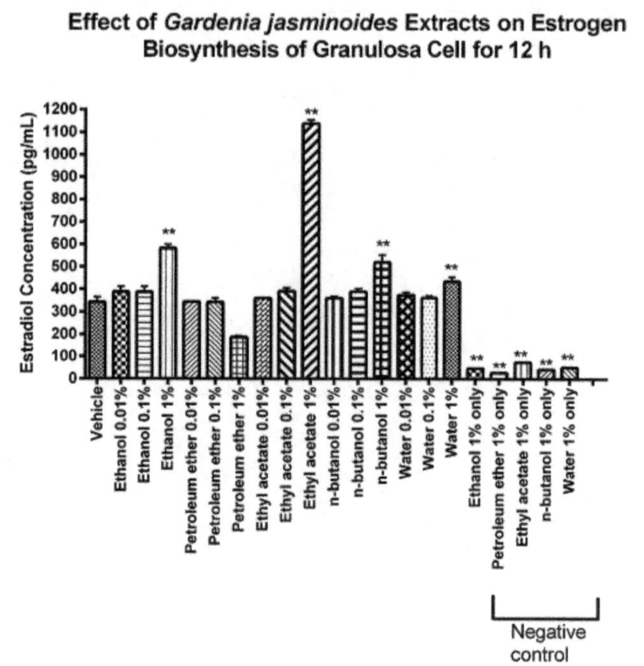

FIGURE 7 | Identification of the GJE- derived bioactive fraction with estrogen stimulating effect using phenotypic screening. Effects of GJE fractions on production of estrogen in granulosa cells after 12 h of treatment were determined by estradiol assay. Each value represents mean ± SEM ($n = 3$), $^{**}p < 0.01$, One-way ANOVA Dunnett's Multiple Comparison Task.

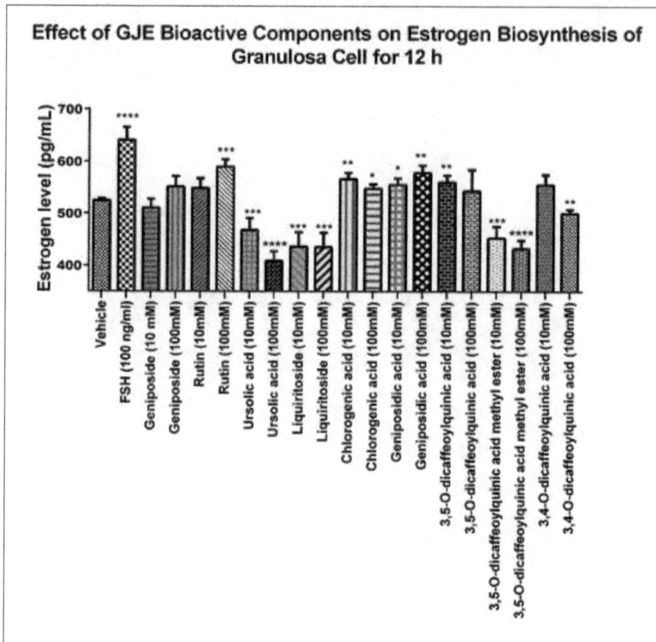

FIGURE 9 | Identification of the GJE-EA derived bioactive components with estrogen stimulating effect using phenotypic screening. Effects of GJE components on production of estrogen in granulosa cells after treatment for 12 h was determined by estradiol assay. Each value represents mean ± SEM ($n = 5$) $^{*}p < 0.05$, $^{**}p < 0.01$, $^{***}p < 0.001$, $^{****}p < 0.0001$ vs. vehicle control group.

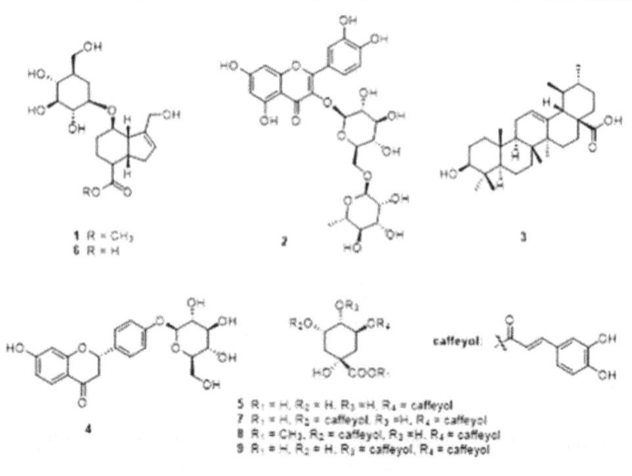

FIGURE 8 | Major compounds 1–9 identified in GJE-EA fraction. The GJE-EA fraction was chromatographed on silica gel column; the fractions were fractionated on Sephadex LH-20; and the compounds were purified by preparative HPLC. (1) geniposide; (2) rutin; (3) ursolic acid; (4) liquiritoside; (5) CGA; (6) GA; (7) 3,5-O-dicaffeoylquinic acid; (8) 3,5-O-dicaffeoylquinic acid methyl ester; and (9) 3,4-O-dicaffeoylquinic acid.

be able to increase StAR levels in ovarian granulosa cells (**Figure 11D**).

Low toxicity and little side effect are the great advantages of GJE (Liu et al., 2013; Chen et al., 2015; Im et al., 2016). The only hepatotoxic and genetoxic properties of GJE reported are due to genipin (Liu et al., 2013), which is excluded by network pharmacology. Importantly, while HT is a conventional approach for relieving postmenopausal syndrome, the long-term use of estrogen in HT imparts an increased risk of breast cancer (Colditz, 1998), and estrogen can be mediated by estrogen receptor alpha (ERα) and estrogen receptor beta (ERβ) (Deroo and Korach, 2006; Jia et al., 2015). However, estrogen interacts with ERα and ERβ downstream pathways in dissimilar ways (Nilsson et al., 2001). ERβ regulates the FSH-aromatase pathway and enhances ovarian steroidogenesis (Deroo et al., 2009; Wang et al., 2017). It has been shown that selective activation of ERβ transcriptional pathways may not promote breast cancer (Paruthiyil et al., 2004). Additionally, ERβ was found to inhibit the proliferation of breast cancer cell line T47D (Ström et al., 2004). However, ERα has a close and positive relationship with breast cancer. ERα gene amplification is frequent in proliferative breast disease, especially breast cancer (Holst et al., 2007). Besides, the presence of high ERα levels in benign breast epithelium may explain the elevated possibility of breast cancer development, which indicates that ERα is crucial in breast cancer cell progression (Ali and Coombes, 2000). In this study, it was found that ERβ was upregulated following treatment with rutin and CGA (**Figure 12B**); and ERα was downregulated after treatment of CGA and GA in granulosa cells (**Figure 12A**). The effect on the ERs could be directly induced by the bioactive compounds in GJE or indirectly as a result of GJE and bioactive compounds increasing estrogen

A

Compound	Rutin	CGA	GA
Binding energy with FSHR (Kcal/mol)	-8.7	-7.8	-7.1
Binding energy with Aromatase (Kcal/mol)	-0.8	-8.5	-7.3

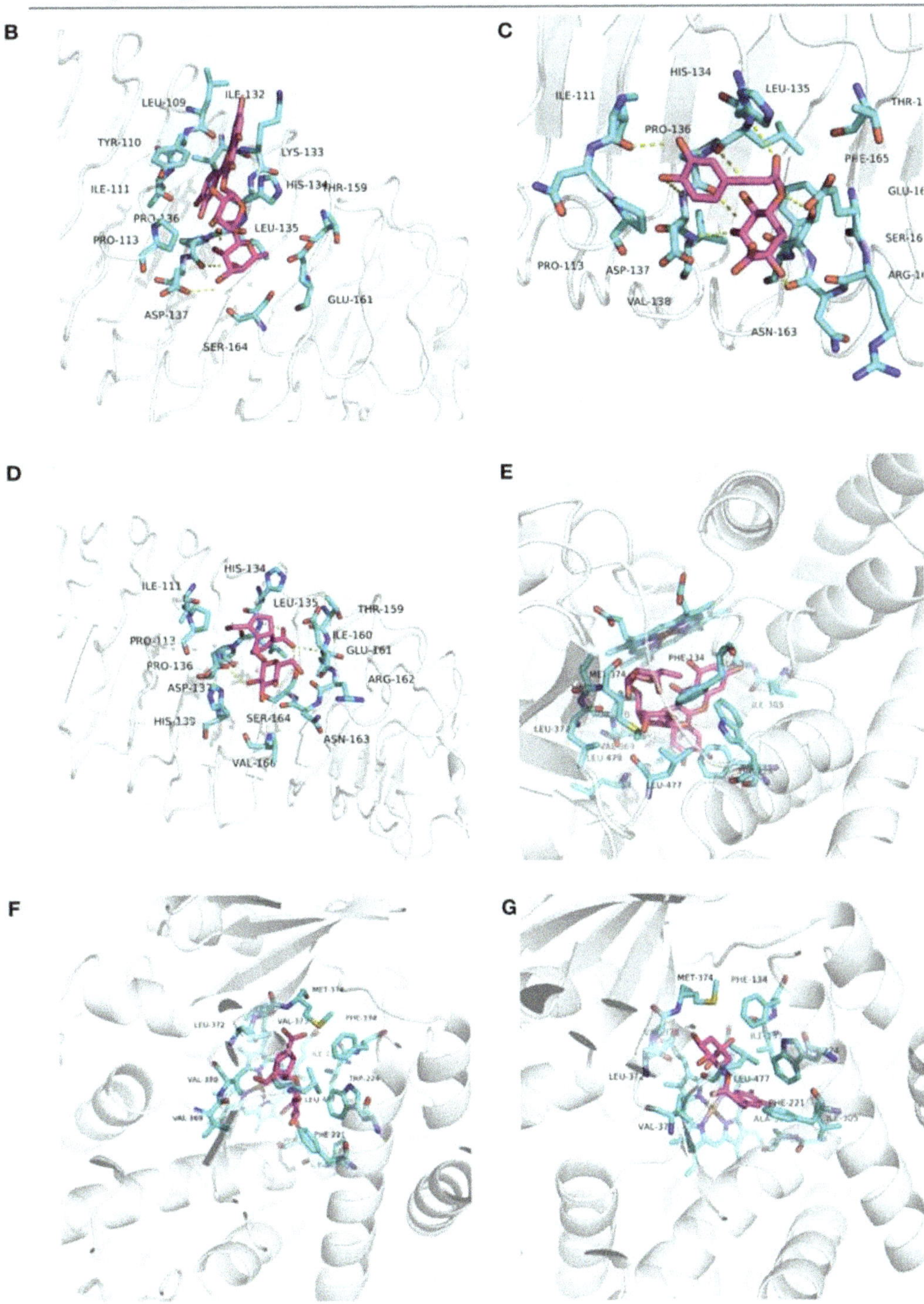

FIGURE 10 | Modes of binding of rutin, CGA and GA with FSHR and aromatase. **(A)** The binding energy of each complex. **(B–D)** The optimal binding conformations of the FSHR-rutin complexes, FSHR-CGA complexes and FSHR-GA complexes. **(E–G)** The optimal binding conformations of the aromatase-rutin complexes, aromatase-CGA complexes and aromatase-GA complexes.

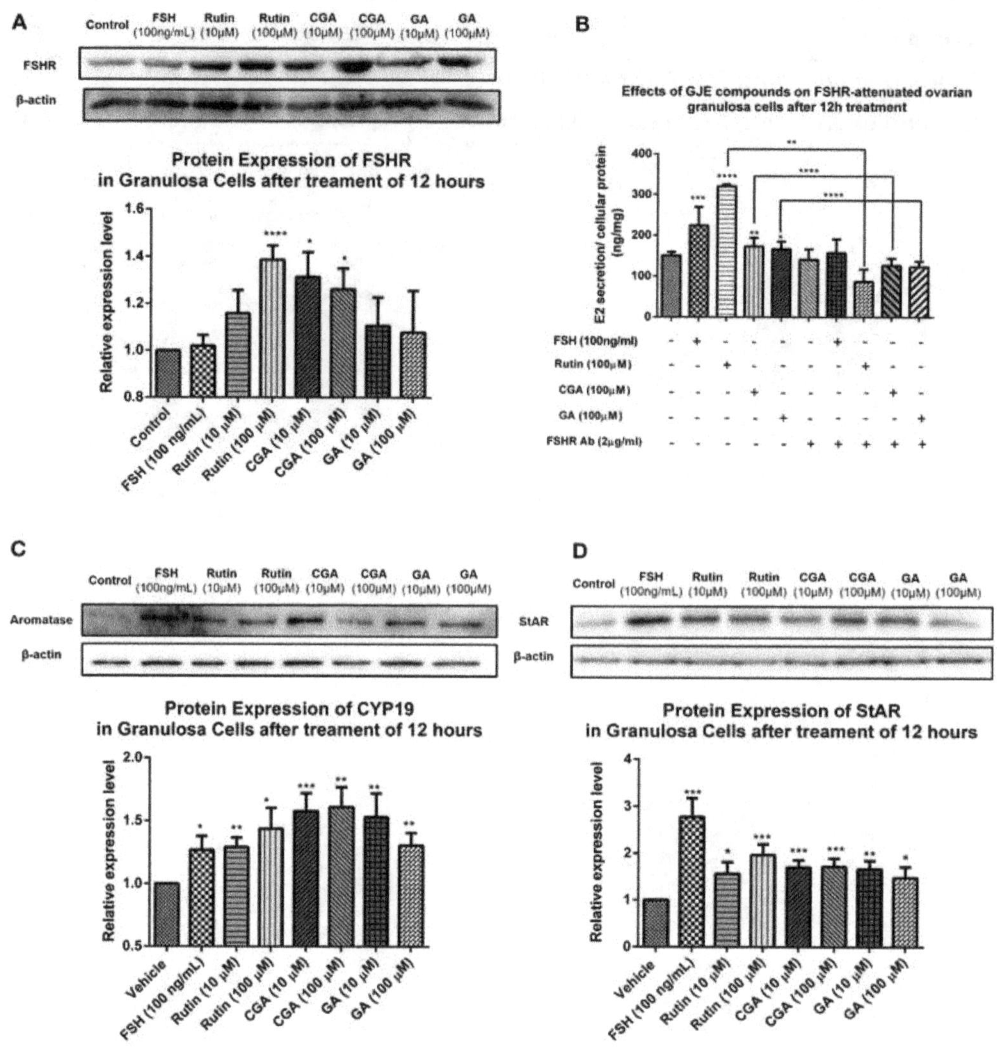

FIGURE 11 | Effects of rutin, CGA, and GA on levels of FSHR, aromatase and StAR in ovarian granulosa cells after 12 h of treatment. **(A,C,D)** Effects of rutin, CGA, and GA on FSHR, aromatase and StAR expression in ovarian granulosa cells. Ovarian granulosa cells of SD rats were treated with various concentrations of rutin, CGA, and GA respectively for 12 h, respectively, and then total cell lysates were extracted for Western blot analysis by using antibodies specific to FSHR, aromatase and StAR. The representative image and the relative expression levels of FSHR, aromatase and StAR are shown. **(B)** Estrogen stimulating effect of rutin, CGA, and GA on ovarian granulosa cells with antibody-blocked FSHR diminished. The data were normalized with the internal control β-actin, each value is the mean ± SEM ($n = 4$), with $^{*}p < 0.05$, $^{**}p < 0.01$, $^{***}p < 0.001$, $^{****}p < 0.0001$ vs. vehicle control group.

levels in ovarian granulosa cells. Furthermore, risk evaluation of active compounds in GJE was performed by investigating the effects of rutin, CGA, and GA on the viability of MCF-7 human breast cancer cell line in the presence or absence of 1×10^{-7} M 17β-estradiol. It was disclosed that 17β-estradiol treatment significantly promoted the proliferation of MCF-7 cells. However, the proliferative response to 17β-estradiol was counteracted by treatment with rutin, CGA, and GA. The anti-human breast cancer activities of rutin, CGA, and GA suggest the safety and potential of GJE as an effective herbal medicine with estrogen-stimulating effects (**Figure 13**). To our knowledge, there is no evidence that reveals the acute or chronic toxicity of rutin, CGA, and GA yet. However, further experiments should be conducted in the future to examine the possibility of GJE and its bioactive compounds on the development of breast cancer *in vivo*, based on the fact that aromatase inhibitors are extensively used by post-menopausal women with estrogen-dependent breast cancer (Brueggemeier et al., 2005).

Different from the traditional approach for TCM study, network pharmacology was exploited to confirm the therapeutic role of GJE in the management of postmenopausal syndrome by constructing the compound-target network in this article. In addition, the possible active compounds were also predicted by network pharmacology in this article. The estrogen screening assay was conducted after the combination of the results from network pharmacology and traditional approach of

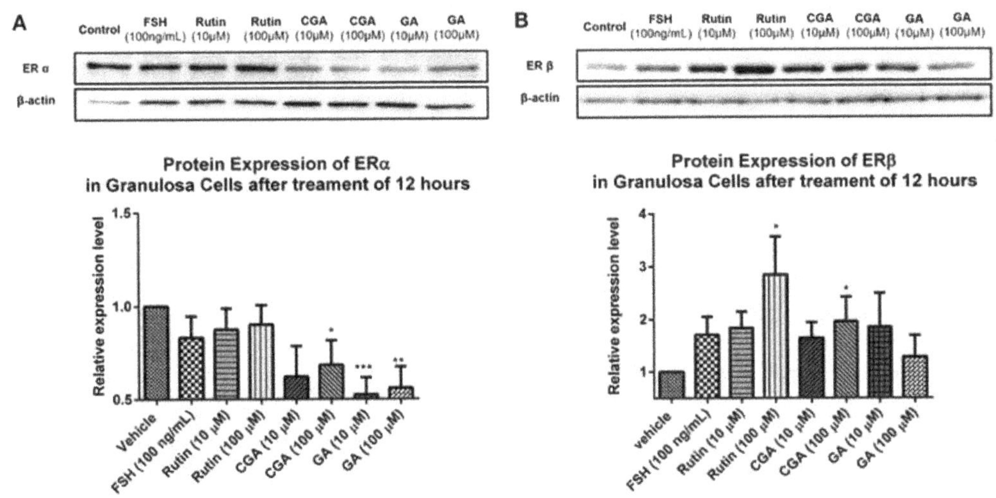

FIGURE 12 | Effects of rutin, CGA, and GA on estrogen receptor expression in ovarian granulosa cells after treatment for 12 h. Ovarian granulosa cells of SD rats were treated with various concentrations of rutin, CGA, and GA for 12 h, respectively, and then total cell lysates were extracted for Western blot analysis by using antibodies specific to ERα and ERβ. The representative image and the relative expression levels analyzed of **(A)** ERα and **(B)** ERβ are shown. The loading control of ERβ is reused from that of StAR since they were from the same membrane. The data were normalized with the internal control β-actin, and each value is the mean ± SEM ($n = 4$), with $^{*}p < 0.05$, $^{**}p < 0.01$, $^{***}p < 0.001$, vs. vehicle control group.

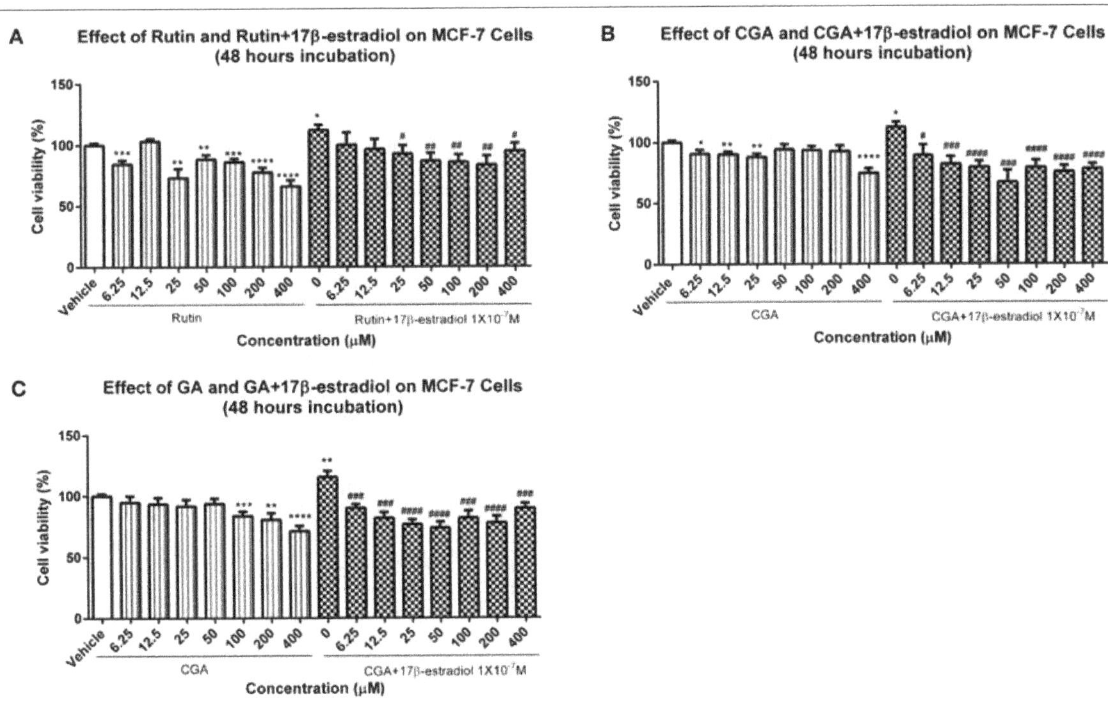

FIGURE 13 | Viability of MCF-7 breast cancer cells. **(A–C)** The proliferation of MCF-7 cells in the presence or absence of 1×10^{-7} M 17β-estradiol was determined by using MTT assay after 12 h treatment with different dosages of rutin, CGA, and GA. Each value represented mean ± SEM ($n = 4$), $^{*}p < 0.05$, $^{**}p < 0.01$, $^{***}p < 0.001$, $^{****}p < 0.0001$, vs. vehicle control group; $^{\#}p < 0.05$, $^{\#\#\#}p < 0.01$, $^{\#\#\#}p < 0.001$, $^{\#\#\#\#}p < 0.0001$ vs. 17β-estradiol group.

isolation of major compounds, which can avoid omission of potential active components and guarantee completeness of the experiment. Importantly, only compounds interacting with the targets that are shared by both the ovary and menopause could be considered for further investigation in this article, indicating the tissue-specificity and disease-specificity of the compounds selected. We hope the scheme in this work will bring new insight into the systematic investigation of TCM and lead to a wide range of applications for the identification and development of the potential novel and safe therapeutic candidates.

CONCLUSION

In summary, we have shown that GJE and its bioactive compounds (rutin, CGA, and GA) exerted estrogen stimulating effects *in vitro* and up-regulated the FSHR-aromatase pathway without increasing the risk of hormone-dependent breast cancer. These data reveal that GJE and its bioactive compounds may be considered as promising candidates for further research and development into therapeutic agents for the treatment of postmenopausal syndrome.

AUTHOR CONTRIBUTIONS

SS, TN, KL, and YZ designed and conceived the study. XW, LZ, H-KW, and G-CW conducted the experiments. XW and SW conducted data analysis. XW and SS wrote the manuscript. JR, KY, TN and YZ provided constructive comments. SS, TN and SS re-wrote parts of manuscript. All authors have read and approved the final version of the manuscript.

ACKNOWLEDGMENTS

This study was partially supported by Innovation and Technology Fund (ITF) awarded by the Innovation and Technology Commission, Government of Hong Kong SAR (project no ITS/262/09FP) and grants from the Seed Funding Programme for Basic Research, the University of Hong Kong (project codes: 201511159306, 201411159213, 200907176203). We thank Mr. Keith Wong, Ms. Cindy Lee, and Mr. Shiwei Wang for their technical assistance.

SUPPLEMENTARY MATERIAL

Figure S1 | Flow chart of extraction procedure for GJE bioactive fractions.

Figure S2 | HPLC standard curve of geniposide. The regression equation of standard constituents is Area = 85.36C-164.88. The standard constituents showed a good linearity (R^2 = 0.999643) with the linear range 62.5–1000 μg/ml.

Figure S3 | 3-D chromatogram of geniposide from sample solution. **(A)** petroleum fractions; **(B)** ethyl acetate fractions; **(C)** n-butanol fractions; **(D)** water fractions; **(E)** ethanol fractions. X-axis as time (min) as, Y-axis as absorbance, Z-axis as wavelength.

Figure S4 | The effect of GJE fractions on CYP19 and FSHR level in granulosa cells was detected by western blot assay. **(A)** Representative western blot results of aromatase, FSHR, and GAPDH levels; **(B)** Densitometric analysis of CYP19 expression levels; **(C)** Densitometric analysis of FSHR expression levels (**p < 0.01).

Table S1 | Forty nine compounds of GJE identified from TCMSP @ Taiwan database.

Table S2 | The 25 significant pathways found by JEPETTO (Cytoscape plugin) with KEGG database.

Table S3 | Precision study of sample solution of geniposide.

Table S4 | Stability study of sample solution of geniposide.

Table S5 | Recovery study of sample solution.

REFERENCES

Al-Azzawi, F., and Wahab, M. (2002). Estrogen and colon cancer: current issues. *Climacteric* 5, 3–14. doi: 10.1080/cmt.5.1.3.14

Ali, S., and Coombes, R. C. (2000). Estrogen receptor alpha in human breast cancer: occurrence and significance. *J. Mammary Gland Biol. Neoplasia* 5, 271–281. doi: 10.1023/A:1009594727358

Al-Safi, Z. A., and Santoro, N. (2014). Menopausal hormone therapy and menopausal symptoms. *Fertil. Steril.* 101, 905–915. doi: 10.1016/j.fertnstert.2014.02.032

An, J., Hu, F., Wang, C., Zhang, Z., Yang, L., and Wang, Z. (2016). Pharmacokinetics and tissue distribution of five active ingredients of Eucommiae cortex in normal and ovariectomized mice by UHPLC-MS/MS. *Xenobiotica* 46, 793–804. doi: 10.3109/00498254.2015.1129470

Avis, N. E., Brambilla, D., Mckinlay, S. M., and Vass, K. (1994). A longitudinal analysis of the association between menopause and depression Results from the Massachusetts women's health study. *Ann. Epidemiol.* 4, 214–220. doi: 10.1016/1047-2797(94)90099-X

Barnabei, V. M., Grady, D., Stovall, D. W., Cauley, J. A., Lin, F., Stuenkel, C. A., et al. (2002). Menopausal symptoms in older women and the effects of treatment with hormone therapy. *Obstetr. Gynecol.* 100, 1209–1218. doi: 10.1016/S0029-7844(02)02369-4

Barzi, A., Lenz, A. M., Labonte, M. J., and Lenz, H.-J. (2013). Molecular pathways: estrogen pathway in colorectal cancer. *Clin. Cancer Res.* 19, 5842–5848. doi: 10.1158/1078-0432.CCR-13-0325

Brueggemeier, R. W., Hackett, J. C., and Diaz-Cruz, E. S. (2005). Aromatase inhibitors in the treatment of breast cancer. *Endocr. Rev.* 26, 331–345. doi: 10.1210/er.2004-0015

Burger, H., Hale, G., Robertson, D., and Dennerstein, L. (2007). A review of hormonal changes during the menopausal transition: focus on findings from the Melbourne Women's Midlife Health Project. *Hum. Reprod. Update* 13, 559–565. doi: 10.1093/humupd/dmm020

Cai, L., Li, R., Tang, W.-J., Meng, G., Hu, X.-Y., and Wu, T.-N. (2015). Antidepressant-like effect of geniposide on chronic unpredictable mild stress-induced depressive rats by regulating the hypothalamus–pituitary–adrenal axis. *Euro. Neuropsychopharmacol.* 25, 1332–1341. doi: 10.1016/j.euroneuro.2015.04.009

Carr, M. C. (2003). The emergence of the metabolic syndrome with menopause. *J. Clin. Endocrinol. Metab.* 88, 2404–2411. doi: 10.1210/jc.2003-030242

Chen, J., Mangelinckx, S., Ma, L., Wang, Z., Li, W., and De Kimpe, N. (2014). Caffeoylquinic acid derivatives isolated from the aerial parts of Gynura divaricata and their yeast α-glucosidase and PTP1B inhibitory activity. *Fitoterapia* 99, 1–6. doi: 10.1016/j.fitote.2014.08.015

Chen, L.-C., Tsao, Y.-T., Yen, K.-Y., Chen, Y.-F., Chou, M.-H., and Lin, M.-F. (2003). A pilot study comparing the clinical effects of Jia-Wey Shiau-Yau San, a traditional Chinese herbal prescription, and a continuous combined hormone replacement therapy in postmenopausal women with climacteric symptoms. *Maturitas* 44, 55–62. doi: 10.1016/S0378-5122(02)00314-6

Chen, L.-C., Wang, B.-R., Chen, I.-C., and Shao, C.-H. (2010). Use of Chinese herbal medicine among menopausal women in Taiwan. *Int. J. Gynecol. Obstetr.* 109, 63–66. doi: 10.1016/j.ijgo.2009.10.014

Chen, Y., Zhang, Y., Li, L., and Hölscher, C. (2015). Neuroprotective effects of geniposide in the MPTP mouse model of Parkinson's disease. *Eur. J. Pharmacol.* 768, 21–27. doi: 10.1016/j.ejphar.2015.09.029

Chuffa, L.. G., Lupi-Júnior L. A., Costa, A. B., De Arruda Amorim, J. P., and Seiva, F. R. F. (2016). The role of sex hormones and steroid receptors on female reproductive cancers. *Steroids* 118, 93–108. doi: 10.1016/j.steroids.2016.12.011

Citraro, R., Gallelli, L., Leo, A., De Fazio, P., Gallelli, P., Russo, E., et al. (2015). Effects of chronic sodium alendronate on depression and anxiety in a menopausal experimental model. *Pharmacol. Biochem. Behav.* 129, 65–71. doi: 10.1016/j.pbb.2014.12.006

Clarke, S., Kelleher, J., Lloyd-Jones, H., Slack, M., and Schofield, P. (2002). A study of hormone replacement therapy in postmenopausal women with ischaemic heart disease: the Papworth HRT atherosclerosis study. *BJOG Int. J. Obstetr. Gynaecol.* 109, 1056–1062. doi: 10.1111/j.1471-0528.2002.01544.x

Colditz, G. A. (1998). Relationship between estrogen levels, use of hormone replacement therapy, and breast cancer. *J. Natl. Cancer Inst.* 90, 814–823. doi: 10.1093/jnci/90.11.814

Constantine, G. D., and Pickar, J. H. (2003). Estrogens in postmenopausal women: recent insights. *Curr. Opin. Pharmacol.* 3, 626–634. doi: 10.1016/j.coph.2003.07.003

Dalal, P. K., and Agarwal, M. (2015). Postmenopausal syndrome. *Ind. J. Psychiatry* 57:S222. doi: 10.4103/0019-5545.161483

Davey, D. A. (2013). HRT: some unresolved clinical issues in breast cancer, endometrial cancer and premature ovarian insufficiency. *Women's Health* 9, 59–67. doi: 10.2217/WHE.12.61

Deroo, B. J., and Korach, K. S. (2006). Estrogen receptors and human disease. *J. Clin. Invest.* 116:561. doi: 10.1172/JCI27987

Deroo, B. J., Rodriguez, K. F., Couse, J. F., Hamilton, K. J., Collins, J. B., Grissom, S. F., et al. (2009). Estrogen receptor β is required for optimal cAMP production in mouse granulosa cells. *Mol. Endocrinol.* 23, 955–965. doi: 10.1210/me.2008-0213

Devi, G., Hahn, K., Massimi, S., and Zhivotovskaya, E. (2005). Prevalence of memory loss complaints and other symptoms associated with the menopause transition: a community survey. *Gend. Med.* 2, 255–264. doi: 10.1016/S1550-8579(05)80055-5

El Bitar, H., Gramain, A., Sévenet, T., and Bodo, B. (2004). Daphcalycinosidines, A., and B, new iridoid-alkaloids from *Daphniphyllum calycinum. Tetrahedron Lett.* 45, 515–518. doi: 10.1016/j.tetlet.2003.11.005

Feng, Y., and Cao, P. (2010). Review on Chinese medical treatment for menopausal syndrome. *J. Liaon. Univ. Trad. Chin. Med.* 4, 125–126.

Folwarczna, J., Pytlik, M., Zych, M., Cegieła, U., Nowinska, B., Kaczmarczyk-Sedlak, I., et al. (2015). Effects of caffeic and chlorogenic acids on the rat skeletal system. *Eur. Rev. Med. Pharmacol. Sci.* 19, 682–693.

Ghose, A. K., Pritchett, A., and Crippen, G. M. (1988). Atomic physicochemical parameters for three dimensional structure directed quantitative structure-activity relationships III: modeling hydrophobic interactions. *J. Comput. Chem.* 9, 80–90. doi: 10.1002/jcc.540090111

Gilbert, I. H. (2013). Drug discovery for neglected diseases: molecular target-based and phenotypic approaches: miniperspectives series on phenotypic screening for antiinfective targets. *J. Med. Chem.* 56, 7719–7726. doi: 10.1021/jm400362b

Greendale, G. A., Reboussin, B. A., Hogan, P., Barnabei, V. M., Shumaker, S., Johnson, S., et al. (1998). Symptom relief and side effects of postmenopausal hormones: results from the Postmenopausal Estrogen/Progestin Interventions Trial. *Obstetr. Gynecol.* 92, 982–988. doi: 10.1097/00006250-199812000-00019

Ha, H., Ho, J., Shin, S., Kim, H., Koo, S., Kim, I.-H., et al. (2003). Effects of Eucommiae Cortex on osteoblast-like cell proliferation and osteoclast inhibition. *Arch. Pharm. Res.* 26, 929–936. doi: 10.1007/BF02980202

Heitman, E., and Ingram, D. K. (2017). Cognitive and neuroprotective effects of chlorogenic acid. *Nutr. Neurosci.* 20, 32–39. doi: 10.1179/1476830514Y.0000000146

Hernandez, C., Beaupre, G., and Carter, D. (2003). A theoretical analysis of the relative influences of peak BMD, age-related bone loss and menopause on the development of osteoporosis. *Osteopor. Int.* 14, 843–847. doi: 10.1007/s00198-003-1454-8

Hoga, L., Rodolpho, J., Gonçalves, B., and Quirino, B. (2015). Women's experience of menopause: a systematic review of qualitative evidence. *JBI Datab. Syst. Rev. Implement. Reports* 13, 250–337. doi: 10.11124/jbisrir-2015-1948

Holst, F., Stahl, P. R., Ruiz, C., Hellwinkel, O., Jehan, Z., Wendland, M., et al. (2007). Estrogen receptor alpha (ESR1) gene amplification is frequent in breast cancer. *Nat. Genet.* 39, 655–660. doi: 10.1038/ng2006

Hoon Lee, C., Kwak, S.-C., Kim, J.-Y., Mee Oh, H., Chual Rho, M., Yoon, K.-H., et al. (2014). Genipin inhibits RANKL-induced osteoclast differentiation through proteasome-mediated degradation of c-Fos protein and suppression of NF-κB activation. *J. Pharmacol. Sci.* 124, 344–353. doi: 10.1254/jphs.13174FP

Hopkins, A. L. (2008). Network pharmacology: the next paradigm in drug discovery. *Nat. Chem. Biol.* 4, 682–690. doi: 10.1038/nchembio.118

Horcajada-Molteni, M. N., Crespy, V., Coxam, V., Davicco, M. J., Rémésy, C., and Barlet, J. P. (2000). Rutin inhibits ovariectomy-induced osteopenia in rats. *J. Bone Min. Res.* 15, 2251–2258. doi: 10.1359/jbmr.2000.15.11.2251

Hsu, H.-Y., Yang, J.-J., Lin, S.-Y., and Lin, C.-C. (1997). Comparisons of geniposidic acid and geniposide on antitumor and radioprotection after sublethal irradiation. *Cancer Lett.* 113, 31–37. doi: 10.1016/S0304-3835(96)04572-7

Huang, C., Zheng, C., Li, Y., Wang, Y., Lu, A., and Yang, L. (2013). Systems pharmacology in drug discovery and therapeutic insight for herbal medicines. *Brief. Bioinform.* 15, 710–733. doi: 10.1093/bib/bbt035

Hughes, J., Rees, S., Kalindjian, S., and Philpott, K. (2011). Principles of early drug discovery. *Br. J. Pharmacol.* 162, 1239–1249. doi: 10.1111/j.1476-5381.2010.01127.x

Hunzicker-Dunn, M., and Maizels, E. T. (2006). FSH signaling pathways in immature granulosa cells that regulate target gene expression: branching out from protein kinase A. *Cell. Signal.* 18, 1351–1359. doi: 10.1016/j.cellsig.2006.02.011

Im, M., Kim, A., and Ma, J. Y. (2016). Ethanol extract of baked Gardeniae Fructus exhibits *in vitro* and *in vivo* anti-metastatic and anti-angiogenic activities in malignant cancer cells: role of suppression of the NF-κB and HIF-1α pathways. *Int. J. Oncol.* 49, 2377–2386. doi: 10.3892/ijo.2016.3742

Janssen, I., Powell, L. H., Crawford, S., Lasley, B., and Sutton-Tyrrell, K. (2008). Menopause and the metabolic syndrome: the Study of Women's Health Across the Nation. *Arch. Intern. Med.* 168, 1568–1575. doi: 10.1001/archinte.168.14.1568

Jia, M., Dahlman-Wright, K., and Gustafsson, J.-Å. (2015). Estrogen receptor alpha and beta in health and disease. *Best Pract. Res. Clin. Endocrinol. Metab.* 29, 557–568. doi: 10.1016/j.beem.2015.04.008

Johnston, B. A. (1997). *One-Third of Nation's Adults Use Herbal Remedies.* Austin, TX: HerbalGram (USA).

Kamaludin, R. (2015). *Apoptotic Mechanism of Apigenin and Rutin in ER+-Breast Cancer Cells, MCF-7.* Shah Alam; Selangor: Universiti Teknologi MARA.

Kamaludin, R., Froemming, G. A., Ibahim, M. J., and Narimah, A. H. H. (2013). Cell apoptotic determination by Annexin V-FITC assay in apigenin and rutin-induced cell death in breast cancer cells. *Open Conf. Proc. J.* 4, 205–205. doi: 10.2174/2210289201304010205

Kaufert, P. A., Gilbert, P., and Tate, R. (1992). The Manitoba Project: a re-examination of the link between menopause and depression. *Maturitas* 14, 143–155. doi: 10.1016/0378-5122(92)90006-P

Kim, E.-S., Jeong, C.-S., and Moon, A. (2012). Genipin, a constituent of *Gardenia jasminoides* Ellis, induces apoptosis and inhibits invasion in MDA-MB-231 breast cancer cells. *Oncol. Rep.* 27:567. doi: 10.3892/or.2011.1508

Kotapalli, S. S., Nallam, S. S. A., Nadella, L., Banerjee, T., Rode, H. B., Mainkar, P. S., et al. (2015). Identification of new molecular entities (NMEs) as potential leads against tuberculosis from open source compound repository. *PLoS ONE* 10:e0144018. doi: 10.1371/journal.pone.0144018

Kuhn, M., Von Mering, C., Campillos, M., Jensen, L. J., and Bork, P. (2008). STITCH: interaction networks of chemicals and proteins. *Nucleic Acids Res.* 36, D684–D688. doi: 10.1093/nar/gkm795

Li, B., Zhang, Y., Shi, B., Chen, Y., Zhang, Z., and Liu, T. (2013). Gardenia oil increases estradiol levels and bone material density by a mechanism associated with upregulation of COX-2 expression in an ovariectomized rat model. *Exp. Ther. Med.* 6, 562–566. doi: 10.3892/etm.2013.1168

Liu, H., Chen, Y.-F., Li, F., and Zhang, H.-Y. (2013). Fructus Gardenia (*Gardenia jasminoides* J. Ellis) phytochemistry, pharmacology of cardiovascular, and safety with the perspective of new drugs development. *J. Asian Natl. Products Res.* 15, 94–110. doi: 10.1080/10286020.2012.723203

Liu, H.-X., Lin, W.-H., Wang, X.-L., and Yang, J.-S. (2005). Flavonoids from preparation of traditional Chinese medicines named Sini-Tang.

J. Asian Nat. Prod. Res. 7, 139–143. doi: 10.1080/10286020420002 04063

Liu, Y., Hua, Q., Lei, H., and Li, P. (2011). Effect of Tong Luo Jiu Nao on Aβ-degrading enzymes in AD rat brains. *J. Ethnopharmacol.* 137, 1035–1046. doi: 10.1016/j.jep.2011.07.031

Liu, Y., Xiao, C., Wang, T., Zhang, L., and Ding, K. (2008). Analyzing characteristics of Chinese herbal medical, symptoms, pattern distribution of traditional Chinese medicine for menopausal syndrome in modern literatures. *J. Beijing Univ. Trad. Chin. Med.* 31, 125–130.

Lobo, R., Davis, S., De Villiers, T., Gompel, A., Henderson, V., Hodis, H., et al. (2014). Prevention of diseases after menopause. *Climacteric* 17, 540–556. doi: 10.3109/13697137.2014.933411

Lu, J., Wong, R., Zhang, L., Wong, R., Ng, T., Lee, K., et al. (2016). Comparative analysis of proteins with stimulating activity on ovarian estradiol biosynthesis from four different dioscorea species *in vitro* using both phenotypic and target-based approaches: implication for treating menopause. *Appl. Biochem. Biotechnol.* 180, 79–93. doi: 10.1007/s12010-016-2084-x

Lufkin, E. G., Wahner, H. W., O'fallon, W. M., Hodgson, S. F., Kotowicz, M. A., Lane, A. W., et al. (1992). Treatment of postmenopausal osteoporosis with transdermal estrogen. *Ann. Intern. Med.* 117, 1–9.

Luo, W., and Wiltbank, M. C. (2006). Distinct regulation by steroids of messenger RNAs for FSHR and CYP19A1 in bovine granulosa cells. *Biol. Reprod.* 75, 217–225. doi: 10.1095/biolreprod.105.047407

Mao, Y., Hao, J., Jin, Z., Niu, Y., Yang, X., Liu, D., et al. (2017). Network pharmacology-based and clinically relevant prediction of the active ingredients and potential targets of Chinese herbs in metastatic breast cancer patients. *Oncotarget.* 8, 27007–27021. doi: 10.18632/oncotarget.15351

Mattingly, C. J., Colby, G. T., Forrest, J. N., and Boyer, J. L. (2003). The Comparative Toxicogenomics Database (CTD). *Environ. Health Perspect.* 111:793. doi: 10.1289/ehp.6028

Meisler, J. G. (2003). Toward optimal health: the experts discuss the use of botanicals by women. *J. Women's Health* 12, 847–852. doi: 10.1089/154099903770948069

Miller, V. M., Garovic, V. D., Kantarci, K., Barnes, J. N., Jayachandran, M., Mielke, M. M., et al. (2013). Sex-specific risk of cardiovascular disease and cognitive decline: pregnancy and menopause. *Biol. Sex Differ.* 4:6. doi: 10.1186/2042-6410-4-6

Nelson, H. D., Humphrey, L. L., Nygren, P., Teutsch, S. M., and Allan, J. D. (2002). Postmenopausal hormone replacement therapy: scientific review. *JAMA* 288, 872–881. doi: 10.1001/jama.288.7.872

Nilsson, S., Mäkelä, S., Treuter, E., Tujague, M., Thomsen, J., Andersson, G., et al. (2001). Mechanisms of estrogen action. *Physiol. Rev.* 81, 1535–1565. doi: 10.1152/physrev.2001.81.4.1535

Noratto, G., Porter, W., Byrne, D., and Cisneros-Zevallos, L. (2009). Identifying peach and plum polyphenols with chemopreventive potential against estrogen-independent breast cancer cells. *J. Agric. Food Chem.* 57, 5219–5226. doi: 10.1021/jf900259m

Oliveira, H., Cai, X., Zhang, Q., De Freitas, V., Mateus, N., He, J., et al. (2017). Gastrointestinal absorption, antiproliferative and anti-inflammatory effect of the major carotenoids of *Gardenia jasminoides* Ellis on cancer cells. *Food Funct.* 8, 1672–1679. doi: 10.1039/C7FO00091J

Papadopoulos, V., and Miller, W. L. (2012). Role of mitochondria in steroidogenesis. *Best Pract. Res. Clin. Endocrinol. Metab.* 26, 771–790. doi: 10.1016/j.beem.2012.05.002

Paruthiyil, S., Parmar, H., Kerekatte, V., Cunha, G. R., Firestone, G. L., and Leitman, D. C. (2004). Estrogen receptor β inhibits human breast cancer cell proliferation and tumor formation by causing a G2 cell cycle arrest. *Cancer Res.* 64, 423–428. doi: 10.1158/0008-5472.CAN-03-2446

Peng, L.-Y., Mei, S.-X., Jiang, B., Zhou, H., and Sun, H.-D. (2000). Constituents from Lonicera japonica. *Fitoterapia* 71, 713–715. doi: 10.1016/S0367-326X(00)00212-4

Phatak, R. S. (2015). Phytochemistry, pharmacological activities and intellectual property landscape of *Gardenia jasminoides* Ellis: a Review. *Pharmacog. J.* 7, 254–265. doi: 10.5530/pj.2015.5.1

Pieroni, L. G., Rezende, F. M. D., Ximenes, V. F., and Dokkedal, A. L. (2011). Antioxidant activity and total phenols from the methanolic extract of Miconia albicans (Sw.) Triana leaves. *Molecules* 16, 9439–9450. doi: 10.3390/molecules16119439

Pollow, D. P., Romero-Aleshire, M. J., Sanchez, J. N., Konhilas, J. P., and Brooks, H. L. (2015). ANG II-induced hypertension in the VCD mouse model of menopause is prevented by estrogen replacement during perimenopause. *Am. J. Physiol. Regul. Integr. Comp. Physiol.* 309, R1546–R1552. doi: 10.1152/ajpregu.00170.2015

Prelevic, G. M., and Jacobs, H. S. (1997). Menopause and post-menopause. *Baillière's Clin. Endocrinol. Metab.* 11, 311–340. doi: 10.1016/S0950-351X(97)80317-5

Qu, J., Zhou, Q., Du, Y., Zhang, W., Bai, M., Zhang, Z., et al. (2014). Retracted: rutin protects against cognitive deficits and brain damage in rats with chronic cerebral hypoperfusion. *Br. J. Pharmacol.* 171, 3702–3715. doi: 10.1111/bph.12725

Ramalingayya, G. V., Nampoothiri, M., Nayak, P. G., Kishore, A., Shenoy, R. R., Rao, C. M., et al. (2016). Naringin and rutin alleviates episodic memory deficits in two differentially challenged object recognition tasks. *Pharmacogn. Mag.* 12, S63. doi: 10.4103/0973-1296.176104

Rassi, C. M., Lieberherr, M., Chaumaz, G., Pointillart, A., and Cournot, G. (2005). Modulation of osteoclastogenesis in porcine bone marrow cultures by quercetin and rutin. *Cell Tiss. Res.* 319, 383–393. doi: 10.1007/s00441-004-1053-9

Ren, L., Tao, W., Zhang, H., Xue, W., Tang, J., Wu, R., et al. (2016). Two standardized fractions of *Gardenia jasminoides* Ellis with rapid antidepressant effects are differentially associated with BDNF up-regulation in the hippocampus. *J. Ethnopharmacol.* 187, 66–73. doi: 10.1016/j.jep.2016.04.023

Ru, J., Li, P., Wang, J., Zhou, W., Li, B., Huang, C., et al. (2014). TCMSP: a database of systems pharmacology for drug discovery from herbal medicines. *J. Cheminform.* 6:13. doi: 10.1186/1758-2946-6-13

Scheid, V. (2007). Traditional Chinese medicine—What are we investigating?: The case of menopause. *Complement. Ther. Med.* 15, 54–68. doi: 10.1016/j.ctim.2005.12.002

Scheid, V., Ward, T., Cha, W.-S., Watanabe, K., and Liao, X. (2010). The treatment of menopausal symptoms by traditional East Asian medicines: review and perspectives. *Maturitas* 66, 111–130. doi: 10.1016/j.maturitas.2009.11.020

Shao, L., and Zhang, B. (2013). Traditional Chinese medicine network pharmacology: theory, methodology and application. *Chin. J. Nat. Med.* 11, 110–120. doi: 10.1016/S1875-5364(13)60037-0

Sheng, L., Qian, Z., Zheng, S., and Xi, L. (2006). Mechanism of hypolipidemic effect of crocin in rats: crocin inhibits pancreatic lipase. *Eur. J. Pharmacol.* 543, 116–122. doi: 10.1016/j.ejphar.2006.05.038

Simpson, E. R., Mahendroo, M. S., Means, G. D., Kilgore, M. W., Hinshelwood, M. M., Graham-Lorence, S., et al. (1994). Aromatase Cytochrome P450, The Enzyme Responsible for Estrogen Biosynthesis*. *Endocr. Rev.* 15, 342–355.

Society, N. A. M. (2006). *Management of Osteoporosis in Postmenopausal Women: 2006 Position Statement of The North American Menopause Society*, Vol. 13. New York, NY: Menopause.

Ström, A., Hartman, J., Foster, J. S., Kietz, S., Wimalasena, J., and Gustafsson, J.-Å. (2004). Estrogen receptor β inhibits 17β-estradiol-stimulated proliferation of the breast cancer cell line T47D. *Proc. Natl. Acad. Sci. U.S.A.* 101, 1566–1571. doi: 10.1073/pnas.0308319100

Su, D., Ti, H., Zhang, R., Zhang, M., Wei, Z., Deng, Y., et al. (2014). Structural elucidation and cellular antioxidant activity evaluation of major antioxidant phenolics in lychee pulp. *Food Chem.* 158, 385–391. doi: 10.1016/j.foodchem.2014.02.134

Su, J.-Y., Xie, Q.-F., Liu, W.-J., Lai, P., Liu, D.-D., Tang, L.-H., et al. (2013). Perimenopause amelioration of a TCM recipe composed of Radix Astragali, Radix Angelicae Sinensis, and Folium Epimedii: an *in vivo* study on natural aging rat model. *Evid. Based Complemen. Altern. Med.* 2013:747240. doi: 10.1155/2013/747240

Sung, Y.-Y., Lee, A. Y., and Kim, H. K. (2014). The *Gardenia jasminoides* extract and its constituent, geniposide, elicit anti-allergic effects on atopic dermatitis by inhibiting histamine *in vitro* and *in vivo*. *J. Ethnopharmacol.* 156, 33–40. doi: 10.1016/j.jep.2014.07.060

Swamidass, S. J., Schillebeeckx, C. N., Matlock, M., Hurle, M. R., and Agarwal, P. (2014). Combined analysis of phenotypic and target-based screening in assay networks. *J. Biomol. Screen.* 19, 782–790. doi: 10.1177/1087057114523068

Sze, S. C. W., Tong, Y., Zhang, Y. B., Zhang, Z. J., Lau, A. S. L., Wong, H. K., et al. (2009). A novel mechanism: Erxian Decoction, a Chinese medicine formula, for relieving menopausal syndrome. *J. Ethnopharmacol.* 123, 27–33. doi: 10.1016/j.jep.2009.02.034

Tattersall, M., Sodergren, J., Sengupta, S., Trites, D., Modest, E., and Frei, E. (1975). Pharmacokinetics of actinomycin 0 in patients with malignant melanoma. *Clin. Pharmacol. Therap.* 17, 701–708. doi: 10.1002/cpt1975176701

Tsai, T.-R., Tseng, T.-Y., Chen, C.-F., and Tsai, T.-H. (2002). Identification and determination of geniposide contained in *Gardenia jasminoides* and in two preparations of mixed traditional Chinese medicines. *J. Chromatogr. A* 961, 83–88. doi: 10.1016/S0021-9673(02)00365-5

Wang, J., Duan, P., Cui, Y., Li, Q., and Shi, Y. (2016). Geniposide alleviates depression-like behavior via enhancing BDNF expression in hippocampus of streptozotocin-evoked mice. *Metab. Brain Dis.* 31, 1113–1122. doi: 10.1007/s11011-016-9856-4

Wang, L., Li, Z., Zhao, X., Liu, W., Liu, Y., Yang, J., et al. (2013). A network study of chinese medicine xuesaitong injection to elucidate a complex mode of action with multicompound, multitarget, and multipathway. *Evid. Based Complement. Altern. Med.* 2013:652373. doi: 10.1155/2013/652373

Wang, S. W., Cheung, H. P., Tong, Y., Lu, J., Ng, T. B., Zhang, Y. B., et al. (2017). Steroidogenic effect of Erxian decoction for relieving menopause via the p-Akt/PKB pathway *in vitro* and *in vivo*. *J. Ethnopharmacol.* 195, 188–195. doi: 10.1016/j.jep.2016.11.018

Wang, S. W., Tong, Y., Ng, T.-B., Lao, L., Lam, J. K. W., Zhang, K. Y., et al. (2015). Network pharmacological identification of active compounds and potential actions of Erxian decoction in alleviating menopause-related symptoms. *Chin. Med.* 10:1. doi: 10.1186/s13020-015-0051-z

Weber, M., and Mapstone, M. (2009). Memory complaints and memory performance in the menopausal transition. *Menopause* 16, 694–700. doi: 10.1097/gme.0b013e318196a0c9

Winterhalter, C., Widera, P., and Krasnogor, N. (2014). JEPETTO: a Cytoscape plugin for gene set enrichment and topological analysis based on interaction networks. *Bioinformatics* 30, 1029–1030. doi: 10.1093/bioinformatics/btt732

Wong, K. L., Lai, Y. M., Li, K. W., Lee, K. F., Ng, T. B., Cheung, H. P., et al. (2015). A novel, stable, estradiol-stimulating, osteogenic yam protein with potential for the treatment of menopausal syndrome. *Sci. Rep.* 5:10179. doi: 10.1038/srep17129

World Health Organization (1996). *Research on the Menopause in the 1990s: Report of a WHO Scientific Group*. World Health Organ Tech Rep Ser.

Xiang, H., Wang, G., Qu, J., Xia, S., Tao, X., Qi, B., et al. (2016). Yin-Chen-Hao Tang attenuates severe acute pancreatitis in rat: an experimental verification of in silico network target prediction. *Front. Pharmacol.* 7:378. doi: 10.3389/fphar.2016.00378

Yang, H. J., Kim, M. J., Kwon, D. Y., Moon, B. R., Kim, A. R., Kang, S., et al. (2016). The combination of *Artemisia princeps* Pamp, *Leonurus japonicas* Houtt, and *Gardenia jasminoides* Ellis fruit attenuates the exacerbation of energy, lipid, and glucose by increasing hepatic PGC-1α expression in estrogen-deficient rats. *BMC Complement. Altern. Med.* 16:137. doi: 10.1186/s12906-016-1109-x

Zhang, G.-B., Li, Q.-Y., Chen, Q.-L., and Su, S.-B. (2013). Network pharmacology: a new approach for chinese herbal medicine research. *Evid. Based Complement. Altern. Med.* 2013:621423. doi: 10.1155/2013/621423

Zhang, H., Lai, Q., Li, Y., Liu, Y., and Yang, M. (2016). Learning and memory improvement and neuroprotection of *Gardenia jasminoides* (Fructus gardenia) extract on ischemic brain injury rats. *J. Ethnopharmacol.* 196, 225–235.. doi: 10.1016/j.jep.2016.11.042

Zhang, H., Xue, W., Wu, R., Gong, T., Tao, W., Zhou, X., et al. (2015). Rapid antidepressant activity of ethanol extract of *Gardenia jasminoides* Ellis is associated with upregulation of BDNF expression in the hippocampus. *Evid. Based Complement. Altern. Med.* 2015:761238. doi: 10.1155/2015/761238

Zhou, R. P., Lin, S. J., Wan, W. B., Zuo, H. L., Yao, F. F., Ruan, H. B., et al. (2016). Chlorogenic acid prevents osteoporosis by Shp2/PI3K/Akt pathway in ovariectomized rats. *PLoS ONE* 11:e0166751. doi: 10.1371/journal.pone.0166751

21

Anti-hyperplasia Effects of Total Saponins from Phytolaccae Radix in Rats with Mammary Gland Hyperplasia via Inhibition of Proliferation and Induction of Apoptosis

Xiaoliang Li[1,2], Zhibin Wang[1], Yu Wang[1], Yanan Zhang[1], Xia Lei[2], Ping Xin[1], Xin Fu[1], Ning Gao[1], Yanping Sun[1], Yanhong Wang[1], Bingyou Yang[1], Qiuhong Wang[3] and Haixue Kuang[1]**

[1] Key Laboratory of Chinese Materia Medica (Ministry of Education), Heilongjiang University of Chinese Medicine, Harbin, China, [2] Science of Chinese Materia Medica, Jiamusi College, Heilongjiang University of Chinese Medicine, Jiamusi, China, [3] Science of Processing Chinese Materia Medica, School of Traditional Chinese Medicine, Guangdong Pharmaceutical University, Guangzhou, China

Correspondence:
Qiuhong Wang
qhwangheb@163.com
Haixue Kuang
hxkuanghlj@163.com

Mammary gland hyperplasia (MGH) is a pathological condition that affects the majority of women at the child-bearing stage. The hormone and endocrinal therapy are typically used to treat MGH. Nevertheless, there are still some certain side effects accompanied with the benefits, which negatively affect the life quality of patients. Therefore, plant-derived agents that are effective against MGH development and with fewer side effects should be developed. The aim of this study was to investigate the protective effects and underlying mechanism of total saponins of Phytolaccae (TSP) against MGH *in vivo*. The results showed that treatment with TSP could significantly correct the disorder of serum sex hormones levels in rats with MGH, and eliminate the formation of MGH. Moreover, TSP significantly protected estrogen and progesterone-induced MGH histological changes, inhibited the swelling of the nipple, and improved the organ coefficient of uterus in rats with MGH. Mechanistically, TSP treatment not only effectively suppressed the mRNA and protein expression of ERα and PR in mammary gland, but also simultaneously up-regulated ERβ expression, and thus blocked sex hormones from interacting with their receptors. TSP treatment markedly suppressed mammary phosphorylation levels of ERK1/2, as well as reduced the mRNA and protein overexpression of VEGF and bFGF in mammary of rats. In addition, TSP treatment substantially down-regulated the expression of Bcl-2 and Ki-67, as well as elevated the expression of Bax. These findings indicated that TSP could potentially be used for effective treatment of MGH.

Keywords: total saponins of Phytolaccae, mammary gland hyperplasia, sex hormones, apoptosis, proliferation

INTRODUCTION

Nowadays, the disease of MGH, especially for women of child-bearing age, is one of the most common and frequently occurring disease and affects people in increasing numbers, which is classified into the category of "Rupi" in Chinese medicine (Zheng et al., 2013; Chen et al., 2015). Without getting any effective control, MGH shows a severe cancerous tendency, and may have been confused and covered with early breast cancer (Wang L. et al., 2011; Wang Z.C. et al., 2011). According to the modern medicine, the occurrence of MGH is closely related to endocrine disorder, and prescription of steroids (Lin et al., 2015) and surgery are the main treatment measures employed. Nevertheless, the potentially severe side effects and complications also emerge and seriously affect the life quality of patients (Henry, 2014), which is therefore prompt us to explore novel, alternative and effective treatments against the disease. Studies have proved that traditional Chinese medicine have the protective effect against MGH via possible regulated mechanism (Li et al., 2017).

Phytolaccae Radix, including *Phytolacca acinosa* and P. Americana, is recorded in Chinese Pharmacopeia (2015 edition) for its important medicinal value. The chemical constituents of Phytolaccae Radix mainly consist of triterpenoid saponins, flavone, phenolic acid, sterol, and polysaccharides. There have been an increasing number of studies focusing on its bio-activities, including diuretic, antibacterial, antiviral, anti-inflammatory anti-tumor and anti-MGH (Wang et al., 2014). It has a long history of use in the treatment of MGH. Patients with MGH achieved good therapeutic effect after taking the tablets which were made by the fresh Phytolaccae Radix (Tian et al., 1985).

The objective of the present study is to investigate the effects and potential mechanisms of TSP to protect against MGH in rats induced by estrogen combined with progestogen. This is first study on anti-MGH effect of TSP *in vivo*.

MATERIALS AND METHODS

Chemicals and Regents

Estradiol (E2) Benzoate Injection and Progesterone (P) Injection was supplied by Ningbo SANSHENG Pharmaceutical Co., Ltd. (Ningbo, Zhejiang, China). Smoothing and moisturizing hair removal was obtained from Watsons. E2, P, luteinizing hormone (LH), follicle stimulating hormone (FSH), prolactin (PRL), and testosterone (T) and T ELISA kits were purchased from Nanjing Jiancheng Bioengineering Institute (Nanjing, Jiangsu, China). The primary antibodies for VEGF, bFGF, p-ERK1/2, ERK1/2, Estrogen Receptor α, Estrogen Receptor β, ki-67, Bax, Bcl-2, GAPDH, and β-actin as well as all of the secondary antibodies were purchased from Cell Signaling Technology (Danvers, MA, United States).

Abbreviations: E2, Estradiol; FSH, follicle stimulating hormone; LH, luteinizing hormone; MGH, Mammary gland hyperplasia; NG, normal group; P, Progesterone; PRL, prolactin; T, testosterone; TSP, total saponins of Phytolaccae.

Total Saponins Extraction and Isolation

The preparation methods of TSP were coincided with the previous study (Wang, 2015). Briefly, the dried Phytolaccae Radix were powdered using an oscillating high speed universal grinder. The power was extracted thrice with water for 1.5 h at each time. The solution was filtered, concentrated, subjected to a HPD100 macroporous adsorption resin column, and then eluted successively with deionized water, 10, 30, and 70% aqueous ethanol. Subsequently, the solutions eluted by water, 10 and 30% aqueous ethanol were discarded. The remaining 70% aqueous ethanol solution was collected and concentrated by a rotary evaporator, and then the concentrated extract of the total saponins was dried in a lyophilizer.

Ultra-Performance Liquid Chromatography-Q/Time-of-Flight Mass Spectrometry (UPLC-Q/TOF-MS) Analysis

Chromatographic analysis was carried out using an Acquity UPLC system (Waters, Milford, MA, United States) with a 3 μL injection volume. Next, Tandem MS was performed using a Q-TOF mass spectrometer (Waters) with an Electron Spray Ionization. The results were analyzed using MassLynx v4.1 and UNIFI v1.8 (Waters).

Animal Experiments

The virgin female Wistar rats weighing 180–220 g (license number: SCXK2015-0001) were commercially obtained from Liaoning Changsheng Biotechnology Co., Ltd. The rats were housed at a controlled room (temperature 23 ± 1 degree Celsius and humidity 60 ± 5%) under a 12 h light-dark cycle, and fed with standard diet and water *ad libitum*. They were acclimated under climate-controlled conditions for 7 days before the experiments began.

After acclimatization to the laboratory conditions, the rats were randomly divided into normal group (NO group) and MGH group (MGH group). The rats in MGH group were injected estrogen (0.5 mg/kg/d) into the muscle of medial side of hind leg for 25 days, and followed with progestogen (5 mg/kg/d) for another 5 days to induce animal model of MGH, meanwhile, the NO group were administered with normal saline intramuscularly for 30 days (Wang L. et al., 2011). From the 31st day, the rats with MGH were further randomly separated into six groups of ten individuals and treated as follows: (1) the vehicle control group (an equal volume of normal saline, i. g.); (2) the MGH model group (an equal volume of normal saline, i. g.); (3) Positive control group (tamoxifen, 1.5 mg/kg bwt, i. g.); (4) total saponins (7.5 mg/kg bwt, i. g.); (5) total saponins (15 mg/kg bwt, i. g.); (6) total saponins (30 mg/kg bwt, i. g.). All drugs were dissolved in distilled water before use and treatments were administered by gastric gavage at 10 ml/kg bodyweight for a total of 30 days continuously. Nipple diameter of rats were measured at the predetermined time during the experiment. At the end of the experimental period, all rats were fasted overnight and anesthetized using

20% urethane 1.0 g/kg body weight injected intraperitoneally. Blood samples were obtained via abdominal aorta, the serum was separated by centrifugation (3000 rpm for 10 min at 4 degree Celsius), and then stored at minus 80 degree Celsius for hormone assays. The tissues of mammary gland were fixed in 10% neutral buffered formalin or kept at minus 80 degree Celsius for subsequent analysis. This study was approved by the Animal Care and Use Committee of Heilongjiang University of Chinese Medicine.

Determination of Nipple Diameter and Organ Coefficients

The diameter of the rat's nipple was measured with vernier caliper on the 1st day, 30th day, 45th day, and the last day of the experiment. The uterus and ovary were completely separated and weighed at the end of the experiment. Then, the organ coefficients were calculated as uterus or ovary weight divided by body weight.

Biochemical Analysis and Enzyme-Linked Immunosorbent Assay (ELISA)

The concentrations of E2, P, LH, FSH, PRL, and T in serum were measured by commercial detection kits according to the procedures recommended by the manufacturer (Nanjing Jiancheng Bioengineering Institute, Nanjing, China).

Real Time PCR Analysis

Real-time PCR was performed to determine gene expression of ERα, ERβ, PR, VEGF, bFGF, Bcl-2, and Bax. Total RNA was extracted from the tissues of mammary gland with Trizol (Invitrogen) following the manufacturer's protocol. The cDNA was synthesized from 1 μg of total RNA using the Reverse Transcription Reagent Kit (TaKaRa, Shiga, Japan) in accordance with instruction manual. The sequences of the primers are listed in **Table 1**. The following thermocycling protocol was used: at 95 degree Celsius for 30 s, 40 cycles at 95 degree Celsius for 5 s and at 60 degree Celsius for 40 s. The relative quantities of the candidate genes and GAPDH mRNA were calculated by comparative CT method. The experiments were repeated for three times. Samples in each experiment were in triplicate.

Western Blot Analysis

The protein samples from the tissues of mammary gland were isolated using a protein extraction kit, and the protein concentrations were determined using a BCA protein assay kit. Equal amounts of proteins (50 μg) were separated by 10% SDS–PAGE and then transferred onto polyvinylidene difluoride (PVDF) membranes. After blocking with 5% nonfat dry milk in Tris-buffered saline Tween (TBS-T) for 2 h at room temperature, the membranes were individually incubated with the primary antibodies overnight at 4 degree Celsius. Following incubation with HRP-conjugated secondary antibody for 2 h at room temperature, the protein bands were visualized by ECL Prime Western Blotting Detection Reagent (Bio-Rad, United States). Chemiluminescent signals were detected and analyzed with the ChemiDoc XRS imaging system (Bio-Rad, United States). The intensity of protein bands was quantified using the Image J Software. The experiments were repeated for three times. Samples in each experiment were in triplicate.

Histological Analysis

The tissues of mammary gland were obtained for histopathological examination. In detail, the specimens of the tissues of mammary gland were fixed in 10% neutral buffered formalin for 48 h. After processed in a series of graded ethanol and dimethyl benzene, the tissues were embedded in paraffin, cut into 4 μm thick sections, and then stained with hematoxylin and eosin (H&E). Finally, we observed pathological changes in the tissues of mammary gland by using an SZX10 microscope (Olympus Corp., Tokyo, Japan).

Immunohistochemistry

Paraffin-embedded sections (4 μm) were dewaxed in xylene, sequentially rehydrated in alcohol and incubated in 3% H_2O_2 for 20 min. The sections were heated twice in a microwave oven for 5 min in 0.01 M citrate buffer at pH 6.0 for antigen retrieval and followed by overnight incubation at 4 degree Celsius with the primary antibodies: Ki-67 at 1:100, Bcl-2 at 1:50 and Bax at 1:50. The sections were washed and incubated with the HRP-conjugated secondary antibody for 30 min at 37 degree Celsius. After staining with DAB, the tissue slides were counterstained with hematoxylin, dehydrated through a graded ethanol series, and sealed with neutral gum in the end. The sections were captured under microscope with a camera (Olympus, Tokyo, Japan).

Statistical Analysis

Statistical analysis was performed with SPSS 18.0 software. All data were presented as mean ± SE. Comparisons of numerical data between two groups were calculated by Student *t*-tests. Differences in mean values of various groups were analyzed by ANOVA. Difference with *P*-value < 0.05 was considered as statistically significant.

TABLE 1 | Primers used in the qRT-PCR study.

Genes	Forward (5′-3′)	Reverse (5′-3′)
ERa	TTGCTCCTAACTTGCT CTTGG	TGCGGAATCGACT TGACG
ERβ	ATTTTCGCTCCCGACCTC	TAACTCACGGAACCTTGACG
PR	CCCAGTTCACAACGCT TCTAT	CTGAGACAAAATGACAC ACCACA
VEGF	CAAAGCCAGCACATAGG AGAGAT	TTTTTGCAGGAACATTTA CACGTC
bFGF	GAAGAGCGACCCACAC GTCAAAC	TCCCTTGATGGACACAAC TCCTCTC
GAPDH	TTCCTACCCCCAATG TATCCG	CCACCCTGTTGCTGTA GCCATA

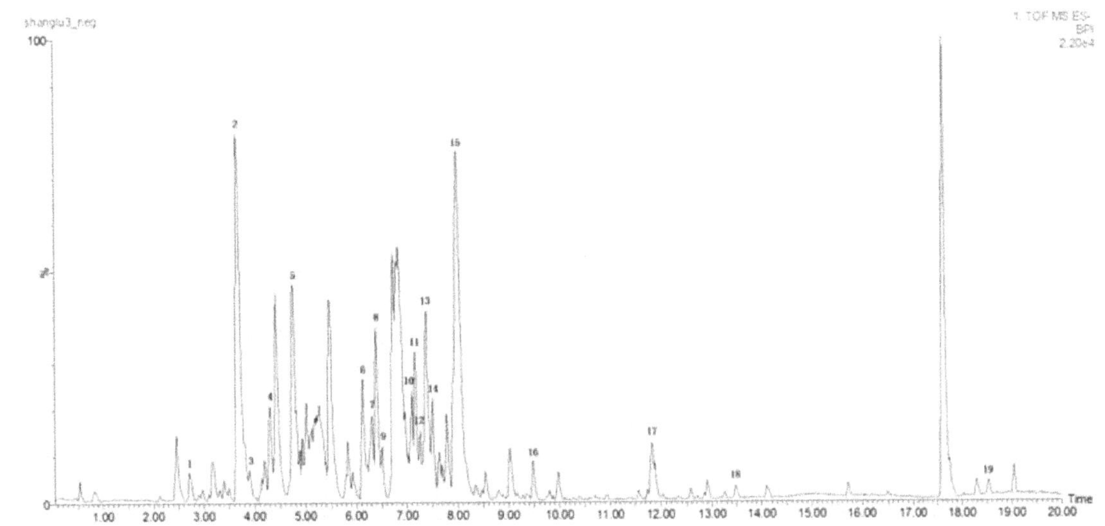

FIGURE 1 | Base peak ion (BPI) chromatogram of TSP in negative ion mode determined by ultra-performance liquid chromatography-Q/-time-of-flight-mass spectrometry (UPLC-Q/TOF-MS).

RESULTS

Identification of the Chemical Composition of TSP by UPLC-Q/TOF-MS

Figure 1 shows the base peak ion (BPI) chromatogram of TSP. A total of 19 compounds were initially identified based on retention time, molecular ions, major fragment ions, and previously published articles and online databases. The identified compounds were mainly classified as triterpene glycoside. The details of the identified compounds are listed in **Table 2**.

TSP Improved the Nipple Diameter of Rats With MGH

As shown in **Figure 2A**, the nipples of MGH model rats were become swelling and larger than those of the normal control. The nipple diameters (Left 2 and Right 2) were markedly increased by intramuscular injection of estrogen and progestin compared with normal control group. After 2 weeks' administration of TSP, the nipple diameters were obviously decreased, and further reduced at the end of the treatment. The change in nipple diameters over time is shown in **Figure 2B**.

TABLE 2 | Chemical composition of TSP determined by UPLC-Q/TOF-MS.

Peak	Component name	RT (min)	Molecular formula	Neutral mass (Da)	Adducts
1	Esculentoside N	2.72	$C_{54}H_{86}O_{26}$	1150.54073	+HCOO, −H
2	Esculentoside K	3.75	$C_{54}H_{86}O_{25}$	1134.54582	+HCOO, −H
3	Phytolaccoside B	3.91	$C_{36}H_{56}O_{11}$	664.38226	+H, +Na, +NH4
4	Esculentoside I	4.31	$C_{49}H_{78}O_{22}$	1018.49847	−H
5	Esculentoside F	4.76	$C_{41}H_{64}O_{16}$	812.41944	+HCOO, −H
6	Esculentoside G	6.10	$C_{48}H_{74}O_{21}$	988.48791	+HCOO
7	Esculentoside H	6.28	$C_{48}H_{76}O_{21}$	988.48791	+HCOO, −H
8	Esculentoside L	6.31	$C_{48}H_{76}O_{20}$	972.49299	+HCOO, −H
9	Phytolaccoside E	6.51	$C_{42}H_{66}O_{16}$	826.43509	+HCOO, −H
10	Phytolaccoside F	7.17	$C_{48}H_{76}O_{19}$	956.49808	+HCOO, −H
11	Esculentoside D	7.27	$C_{37}H_{58}O_{12}$	694.39283	+HCOO, −H
12	Phytolaccoside D	7.38	$C_{42}H_{66}O_{15}$	810.44017	+HCOO, −H
13	2-hydroxyl esculentic acid	7.44	$C_{30}H_{46}O_{7}$	518.32435	−H, +HCOO
14	Esculentoside A	7.51	$C_{42}H_{66}O_{16}$	826.43509	+HCOO, −H
15	Esculentoside B	7.99	$C_{36}H_{56}O_{11}$	664.38226	+HCOO, −H
16	Esculentoside C	9.48	$C_{42}H_{66}O_{15}$	810.44017	+HCOO, −H
17	Phytolaccagenin	11.84	$C_{31}H_{48}O_{7}$	532.34000	+NH4, +Na, −e
18	Esculentoside E	13.49	$C_{35}H_{54}O_{11}$	650.36661	−H
19	Phytolaccagenic acid	18.54	$C_{31}H_{48}O_{6}$	516.34509	−H

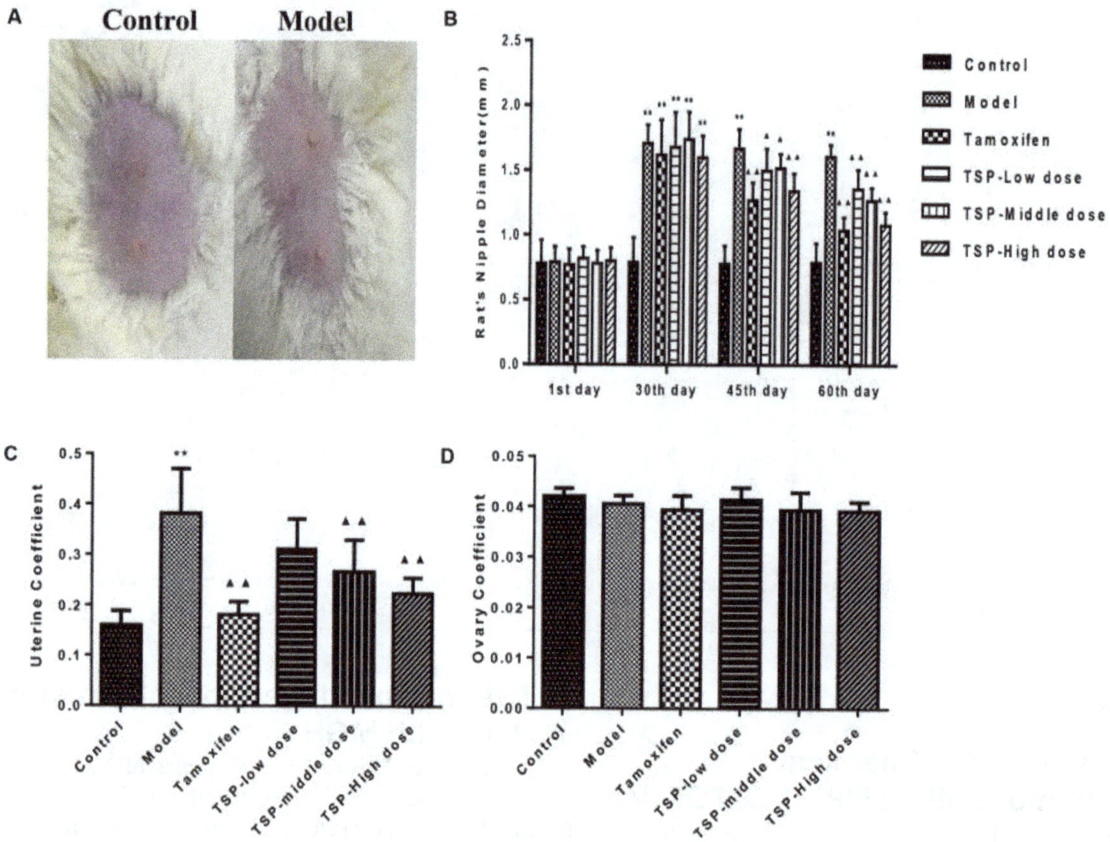

FIGURE 2 | Effects of TSP on the nipple diameters and organ coefficients of uterus and ovary index in rats with MGH. **(A)** Representative photograph of rat breasts. **(B)** Comparison of nipples diameter in rats. **(C)** Coefficient of uterus. **(D)** Coefficient of ovary in rats. Data were shown as mean ± SE (n = 10), $^{**}P < 0.01$ vs. control group; $^{▲}P < 0.05$ and $^{▲▲}P < 0.01$ vs. model group.

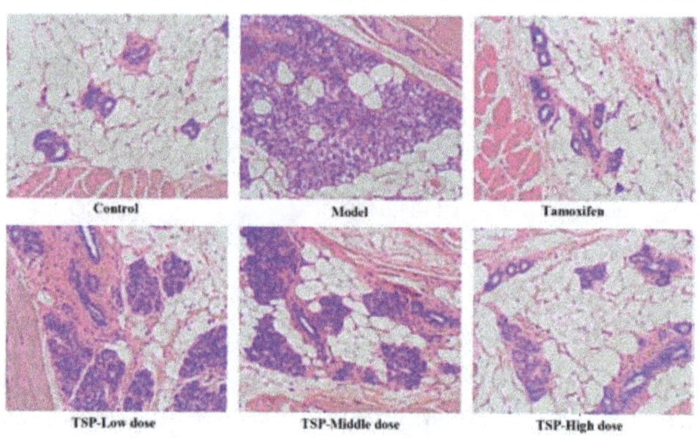

FIGURE 3 | Morphology of mammary gland tissue was observed by microscope (original magnification, 100×).

Effects of TSP on Organ Coefficients of Uterus and Ovary in Rats With MGH

To further investigate the effects of TSP on MGH, the organ coefficients of uterus and ovary in rats of each group were obtained. Results showed that compared with normal control group, the organ coefficient of uterus in MGH model group were obviously increased. However, the organ coefficient of uterus was markedly decreased by TSP-Middle and -High dose treatment as compared with MGH model group. There were no outstanding differences in the organ coefficients of the ovary between all the groups (**Figure 2**).

Effect of TSP on Pathomorphology of Mammary Gland Tissue in MGH Model Rats

To verify the effectiveness of TSP in mitigating MGH, H&E staining was conducted and histological variation was observed. As can be seen from **Figure 3**, there were no histopathological alterations in the mammary gland of the control group rats. In contrast in the model group, mammary epithelial cell tissue had significantly proliferative lesions, including hyperplasia in most lobules, increased numbers of acini and ducts, and thickened glandular epithelium. Administration of tamoxifen and TSP-High dose for four consecutive weeks significantly suppressed these typical histological patterns. The proliferative degree of mammary lobules and the number of acini and ducts markedly decreased. While daily treatment of TSP-Low and -Middle dose for 4 weeks, compared to the model group, were also capable to decrease the lumen area and numbers of mammary acini and ducts in different degree. These results illustrated that TSP had therapeutic effect on the rats with MGH induced by estrogen and progestogen.

TSP Ameliorated the Levels of Serum Sex Hormones in Rats With MGH

After injection of estrogen and progestogen, as shown in **Figure 4**, E2 and PRL contents were obviously increased ($P < 0.01$ for both cases), while P ($P < 0.01$) and T ($P < 0.05$) contents were notably decreased when compared to the control group, and most noticeably, there was no significant changes in LH and FSH contents in each group. However, the administration of TSP at different concentrations decreased the level of E2 and increased the level of P, but only TSP at a high dose reduced the contents of PRL and elevated contents of T. Our results suggested that TSP could adjust the serum E2, P, PRL, and T level of rats with MGH to play anti-MGH function.

TSP Modulated the mRNA and Protein Expression of ERα, ERβ, and PR in Mammary Gland of Rats With MGH

ER is an important nuclear transcription factor activated by ligand. As two kinds of subtypes, ERα and ERβ mediate estrogen and make it work. Meanwhile, PR is depending on the existence of ER, which is regulated and controlled by estrogen (Guo et al., 2017). To investigate the effect of TSP on ERα, ERβ and PR, the levels of related protein and mRNA were detected. As shown in **Figure 5**, The protein and mRNA expressions of ERα and PR were elevated in comparison with control group, while protein and mRNA expressions of ERβ were reduced in mammary gland of rats with MGH. However, TSP, at any dose, showed significant inhibitory effects on the protein and mRNA expressions of ERα and remarkable promoting effects on the protein and mRNA expressions of ERβ. Moreover, TSP treatment also exhibited the decrease in PR protein expressions in mammary gland of rats with MGH. Compared with that of model group, the mRNA levels of PR in mammary gland of rats with MGH were notably decreased after the administration of these MGH rats with TSP middle-($P < 0.05$) and high-doses ($P < 0.01$).

TSP Reduced the mRNA and Protein Expression of VEGF and bFGF, and Inhibited the Phosphorylation of ERK1/2 in Mammary Gland of Rats With MGH

The effects of TSP on the expression of VEGF and bFGF were determined by qPCR and western blot in mammary gland. The results showed that the mRNA and protein expressions of VEGF and bFGF were increased in MGH rats induced by estrogen and progesterone. TSP treatment inhibited the protein and mRNA

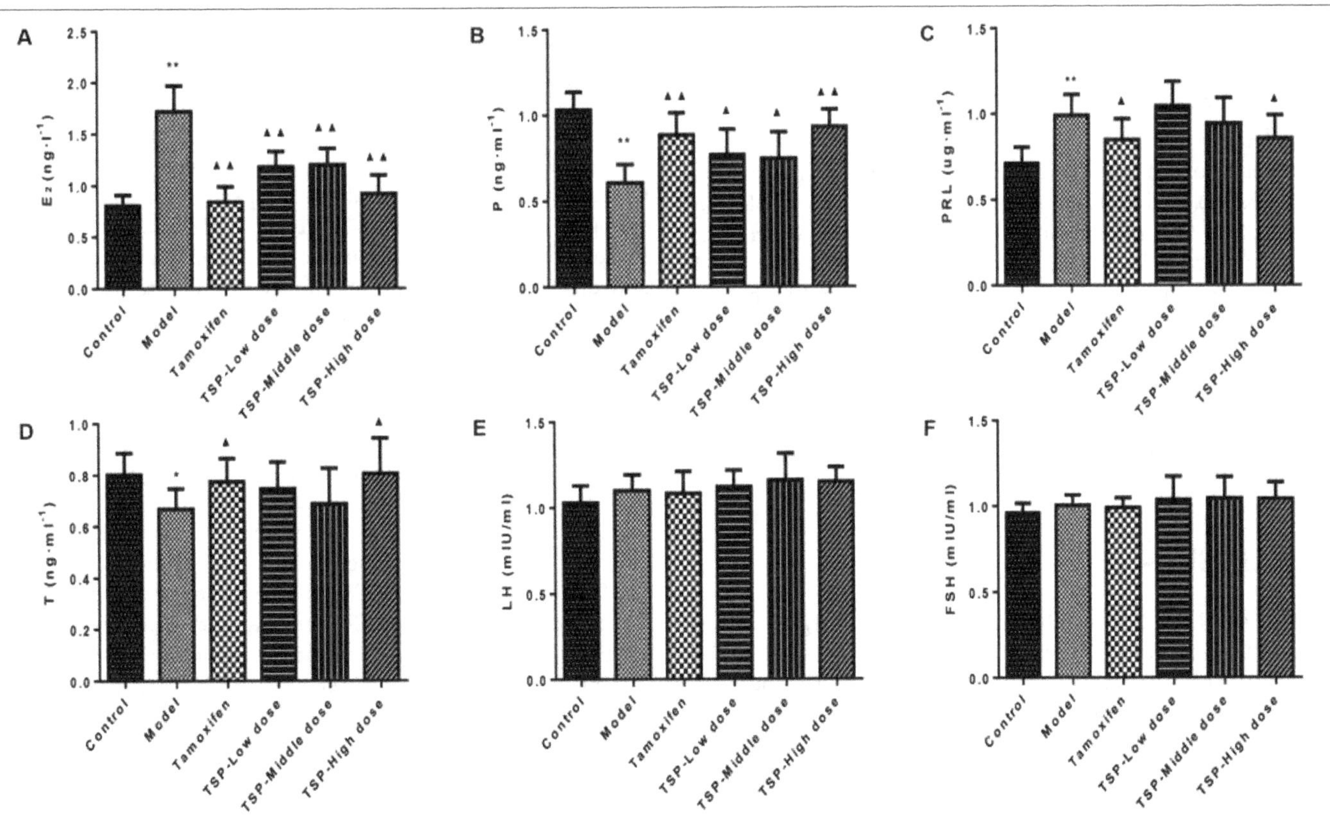

FIGURE 4 | Effects of TSP on sex hormones levels in rat's serum. **(A)** E2, **(B)** P, **(C)** PRL, **(D)** T, **(E)** LH, and **(F)** FSH in rat's serum. Values are expressed as mean ± SE ($n = 10$). *$P < 0.05$, and **$P < 0.01$ vs. control group; ▲$P < 0.05$ and ▲▲$P < 0.01$ vs. model group.

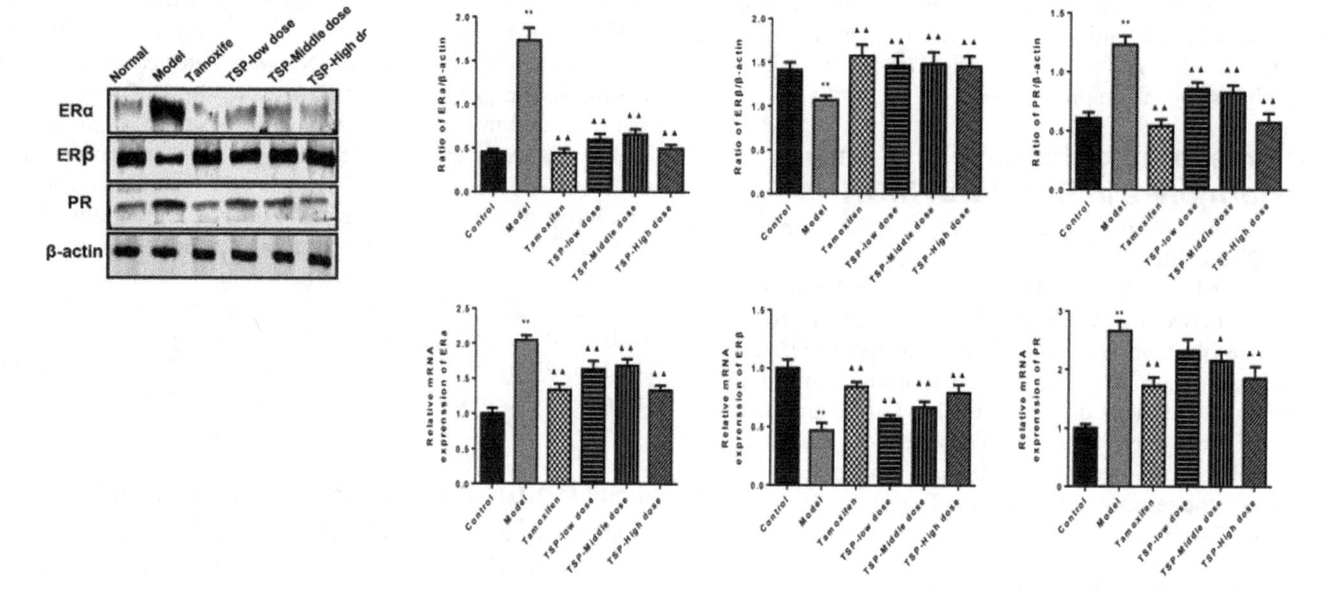

FIGURE 5 | Effects of TSP on the mRNA and protein expression of ERα, ERβ, and PR in mammary gland of rats with MGH. Data were shown as mean ± SE from three independent experiments, *$P < 0.05$, and **$P < 0.01$ vs. control group; ▲$P < 0.05$ and ▲▲$P < 0.01$ vs. model group.

expressions of VEGF and bFGF in a dose-dependent manner in mammary gland. ($P < 0.01$, **Figure 6A**). The phospho-ERK1/2 levels were also altered after estrogen and progesterone induction, and the application of TSP reduced ERK1/2 activation in a dose-dependent manner in mammary gland. ($P < 0.01$, **Figure 6B**).

TSP Induced Apoptosis in Rats With MGH

The expression of Bcl-2, Bax, and ki-67 in mammary gland were detected by immunohistochemistry and western blotting, so that the action mechanism of TSP in rats with MGH could be investigated. The results could be seen in **Figures 7A–E**, which showed that TSP at a middle-($P < 0.05$) and high-doses ($P < 0.01$) significantly down-regulated the levels of Bcl-2 and ki-67 compared with those in the model group, but had no effect at low dose. In addition, treatment of MGH rats with TSP also up-regulated level of Bax ($P < 0.01$) in MGH rat's mammary gland. These findings indicated that TSP could significantly promote apoptosis in rats with MGH.

DISCUSSION

Modern medicine believes that the breast is the target organ of the sex hormones, and the main cause leading to the MGH is the disorder of hormones metabolism in the body. The increased E2 in the absolute or relative terms and a persistent lack of P make the breast excessive hyperplasia and incomplete restoration (Schindler, 2011). PRL which is produced by eosinophilic cells in the distal part of the adenohypophysis promotes the growth and development of the mammary gland under the combined action of E2 and P. T is mainly secreted by the ovary and adrenal cortex in women. A small amount of T promotes the development of mammary glands. On the contrary, a large number of T plays an inhibitory effect (Han et al., 2015). In the present study, the continuous stimulation of exogenous hormones eventually leads to abnormal secretion of serum sex hormones in female rats. The treatment of TSP for consecutive 30 days could effectively regulate the levels of E2, P, PRL, and T hormones in serum of rats with MGH.

The effect of sex hormones on the body is mediated through the specific binding of the receptor. Estrogen action in target tissues is achieved by binding to specific nuclear receptors, estrogen receptors α and β (Higa and Fell, 2013). These receptors play a critical role in the regulation of cell proliferation and differentiation in the mammary glands, uterus, and other tissues (Jonsson et al., 2014). Activation of ERα supports cell proliferation and differentiation in the breast and other tissues. And recent studies suggest that high ERβ content can down-regulate the expression of ERα (Stope et al., 2010; Mehta et al., 2014). PR is regulated by estrogen, and its synthesis in normal mammary cells requires the combination of estrogen and estrogen receptor (Savouret et al., 1991; Lian et al., 2017). The increase of ERα and PR will definitely increase the sensitivity of breast epithelial to estrogen, and induce the occurrence of MGH. Here, we found that TSP effectively suppressed the mRNA and protein expression of ERα and PR, and simultaneously up-regulated ERβ expression in mammary gland of rats.

VEGF is a specific mitogen and angiogenic factor which stimulates endothelial cell growth and proliferation, promotes the generation of new blood vessels and regulates vascular permeability (Queiroga et al., 2010; Anadol et al., 2017). bFGF can promote mitosis, especially for the proliferation and differentiation of mesoderm cells. Although VEGF and bFGF have different mechanisms for promoting angiogenesis, there is a good synergy between them. As the degree of MGH increases,

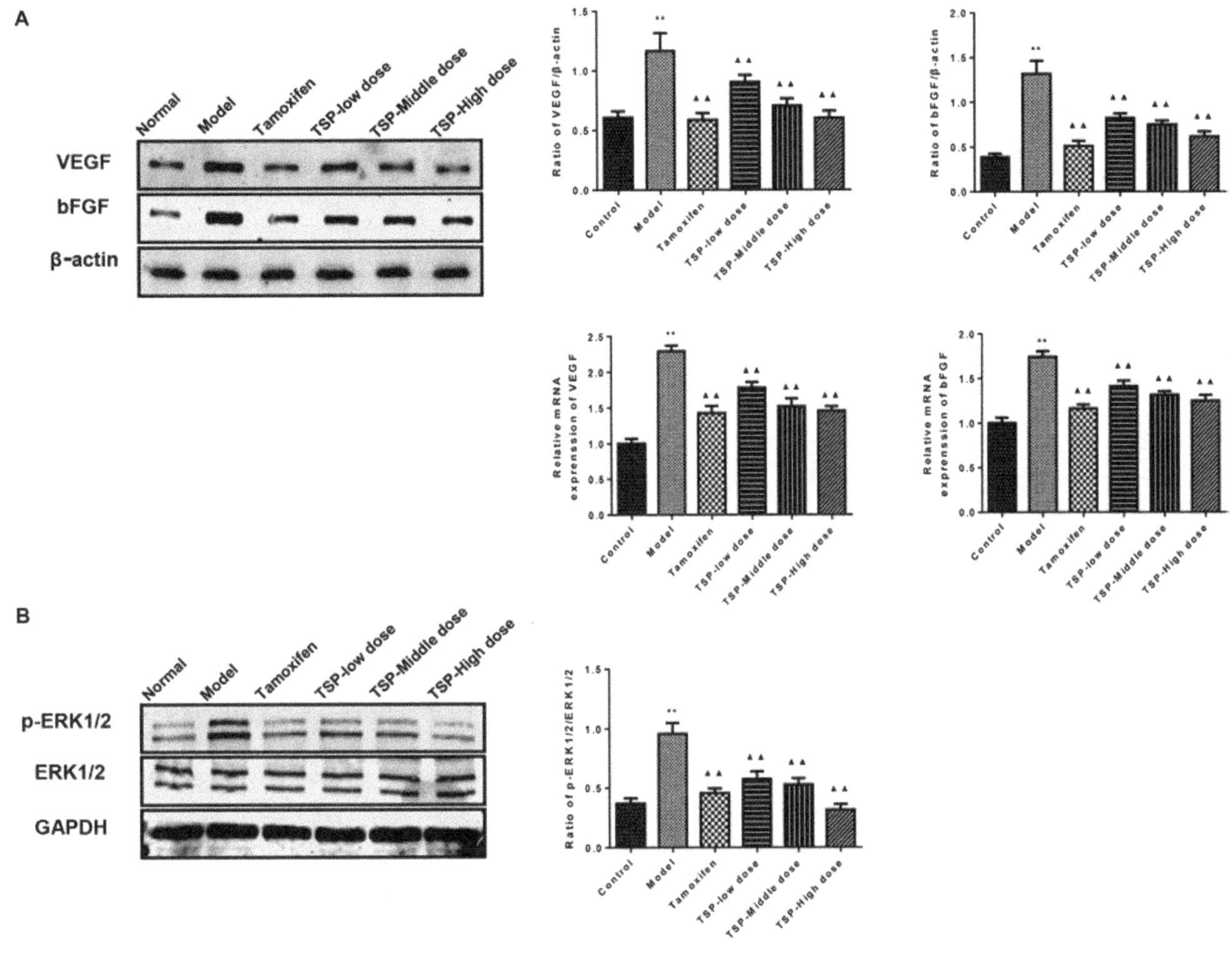

FIGURE 6 | Effects of TSP on the mRNA and protein expression of VEGF and bFGF and the phosphorylation of ERK1/2 in mammary gland of rats with MGH. **(A)** The mRNA and protein expression of VEGF and bFGF in different groups were determined respectively by reverse transcription quantitative polymerase chain reaction and western blot. **(B)** ERK1/2 phosphorylation in different groups were detected by western blot. Representative western blots images are displayed. Data were presented as mean ± SE from three independent experiments, $^{*}P < 0.05$, and $^{**}P < 0.01$ vs. control group; $^{▲}P < 0.05$ and $^{▲▲}P < 0.01$ vs. model group.

the activity of new blood vessels increased in tissues (Tao et al., 2017). ERK is an important member of mitogen activated protein kinase (mitogen activated protein kinase, MAPK) family. The combination of growth factors and hormones with neurotransmitter receptors will lead to the phosphorylation of ERK, promote the activated factor into the nucleus, and then participate in cell proliferation and differentiation (Feng et al., 2015; An et al., 2017). One study showed that estrogen activated the ERK1/2 pathway and increased the expression of VEGF. The higher the expression of VEGF, the more abundant the new blood vessel were produced and hence hyperplasia will be aggravated (Shan et al., 2013; Lin et al., 2015). These are consistent with the phenomena in our present study. 30 continuous days' administration of TSP markedly attenuated the MGH rat induced by estrogen combined with progestogen through suppressing mammary phosphorylation levels of ERK1/2, as well as reducing the mRNA and protein expression of VEGF and bFGF.

Apoptosis, also known as programmed cell death, refers to an active and ordered form of cell death, which are mainly genetically controlled (Zaman et al., 2014; Wei et al., 2017). The Bcl-2 protein family includes key regulatory factors for apoptosis, such as anti-apoptotic protein Bcl-2 and pro-apoptotic protein Bax, both of which are generally considered as important molecular proteins for apoptosis (Zhang and Saghatelian, 2013; Zhao et al., 2017). Ki-67 was found by Gerdes et al. (1984), and increased in mitotic stage, especially in the M phase of tumor active stage, and then decreased rapidly after mitotic cycle (Ding et al., 2004). With the development of science and technology, there are more and more researches on the influence of Chinese medicine treatment on the biological behavior of Ki-67. Many studies have found that Ki-67 is highly expressed in the tissue of MGH (Chen et al., 2014; Zhou and Wu, 2016). In concert with these findings, we found in this study that TSP substantially down-regulated the expression of Bcl-2 and Ki-67, as well as elevated the expression of Bax.

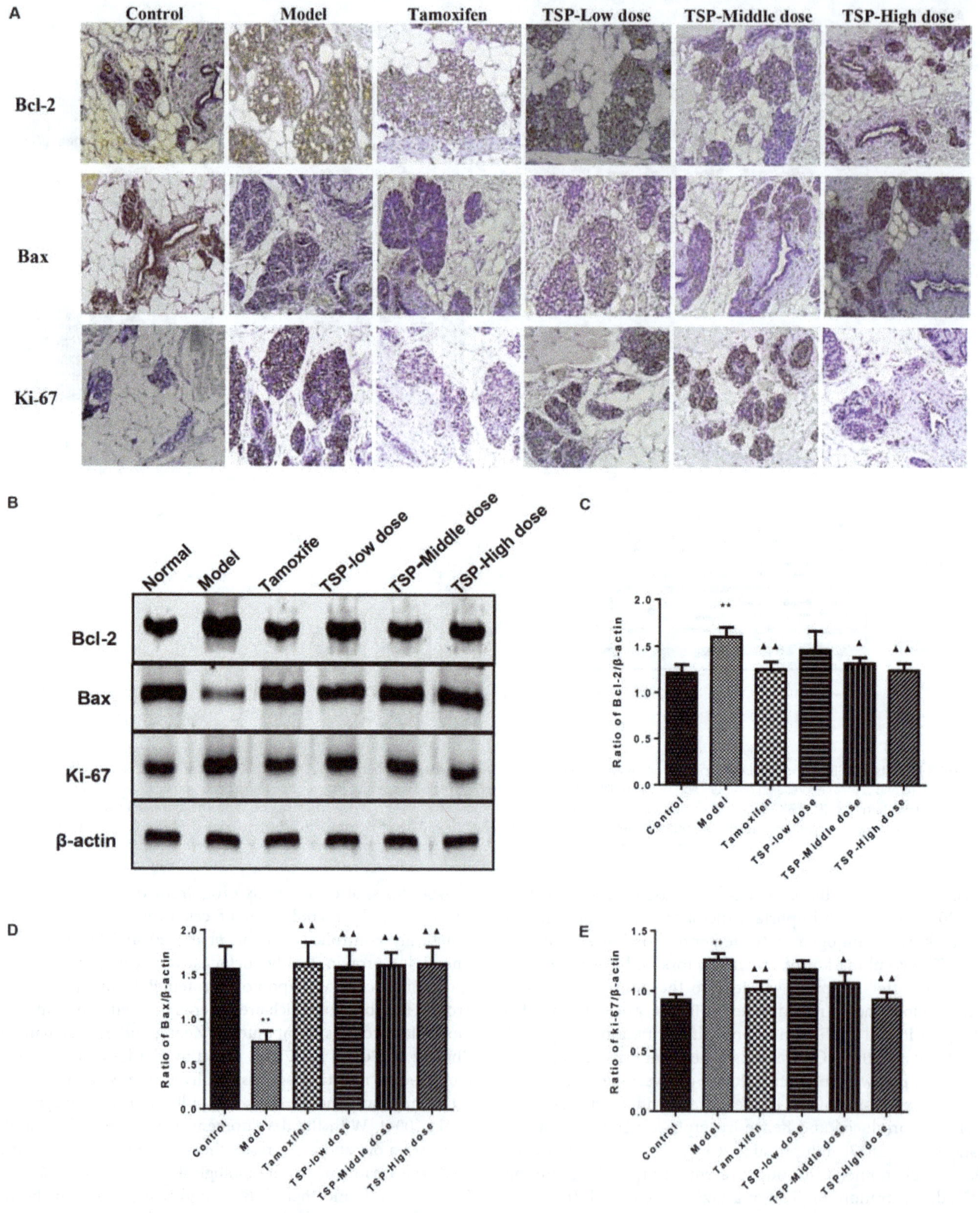

FIGURE 7 | Effects of TSP on level of Bcl-2, Bax and ki-67 in mammary gland of rats with MGH. **(A)** Immunohistochemistry findings of Bcl-2, Bax and ki-67 in each group. Tissue sections from mammary gland in each group were stained with anti-Bcl-2, anti-Bax, and anti-ki-67. Original magnification 100×. **(B–E)** The expression was detected by western-blot. Representative western blots images are displayed. Data were presented as mean ± SE from three independent experiments, *$P < 0.05$, and **$P < 0.01$ vs. control group; ▲$P < 0.05$ and ▲▲$P < 0.01$ vs. model group.

CONCLUSION

The whole results confirmed that TSP markedly attenuated MGH through rectifying the disorder of sex hormone, regulating the expression of hormone receptor, inhibiting the proliferation of mammary tissue cells, promoting apoptosis and inhibiting angiogenesis. Based on the results of this study, additional clinical studies are needed for patients with MGH.

AUTHOR CONTRIBUTIONS

XLi designed the study and drafted the manuscript. YuW contributed to the analysis of TSP components. XLi, YZ, ZW, and XLei conducted the experiments, analyzed data, and interpreted results. PX, XF, NG, YS, BY, and YanW provided suggestions and material support. QW and HK designed the study, supervised the whole research work, and revised the manuscript. All authors approved the version of the manuscript.

FUNDING

This work was supported by the Major State Basic Research Development Program (973 Program) of China (2013CB531800), and the National Natural Science Foundation of China (81473351, 81503271, and 81773904).

REFERENCES

An, H. Y., Xiang, C. N., Yu, X. L., Tang, L., Li, Y., Tang, X. P., et al. (2017). Mechanisms of apoptosis of human breast cancer cell line MCF-7 induced by baicalein and U0126. *China J. Mod. Med.* 27, 6–13. doi: 10.3969/j.issn.1005-8982.2017.10.002

Anadol, E., Yar Saglam, A. S., Gultiken, N., Karakas, K., Alcigir, E., Alkan, H., et al. (2017). Expression of inos, cox-2 and vegf in canine mammary tumours and non-neoplastic mammary glands: association with clinicopathological features and tumour grade. *Acta Vet. Hung.* 65, 382–393. doi: 10.1556/004.2017.036

Chen, T., Li, J. J., Chen, J. L., Song, H. P., and Yang, C. H. (2015). Anti-hyperplasia effects of *Rosa rugosa* polyphenols in rats with hyperplasia of mammary gland. *Environ. Toxicol. Pharmacol.* 39, 990–996. doi: 10.1016/j.etap.2015.02.014

Chen, X. Y., Ma, Z. R., Guo, J. F., and Zhao, H. J. (2014). Effect of Tianding Granules on immunohistochemical expression of CerbB-2 and Ki-67 in breast hyperplasia enclosed mass. *Mod. J. Integr. Tradit. Chin. West. Med.* 23, 168–169.

Ding, S. L., Sheu, L. F., Yu, J. C., Yang, T. L., Chen, B., Leu, F. J., et al. (2004). Expression of estrogen receptor-alpha and Ki-67 in relation to pathological and molecular features in early-onset infiltrating ductal carcinoma. *J. Biomed. Sci.* 11, 911–919. doi: 10.1007/BF02254376

Feng, D., Wang, B., Ma, Y., Shi, W., Tao, K., Zeng, W., et al. (2015). The Ras/Raf/Erk pathway mediates the subarachnoid hemorrhage-induced apoptosis of hippocampal neurons through phosphorylation of p53. *Mol. Neurobiol.* 53, 5737–5748. doi: 10.1007/s12035-015-9490-x

Gerdes, J., Lemke, H., Baisch, H., Wacker, H. H., Schwab, U., and Stein, H. (1984). Cell cycle analysis of a cell proliferation-associated human nuclear antigen defined by the monoclonal antibody ki-67. *J. Immunol.* 133, 1710–1715.

Guo, Y. F., Lv, J., and Wang, S. Q. (2017). Effect of Yanlurukang capsules on breast tissue and expressions of ER and PR in rats with hyperplasia of mammary glands. *China J. Mod. Med.* 27, 14–18. doi: 10.3969/j.issn.1005-8982.2017.13.003

Han, R., Li, R. T., and Wang, H. (2015). Effect of ruxianning tablets on mammary gland hyperplasia rats and hormone level. *J. Sichuan Tradit. Chin. Med.* 33, 40–42.

Henry, N. L. (2014). Endocrine therapy toxicity: management options. *Am. Soc. Clin. Oncol. Educ. Book* 34, e25–e30. doi: 10.14694/EdBook_AM.2014.34.e25

Higa, G. M., and Fell, R. G. (2013). Sex hormone receptor repertoire in breast cancer. *Int. J. Breast Cancer* 2013:284036. doi: 10.1155/2013/284036

Jonsson, P., Katchy, A., and Williams, C. (2014). Support of a bi-faceted role of estrogen receptor β (ERβ) in ERα-positive breast cancer cells. *Endocr. Relat. Cancer* 21, 143–160. doi: 10.1530/ERC-13-0444

Li, X. L., Xin, P., Wang, C. F., Wang, Z. B., Wang, Q. H., and Kuang, H. X. (2017). Mechanisms of traditional Chinese medicine in the treatment of mammary gland hyperplasia. *Am. J. Chin. Med.* 45, 443–458. doi: 10.1142/S0192415X17500276

Lian, X. L., Zhao, M., Han, Y., Wang, Q. L., and Han, T. (2017). Effect of Xihuang pills on the antioxidant capacity and the expression of ER and PR in rats with mammary gland hyperplasia. *Pharmacol. Clin. Chin. Mater. Med.* 33, 9–12. doi: 10.13412/j.cnki.zyyl.2017.05.003

Lin, N., Qiu, Y. W., and Guan, N. (2015). Effects of litchi chinensis seed saponins on the expression of ERα, ERβ, ERK and VEGF in rats with mammary gland hyperplasia. *J. Chin. Med. Mater.* 39, 659–662.

Mehta, R. G., Hawthorne, M., Mehta, R. R., Torres, K. E., Peng, X. J., McCormick, D. L., et al. (2014). Differential roles of ERα and ERβ in normal and neoplastic development in the mouse mammary gland. *PLoS One* 9:e113175. doi: 10.1371/journal.pone.0113175

Queiroga, F. L., Pires, I., Lobo, L., and Lopes, C. S. (2010). The role of COX-2 expression in the prognosis of dogs with malignant mammary tumours. *Res. Vet. Sci.* 88, 441–445. doi: 10.1016/j.rvsc.2009.10.009

Savouret, J. F., Bailly, A., Misrahi, M., Rauch, C., Redeuilh, G., Chauchereau, A., et al. (1991). Characterization of the hormone responsive element involved in the regulation of the progesterone receptor gene. *EMBO J.* 10, 1875–1883.

Schindler, A. E. (2011). Dydrogesterone and other progestins in benign breast disease: an overview. *Arch. Gynecol. Obstet.* 283, 369–371. doi: 10.1007/s00404-010-1456-7

Shan, B., Li, W., Yang, S. Y., and Li, Z. R. (2013). Estrogen up-regulates MMP2/9 expression in endometrial epithelial cell via VEGF-ERK1/2 pathway. *Asian Pac. J. Trop. Med.* 6, 826–830. doi: 10.1016/S1995-7645(13)60146-7

Stope, M. B., Popp, S. L., Knabbe, C., and Buck, M. B. (2010). Estrogen receptor alpha attenuates transforming growth factor beta signaling in breast cancer cells independent from agonistic and antagonistic ligands. *Breast Cancer Res. Treat.* 120, 357–367. doi: 10.1007/s10549-009-0393-2

Tao, C. J., Hu, J. N., and Chen, R. (2017). Effects of Xiaojin capsule, Xiaoyao Pill and Shu er jing capsule in patients with hyperplasia of mammary glands and its effects on vascular endothelial growth factor and basic fibroblast growth factor. *Chin. J. Biochem. Pharm.* 37, 90–92. doi: 10.3969/j.issn.1005-1678.2017.02.027

Tian, P. Y., Liu, X. C., Li, J. G., He, X. H., and Ni, J. Y. (1985). Clinical observation of 253 cases of hyperplasia of mammary glands treated with *Phytolacca*. *Med. J. NDFNC* 6, 235–236.

Wang, L., Zhao, D., Di, L., Cheng, D., Zhou, X., Yang, X., et al. (2011). The anti-hyperplasia of mammary gland effect of *Thladiantha dubia*, root ethanol extract in rats reduced by estrogen and progestogen. *J. Ethnopharmacol.* 134, 136–140. doi: 10.1016/j.jep.2010.11.071

Wang, Z. C., E, D., Batu, D. L., Saixi, Y. L., Zhang, B., and Ren, L. Q. (2011). 2D-DIGE proteomic analysis of changes in estrogen/progesterone-induced rat breast hyperplasia upon treatment with the mongolian remedy RuXian-I. *Molecules* 16, 3048–3065. doi: 10.3390/molecules16043048

Wang, P. C. (2015). *Studies on Nature and Flavor of Radix Phytolacca*. Heilongjiang: Heilongjiang University of Chinese Medicine.

Wang, P. C., Wang, Q. H., Zhao, S., Sun, X., and Kuang, H. X. (2014). Research progress on chemical constituents, pharmacological effects, and clinical applications of Phytolaccae Radix. *Chin. Tradit. Herb. Drugs* 45, 2722–2731. doi: 10.7501/j.issn.0253-2670.2014.18.028

Wei, L. Q., Li, W. T., Li, T., Xu, C. F., Tang, S. Y., and Gan, J. L. (2017). Effects of genistein on apoptosis and EGFR/PI3K/Akt signal transduction pathway in triple-negative breast cancer MDA-MB-231 cells. *Chin. Pharmacol. Bull.* 33, 1376–1381. doi: 10.3969/j.issn.1001-1978.2017.10.010

Zaman, S., Wang, R., and Gandhi, V. (2014). Targeting the apoptosis pathway in hematologic malignancies. *Leuk. Lymphoma* 55, 1980–1992. doi: 10.3109/10428194.2013.855307

Zhang, T., and Saghatelian, A. (2013). Emerging roles of lipids in BCL-2 family-regulated apoptosis. *Biochim. Biophys. Acta* 1831, 1542–1554. doi: 10.1016/j.bbalip.2013.03.001

Zhao, Z. D., Fang, C. S., Xie, X. X., Xia, J., and Yang, Y. J. (2017). Physalin B inhibit cell proliferation in MDA-MB-231 human breast cancer cells. *Chin. Tradit. Pat. Med.* 39, 1502–1506.

Zheng, J. J., Zhao, Y., Wang, Y. F., Hu, S. F., Lu, P., and Shen, X. Y. (2013). The infrared radiation temperature characteristic of acupoints of mammary gland hyperplasia patients. *J. Evid. Based Complement. Altern. Med.* 2013:567987. doi: 10.1155/2013/567987

Zhou, D. W., and Wu, L. J. (2016). Effect of compound *Centella asiatica* tablets combined with western medicine on expression of ER, PR and Ki-67 of patients with galactophore lobule hyperplasia. *J. New Chin. Med.* 23, 168–169. doi: 10.13457/j.cnki.jncm.2016.07.061

Permissions

All chapters in this book were first published by Frontiers; hereby published with permission under the Creative Commons Attribution License or equivalent. Every chapter published in this book has been scrutinized by our experts. Their significance has been extensively debated. The topics covered herein carry significant findings which will fuel the growth of the discipline. They may even be implemented as practical applications or may be referred to as a beginning point for another development.

The contributors of this book come from diverse backgrounds, making this book a truly international effort. This book will bring forth new frontiers with its revolutionizing research information and detailed analysis of the nascent developments around the world.

We would like to thank all the contributing authors for lending their expertise to make the book truly unique. They have played a crucial role in the development of this book. Without their invaluable contributions this book wouldn't have been possible. They have made vital efforts to compile up to date information on the varied aspects of this subject to make this book a valuable addition to the collection of many professionals and students.

This book was conceptualized with the vision of imparting up-to-date information and advanced data in this field. To ensure the same, a matchless editorial board was set up. Every individual on the board went through rigorous rounds of assessment to prove their worth. After which they invested a large part of their time researching and compiling the most relevant data for our readers.

The editorial board has been involved in producing this book since its inception. They have spent rigorous hours researching and exploring the diverse topics which have resulted in the successful publishing of this book. They have passed on their knowledge of decades through this book. To expedite this challenging task, the publisher supported the team at every step. A small team of assistant editors was also appointed to further simplify the editing procedure and attain best results for the readers.

Apart from the editorial board, the designing team has also invested a significant amount of their time in understanding the subject and creating the most relevant covers. They scrutinized every image to scout for the most suitable representation of the subject and create an appropriate cover for the book.

The publishing team has been an ardent support to the editorial, designing and production team. Their endless efforts to recruit the best for this project, has resulted in the accomplishment of this book. They are a veteran in the field of academics and their pool of knowledge is as vast as their experience in printing. Their expertise and guidance has proved useful at every step. Their uncompromising quality standards have made this book an exceptional effort. Their encouragement from time to time has been an inspiration for everyone.

The publisher and the editorial board hope that this book will prove to be a valuable piece of knowledge for researchers, students, practitioners and scholars across the globe.

List of Contributors

Hirai Kuniaki, Tanaka Akihiko, Homma Tetsuya, Mikuni Hatsuko, Kawahara Tomoko, Ohta Shin, Kusumoto Sojiro, Yamamoto Mayumi, Yamaguchi Fumihiro, Suzuki Shintaro, Ohnishi Tsukasa and Sagara Hironori
Division of Allergology and Respiratory Medicine, Department of Internal Medicine, Showa University School of Medicine, Tokyo, Japan

Kanako Miyano, Miki Nonaka and Miaki Uzu
Division of Cancer Pathophysiology, National Cancer Center Research Institute, Tokyo, Japan

Kaori Ohshima
Division of Cancer Pathophysiology, National Cancer Center Research Institute, Tokyo, Japan
Faculty of Pharmaceutical Sciences, Tokyo University of Science, Chiba, Japan

Yasuhito Uezono
Division of Cancer Pathophysiology, National Cancer Center Research Institute, Tokyo, Japan
Division of Supportive Care Research, Exploratory Oncology Research and Clinical Trial Center, National Cancer Center, Tokyo, Japan
Innovation Center for Supportive, Palliative and Psychosocial Care, National Cancer Center Hospital, Tokyo, Japan
Department of Comprehensive Oncology, Nagasaki University Graduate School of Biomedical Sciences, Nagasaki, Japan

Tomoki Ito, Akiko Konishi, Yukie Tsubokura, Yoshiko Azuma, Masaaki Hotta, Hideaki Yoshimura, Takahisa Nakanishi, Shinya Fujita, Aya Nakaya, Atsushi Satake, Kazuyoshi Ishii and Shosaku Nomura
First Department of Internal Medicine, Kansai Medical University, Hirakata, Japan

Wayne Balkan and Joshua M. Hare
Interdisciplinary Stem Cell Institute, University of Miami Miller School of Medicine, Miami, FL, United States

Ivonne Hernandez Schulman
Interdisciplinary Stem Cell Institute, University of Miami Miller School of Medicine, Miami, FL, United States
Katz Family Division of Nephrology and Hypertension, University of Miami Miller School of Medicine, Miami, FL, United States

Naoya Sakisaka
Sakisaka Clinic, Osaka, Japan

Kazuo Mitani
Mitani Family Clinic, Osaka, Japan

Sadahiro Sempuku
Sempuku Clinic, Osaka, Japan

Tamaki Imai
Imai Clinic, Osaka, Japan

Yoshinori Takemoto
Takemoto Clinic, Nara, Japan

Hiroaki Shimomura
Shimomura Clinic of Internal Medicine, Osaka, Japan

Takahisa Ushiroyama
Osaka Medical College Health Science Clinic, Osaka, Japan

Hajime Nakae
Department of Emergency and Critical Care Medicine, Akita University Graduate School of Medicine, Akita, Japan
Department of Traditional Japanese Medicine, Akita University Hospital, Akita, Japan

Yuko Hiroshima and Miwa Hebiguchi
Department of Traditional Japanese Medicine, Akita University Hospital, Akita, Japan

Katsuyoshi Matsunami
Department of Pharmacognosy, Graduate School of Biomedical and Health Sciences, Hiroshima University, Hiroshima, Japan

Shin Takayama, Ryutaro Arita, Akiko Kikuchi, Minoru Ohsawa, Soichiro Kaneko and Tadashi Ishii
Department of Education and Support for Regional Medicine, Department of Kampo Medicine, Tohoku University Hospital, Sendai, Japan

Meiling Zhang, Bo Yu and Yao Zhang
Key Laboratory of Myocardial Ischemia Mechanism and Treatment, Ministry of Education, Harbin Medical University, Harbin, China
Department of Cardiology, The Second Affiliated Hospital of Harbin Medical University, Harbin, China

Yan Zhang, Hangfei Liang, Huqiang Cai, Xueling Hu, Yu Bian, Xin Li, Lei Dong and Lili Ding
State Province Key Laboratories of Biomedicine - Pharmaceutics of China, Key Laboratory of Cardiovascular Medicine Research, Ministry of Education, Department of Pharmacology, College of Pharmacy, Harbin Medical University, Harbin, China

Libo Wang
Department of Medicinal Chemistry and Natural Medicine Chemistry, College of Pharmacy, Harbin Medical University, Harbin, China

Shizhang Wei, Yuxue Yang, Yingying Wang, Lu Zhang, Xuelin Zhou, Haotian Li, Kun Li and Yanling Zhao
Department of Pharmacy, 302 Hospital of People's Liberation Army, Beijing, China

Ruilin Wang and Liqi Qian
Department of Traditional Chinese Medicine, First Affiliated Hospital of Chinese PLA General Hospital, Beijing, China

Ming Niu
China Military Institute of Chinese Medicine, 302 Hospital of People's Liberation Army, Beijing, China

Honghong Liu
Department of Integrative Medical Center, 302 Hospital of People's Liberation Army, Beijing, China

Xin Hua, Qin Yang, Wanjiang Zhang, Shenye Yu and Siguo Liu
Division of Bacterial Diseases, State Key Laboratory of Veterinary Biotechnology, Harbin Veterinary Research Institute, Chinese Academy of Agricultural Sciences, Harbin, China

Zhimin Dong
Tianjin Animal Science and Veterinary Research Institute, Tianjin, China

Stefan Schwarz
Institute of Microbiology and Epizootics, Department of Veterinary Medicine, Freie Universität Berlin, Berlin, Germany

Yi-Hsin Wang and Jinghua T. Chang
Institute of Medicine, Chung Shan Medical University, Taichung, Taiwan

Shun-An Li
Superintendent Office, Yuanli Lee's General Hospital, Lee's Medical Corporation, Miaoli, Taiwan

Chao-Hsin Huang
Department of Internal Medicine, Dajia Lee's General Hospital, Lee's Medical Corporation, Taichung, Taiwan

Hsing-Hui Su
Department and Institute of Pharmacology, School of Medicine, National Yang-Ming University, Taipei, Taiwan

Yi-Hung Chen
Graduate Institute of Acupuncture Science and Research Center for Chinese Medicine and Acupuncture, China Medical University, Taichung, Taiwan
Department of Photonics and Communication Engineering, Asia University, Taichung, Taiwan

Shiang-Suo Huang
Department of Pharmacology and Institute of Medicine, Chung Shan Medical University, Taichung, Taiwan
Department of Pharmacy, Chung Shan Medical University Hospital, Taichung, Taiwan

Wenting Wan, Hongxiang Li, Jiamei Xiang, Lijia Xu, Baoping Jiang and Peigen Xiao
Institute of Medicinal Plant Development, Chinese Academy of Medical Sciences and Peking Union Medical College, Beijing, China
Key Laboratory of Bioactive Substances and Resources Utilization of Chinese Herbal Medicine, Ministry of Education, Beijing, China

Fan Yi
School of Sciences/Key Laboratory of Cosmetic, China National Light Industry, Beijing Technology and Business University, Beijing, China

Zhenyan Hou, Lei Chen, Pingfei Fang, Hualin Cai, Lingjuan Cao, Huande Li, Bikui Zhang and Miao Yan
Department of Pharmacy, The Second Xiangya Hospital, Central South University, Changsha, China
Institute of Clinical Pharmacy, Central South University, Changsha, China

Huaibo Tang
Department of Pharmacy, Chemistry College, Xiangtan University, Xiangtan, China

Yongbo Peng
Molecular Science and Biomedicine Laboratory, College of Life Sciences, State Key Laboratory of Chemo, Bio-Sensing and Chemometrics, Hunan University, Changsha, China

Yang Deng
School of Pharmacy, Hunan University of Chinese Medicine, Changsha, China

Yingqiu Liu, Zengyuan Liu, Yuanyuan Li, Taotao He, Weimin Zhang, Yunpeng Fan Xiaoping Song and Wuren Ma
Laboratory of Traditional Chinese Veterinary Medicine, College of Veterinary Medicine, Northwest A&F University, Yangling, China

Tianyi Liu
Department of Neurosurgery, The First Hospital of Jilin University, Changchun, China

Kevin Ding
University of Illinois at Urbana–Champaign, Urbana, IL, United States

Li Cui
Department of Neurosciences, University of California, San Diego School of Medicine, La Jolla, CA, United States

Kenta Murata, Nina Fujita and Ryuji Takahashi
Kampo Research Laboratories, Kracie Pharma, Ltd., Tokyo, Japan

Akio Inui
Pharmacological Department of Herbal Medicine, Kagoshima University Graduate School of Medical and Dental Sciences, Kagoshima, Japan

Xinxin Dai, Shulan Su, Hongdie Cai, Dandan Wei, Hui Yan, Tianyao Zheng, Zhenhua Zhu, Er-xin Shang, Sheng Guo, Dawei Qian and Jin-ao Duan
Jiangsu Collaborative Innovation Center of Chinese Medicinal Resources Industrialization, State Key Laboratory Cultivation Base for TCM Quality and Efficacy, Nanjing University of Chinese Medicine, Nanjing, China

Asha Jose
Department of Pharmacology, JSS College of Pharmacy, JSS Academy of Higher Education and Research, Udhagamandalam, India

Motamari V. N. L. Chaitanya
Department of Pharmacognosy and Phytopharmacy, JSS College of Pharmacy, Udhagamandalam, India

Elango Kannan
Department of Pharmacology, JSS College of Pharmacy, Udhagamandalam, India

Subba Rao V. Madhunapantula
Center of Excellence in Molecular Biology and Regenerative Medicine, JSS Medical College, JSS Academy of Higher Education and Research, Mysore, India

Wen-Bei Han
Department of Traditional Chinese Medicine, Nanjing Drum Tower Hospital Clinical College of Traditional Chinese and Western Medicine, Nanjing University of Chinese Medicine, Nanjng, China

Ying-Lu Liu and Wei Wu
Department of Traditional Chinese Medicine, Nanjing Drum Tower Hospital Clinical College of Traditional Chinese and Western Medicine, Nanjing University of Chinese Medicine, Nanjng, China
Department of Traditional Chinese Medicine, Nanjing Drum Tower Hospital, The Affiliated Hospital of Nanjing University Medical School, Nanjing, China

Hai-Ming Yang, Qi-Jun Fang, Mo-Yi Zhou and Yi-Gang Wan
Department of Traditional Chinese Medicine, Nanjing Drum Tower Hospital, The Affiliated Hospital of Nanjing University Medical School, Nanjing, China

Wei Hu
Department of Pharmacy, Nanjing Drum Tower Hospital, The Affiliated Hospital of Nanjing University Medical School, Nanjing, China

Yue Tu
Department of TCM Health Preservation, Second Clinic Medical School, Nanjing University of Chinese Medicine, Nanjing, China

Zi-Yue Wan
Department of Social Work, Meiji Gakuin University, Tokyo, Japan

Ren-Mao Tang and Hai-Tao
Institute of Huanghui, Suzhong Pharmaceutical Group Co., Ltd., Taizhou, China

Xueyu Wang, Jianhui Rong, Shi Wei Wang, Yan Bo Zhang, Lin Zheng and Hei-Kiu Wong
School of Chinese Medicine, LKS Faculty of Medicine, The University of Hong Kong, Hong Kong, China

Guo-Cai Wang
Institute of Traditional Chinese Medicine and Natural Products, College of Pharmacy, Jinan University, Guangzhou, China

Tzi Bun Ng
School of Biomedical Sciences, Faculty of Medicine, The Chinese University of Hong Kong, Hong Kong, China

Kai Fai Lee
Department of Obstetrics and Gynaecology, LKS Faculty of Medicine, The University of Hong Kong, Hong Kong, China

Ken Kin Lam Yung and Stephen Cho Wing Sze
Department of Biology, Faculty of Science, Hong Kong Baptist University, Hong Kong, China

Zhibin Wang, Yu Wang, Yanan Zhang, Ping Xin, Xin Fu, Ning Gao, Yanping Sun, Yanhong Wang, ingyou Yang and Haixue Kuang
Key Laboratory of Chinese Materia Medica (Ministry of Education), Heilongjiang University of Chinese Medicine, Harbin, China

Xiaoliang Li
Key Laboratory of Chinese Materia Medica (Ministry of Education), Heilongjiang University of Chinese Medicine, Harbin, China
Science of Chinese Materia Medica, Jiamusi College, Heilongjiang University of Chinese Medicine, Jiamusi, China

Qiuhong Wang
Science of Processing Chinese Materia Medica, School of Traditional Chinese Medicine, Guangdong Pharmaceutical University, Guangzhou, China

Yunping Bai, Jiansheng Li, Peng Zhao, Suxiang Feng, Yanqin Qin, Yange Tian and Tiqiang Zhou
Henan Key Laboratory of Chinese Medicine for Respiratory Disease, Henan University of Chinese Medicine, Zhengzhou, China
Collaborative Innovation Center for Respiratory Disease Diagnosis and Treatment - Chinese Medicine Development of Henan Province, Zhengzhou, China

Index

A

Alzheimer's Disease, 3-4, 6, 8-11, 34-35, 39, 41, 46, 140-141, 149
Anthraquinones, 53-56, 58-61, 63
Anti-cancer Activity, 75, 166-169, 172, 174, 179, 208
Anticancer Agents, 166-167, 173, 180-181
Apoptosis, 8, 10-11, 24, 85-87, 91-93, 95-99, 122, 137, 139, 152, 163, 166-167, 171, 177-181, 208, 215, 218, 224-225, 227-228
Aqueous Extract Of Black Maca, 100, 102-105, 107, 110, 112
Atherosclerotic Cardiovascular Disease, 101

C

Carcinoma Cells, 10, 169-170, 173-174, 176-177
Cell Culture, 75, 116, 142, 167, 174, 186, 202-204
Cell Viability Assay, 116, 203
Chromatographic Separation, 117
Chromatography, 61, 63, 66, 115, 124, 141, 164, 168, 173, 181, 183-184, 198, 201-202, 219, 221
Chronic Obstructive Pulmonary Disease, 1, 4, 46, 51
Cytoplasm, 57-58, 60, 130

D

Delirium, 42, 50
Dementia, 8-10, 23, 41-42, 44-46, 48, 51

E

Estradiol Biosynthesis, 205, 209, 216

F

Fasting Blood Glucose, 53-57, 152
Fasting Serum Insulin, 53-55, 57, 61
Fibroblast, 142, 227
Food Utilization, 103, 108
Fractionation, 167, 172-173
Functional Dyspepsia, 44-46, 50

G

Gastro-intestinal Dysfunction, 42, 44
Gluconeogenesis, 61, 100-101, 106, 108-111
Gluconeogenic Flux, 109-110
Glucose Homeostasis, 37, 61, 63, 106, 108, 112-113
Glucose Metabolism Disorder, 101, 108, 111
Glucose Transporters, 57, 60
Glucosinolates, 104, 106, 112
Glycolysis, 100-101, 106, 108-111

H

Hepatocellular Carcinoma, 9, 11
Hepatotoxicity, 73, 114-116, 118-119, 121, 123-128
High-fructose Diet, 100-101
Histone Deacetylase, 87, 167, 170, 180-181
Hyperglycaemia, 53-54, 59-61
Hyperinsulinemia, 100, 104, 108, 111
Hyperlipidemia, 63, 100, 104, 108, 111, 113, 130, 152, 157
Hyperplasia, 64-65, 72-73, 104, 154, 218-219, 222, 224-225, 227-228
Hypertension, 2, 16, 18, 32, 46-48, 51, 59, 98, 164, 198, 216
Hypolipidaemic Effect, 58, 60

I

Immune Function, 20
Insulin Resistance, 7, 10-11, 56-57, 59-60, 62-63, 100-102, 104, 111-113, 152, 163, 165
Insulin Stimulation, 57
Intraperitoneal Injection, 53, 55, 151, 154, 182-183, 202
Irritable Bowel Syndrome, 44-46, 50
Isoliquiritigenin, 114-115, 118, 120, 125-127

K

Kampo Medicine, 1-2, 4-6, 8-9, 31-32, 35, 42-52, 150

L

Laxmitaru, 166, 181
Lipid Metabolism, 33, 58, 101, 106, 109, 111, 113, 127, 152

M

Mammary Gland Hyperplasia, 72-73, 218-219, 227-228
Metabolism Disorder, 59-60, 100-101, 106, 108, 111, 113
Metabolites, 6, 18, 64, 66-73, 100-101, 106, 108, 110, 114-115, 124, 126-127, 151-152, 154, 156-157, 160, 162, 164, 181
Metabolomic Analysis, 100, 102, 106
Molecular Docking, 169, 175, 181, 203, 205, 209

N

Nuclear Fraction, 170

O

Oral Glucose Tolerance, 53-55
Oxidative Stress, 8, 10, 23, 35, 39, 72, 84, 90-91, 93, 95-99, 114-115, 124, 126, 152, 164-165, 180, 184, 198

P

Pharmacodynamics, 101, 127, 130, 156
Pharmacognosy, 36, 51, 54, 59, 166
Pharmacology, 10, 35, 53, 61-62, 64-66, 69, 71-73, 86, 127, 166, 180, 198-208, 210, 212, 215-217
Phosphorylation, 57, 60, 62, 110, 131, 133-135, 139, 182-183, 189, 191, 195-196, 218, 223, 225, 227
Phytochemicals, 166, 179, 203
Plasma Membrane, 58, 60
Postmenopausal Syndrome, 199-200, 208, 210, 212, 214-215
Proliferation, 8, 10, 19-20, 24, 85, 140, 142-143, 145-149, 152, 163, 166-167, 169, 179, 187, 192, 197, 206, 208, 210, 212-213, 215-216, 218, 224-225, 227-228
Pulmonary Fibrosis, 72
Purification, 98, 167, 173, 180

R

Renal Dysfunction, 32, 183, 192

S

Semen Cassiae Extract, 53-54, 56-57, 60-61, 63
Serum Lipid Determination, 55
Sex Hormones, 215, 218, 223-224
Simarouba Glauca, 166, 168, 170, 172, 179-181
Standard Error, 88, 118, 143, 203
Structural Elucidation, 168, 216

T

Traditional Medicine, 51, 54, 166, 179
Tricaproin, 166-174, 177, 179-180
Triptolide, 114-115, 118, 120, 125-128

U

Urinary Dysfunction, 42, 44

V

Virtual Screening, 100-101, 103, 108, 111-113

W

Western Blot, 56, 58-59, 88, 91, 93-94, 117, 119-120, 122-123, 131, 183, 186, 199-200, 203, 206, 208, 212-214, 220, 223, 225